Pocket
MEDICINE

Sixth Edition

Edited by
MARC S. SABATINE, MD, MPH
Professor of Medicine
Harvard Medical School

*The Massachusetts General Hospital
Handbook of Internal Medicine*

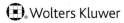 Wolters Kluwer

Philadelphia • Baltimore • New York • London
Buenos Aires • Hong Kong • Sydney • Tokyo

Executive Editor: Rebecca Gaertner
Product Manager: Kristina Oberle
Vendor Manager: Bridgett Dougherty
Manufacturing Coordinator: Beth Welsh
Marketing Manager: Rachel Mante Leung
Creative Director: Teresa Mallon
Production Service: Aptara, Inc.

Library of Congress Cataloging-in-Publication Data

Names: Sabatine, Marc S., author.
Title: Pocket medicine : the Massachusetts General Hospital handbook of
    internal medicine / edited by Marc S. Sabatine.
Other titles: Pocket medicine (Sabatine) | Pocket notebook.
Description: Sixth edition. | Philadelphia : Wolters Kluwer, [2017] | Series:
    Pocket notebook | Includes bibliographical references and index.
Identifiers: LCCN 2016037021 | ISBN 9781496349484 (loose-leaf)
Subjects: | MESH: Internal Medicine | Clinical Medicine | Handbooks
Classification: LCC RC55 | NLM WB 39 | DDC 616—dc23
LC record available at https://lccn.loc.gov/2016037021

CCS1016

CONTENTS

NEPHROLOGY
Jacob Stevens, Andrew S. Allegretti, Hasan Bazari

HEMATOLOGY-ONCOLOGY
Edmond M. Chan, Tanya E. Keenan, Andrew M. Brunner, Sheheryar K. Kabraji, Jean M. Connors, Daniel J. DeAngelo, David P. Ryan

INFECTIOUS DISEASES
Michael S. Abers, Ana A. Weil, Nesli Basgoz

CONTRIBUTING AUTHORS

Michael S. Abers, MD
Internal Medicine Resident, Massachusetts General Hospital

Andrew S. Allegretti, MD, MSc
Nephrology Fellow, BWH/MGH Joint Nephrology Fellowship Program

Elias N. Baedorf Kassis, MD
Pulmonary Fellow, Massachusetts General Hospital

Jessica M. Baker, MD
Neurology Resident, Partners Neurology Residency

Nesli Basgoz, MD
Associate Chief and Clinical Director, Infectious Disease Division,
 Massachusetts General Hospital
Associate Professor of Medicine, Harvard Medical School

Hasan Bazari, MD
Program Director Emeritus, Internal Medicine Residency, Massachusetts
 General Hospital
Attending Physician, Nephrology Unit, Massachusetts General Hospital
Associate Professor of Medicine, Harvard Medical School

Andrew M. Brunner, MD
Hematology-Oncology Fellow, Dana-Farber/Partners CancerCare
Hematology/Oncology Program

Sarah J. Carlson, MD
Surgical Resident, Beth Israel Deaconess Medical Center

Edmond M. Chan, MD
Internal Medicine Resident, Massachusetts General Hospital

Katherine T. Chen, MD, MPH
Professor of Obstetrics, Gynecology, and Reproductive Science
Professor of Medical Education
Vice-Chair of Ob/Gyn Education, Career Development, and Mentorship
Icahn School of Medicine at Mount Sinai, New York

Tracey A. Cho, MD
Associate Program Director, Partners-Harvard Neurology Residency
Assistant Neurologist, Massachusetts General Hospital
Assistant Professor of Neurology, Harvard Medical School

Jean M. Connors, MD
Medical Director, Anticoagulation Management Services
Hematology Division, Brigham and Women's Hospital & Dana-Farber
 Cancer Institute
Assistant Professor of Medicine, Harvard Medical School

Daniel J. DeAngelo, MD, PhD
Director of Clinical and Translational Research, Adult Leukemia Program
Dana-Farber Cancer Institute and Brigham and Women's Hospital
Associate Professor of Medicine, Harvard Medical School

Michael G. Erkkinen, MD
Neurology Resident, Partners Neurology Residency

Mark R. Etherton, MD, PhD
Neurology Resident, Partners Neurology Residency

Robert P. Friday, MD, PhD
Chief of Rheumatology, Newton-Wellesley Hospital Affiliate Physician, Rheumatology Unit, Massachusetts General Hospital
Instructor in Medicine, Harvard Medical School

Lawrence S. Friedman, MD
Anton R. Fried, MD, Chair, Department of Medicine, Newton-Wellesley Hospital
Assistant Chief of Medicine, Massachusetts General Hospital
Professor of Medicine, Harvard Medical School
Professor of Medicine, Tufts University School of Medicine

J. Sawalla Guseh, II, MD
Cardiology Fellow, Massachusetts General Hospital

William J. Hucker, MD, PhD
Cardiology Fellow, Massachusetts General Hospital

Sheheryar K. Kabraji, BM, BCh
Hematology-Oncology Fellow, Dana-Farber/Partners CancerCare Hematology/Oncology Program

Sarah Keller, MD
Internal Medicine Resident, Massachusetts General Hospital

Tanya E. Keenan, MD, MPH
Internal Medicine Resident, Massachusetts General Hospital

Stella K. Kim, MD
Joe M. Green Jr. Professor of Clinical Ophthalmology
Ruiz Department of Ophthalmology and Visual Sciences
Robert Cizik Eye Clinic
University of Texas McGovern School of Medicine

Michael Mannstadt, MD
Chief, Endocrine Unit, Massachusetts General Hospital
Assistant Professor of Medicine, Harvard Medical School

Nino Mihatov, MD
Internal Medicine Resident, Massachusetts General Hospital

Vanessa Mitsialis, MD
Internal Medicine Resident, Massachusetts General Hospital

Taher Modarressi, MD
Internal Medicine Resident, Massachusetts General Hospital

Khaled Moussawi, MD, PhD
Neurology Resident, Partners Neurology Residency

Walter J. O'Donnell, MD
Clinical Director, Pulmonary/Critical Care Unit, Massachusetts General Hospital
Assistant Professor of Medicine, Harvard Medical School

Michelle L. O'Donoghue, MD, MPH
Investigator, TIMI Study Group
Associate Physician, Cardiovascular Division, Brigham and Women's Hospital
Affiliate Physician, Cardiology Division, Massachusetts General Hospital
Assistant Professor of Medicine, Harvard Medical School

Kelly Lauter Roszko, MD, PhD
Endocrinology Fellow, Massachusetts General Hospital

David P. Ryan, MD
Clinical Director, Massachusetts General Hospital Cancer Center
Chief of Hematology/Oncology, Massachusetts General Hospital
Professor of Medicine, Harvard Medical School

Marc S. Sabatine, MD, MPH
Chairman, TIMI Study Group
Lewis Dexter, MD, Distinguished Chair in Cardiovascular Medicine, Brigham and Women's Hospital
Affiliate Physician, Cardiology Division, Massachusetts General Hospital
Professor of Medicine, Harvard Medical School

Alyssa Sclafani, MD
Internal Medicine Resident, Massachusetts General Hospital

John D. Serfas, MD
Internal Medicine Resident, Massachusetts General Hospital

Jacob Stevens, MD
Internal Medicine Resident, Massachusetts General Hospital

Jennifer F. Tseng, MD, MPH
Chief, Division of Surgical Oncology, Beth Israel Deaconess Medical Center
Associate Professor of Surgery, Harvard Medical School

Nneka N. Ufere, MD
Gastroenterology Fellow, Massachusetts General Hospital

Zachary S. Wallace, MD
Rheumatology Fellow, Massachusetts General Hospital

Ana A. Weil, MD, MPH
Infectious Disease Fellow, Massachusetts General Hospital

FOREWORD

To the 1st Edition

It is with the greatest enthusiasm that I introduce *Pocket Medicine*. In an era of information glut, it will logically be asked, "Why another manual for medical house officers?" Yet, despite enormous information readily available in any number of textbooks, or at the push of a key on a computer, it is often that the harried house officer is less helped by the description of differential diagnosis and therapies than one would wish.

    Pocket Medicine is the joint venture between house staff and faculty expert in a number of medical specialties. This collaboration is designed to provide a rapid but thoughtful initial approach to medical problems seen by house officers with great frequency. Questions that frequently come from faculty to the house staff on rounds, many hours after the initial interaction between patient and doctor, have been anticipated and important pathways for arriving at diagnoses and initiating therapies are presented. This approach will facilitate the evidence-based medicine discussion that will follow the workup of the patient. This well-conceived handbook should enhance the ability of every medical house officer to properly evaluate a patient in a timely fashion and to be stimulated to think of the evidence supporting the diagnosis and the likely outcome of therapeutic intervention. *Pocket Medicine* will prove to be a worthy addition to medical education and to the care of our patients.

DENNIS A. AUSIELLO, MD
Physician-in-Chief, Massachusetts General Hospital
Jackson Professor of Clinical Medicine, Harvard Medical School

PREFACE

To my parents, Matthew and Lee Sabatine, to their namesake grandchildren Matteo and Natalie, and to my wife Jennifer

Written by residents, fellows, and attendings, the mandate for *Pocket Medicine* was to provide, in a concise a manner as possible, the key information a clinician needs for the initial approach to and management of the most common inpatient medical problems.

The tremendous response to the previous editions suggests we were able to help fill an important need for clinicians. With this sixth edition come several major improvements. We have updated every topic thoroughly. In particular, we have included the latest pharmacotherapy for acute coronary syndromes, heart failure, pulmonary hypertension, hepatitis C, HIV, and diabetes, as well as the latest device-based treatments for valvular heart disease, atrial fibrillation, and stroke. Recent paradigm shifts in the guidelines for hypertension and cholesterol have been distilled and incorporated. We have expanded coverage of the molecular classification of malignancies and the corresponding biologic therapies. We have added new sections on mechanical circulatory support, angioedema, non-invasive ventilation, toxicology, lung transplantation, GI motility disorders, and the cardiorenal syndrome, just to name a few. We have also updated the section on Consults in which non-internal medicine specialists provide expert guidance in terms of establishing a differential diagnosis for common presenting symptoms and initiating an evaluation in anticipation of calling a consult. As always, we have incorporated key references to the most recent high-tier reviews and important studies published right up to the time *Pocket Medicine* went to press. We welcome any suggestions for further improvement.

Of course medicine is far too vast a field to ever summarize in a textbook of any size. Long monographs have been devoted to many of the topics discussed herein. *Pocket Medicine* is meant only as a starting point to guide one during the initial phases of diagnosis and management until one has time to consult more definitive resources. Although the recommendations herein are as evidence-based as possible, medicine is both a science and an art. As always, sound clinical judgement must be applied to every scenario.

I am grateful for the support of the house officers, fellows, and attendings at the Massachusetts General Hospital. It is a privilege to work with such a knowledgeable, dedicated, and compassionate group of physicians. I always look back on my time there as Chief Resident as one of the best experiences I have ever had. I am grateful to several outstanding clinical mentors, including Hasan Bazari, Larry Friedman, Nesli Basgoz, Eric Isselbacher, Bill Dec, Mike Fifer, and Roman DeSanctis, as well as the late Charlie McCabe, Mort Swartz, and Peter Yurchak.

This edition would not have been possible without the help of Melinda Cuerda, my academic coordinator. She shepherded every aspect of the project from start to finish, with an incredible eye to detail to ensure that each page of this book was the very best it could be.

Lastly, special thanks to my parents for their perpetual encouragement and love and, of course, to my wife, Jennifer Tseng, who, despite being a surgeon, is my closest advisor, my best friend, and the love of my life.

I hope that you find *Pocket Medicine* useful throughout the arduous but incredibly rewarding journey of practicing medicine.

MARC S. SABATINE, MD, MPH

Approach (a systematic approach is vital)
- **Rate** (? tachy or brady) and **rhythm** (? P waves, regularity, P & QRS relationship)
- **Intervals** (PR, QRS, QT) and **axis** (? LAD or RAD)
- **Chamber abnormality** (? LAA and/or RAA, ? LVH and/or RVH)
- **QRST changes** (? Q waves, poor R-wave progression V_1–V_6, ST ↑/↓ or T-wave Δs)

Figure 1-1 QRS axis

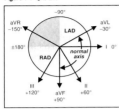

Left axis deviation (LAD)
- **Definition:** axis beyond −30° (S > R in lead II)
- **Etiologies:** LVH, LBBB, inferior MI, WPW
- **Left anterior fascicular block (LAFB):** LAD (−45 to −90°) and qR in aVL and QRS <120 msec and no other cause of LAD (eg, IMI)

Right axis deviation (RAD)
- **Definition:** axis beyond +90° (S > R in lead I)
- **Etiologies:** RVH, PE, COPD (usually not > +110°), septal defects, lateral MI, WPW
- **Left posterior fascicular block (LPFB):** RAD (90–180°) and rS in I & aVL and qR in III & aVF and QRS < 120 msec and no other cause of RAD

		Bundle Branch Blocks (Circ 2009;119:e235)
Normal	V_1 V_6	Initial depol. left-to-right across septum (r in V_1 & q in V_6; nb, absent in LBBB) followed by LV & RV free wall, with LV dominating (nb, RV depol. later and visible in RBBB).
RBBB		1. QRS ≥120 msec (110–119 = IVCD or "incomplete") 2. rSR' in R precordial leads (V_1,V_2) 3. Wide S wave in I and V_6 4. ± ST↓ or TWI in R precordial leads
LBBB		1. QRS ≥120 msec (110–119 = IVCD or "incomplete") 2. Broad, slurred, monophasic R in I, aVL, V_5–V_6 (± RS in V_5–V_6 if cardiomegaly) 3. Absence of Q in I, V_5 and V_6 (may have narrow q in aVL) 4. Displacement of ST & Tw opposite major QRS deflection 5. ± PRWP, LAD, Qw's in inferior leads

Bifascicular block: RBBB + LAFB/LPFB. "Trifascicular block": bifascicular block + 1° AVB.

Prolonged QT interval (NEJM 2008;358:169; www.torsades.org)
- QT measured from beginning of QRS complex to end of T wave (measure longest QT)
- QT varies w/ HR → corrected w/ Bazett formula: QTc = QT/$\sqrt{RR}$ (RR in sec), overcorrects at high HR, undercorrects at low HR (nl QTc <440 msec ♂, <460 msec ♀)
- Fridericia's formula preferred at very high or low HR: QTc = QT/$\sqrt[3]{RR}$
- QT prolongation a/w ↑ risk TdP (espec >500 msec); establish baseline QT and monitor if using QT prolonging meds, no estab guidelines for stopping Rx if QT prolongs
- Etiologies:
  Antiarrhythmics: class Ia (procainamide, disopyramide), class III (amio, sotalol, dofet)
  Psych drugs: antipsychotics (phenothiazines, haloperidol, atypicals), Li, ? SSRI, TCA
  Antimicrobials: macrolides, quinolones, azoles, pentamidine, atovaquone, atazanavir
  Other: antiemetics (droperidol, 5-HT₃ antagonists), alfuzosin, methadone, ranolazine
  Electrolyte disturbances: hypoCa (nb, hyperCa a/w ↓ QT), ± hypoK, ? hypoMg
  Autonomic dysfxn: ICH (deep TWI), Takotsubo, stroke, CEA, neck dissection
  Congenital (long QT syndrome): K, Na, & Ca channelopathies (Circ 2013;127:126)
  Misc: CAD, CMP, bradycardia, high-grade AVB, hypothyroidism, hypothermia, BBB

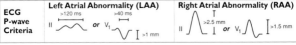

ECG P-wave Criteria	Left Atrial Abnormality (LAA)	Right Atrial Abnormality (RAA)

Left ventricular hypertrophy (LVH) (Circ 2009;119:e251)
- Etiologies: HTN, AS/AI, HCM, coarctation of aorta
- Criteria (all w/ Se <50%, Sp >85%; accuracy affected by age, sex, race, BMI)
  Romhilt-Estes point-score system (4 points = probable; 5 points = diagnostic):
  ↑ volt: limb lead R or S ≥20 mm or S in V_1 or V_2 ≥30 mm or R in V_5 or V_6 ≥30 mm (3 pts)

ST displacement opposite to QRS deflection: w/o dig (3 pts); w/ dig (1 pt)

LAA (2 pts); LAD (2 pts); QRS duration ≥90 msec (1 pt)

Intrinsicoid deflection (QRS onset to peak of R) in V_5 or V_6 ≥50 msec (1 pt)

Sokolow-Lyon: S in V_1 + R in V_5 or V_6 ≥35 mm or R in aVL ≥11 mm (↓ Se w/ ↑ BMI)

Cornell: R in aVL + S in V_3 >28 mm in men or >20 mm in women

If LAFB present: S in III + max (R+S) in any lead ≥30 mm in men or ≥28 mm in women

Right ventricular hypertrophy (RVH) (Circ 2009;119:e251; JACC 2014;63:672)

- Etiologies: cor pulmonale, congenital (tetralogy, TGA, PS, ASD, VSD), MS, TR
- Criteria [all insensitive, but specific (except in COPD); all w/ poor PPV in general population]

  R > S in V_1, R in V_1 ≥6 mm, S in V_5 ≥10 mm, S in V_6 ≥3 mm, R in aVR ≥4 mm

  RAD ≥110° (LVH + RAD or prominent S in V_5 or V_6 → consider biventricular hypertrophy)

Ddx of dominant R wave in V_1 or V_2

- Ventricular enlargement: RVH (RAD, RAA, deep S waves in I, V_5, V_6); HCM
- Myocardial injury: posterior MI (anterior R wave = posterior Q wave; often with IMI)
- Abnormal depolarization: RBBB (QRS >120 msec, rSR′); WPW (↓ PR, δ wave, ↑ QRS)
- Other: dextroversion; counterclockwise rotation; Duchenne's; lead misplacement; nl variant

Poor R wave progression (PRWP) (Am Heart J 2004;148:80)

- Definition: loss of anterior forces w/o frank Q waves (V_1–V_3); R wave in V_3 ≤3 mm
- Possible etiologies (nonspecific):

  old anteroseptal MI (usually w/ R wave V_3 ≤1.5 mm, ± persistent ST ↑ or TWI V_2 & V_3)

  LVH (delayed RWP w/ ↑ left precordial voltage), RVH (may also have RAA,

  RAD, limb lead QRS amplitude ≤5, $S_IS_{II}S_{III}$ w/ R/S ratio <1 in those leads)

  LBBB; WPW; clockwise rotation of the heart; lead misplacement; CMP; PTX

Pathologic Q waves

- Definition: ≥30 msec (≥20 msec V_2–V_3) or >25% height of R in that QRS complex
- Small (septal) q waves in I, aVL, V_5 & V_6 are nl, as can be isolated Qw in III, aVR, V_1
- "Pseudoinfarct" pattern may be seen in LBBB, infiltrative dis., HCM, COPD, PTX, WPW

ST elevation (STE) (NEJM 2003;349:2128; Circ 2009;119:e241 & e262)

- **Acute MI:** upward convexity STE (ie, a "frown") ± TWI (or prior MI w/ persistent STE)
- **Coronary spasm:** Prinzmetal's angina; transient STE in a coronary distribution
- **Pericarditis:** diffuse, upward concavity STE (ie, a "smile"); a/w PR ↓; Tw usually upright
- **HCM, Takotsubo CMP, ventricular aneurysm,** cardiac contusion
- **Pulmonary embolism:** occ. STE V_1–V_3; classically a/w TWI V_1–V_4, RAD, RBBB, $S_1Q_3T_3$
- **Repolarization abnormalities:**

  LBBB (↑ QRS duration, STE discordant from QRS complex; see "ACS" for dx MI in LBBB)

  LVH (↑ QRS amplitude); Brugada syndrome (rSR′, downsloping STE V_1–V_2); pacing

  Hyperkalemia (↑ QRS duration, tall Ts, no Ps)
- **aVR:** STE >1 mm a/w ↑ mortality in STEMI; STE aVR > V_1 a/w left main disease
- **Early repolarization:** most often seen in V_2–V_5 in young adults (JACC 2015;66:470)

  1–4 mm elev of peak of notch or start of slurred downstroke of R wave (ie, J point); ± up
  concavity of ST & large Tw (∴ ratio of STE/T wave <25%; may disappear w/ exercise)

  ? early repol in inf leads may be a/w ↑ risk of VF (NEJM 2009;361:2529; Circ 2011;124:2208)

ST depression (STD)

- **Myocardial ischemia** (± Tw abnl)
- **Acute true posterior MI:** posterior STE appearing as anterior STD (± ↑ R wave) in V_1–V_3

  ✓ posterior ECG leads; manage as a STEMI with rapid reperfusion (see "ACS")
- **Digitalis effect** (downsloping ST ± Tw abnl, does not correlate w/ dig levels)
- **Hypokalemia** (± U wave)
- **Repolarization abnl** a/w LBBB or LVH (usually in leads V_5, V_6, I, aVL)

T wave inversion (TWI; generally ≥1 mm; deep if ≥5 mm) (Circ 2009;119:e241)

- Ischemia or infarct; Wellens' sign (deep, symm precordial TWI) → critical prox LAD lesion
- Myopericarditis; CMP (Takotsubo, ARVC, apical HCM); MVP; PE (espec if TWI V_1–V_4)
- Repolarization abnl a/w LVH/RVH ("strain pattern"), BBB
- Posttachycardia or postpacing ("memory" T waves)
- Electrolyte, digoxin, PaO_2, $PaCO_2$, pH or core temperature disturbances
- Intracranial bleed ("cerebral T waves," usually w/ ↑ QT)
- Normal variant in children (V_1–V_4) and leads in which QRS complex predominantly ⊖

Low voltage

- QRS amplitude (R + S) <5 mm in all limb leads & <10 mm in all precordial leads
- Etiol: COPD, pericard./pleural effusion, myxedema, ↑ BMI, amyloid, diffuse CAD

Electrolyte abnormalities

- ↑ **K:** tented Tw, ↓ QT, ↑ PR, AVB, wide QRS, STE; ↓ **K:** flattened Tw, U waves, ↑ QT
- ↑ **Ca:** ↓ QT, flattened Tw & Pw, J point elevation; ↓ **Ca:** ↑ QT; Tw Δs

Disorder	Typical Characteristics & Diagnostic Studies
Cardiac Causes	
ACS (15–25% of chest pain in ED)	Substernal "pressure" (⊕ LR 1.3) → neck, jaw, arm (⊕ LR 1.3–2.6) Sharp, pleuritic, positional, or reprod. w/ palp all w/ ⊖ LR ≤0.35 Diaphoresis (⊕ LR 1.4), dyspnea (⊕ LR 1.2), a/w exertion (⊕ LR 1.5–1.8) ≈ prior MI (⊕ LR 2.2); ↓ w/ NTG/rest (but not reliable; *Annals EM* 2005;45:581) ± ECG Δs: STE, STD, TWI, Qw. ± ↑ Troponin.
Pericarditis & myo-pericarditis	Sharp pain → trapezius, ↑ w/ respiration, ↓ w/ sitting forward. ± Pericardial friction rub. ECG Δs (diffuse STE & PR ↓, opposite in aVR) ± pericardial effusion. If myocarditis, same as above + ↑ Tn and ± s/s HF and ↓ EF.
Aortic dissection	Sudden severe tearing pain (absence ⊖ LR 0.3). ± Asymm (>20 mmHg) BP or pulse (⊕ LR 5.7), focal neuro deficit (⊕ LR >6), AI, widened mediast. on CXR (absence ⊖ LR 0.3); false lumen on imaging. (*JAMA* 2002;287:2262)
Pulmonary Causes	
Pneumonia	Pleuritic; dyspnea, fever, cough, sputum. ↑ RR, crackles. CXR infiltrate.
Pleuritis	Sharp, pleuritic pain. ± Pleuritic friction rub.
PTX	Sudden onset, sharp pleuritic pain. Hyperresonance, ↓ BS. PTX on CXR.
PE	Sudden onset pleuritic pain. ↑ RR & HR, ↓ S_aO_2, ECG Δs (sinus tach, RAD, RBBB, $S_IQ_{III}T_{III}$, TWI V_1–V_4, occ STE V_1–V_3), ⊕ CTA or V/Q, ± ↑ Tn
Pulm HTN	Exertional pressure, DOE. ↓ S_aO_2, loud P_2, RV heave, right S_3 and/or S_4.
GI Causes	
Esophageal reflux	Substernal burning, acid taste in mouth, water brash. ↑ by meals, recumbency; ↓ by antacids. EGD, manometry, pH monitoring.
Esoph spasm	Intense substernal pain. ↑ by swallowing, ↓ by NTG/CCB. Manometry.
Mallory-Weiss	Esoph tear precipitated by vomiting. ± Hematemesis. Dx w/ EGD.
Boerhaave	Esoph rupture. Severe pain, ↑ w/ swallow. Mediastinal air palpable & on CT.
PUD	Epigastric pain, relieved by antacids. ± GIB. EGD, ± *H. pylori* test.
Biliary dis.	RUQ pain, N/V. ↑ by fatty foods. RUQ U/S; ↑ LFTs.
Pancreatitis	Epigastric/back discomfort. ↑ amylase & lipase; abd CT.
Musculoskeletal and Miscellaneous Causes	
Costochond	Localized sharp pain. ↑ w/ movement. Reproduced by palpation.
Zoster	Intense unilateral pain. Pain may precede dermatomal rash.
Anxiety	"Tightness," dyspnea, palpitations, other somatic symptoms

(*Braunwald's Heart Disease*, 10th ed, 2014; *JAMA* 2015;314:1955)

Initial approach

- **Focused history:** quality, severity, location, radiation; provoking/palliating factors; intensity at onset; duration, freq & pattern; setting; assoc sx; cardiac hx & risk factors
- **Targeted exam:** VS (incl. BP in both arms); gallops, murmurs, rubs; signs of vascular dis. (carotid/femoral bruits, ↓ pulses) or CHF; lung & abd. exam; chest wall for reproducibility
- **12-lead ECG:** obtain w/in 10 min; c/w priors & obtain serial ECGs; consider *posterior* leads (V₇–V₉) to ✓ for posterior STEMI if hx c/w ACS but stnd ECG unrevealing or ST ↓ V_1–V_3 (ant ischemia vs. post STEMI) and angina that is hard to relieve or R/S >1 in V_1–V_2
- **CXR;** other imaging (echo, PE CTA, etc.) as indicated based on H&P and initial testing
- **Troponin:** ✓ at baseline & 3–6 h after sx onset; repeat 6 h later if clinical or ECG Δs; level >99th %ile w/ rise & fall in appropriate setting is dx of MI; >95% Se, 90% Sp detectable 1–6 h after injury, peaks 24 h, may be elevated for 7–14 d in STEMI high-sens. assays (not yet available in U.S.) offer NPV >99% at 1 h (*Lancet* 2015;386:2481) Causes for ↑ Tn other than plaque rupture (= "type 1 MI"): (1) Supply-demand mismatch not due to Δ in CAD (= "type 2 MI"; eg, ↑↑ HR, shock, HTN crisis, spasm, severe AS), (2) non-ischemic injury (myocarditis/toxic CMP, cardiac contusion) or (3) multifactorial (PE, sepsis, severe HF, renal failure, Takotsubo, infilt. dis.) (*Circ* 2012;126:2020)
- **CK-MB:** less Se & Sp than Tn (other sources: skel. muscle, intestine, etc); CK-MB/CK ratio >2.5 → cardiac source. Useful for dx of post-PCI/CABG MI or (re)MI if Tn already high.

Early noninvasive imaging

- If low prob of ACS (eg, ⊖ ECG & Tn) & stable → outPt or inPt noninvasive fxnal or imaging test (qv). CCTA w/ high NPV but low PPV; ↓ LOS c/w fxnal testing (*NEJM* 2012;366:1393).
- "Triple r/o" CT angiogram sometimes performed to r/o CAD, PE, AoD if dx unclear

Stress testing (Circ 2007;115:1464; JACC 2012;60:1828)
- **Indications:** dx CAD, evaluate Δ in clinical status in Pt w/ known CAD, risk stratify after ACS, evaluate exercise tolerance, localize ischemia (imaging required)
- **Contraindications** (Circ 2002;106:1883; & 2012;126:2465)
  Absolute: AMI w/in 48 h, high-risk UA, acute PE, severe sx AS, uncontrolled HF, uncontrolled arrhythmias, myopericarditis, acute aortic dissection
  Relative (discuss with stress lab): left main CAD, mod valvular stenosis, severe HTN, HCMP, high-degree AVB, severe electrolyte abnl

Exercise tolerance test (w/ ECG alone)
- Generally preferred if Pt can meaningfully exercise; ECG Δs w/ Se ~65%, Sp ~80%
- Typically use treadmill w/ Bruce protocol (modified Bruce if decond. or recent MI)
- Hold anti-isch. meds (eg, nitrates, βB) if dx'ing CAD but give to assess adequacy of meds

Pharmacologic stress test (nb, requires imaging as ECG not interpretable)
- Use if unable to exercise, low exercise tolerance, or recent MI. Se & Sp ≈ exercise.
- Preferred if LBBB or V-paced, as higher prob of false ⊕ imaging with exercise
- *Coronary vasodilator:* diffuse vasodilation → relative "coronary steal" from vessels w/ fixed epicardial disease. Reveals CAD, *but not if Pt ischemic w/ exercise.* Regadenoson, dipyridamole, adenosine. Side effects: flushing, ↓ HR & AVB, dyspnea & bronchospasm.
- *Chronotropes/inotropes* (dobuta): more physiologic, but longer test; may precip arrhythmia

Imaging for stress test
- Use if uninterpretable ECG (V-paced, LBBB, resting ST ↓ >1 mm, digoxin, LVH, WPW), after indeterminate ECG test, or if pharmacologic test
- Use when need to localize ischemia (often used if prior coronary revasc)
- **Radionuclide myocardial perfusion imaging** w/ images obtained at rest & w/ stress
  SPECT (eg, ^{99m}Tc-sestamibi): Se ~85%, Sp ~80%
  PET (rubidium-82): Se ~90%, Sp ~85%; requires pharmacologic stress not exercise
  ECG-gated imaging allows assessment of regional LV fxn (sign of ischemia/infarction)
- **Echo** (exercise or dobuta): Se ~85%, Sp ~85%; no radiation; operator-dependent
- **Cardiac MRI** (w/ pharmacologic stress) another option with excellent Se & Sp

Test results
- **HR** (must achieve ≥85% of max predicted HR [220-age] for exer. test to be dx), **BP** response, peak **double product** (HR × BP; nl >20k), HR recovery (HR$_{peak}$ – HR$_{1 min later}$; nl >12)
- **Max exercise capacity** achieved (METS or min); **occurrence of symptoms**
- **ECG Δs:** downsloping or horizontal ST ↓ (≥1 mm) 60–80 ms after QRS predictive of CAD (but does not localize ischemic territory); however, STE highly predictive & localizes
- Duke treadmill score = exercise min – (5 × max ST dev) – (4 × angina index) [0 none, 1 nonlimiting, 2 limiting); score ≥5 → <1% 1-y mort; –10 to + 4 → 2–3%; ≤–11 → ≥5%
- **Imaging:** radionuclide defects or echocardiographic regional wall motion abnormalities reversible defect = ischemia; fixed defect = infarct; transient isch dilation → ? severe 3VD false ⊕: breast → ant defect; diaphragm → inf defect. False ⊖: balanced (3VD) ischemia.

High-risk test results (PPV ~50% for LM or 3VD, ∴ consider coronary angio)
- ECG: ST ↓ ≥2 mm or ≥1 mm in stage 1 or in ≥5 leads or ≥5 min in recovery; ST ↑; VT
- Physiologic: ↓ or fail to ↑ BP, <4 METS, angina during exercise, Duke score ≤–11; ↓ EF
- Radionuclide: ≥1 lg or ≥2 mod. reversible defects, transient LV cavity dilation, ↑ lung uptake

Myocardial viability (Circ 2008;117:103; Eur Heart J 2011;31:2984 & 2011;32:810)
- Goal: identify hibernating myocardium that could regain fxn after revascularization
- Options: **MRI** (Se ~85%, Sp ~75%), **PET** (Se ~90%, Sp ~65%), **dobutamine stress echo** (Se ~80%, Sp ~80%); **SPECT/rest-redistribution** (Se ~85%, Sp ~60%)
  In Pts w/ LV dysfxn, viabil. doesn't predict ↑ CABG benefit vs. med Rx (NEJM 2011;364:1617)

Coronary CT/MR angio (NEJM 2008;359:2324; Circ 2010;121:2509; Lancet 2012;379:453)
- In Pts w/ CP, CCTA 100% Se, 54% Sp for ACS, ∴ NPV 100%, PPV 17% (JACC 2009;53: 1642). ↓ LOS, but ↑ cath/PCI, radiation vs. fxnal study (NEJM 2012;367:299; JACC 2013;61:880).
- In sx outPt, CCTA vs. fxnal testing → ↑ radiation, cath/PCI, ≈ outcomes (NEJM 2015;372:1291)
- Unlike CCTA, MR does not require iodinated contrast, HR control or radiation. Can assess LV fxn, enhancement (early = microvasc obstr.; late = MI). Grossly ≈ Se/Sp to CCTA.

Coronary artery calcium score (CACS; NEJM 2012;366:294; JAMA 2012;308:788)
- Quantifies extent of calcium; thus *estimates* plaque burden (but *not* % coronary stenosis)
- CAC sensitive (91%) but not specific (49%) for presence of CAD; high NPV to r/o CAD
- May provide incremental value to clinical scores for risk stratification (JAMA 2004;291:210). ACC/AHA guidelines note CAC assessment is reasonable in asx Pts w/ intermed risk (10–20% 10-y Framingham risk; ? value if 6–10% 10-y risk) (Circ 2010;122:e584).

Indications for coronary angiography in stable CAD or asx Pts

- CCS class III–IV angina despite med Rx, angina + systolic dysfxn, or unexplained low EF
- High-risk stress test findings (qv) or uncertain dx after noninv testing (& info will Δ mgmt)
- Occupational need for definitive dx (eg, pilot) or inability to undergo noninvasive testing
- Survivor of SCD, polymorphic VT, sustained monomorphic VT
- Suspected spasm or nonatherosclerotic cause of ischemia (eg, anomalous coronary)

Precath checklist & periprocedural pharmacotherapy

- Document peripheral arterial exam (radial, femoral, DP, PT pulses; bruits). For radial access, ✓ palmar arch intact (eg, w/ pulse oximetry & plethysmography). Ensure can lie flat for several hrs. NPO >6 h. Ensure blood bank sample.
- ✓ CBC, PT & Cr; IVF (? NaHCO₃), ± acetylcysteine (see "CIAKI"), hold ACEI/ARB
- ASA 325 mg × 1. Timing of P2Y₁₂ inhib debated. ASAP for STEMI. ? preRx NSTEACS if clopi (JAMA 2012;308:2507) or ticag (PLATO), not prasugrel. Cangrelor (IV P2Y₁₂ inhib) ↓ peri-PCI events vs. clopi w/o preload (NEJM 2013;368:1303). ? statin preRx (Circ 2011;123:1622).

Coronary revascularization in stable CAD (Circ 2011;124:e574; NEJM 2016;374:1167)

- Optimal med Rx (**OMT**) should be initial focus if stable, w/o critical anatomy, & w/o ↓ EF
- **PCI:** ↓ angina vs OMT; does *not* ↓ D/MI (NEJM 2007;356:1503 & 2015;373:1204); if ≥1 stenosis w/ FFR (qv) ≤0.8, ↓ urg revasc & ? D/MI c/w OMT (NEJM 2014;371:1208); ? noninf to CABG in unprot LM dz. (NEJM 2011;364:1718)
- **CABG** (NEJM 2016;374:1954): in older studies, ↓ mort. c/w OMT if 3VD, LM, 2VD w/ crit. prox LAD, esp. if ↓ EF; recently confirmed if multivessel dis. & EF <35% (NEJM 2016;374:1511); in diabetics w/ ≥2VD, ↓ D/MI, but ↑ stroke c/w PCI (NEJM 2012;367:2375)
- If revasc deemed necessary, *PCI* if limited # of discrete lesions, nl EF, no DM, poor operative candidate; *CABG* if extensive or diffuse disease, ↓ EF, DM or valvular disease; if 3VD/LM: CABG ↓ D/MI & revasc but trend toward ↑ stroke c/w PCI (Lancet 2013;381:629); SYNTAX score II helps identify Pts who benefit most from CABG (Lancet 2013;381:639)

PCI and peri-PCI interventions

- **Access:** radial vs femoral, w/ former → ↓ bleeding and MACE (JACC Intv 2016;9:1419)
- **Fractional flow reserve** (FFR): ratio of max flow (induced by IV or IC adenosine) distal vs. prox to stenosis; help ID lesions that are truly hemodyn. significant
- Balloon angioplasty by itself rare b/c elastic recoil; reserved for lesions too narrow to stent
- **Bare metal stents (BMS):** ↓ restenosis & repeat revasc c/w angioplasty alone
- **Drug-eluting stents (DES):** ↓ neointimal hyperplasia → ~75% ↓ restenosis, ~50% ↓ repeat revasc (<5% by 1 y), ? ↑ late stent thrombosis, no Δ D/MI c/w BMS (NEJM 2013;368:254); latest gen. DES w/ very low rates of restenosis, repeat revasc & stent thrombosis
- **Bioresorbable stent:** resorbs over yrs, but ? ↑ MACE & stent thromb. (NEJM 2015;373:1905)
- Duration of DAPT: ASA (81 mg) lifelong. If SIHD, P2Y₁₂ inhib × 4 wk (BMS) or ≥6 mo (DES). If ACS, P2Y₁₂ >12 mo → ~20% ↓ MACE, ↑ bleeding and ~15% ↓ CV death (NEJM 2014;371:2155 & 2015;372:1791). If need oral anticoag, consider clopi + NOAC ± ASA.

Post-PCI complications

- Postprocedural ✓ vascular access site, distal pulses, ECG, CBC, Cr
- **Bleeding**
  hematoma/overt bleeding: **manual compression**, reverse/stop anticoag
  retroperitoneal bleed: may p/w ↓ Hct ± back pain; ↑ HR & ↓ BP late; Dx w/ abd/pelvic CT (I⁻); Rx: reverse/stop anticoag (d/w interventionalist), IVF/PRBC/plts as required if bleeding uncontrolled, consult performing interventionalist or surgery
- **Vascular damage** (~1% of dx angio, ~5% of transfemoral PCI; Circ 2007;115:2666)
  pseudoaneurysm: triad of pain, expansile mass, systolic bruit; Dx: U/S; Rx (if pain or >2 cm): manual or U/S-directed compression, thrombin injection or surgical repair
  AV fistula: continuous bruit; Dx: U/S; Rx: surgical repair if large or sx
  LE ischemia (emboli, dissection, clot): cool, mottled extremity, ↓ distal pulses; Dx: pulse volume recording (PVR), angio; Rx: percutaneous or surgical repair
- **Peri-PCI MI:** >5× ULN of Tn/CK-MB + either sx or ECG/angio Δs; Qw MI in <1%
- **Contrast-induced acute kidney injury:** manifests w/in 48 h, peaks 3–5 d (see "CIAKI")
- **Cholesterol emboli syndrome** (typically in middle-aged & elderly and w/ Ao atheroma) renal failure and progressive, ± eos in urine); mesenteric ischemia (abd pain, LGIB, pancreatitis); intact distal pulses but livedo pattern and toe necrosis
- **Stent thrombosis:** mins to yrs after PCI, typically p/w AMI. Due to mech prob. (stent underexpansion or unrecognized dissection, typically presents early) or **d/c of antiplt Rx** (espec if d/c both ASA & P2Y₁₂ inhib; JAMA 2005;293:2126).
- **In-stent restenosis:** mos after PCI, typically p/w gradual ↑ angina (10% p/w ACS). Due to combination of elastic recoil and neointimal hyperplasia; ↓ w/ DES vs. BMS.

ACUTE CORONARY SYNDROMES

Spectrum of Acute Coronary Syndromes			
Dx	UA	NSTEMI	STEMI
Coronary thrombosis	Subtotal occlusion		Total occlusion
History	angina that is new-onset, crescendo or at rest; usually <30 min		angina at rest
ECG	± ST depression and/or TWI		ST elevations
Troponin/CK-MB	⊖	⊕	⊕⊕

Ddx (causes of myocardial ischemia/infarction other than atherosclerotic plaque rupture)
• **Nonatherosclerotic coronary artery disease**
  Spasm: Prinzmetal's variant, cocaine-induced (6% of chest pain + cocaine use r/i for MI)
  Dissection: spontaneous (vasculitis, CTD, pregnancy), aortic dissection with retrograde extension (usually involving RCA → IMI) or mechanical (PCI, surgery, trauma)
  Embolism (*Circ* 2015;132:241): AF, thrombus/myxoma, endocard., prosth valve thrombosis
  Vasculitis: Kawasaki syndrome, Takayasu arteritis, PAN, Churg-Strauss, SLE, RA
  Congenital: anomalous origin from aorta or PA, myocardial bridge (intramural segment)
• **Ischemia w/o plaque rupture** ("type 2" MI): ↑ demand (eg, ↑ HR), ↓ supply (eg, HoTN)
• **Direct myocardial injury:** myocarditis; Takotsubo/stress CMP; toxic CMP; cardiac contusion

Clinical manifestations (*JAMA* 2015;314:1955)
• **Typical angina:** retrosternal pressure/pain/tightness ± radiation to neck, jaw, arms; precip. by exertion, relieved by rest/ NTG. In ACS: new-onset, crescendo or at rest.
• **Associated symptoms:** dyspnea, diaphoresis, N/V, palpitations or light-headedness
• Many MIs (~20% in older series) are initially unrecognized b/c silent or atypical sx
• **Atypical sxs** (incl N/V & epig pain) ? more common in ♀, elderly, diabetes, inferior ischemia

Physical exam
• Signs of ischemia: S₄, new MR murmur 2° pap. muscle dysfxn, paradoxical S₂, diaphoresis
• Signs of heart failure: ↑ JVP, crackles in lung fields, ⊕ S₃, HoTN, cool extremities
• Signs of other vascular disease: asymmetric BP, carotid or femoral bruits, ↓ distal pulses

Diagnostic studies
• **ECG:** ST ↓/↑, TWI, new LBBB, hyperacute Tw; Qw/PRWP may suggest prior MI & ∴ CAD
  ✓ ECG w/in 10 min of presentation, with any Δ in sx & at 6–12 h; compare w/ baseline
  STEMI dx if old LBBB: ≥1 mm STE *concordant* w/ QRS (Se 73%, Sp 92%), STD ≥1 mm V₁–V₃ (Se 25%, Sp 96%), STE ≥5 mm *discordant* w/ QRS (Se 31%, Sp 92%)

Localization of MI		
Anatomic area	ECG leads w/ STE	Coronary artery
Septal	V₁–V₂ ± aVR	Proximal LAD
Anterior	V₃–V₄	LAD
Apical	V₅–V₆	Distal LAD, LCx, or RCA
Lateral	I, aVL	LCx
Inferior	II, III, aVF	RCA (~85%), LCx (~15%)
RV	V₁–V₂ & V₄R (most Se)	Proximal RCA
Posterior	ST *depression* V₁–V₃ (= STE V₇–V₉ posterior leads, ✓ if clinical suspicion)	RCA or LCx

If ECG non-dx & suspicion high, ✓ leads V₇–V₉ to assess distal LCx/RCA territory. ✓ R-sided precordial leads in IMI to help detect RV involvement (STE in V₄R most Se). STE in III > STE in II and lack of STE in I or aVL suggest RCA rather than LCx culprit in IMI. STE in aVR suggests LM or prox LAD occlusion or diffuse ischemia.

• **Cardiac biomarkers:** ✓ Tn (preferred over CK-MB) at presentation & 3–6 h after sx onset; repeat 6 h later if clinical or ECG Δs; rise to >99th %ile in appropriate clinical setting dx of MI (see "Chest Pain"); rise in Tn in CKD still portends poor prognosis (*NEJM* 2002;346:2047)
• If low prob, **stress test, CT angio** to r/o CAD; new wall motion abnl on TTE suggests ACS
• **Coronary angio** gold standard for CAD

Prinzmetal's (variant) angina
• Coronary spasm → transient STE usually w/o MI (*but* MI, AVB, VT can occur)
• Pts usually young, smokers, ± other vasospastic disorders (eg, migraines, Raynaud's)
• Angiography: nonobstructive CAD (spasm can be provoked during cath but rarely done)
• Treatment: high-dose CCB ± long-acting nitrates (+SL prn), ↑ nitroglycerin; d/c smoking; avoid high-dose ASA (can inhibit prostacyclin and worsen spasm), nonselect βB, triptans
• Cocaine-induced vasospasm: CCB, nitrates, ASA; ? avoid βB, but labetalol appears safe

Likelihood of ACS (Circ 2007;116:e148)

Feature	High (any of below)	Intermediate (no high features, any of below)	Low (no high/inter. features, may have below)
History	Chest or L arm pain like prior angina, h/o CAD (incl MI)	Chest or arm pain, age >70 y, male, diabetes	Atypical sx (eg, pleuritic, sharp or positional pain)
Exam	HoTN, diaphoresis, HF, transient MR	PAD or cerebrovascular disease	Pain reproduced on palp.
ECG	New STD (≥1 mm) TWI in mult leads	Old Qw, STD (0.5–0.9 mm), TWI (>1 mm)	TWF/TWI (<1 mm) in leads w/ dominant R wave
Biomarkers	⊕ Tn or CK-MB	Normal	Normal

Approach to triage
- If hx and initial ECG & Tn non-dx, repeat ECG q15–30min × 1 h & Tn 3–6 h after sx onset
- If remain nl and low likelihood of ACS, search for alternative causes of chest pain
- If remain nl, have ruled out MI, *but* if suspicion for ACS based on hx, then still need to r/o UA w/ stress test to assess for inducible ischemia (or CTA to r/o CAD);
  if low risk (eg, age ≤70; ∅ prior CAD, CVD, PAD; ∅ rest angina) can do before d/c from ED or as outPt w/in 72 h (0% mortality, <0.5% MI; Ann Emerg Med 2006;47:427)
  if not low risk, admit and initiate Rx for possible ACS and consider stress test or cath

Acute Anti-Ischemic and Analgesic Treatment

Nitrates (SL or IV) 0.3–0.4 mg SL q5min × 3, then consider IV if still sx	Use for relief of sx, Rx for HTN or HF. No clear ↓ in mortality. *Caution* if preload-sensitive (eg, HoTN, AS, sx RV infarct); contraindicated if recent PDE5 inhibitor use.
β-blockers eg, metop 25–50 mg PO q6h titrate slowly to HR 50–60 IV only if HTN and no HF	↓ ischemia & progression of UA to MI (JAMA 1988:260:2259) STEMI: ↓ arrhythmic death & reMI, but ↑ cardiogenic shock early (espec if signs of HF) (Lancet 2005;366:1622). IV βB prior to 1° PCI ↓ infarct size and ↑ EF (Circ 2013;128:1495). *Contraindic.* PR >0.24 sec, HR <60, 2°/3° AVB, severe bronchospasm, s/s HF or low output, risk factors for shock (eg, >70 y, HR >110, SBP <120, late presentation STEMI)
CCB (nondihydropyridines)	If cannot tolerate βB b/c bronchospasm
Morphine	Relieves pain/anxiety; venodilation ↓ preload. Do not mask refractory sx. May delay antiplt effects of P2Y₁₂ inhib.
Oxygen	Use prn for resp distress or to keep S₂O₂ >90% ? ↑ infarct size in STEMI w/o hypoxia (Circ 2015;131:2143)

Other early adjunctive therapy
- **High-intensity statin therapy** (eg, atorva 80 mg qd; PROVE-IT TIMI 22 NEJM 2004;350:1495)
  ↓ ischemic events w/ benefit emerging w/in wks (JAMA 2001;285:1711 & JACC 2005;46:1405)
  ↓ peri-PCI MI (JACC 2010;56:1099); ↓ contrast-induced nephropathy (JACC 2014;63:71)
- **ACEI/ARB:** start once hemodynamics and renal function stable
  Strong indication for ACEI if heart failure, EF <40%, HTN, DM, CKD; ~10% ↓ mortality, greatest benefit in STEMI or prior MI (Lancet 1994;343:1115 & 1995;345:669)
  ARB appear ≈ ACEI (NEJM 2003;349:20); give if contraindic to ACEI
- Ezetimibe, aldosterone blockade, and ranolazine discussed later (long-term Rx)
- **IABP:** can be used for refractory angina when PCI not available

NSTE-ACS (Circ 2014;130:e344)

Key issues are antithrombotic regimen and invasive vs. conservative strategy

Antiplatelet Therapy

Aspirin 162–325 mg × 1, then 81 mg qd (non–enteric-coated, chewable)	50–70% ↓ D/MI (NEJM 1988;319:1105) Low dose (~81 mg) pref long term (NEJM 2010;363:930) If allergy, use clopi and/or desensitize to ASA
P2Y₁₂ (ADP receptor) inhibitor (choose one of the following in addition to ASA) Timing remains controversial. European guidelines recommend P2Y₁₂ inhibitor as soon as possible (except prasugrel; EHJ 2011;32:2999). See below for specific recommendations.	
• **Ticagrelor** (preferred over clopi) 180 mg × 1 → 90 mg bid Reversible, but wait 3–5 d prior to surg Use only with ASA <100 mg qd	More rapid and potent plt inhib c/w clopi 16% ↓ CVD/MI/stroke & 21% ↓ CV death c/w clopi; ↑ non-CABG bleeding (NEJM 2009;361:1045) Given upstream or at time of PCI Dyspnea (but S₂O₂ & PFTs nl) & ventricular pauses

• **Prasugrel** (preferred over clopi) 60 mg × 1 at PCI → 10 mg qd (consider 5 mg/d if <60 kg) Wait 7 d prior to surgery	More rapid and potent plt inhib c/w clopi 19% ↓ CVD/MI/stroke in ACS w/ planned PCI vs. clopi, but ↑ bleeding (*NEJM* 2007:359:2001), incl fatal bleeds Not sup to clopi if med mgmt w/o PCI (*NEJM* 2012:367:1297) In NSTE-ACS, should be given at time of PCI and not upstream due to ↑ bleeding (*NEJM* 2013:369:999) Contraindic. if h/o TIA/CVA; ? avoid if >75 y
• **Clopidogrel*** 300–600 mg × 1 → 75 mg qd Requires ~6 h to steady state	ASA+clopi → 20% ↓ CVD/MI/stroke vs. ASA alone ↑ benefit if given hrs *prior* to PCI (*JAMA* 2012:308:2507), but if require CABG, need to wait >5 d after d/c clopi
• **Cangrelor** Only IV P2Y₁₂ inhibitor Rapid onset/offset; t½ 3–5 min	22% ↓ CV events (mostly peri-PCI MI and stent thrombosis) vs. clopi 300 mg at time of PCI; no significant ↑ bleeding (*NEJM* 2013:368:1303) Unclear benefit if upstream clopi administered (*NEJM* 2009:361:2318) and no data vs. prasugrel or ticagrelor
GP IIb/IIIa inhibitors (GPI) abciximab; eptifibatide; tirofiban Infusions given ≤24 h peri & post PCI; shorter (~2 h) as effective w/ ↓ bleeding (*JACC* 2009:53:837)	No clear benefit for routinely starting prior to PCI and ↑ bleeding (*NEJM* 2009:360:2176) Consider if refractory ischemia or to maintain optimal Rx while awaiting angio or in high-risk Pts (eg, large clot burden) at time of PCI, espec if using clopi and no preRx.

*~30% pop has ↓ fxn *CYP2C19* → ↑ CV events if PCI on clopi (*NEJM* 2009:360:354)

Anticoagulant Therapy (choose one)	
UFH: 60 U/kg IVB (max 4000 U) then 12 U/kg/h (max 1000 U/h initially) × 48 h or until end of PCI	24% ↓ D/MI (*JAMA* 1996:276:811) Titrate to aPTT 1.5–2× control (~50–70 sec) Hold until INR <2 if already on warfarin
Enoxaparin (low-molec-wt heparin) 1 mg/kg SC bid (± 30 mg IVB) (qd if CrCl <30) × 2–8 d or until PCI	~10% ↓ D/MI vs. UFH (*JAMA* 2004:292:45,89). Can perform PCI on enox (*Circ* 2001:103:658), but ↑ bleeding if switch b/w enox and UFH.
Bivalirudin (direct thrombin inhibitor) 0.75 mg/kg IVB at → 1.75 mg/kg/h	↓ bleeding (espec vs. UFH + GPI), ↑ ↑ early MI (*Lancet* 2014:384:599). Use instead of UFH if HIT.
Fondaparinux (Xa inhibitor) 2.5 mg SC qd × 2–8 d	C/w enox, 17% ↓ death & 38% ↓ bleeding (*NEJM* 2006:354:1464). However, ↑ risk of catheter thrombosis; ∴ must supplement w/ UFH if PCI.

Coronary angiography (*Circ* 2014;130:e344)
• **Immediate/urgent coronary angiography** (w/in 2 h) if refractory/recurrent angina or hemodynamic or electrical instability
• **Invasive (INV) strategy** = routine angiography w/in 72 h
 Early (w/in 24 h) if: ⊕ Tn, ST Δ, GRACE risk score (www.outcomes-umassmed.org/grace) >140 (*NEJM* 2009:360:2165)
 Delayed (ie, w/in 72 h) acceptable if w/o above features but w/: diabetes, EF <40%, GFR <60, post-MI angina, TRS ≥3, GRACE score 109–140, PCI w/in 6 mo, prior CABG
 32% ↓ rehosp for ACS, nonsignif 16% ↓ MI, no Δ in mortality c/w cons. (*JAMA* 2008:300:71)
 ↑ peri-PCI MI counterbalanced by ↓↓ in spont. MI
 mortality benefit seen in some studies, likely only if cons. strategy w/ low rate of angio
• **Conservative (CONS) strategy** = selective angio. Med Rx w/ pre-d/c stress test; angio only if recurrent ischemia or strongly ⊕ ETT. Indicated for: low TIMI Risk Score, Pt or physician pref in absence of high-risk features, or low-risk women (*JAMA* 2008:300:71).

TIMI Risk Score (TRS) for UA/NSTEMI (*JAMA* 2000:284:835)				
Calculation of Risk Score		**Application of Risk Score**		
Characteristic	**Point**	**Score**	**D/MI/UR by 14 d**	
Historical		0–1	5%	
Age ≥65 y	1	2	8%	
≥3 Risk factors for CAD	1	3	13%	
Known CAD (stenosis ≥50%)	1	4	20%	
ASA use in past 7 d	1	5	26%	
Presentation		6–7	41%	
Severe angina (≥2 episodes w/in 24 h)	1	Higher risk Pts (TRS ≥3) derive ↑ benefit from LMWH, GP IIb/IIIa inhibitors and early angiography (*JACC* 2003:41:89S)		
ST deviation ≥0.5 mm	1			
⊕ cardiac marker (troponin, CK-MB)	1			
RISK SCORE = Total points	**(0–7)**			

Figure 1-2 Approach to UA/NSTEMI

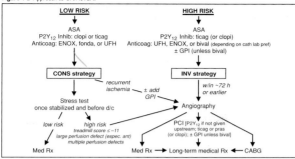

STEMI

Requisite STE (at J point)
- ≥2 contiguous leads w/ ≥1 mm (except for V_2–V_3: ≥2 mm in ♂ and ≥1.5 mm in ♀), or
- New or presumed new LBBB w/ compelling H&P, or
- True posterior MI: ST depression V_1–V_3 ± tall Rw w/ STE on posterior leads (V_7–V_9)

Reperfusion ("time is muscle")
- Immediate reperfusion (ie, opening occluded culprit coronary artery) is critical
- In PCI-capable hospital, goal should be **primary PCI w/in 90 min** of 1st medical contact
- In non-PCI-capable hospital, consider *transfer* to PCI-capable hospital (see below), o/w **fibrinolytic therapy** w/in 30 min of hospital presentation
- Do not let decision regarding *method* of reperfusion delay *time* to reperfusion

Primary PCI (NEJM 2007;356:47; JACC 2013;61:e78 & 2016;67:1235)
- Definition: immediate PCI upon arrival to hospital or transfer for immediate PCI
- Indic: STE + sx onset w/in <12 h; ongoing ischemia 12–24 h after sx onset; shock
- Superior to lysis: 27% ↓ death, 65% ↓ reMI, 54% ↓ stroke (Lancet 2003;361:13)
- *Transfer* to center for 1° PCI superior to lysis (NEJM 2003;349:733), see below
- Routine thrombus aspiration: no benefit, ↑ stroke (Lancet 2015;387:127; 2015;372:1389)
- Complete revasc: ↓ MACE vs. culprit artery alone (NEJM 2013; 369:1115; JACC 2015;65:963); alternatively, assess ischemia due to residual lesions w/ imaging stress (Circ 2011;124:e574)

Fibrinolysis vs. Hospital Transfer for Primary PCI: Assess Time and Risk
1. **Time required for transport to skilled PCI lab:** door-to-balloon <120 min & [door-to-balloon]–[door-to-needle] <1 h favors transfer for PCI
2. **Risk from STEMI:** high-risk Pts (eg, shock) fare better with mechanical reperfusion
3. **Time to presentation:** efficacy of lytics ↓ w/ ↑ time from sx onset, espec >3 h
4. **Risk of fibrinolysis:** if high risk of ICH or bleeding, PCI safer option

Adapted from ACC/AHA 2013 STEMI Guidelines (Circ 2013;127:529)

Fibrinolysis
- Indic: STE/LBBB + sx <12 h (& >120 min before PCI can be done); benefit if sx >12 h less clear; reasonable if persist. sx & STE or hemodynamic instability or large territory at risk
- Mortality ↓ ~20% in anterior MI or LBBB and ~10% in IMI c/w ∅ reperfusion Rx
- Prehospital lysis (ie, ambulance): further 17% ↓ in mortality (JAMA 2000;283:2686)
- ~1% risk of ICH; high risk incl elderly (~2% if >75 y), ♀, low wt. ∴ PCI more attractive

Contraindications to Fibrinolysis	
Absolute contraindications	**Relative contraindications**
• Any prior ICH	• H/o severe HTN, SBP >180 or DBP >110
• Intracranial neoplasm, aneurysm, AVM	on presentation (? absolute if low-risk MI)
• Ischemic stroke or closed head trauma	• Ischemic stroke >3 mo prior
w/in 3 mo; head/spinal surg. w/in 2 mo	• CPR >10 min; trauma/major surg. w/in 3 wk
• Active internal bleeding or known	• Internal bleed w/in 2–4 wk; active PUD
bleeding diathesis	• Noncompressible vascular punctures
• Suspected aortic dissection	• Pregnancy
• Severe uncontrollable HTN	• Current use of anticoagulants
• For SK, SK Rx w/in 6 mo	• For SK, prior SK exposure

Nonprimary PCI

- Rescue PCI if shock, unstable, failed reperfusion or persistent sx (NEJM 2005;353:2758)
- Routine angio ± PCI w/in 24 h of successful lysis: ↓ D/MI/revasc (Lancet 2004;364:1045) and w/in 6 h ↓ reMI, recurrent ischemia, & HF compared to w/in 2 wk (NEJM 2009;360:2705); ∴ if lysed at non-PCI-capable hosp., consider transfer to PCI-capable hosp. ASAP esp if hi-risk (eg, ant. MI, IMI w/ ↓ EF or RV infarct, extensive STE/LBBB, HF, ↓ BP or ↑ HR)
- Late PCI (median day 8) of occluded infarct-related artery: no benefit (NEJM 2006;355:2395)

Antiplatelet Therapy	
Aspirin 162–325 mg × 1 (crushed/chewed) then 81 mg qd	23% ↓ in death (Lancet 1988;ii:349) Should not be stopped if CABG required
P2Y₁₂ inhibitor Give ASAP (do not wait for angio) b/c onset inhib delayed in STEMI pts Ticagrelor or prasugrel (if PCI as detailed above) Clopidogrel: 600 mg pre-PCI; 300 mg if lysis (no LD if >75 y) → 75 mg qd	Lysis: clopidogrel 41% ↑ in patency, 7% ↓ mort, no Δ major bleed or ICH (NEJM 2005;352:1179; Lancet 2005;366:1607); no data for pras or ticag w/ lytic PCI: prasugrel and ticagrelor ↓ CV events c/w clopi (Lancet 2009;373:723 & Circ 2010;122:2131) Prehospital ticagrelor may be safe & ? ↓ rate of stent thrombosis (NEJM 2014;371:1016)
GP IIb/IIIa inhibitors abciximab, eptifibatide, tirofiban	Lysis: no indication (Lancet 2001;357:1905) Peri-PCI: 60% ↓ D/MI/UR (NEJM 2001;344:1895)

Adapted from ACC/AHA 2013 STEMI Guidelines Update (Circ 2013;127:529; Lancet 2013;382:633)

Anticoagulant Therapy (choose one)	
UFH 60 U/kg IVB (max 4000 U) 12 U/kg/h (max 1000 U/h initially)	No demonstrated mortality benefit ↑ patency with fibrin-specific lytics Titrate to aPTT 1.5–2× control (~50–70 sec)
Enoxaparin Lysis: 30 mg IVB → 1 mg/kg SC bid (adjust for age >75 & CrCl) PCI: 0.5 mg/kg IVB	Lysis: 17% ↓ D/MI w/ ENOX × 7 d vs. UFH × 2 d (NEJM 2006;354:1477) PCI: ↓ D/MI/revasc and ≈ bleeding vs. UFH (Lancet 2011;378:693)
Bivalirudin 0.75 mg/kg IVB → 1.75 mg/kg/hr IV	PCI: ↓ bleeding (espec vs. UFH + GP IIb/IIIa inhib), ± ↑ MI, ↑ stent thromb, ? ↓ mortality (Lancet 2014;384:599; JAMA 2015;313:1336; NEJM 2015;373:997)

Fondaparinux can be used (if CrCl >30 mL/min) in setting of lysis, where superior to UFH w/ less bleeding (JAMA 2006;295:1519). Adapted from ACC/AHA 2013 STEMI Guidelines (Circ 2013;127:529; Lancet 2013;382:633)

Intraaortic Balloon Pump (IABP) Counterpulsation

- Routine use in high-risk STEMI → ↑ stroke/bleeds w/o Δ in survival (JAMA 2011;306:1329)
- In cardiogenic shock, no survival benefit w/ IABP if early revasc (NEJM 2012;367:1287); 18% ↓ death in Pts w/ cardiogenic shock treated with lytic (EHJ 2009;30:459)

LV failure (~25%)

- Diurese to achieve PCWP ~14 → ↓ pulmonary edema, ↓ myocardial O₂ demand
- ↓ Afterload → ↑ stroke volume & CO, ↓ myocardial O₂ demand can use IV NTG or nitroprusside (risk of coronary steal) → short-acting ACEI
- Inotropes if HF despite diuresis & ↓ afterload; use dopamine, dobutamine, or milrinone
- **Cardiogenic shock** (~7%) = MAP <60 mmHg, CI <2 L/min/m², PCWP >18 mmHg; inotropes, mech circulatory support to keep CI >2; pressors to keep MAP >60; if not done already, coronary revasc (NEJM 1999;341:625)

IMI complications (Circ 1990;81:401; NEJM 1994;330:1211; JACC 2003;41:1273)

- **Heart block:** ~20%, occurs in part because RCA typically supplies AV node 40% on present., 20% w/in 24 h, rest by 72 h; high-grade AVB can develop abruptly Rx: atropine, epi, aminophylline (100 mg/min × 2.5 min), temp pacing wire
- **RV infarct** (proximal RCA occlusion → compromised flow to RV marginal branch) Angiographically present in 30–50%, but only ½ of those clinically signif. HoTN; ↑ JVP; ⊕ Kussmaul's; ≥1 mm STE in V₄R; RA/PCWP ≥0.8; RV dysfxn on TTE Rx: optimize preload (RA goal 10–14; BHJ 1990;63:98); ↑ contractility (dobutamine; maintain AV synchrony (pacing as necessary); reperfusion (NEJM 1998;338:933); mechanical support (IABP or RVAD); pulmonary vasodilators (eg, inhaled NO)

Mechanical complications (incid. <1% for each; typically occur a few days post-MI)

- **Free wall rupture:** ↑ risk w/ lysis, large MI, ↑ age, ♀, HTN; p/w PEA or hypoTN, pericardial sx, tamponade; Rx: volume resusc., ? pericardiocentesis, inotropes, **surgery**
- **VSD:** large MI in elderly; AMI → apical VSD, IMI → basal septum; 90% w/ harsh murmur ± thrill (NEJM 2002;347:1426); Rx: diuretics, vasodil., inotropes, IABP, **surgery**, perc. closure
- **Papillary muscle rupture:** more common after IMI (PM pap m. supplied by PDA a lone) than AMI (AL supplied by OMs & diags); 50% w/ new murmur; ↑ v wave in PCWP tracing;

asymmetric pulmonary edema on CXR. Rx: diuretics, vasodilators, IABP, **surgery**.

Arrhythmias post-MI (treat all per ACLS protocols if unstable or symptomatic)

- **AF** (10–16% incidence): βB or amio, ± digoxin (particularly if HF), heparin
- **VT/VF:** lido or amio × 6–24 h, then reassess; ↑ βB as tol., replete K & Mg, r/o ischemia; monomorphic VT <48 h post-MI does *not* worsen prognosis; >48 h, consider ICD (? wearable; see below)
- Accelerated idioventricular rhythm (AIVR): slow VT (<100 bpm), often seen after successful reperfusion; typically asx, self-terminates, and does not require treatment
- May consider **backup transcutaneous pacing** (TP) if: 2° AVB type I, BBB
- **Backup TP or initiate transvenous pacing** if: 2° AVB type II; BBB + AVB
- **Transvenous pacing** (TV) if: 3° AVB; new BBB + 2° AVB type II; alternating LBBB/RBBB (can bridge w/ TP until TV, which is best accomplished with fluoroscopic guidance)

Other Post-MI Complications		
Complication	**Clinical features**	**Treatment**
LV thrombus	~30% incid. (espec lg antero-apical MI)	Anticoagulate × 3–6 mo
Ventricular aneurysm	Noncontractile pouching of LV; 8–15% incid. (espec ant) persist STE	Surgery or perc implant if HF, thromboembol, arrhythmia
Ventricular pseudoaneurysm	Rupture (narrow neck) → sealed by thrombus and pericardium (esp in inf.)	Urgent surgery (or percutaneous repair)
Pericarditis	10–20% incid.; 1–4 d post-MI ⊕ pericardial rub; ECG Δs rare	High-dose ASA, colchicine, narcotics; minimize anticoag
Dressler's syndrome	<4% incid.; 2–10 wk post-MI fever, pericarditis, pleuritis	High-dose aspirin, NSAIDs

Prognosis
- In registries, in-hospital mortality is 6% w/ reperfusion Rx (lytic or PCI) and ~20% w/o
- TIMI Risk Score for STEMI (includes age, time to Rx, anterior MI or LBBB, Killip class, tachycardia, HoTN) defines 30-d mortality after STEMI (*JAMA* 2001;286:1356)

Checklist and Long-Term Post-ACS Management
Risk stratification
- Stress test if anatomy undefined; consider stress if signif residual CAD post-PCI of culprit
- Assess LVEF prior to d/c; EF ↑ ~6% in STEMI over 6 mo (*JACC* 2007;50:149)

Medications (barring contraindications)
- **Aspirin:** 81 mg daily (no clear benefit to higher doses)
- **P2Y₁₂ inhib** (ticagrelor or prasugrel preferred over clopi): treat for *at least* 12 mo Prolonged Rx >12 mo → ↓ MACE & CV death, ↑ in bleeding, but no ↑ ICH. Beyond 1ˢᵗ 12 mo, ticag 60 bid preferred to 90, as better tolerability (*NEJM* 2015;372:1791; *EHJ* 2016;37:390). PPIs ↓ GI complic; some PPIs ↓ antiplt effect, but no clear ↑ in CV risk (*NEJM* 2010;363:1909)
- **β-blocker:** 23% ↓ mortality after MI
- **Statin:** high-intensity lipid-lowering (eg, atorva 80 mg, PROVE-IT TIMI 22, *NEJM* 2004;350:1495)
- **Ezetimibe:** ↓ CV events when added to statin (IMPROVE-IT, *NEJM* 2015;372:1500)
- **ACEI:** lifelong if HF, ↓ EF, HTN, DM; 4–6 wk or at least until hosp. d/c in all STEMI ? long-term benefit in CAD w/o HF (*NEJM* 2000;342:145 & 2004;351:2058; *Lancet* 2003;362:782)
- **Aldosterone antag:** 15% ↓ mort. if EF <40% & either s/s of HF or DM (*NEJM* 2003;348:1309)
- Nitrates: standing if symptomatic; SL NTG prn for all
- Ranolazine: ↓ recurrent ischemia, no impact on CVD/MI (*JAMA* 2007;297:1775)
- Oral anticoag: if needed (eg, AF or LV thrombus), warfarin w/ target INR 2–2.5 or NOAC. Clopi (not ticag or pras) and ? stop ASA if at high bleeding risk (*Lancet* 2013;381:1107). Not FDA approved: low-dose rivaroxaban (2.5 mg bid) in addition to ASA & clopi in patients *without* an indication for anticoag → 16% ↓ D/MI/stroke and 32% ↓ all-cause death, but ↑ major bleeding and ICH (*NEJM* 2012;366:9).

ICD (*NEJM* 2008;359:2245; *Circ* 2014;130:94)
- If sust. VT/VF >2 d post-MI not due to reversible ischemia; consider wearable defib
- Indicated in 1° prevention of SCD if post-MI w/ EF ≤30–40% (NYHA II–III) or ≤35% (NYHA I); need to wait ≥40 d after MI (*NEJM* 2004;351:2481 & 2009;361:1427)

Risk factors and lifestyle modifications (*Circ* 2014;129(Suppl 2):S1 & S76)
- Low chol. (<200 mg/d) & fat (<7% saturated) diet; ? Ω-3 FA
- Traditional LDL-C goal <70 mg/dL; current recs w/o target; given IMPROVE-IT, ? mid 50s
- BP <140/90 & ? 120–130/80 mmHg (HTN 2015;65:1372; *NEJM* 2015;373:2103); quit smoking
- If diabetic, tailor HbA1c goal based on Pt (avoid TZDs if HF); in Pts w/ CAD, empagliflozin (*NEJM* 2015; 373:2117) and liraglutide (*NEJM* 2016;375:311) ↓ cardiovascular events
- Exercise (30–60 min 5–7×/wk); cardiac rehab; BMI goal 18.5–24.9 kg/m²
- Influenza & *S. pneumo* vaccines (*Circ* 2006;114:1549; *JAMA* 2013;310:1711); ✓ for depression

Rationale

- Cardiac output (CO) = SV × HR; optimize SV (and thereby CO) by manipulating preload/LVEDV (w/ IVF, diuretics), contractility (w/ inotropes), & afterload (w/ vasodilators)
- Balloon at catheter tip inflated → floats into "wedge" position. Column of blood extends from tip of catheter, through pulm venous circulation to a point just prox to LA. Under conditions of no flow, PCWP ≈ LA pressure ≈ LVEDP, which is proportional to LVEDV.
- Situations in which these basic assumptions fail:
  (1) Catheter tip not in West lung zone 3 (and ∴ PCWP = alveolar pressure ≠ LA pressure); clues include lack of *a* & *v* waves and if PA diastolic pressure < PCWP
  (2) PCWP > LA pressure (eg, mediastinal fibrosis, pulmonary VOD, PV stenosis)
  (3) Mean LA pressure > LVEDP (eg, MR, MS)
  (4) Δ LVEDP-LVEDV relationship (ie, abnl compliance, ∴ "nl" LVEDP may not be optimal)

Indications (Circ 2009;119:e391; NEJM 2013;369:e35)

- **Diagnosis and evaluation**
  Ddx of shock (cardiogenic vs. distributive; espec if trial of IVF failed or is high risk) and of pulmonary edema (cardiogenic vs. not; espec if trial of diuretic failed or is high risk)
  Evaluation of CO, intracardiac shunt, pulm HTN, MR, tamponade, cardiorenal syndrome
  Evaluation of unexplained dyspnea (PAC during provocation w/ exercise, vasodilator)
- **Therapeutics** (Circ 2006;113:1020)
  Tailored therapy to optimize PCWP, SV, $S_{MV}O_2$, RAP, PVR in heart failure or shock
  Guide to vasodilator therapy (eg, inhaled NO, nifedipine) in PHT, RV infarction
  Guide periop mgmt in some high-risk Pts, candidacy for mech circ support & transplant
- **Contraindications**
  Absolute: right-sided endocarditis, thrombus/mass or mechanical valve; proximal PE
  Relative: coagulopathy (reverse), recent PPM or ICD (place under fluoroscopy), LBBB (~5% risk of RBBB → CHB, place under fluoro), bioprosthetic R-sided valve

Efficacy concerns (NEJM 2006;354:2213; JAMA 2005;294:1664)

- No benefit to routine PAC use in high-risk surgery, sepsis, ARDS
- No benefit in decompensated HF (JAMA 2005;294:1625); untested in cardiogenic shock
- But: ~½ of clinical CO & PCWP estimates incorrect; CVP & PCWP not well correl.; ∴ use PAC to (a) answer hemodynamic ? and then remove, or (b) manage cardiogenic shock

Placement (NEJM 2013;369:e35)

- Insertion site: **R internal jugular** or **L subclavian** veins for "anatomic" flotation into PA
- **Inflate** balloon (max 1.5 mL) when **advancing** and to **measure PCWP**
- Use resistance to inflation and pressure tracing to avoid overinflation & risk of PA rupture
- **Deflate** the balloon when **withdrawing** and at all other times
- CXR should be obtained after placement to assess for catheter position and PTX
- If catheter cannot be floated (i.e., severe TR, RV dilatation), consider fluoroscopic guidance

Complications

- **Central venous access:** pneumo/hemothorax (~1%), arterial puncture (if inadvertent cannulation w/ dilation → surgical/endovasc eval), air embolism, thoracic duct injury
- **Advancement:** atrial or ventricular arrhythmias (3% VT; 20% NSVT or >50% PVC), RBBB (5%), catheter knotting, cardiac perforation/tamponade, PA rupture
- **Maintenance:** infection (espec if catheter >3 d old), thrombus, pulm infarction (≤1%), valve/chordae damage, PA rupture/pseudoaneurysm (espec w/ PHT), balloon rupture

Intracardiac pressures

- Transmural pressure (≈ preload) = measured intracardiac pressure − intrathoracic pressure
- Intrathoracic pressure (usually slightly ⊖) is transmitted to vessels and heart
- **Always measure intracardiac pressure at end-expiration,** when intrathoracic pressure closest to 0 ("high point" in spont. breathing Pts; "low point" in Pts on ⊕ pressure vent.)
- If ↑ intrathoracic pressure (eg, PEEP), measured PCWP overestimates true transmural pressures. Can approx by subtracting ~½ PEEP (× ¾ to convert cm H_2O to mmHg).
- PCWP: LV preload best estimated at *a* wave; risk of pulmonary edema from avg PCWP

Cardiac output

- **Thermodilution:** saline injected in RA or prox thermal filament. Δ in temp over time measured at thermistor (in PA) used to calc CO. Inaccurate if ↓ CO, sev TR, or shunt.
- **Fick method:** O_2 consumption ($\dot{V}O_2$)(L/min) = CO (L/min) × Δ arteriovenous O_2 content
  ∴ $CO = \dot{V}O_2 / C(a\text{-}v)O_2$
  $\dot{V}O_2$ ideally measured (esp. if ↑ metab demands), but freq estimated (125 mL/min/m²)
  $C(a\text{-}v)O_2 = [10 × 1.36$ mL O_2/g of Hb × Hb g/dL × ($S_aO_2 − S_{MV}O_2$)]. $S_{MV}O_2$ is key variable that Δs.
  If $S_{MV}O_2$ >80%, consider if the PAC is "wedged" (ie, pulm vein sat), L→R shunt, impaired O_2 utilization (severe sepsis, cyanide, carbon monoxide), ↑↑ FiO_2.

PA Catheter Waveforms

Location	RA	RV	PA	PCWP
Distance	~20 cm	~30 cm	~40 cm	~50 cm
Normal Pressure (mmHg)	mean ≤6	syst 15–30 diast 1–8	syst 15–30 mean 9–18 diast 6–12	mean ≤12
Waves			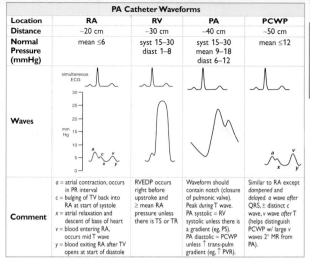	
Comment	a = atrial contraction, occurs in PR interval; c = bulging of TV back into RA at start of systole; x = atrial relaxation and descent of base of heart; v = blood entering RA, occurs mid T wave; y = blood exiting RA after TV opens at start of diastole	RVEDP occurs right before upstroke and ≥ mean RA pressure unless there is TS or TR	Waveform should contain notch (closure of pulmonic valve). Peak during T wave. PA systolic = RV systolic unless there is a gradient (eg, PS). PA diastolic ≈ PCWP unless ↑ trans-pulm gradient (eg, ↑ PVR).	Similar to RA except dampened and delayed. a wave after QRS, ± distinct c wave, v wave after T (helps distinguish PCWP w/ large v waves 2° MR from PA).

PCWP waveform abnormalities: large a wave → ? mitral stenosis; large v wave → ? mitral regurgitation; blunted y descent → ? tamponade; steep x & y descents → ? constriction.

Hemodynamic Profiles of Various Forms of Shock (NEJM 2013;369:1726)

Type of shock	RA	PCWP	CO	SVR
Hypovolemic	↓	↓	↓	↑
Cardiogenic	nl or ↑	↑	↓	↑
RV infarct/massive PE	↑	nl or ↓	↓	↑
Tamponade	↑	↑	↓	↑
Distributive	variable	variable	usually ↑ (can be ↓ in sepsis)	↓

Surrogates: RA ≈ JVP (1 mmHg = 1.36 cm H$_2$O); pulmonary edema on CXR implies ↑ PCWP; UOP ∝ CO (barring AKI); delayed capillary refill (ie, >2–3 sec) implies ↑ SVR.

Tailored therapy in cardiogenic shock (Circ 2009;119:e391)
• **Goals:** optimize both MAP and CO while ↓ risk of pulmonary edema
  MAP = CO × SVR; CO = HR × SV (which depends on preload, afterload and contractility)
  pulmonary edema when PCWP >20–25 (↑ levels may be tolerated in chronic HF)
  hepatic and renal congestion when CVP/RAP >15 mmHg
• **Optimize preload** = LVEDV ≈ LVEDP ≈ LAP ≈ PCWP (NEJM 1973;289:1263)
  goal **PCWP ~14–18 in acute MI, ≤14 in acute decompensated HF**
  optimize in individual Pt by measuring SV w/ different PCWP to create Starling curve
  ↑ by giving NS (albumin w/o clinical benefit over NS; PRBC if significant anemia)
  ↓ by diuresis (qv), ultrafiltration or dialysis if refractory to diuretics
• **Optimize afterload** ≈ wall stress during LV ejection = [(~SBP × radius) / (2 × wall thick.)]
  and ∴ ∝ MAP and ∝ SVR = (MAP – CVP / CO); goals: **MAP >60, SVR 800–1200**
  MAP >60 & SVR ↑: vasodilators (eg, nitroprusside, NTG, ACEI, hydral.) or wean pressors
  MAP <60 & SVR ↑ (& ∴ CO ↓): temporize w/ pressors until can ↑ CO (see below)
  MAP <60 & SVR low/nl (& ∴ inappropriate vasoplegia): vasopressors (eg, norepinephrine [α, β], dopamine [D, α, β], phenylephrine [α] or vasopressin [V₁] if refractory);
  better outcomes w/ norepi than dopa even in cardiogenic shock (NEJM 2010;362:779)
• **Optimize contractility** ∝ CO for given preload & afterload; **goal CI = (CO / BSA) >2.2**
  if too low despite optimal preload & vasodilators (as MAP permits):
  ⊕ inotropes: eg, dobutamine (mod inotrope & mild vasodilator) or milrinone (strong
  inotrope & vasodilator, incl pulm), both proarrhythmic, or epi (strong inotrope & pressor)
  mech circulatory support (L/min): IABP (0.5), Impella (2–5), TandemHeart (5), VAD
  (L-sided, R-sided or both; temp or perm; 10) or ECMO (6) (JACC 2015;65:e7 & 2542)

Definitions (Braunwald's Heart Disease, 10th ed., 2014)
- Failure of heart to pump blood forward at rate sufficient to meet metabolic demands of peripheral tissues, or ability to do so only at abnormally high cardiac filling pressures
- Low output (↓ cardiac output) vs. high output (↑ stroke volume ± ↑ cardiac output)
- Left-sided (pulmonary edema) vs. right-sided (↑ JVP, hepatomegaly, peripheral edema)
- Backward (↑ filling pressures, congestion) vs. forward (impaired systemic perfusion)
- Systolic (inability to expel sufficient blood) vs. diastolic (failure to relax and fill normally)
- Reduced (HFrEF, EF <40%), mid-range (HFmrEF, EF 40–49%), & preserved (HFpEF, EF >50%); combination of systolic and diastolic dysfxn may occur regardless of EF

Figure 1-3 Approach to left-sided heart failure

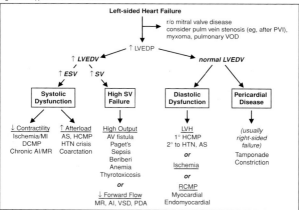

History
- Low output: fatigue, weakness, exercise intolerance, Δ MS, anorexia
- Congestive: left-sided → dyspnea, orthopnea, paroxysmal nocturnal dyspnea
  right-sided → peripheral edema, RUQ discomfort, bloating, satiety

Functional classification (New York Heart Association class)
- Class I: no sx w/ ordinary activity; class II: sx w/ ordinary activity;
  class III: sx w/ minimal activity; class IV: sx at rest

Physical exam ("2-minute" hemodynamic profile; JAMA 1996;275:630 & 2002;287:628)
- **Congestion ("dry" vs. "wet"):** ↑ JVP (~80% of the time JVP >10 → PCWP >22)
  ⊕ hepatojugular reflux: ≥4 cm ↑ in JVP for ≥15 sec w/ abdominal pressure
  Se/Sp 73/87% for RA >8 and Se/Sp 55/83% for PCWP >15 (AJC 1990;66:1002)
  Abnl Valsalva response: square wave (↑ SBP w/ strain), no overshoot (no ↑ BP after strain)
  S_3 (in Pts w/ HF → ~40% ↑ risk of HF hosp. or pump failure death; NEJM 2001;345:574)
  rales, dullness at base 2° pleural effus. (often absent in chronic HF due to lymphatic compensation) ± hepatomegaly, ascites and jaundice, peripheral edema
- **Perfusion ("warm" vs. "cold")**
  narrow pulse pressure (<25% of SBP) → CI <2.2 (91% Se, 83% Sp; JAMA 1989;261:884);
  soft S_1 (↓ dP/dt), pulsus alternans, cool & pale extremities, ↓ UOP, muscle atrophy
- ± Other: Cheyne-Stokes resp., abnl PMI (diffuse, sustained or lifting depending on cause of HF), S_4 (diast. dysfxn), murmur (valvular dis., ↑ MV annulus, displaced papillary muscles)

Evaluation for the presence of heart failure
- CXR (see Radiology insert): pulm edema, pleural effusions ± cardiomegaly, cephalization, Kerley B-lines; lung U/S better than CXR (PPV & NPV 92% vs. 77%; Chest 2015;148:202)
- BNP/NT-proBNP can help exclude HF; levels ↑ w/ age, renal dysfxn, AF; ↓ w/ obesity
  Se ≥95%, Sp: ~50%, PPV ~65%, NPV ≥ 94% for HF in Pts p/w SOB (BMJ 2015;350:h910)
- Evidence of ↓ organ perfusion: ↑ Cr, ↓ Na, abnl LFTs
- Echo (see inserts): ↓ EF & ↑ chamber size → systolic dysfxn; hypertrophy, abnl MV inflow, abnl tissue Doppler → ? diastolic dysfxn; abnl valves or pericardium; ↑ estimated RVSP
- PA catheterization: ↑ PCWP, ↓ CO, and ↑ SVR (in low-output failure)

Evaluation for the potential causes of heart failure
- **ECG**: evidence for CAD, LVH, LAE, heart block or low voltage (? infiltrative CMP/DCMP)
- **TTE**: LV & RV size & fxn, valve abnl (cause or consequence?), infiltrative or pericardial dis.
- **Cardiac MRI**: distinguishes ischemic vs. nonischemic and can help determine etiol. of latter
- **Coronary angio** (or noninvasive imaging, eg, CT angio); if no CAD, w/u for NICM

Precipitants of acute heart failure
- **Dietary indiscretion or medical nonadherence** (~40% of cases)
- **Myocardial ischemia or infarction** (~10–15% of cases); **myocarditis**
- **Renal failure** (acute, progression of CKD, or insufficient dialysis) → ↑ preload
- **Hypertensive crisis** (incl. from RAS), **worsening AS** → ↑ left-sided afterload
- **Drugs** (βB, CCB, NSAIDs, TZDs), **chemo** (anthracyclines, trastuzumab), or **toxins** (EtOH)
- **Arrhythmias**; **valvular dysfxn** (eg, endocarditis), espec mitral or aortic regurgitation
- **COPD/PE** → ↑ right-sided afterload; extreme stress, anemia, systemic infxn, thyroid dis.

Treatment of acute decompensated heart failure
- Assess degree of congestion & adequacy of perfusion
- For congestion: **"LMNOP"**

		Congestion?	
		No	Yes
Low perfusion?	No	Warm & Dry OutPt Rx	Warm & Wet Diuresis
	Yes	Cold & Dry inotropes (CCU)	Cold & Wet Diuresis, inotropes and/or vasodil (CCU)

  Lasix IV; total daily dose 2.5× usual daily PO dose → ↑ UOP, but transient ↑ in Cr vs. 1× usual dose; ∅ clear diff between contin. gtt vs. q12h (NEJM 2011;364:797)
  Morphine (↓ sx, venodilator, ↓ afterload)
  Nitrates (venodilator)
  Oxygen ± noninvasive vent (↓ sx, ↑ P_aO_2; no Δ mortality; see "Mechanical Ventilation")
  Position (sitting up & legs dangling over side of bed → ↓ preload)
- For **low perfusion**, see below
- Adjustment of oral meds
  ACEI/ARB: hold if HoTN, consider Δ to hydralazine & nitrates if renal decompensation
  βB: reduce dose by at least ½ if mod HF, d/c if severe HF and/or need inotropes

Treatment of acute advanced heart failure (Circ 2009;119:e391)
- Consider PAC if not resp to Rx, unsure re: vol status, HoTN, ↑ Cr, need inotropes
- Tailored Rx w/ PAC (qv); goals of MAP >60, CI >2.2 (MVO_2 >60%), SVR <800, PCWP <18
- **IV vasodilators**: NTG, nitroprusside (risk of coronary steal if CAD; prolonged use → cyanide/thiocyanate toxicity); nesiritide (rBNP) not rec for routine use (NEJM 2011;365:32)
- **Inotropes** (properties in addition to ↑ inotropy listed below)
  dobutamine: vasodilation at doses ≤5 μg/kg/min; mild ↑ PVR; desensitization over time
  dopamine: splanchnic vasodil. → ↑ GFR & natriuresis; vasoconstrictor at ≥5 μg/kg/min
  milrinone: prominent systemic & pulmonary vasodilation; ↓ dose by 50% in renal failure
- **Ultrafiltration**: similar wt loss to aggressive diuresis, but ↑ renal failure (NEJM 2012;367:2296)
- **Mechanical circulatory support** (also see "Tailored Therapy") (JACC 2015;65:e7 & 2542)
  Temporary: bridge to recovery, transplant, or durable MCS; periprocedural support
    Intra-aortic balloon pump (IABP): inflates in diastole & deflates in systole to ↓ impedance to LV ejection, ↓ myocardial O_2 demand & ↑ coronary perfusion. +0.5 L/min CO
    Axial flow pumps (eg, Impella): Archimedes screw principle in LV; +2.5–5 L/min
    Extracorporeal centrifugal pumps: TandemHeart (+5 L/min, percutaneous) & CentriMag (10 L/min, surgical).
    Extracorporeal membrane oxygenation (ECMO): 6 L/min (Circ 2015;131:676)
  Durable: surgically placed LVAD ± RVAD as bridge to recovery (HeartMate II or HeartWare LVAD or Total Artificial Heart if BiV failure), or as destination Rx (>50% ↓ 1-y mort. vs. med Rx; NEJM 2001;345:1435 & 2009;361:2241).
- Cardiac transplantation: ~2500/yr in U.S. 10% mort. in 1st y, median survival ~10 y

Recommended Chronic Therapy by HF Stage (Circ 2009;119:e391)

Stage (not NYHA Class)		Therapy
A	At risk for HF (eg HTN, FHx CMP); but asx & w/o struct. heart dis.	Rx HTN, lipids, DM. Stop smoking, EtOH. ↑ exercise. ACEI/ARB if HTN/DM/CAD/PAD
B	⊕ Struct. heart dis. (eg CMP, LVH), but asx	As per stage A + ACEI/ARB & βB if MI/CAD or ↓ EF. ? ICD.
C	⊕ Struct. heart dis. ⊕ Any h/o Sx of HF	As per stage A + diuretics, ↓ Na. If ↓ EF: ACEI, ARB or ARNI; βB; aldo antag; ICD; ? CRT; nitrate/hydral; dig.
D	Refractory HF requiring specialized interventions	All measures for stages A–C. Consider IV inotropes, VAD, transplant, end-of-life care (4-y mortality >50%)

- Utility of BNP-guided Rx remains debated *(Eur Heart J* 2014;35:16)
- Implantable PA pressure sensor in NYHA III → ~33% ↓ risk of hosp *(Lancet* 2016;387:453)

Treatment of Chronic Heart Failure with Reduced Ejection Fraction	
Diet, exercise	Na <2 g/d, fluid restriction, exercise training in ambulatory Pts
ACEI	↓ mortality: 40% in NYHA IV, 16% in NYHA II/III, 20–30% in asx but ↓ EF *(NEJM* 1992;327:685 & *Lancet* 2000;355:1575) High-dose more effic. than low. Watch for ↑ Cr, ↑ K (ameliorate by low-K diet, diuretics, K binders), cough, angioedema.
ATII receptor blockers (ARBs)	*Consider as alternative if cannot tolerate ACEI (eg, b/c cough)* Noninferior to ACEI *(Lancet* 2000;355:1582 & 2003;362:772) As with ACEI, higher doses more efficacious *(Lancet* 2009;374:1840) Adding to ACEI → ↑ risk of ↑ K and ↑ Cr *(BMJ* 2013;346:f360)
ARNi (ARB + neprilysin inhib) *(do not use w/ ACEI, allow 36-h washout)*	*Alternative to ACEI/ARB, espec if sx despite ACEI/ARB.* Neutral endopeptidase (NEP, aka neprilysin) degrades natriuretic peptides, bradykinin & angiotensins. Valsartan + sacubitril (NEPi) ↓ CV mort & HF hosp c/w ACEI; ↑ HoTN, AKI, ? angioedema *(NEJM* 2014;371:993).
Hydralazine + nitrates	*Consider if cannot tolerate ACEI/ARB or in blacks w/ class III/IV* 25% ↓ mort. *(NEJM* 1986;314:1547); infer. to ACEI *(NEJM* 1991;325:303) 40% ↓ mort. in blacks on standard Rx (A-HEFT, *NEJM* 2004;351:2049)
β-blocker (data for carvedilol, metoprolol, bisoprolol)	*EF will transiently ↓, then ↑. Contraindic. in decompensated HF.* 35% ↓ mort. & 40% ↓ rehosp. in NYHA II–IV *(JAMA* 2002;287:883) Carvedilol superior to low-dose metop in 1 trial *(Lancet* 2003;362:7), but meta-analysis suggests no diff between βB *(BMJ* 2013;346:f55).
Aldosterone antagonists	*Consider if adeq. renal fxn and w/o hyperkalemia; watch for ↑ K* 25–30% ↓ mort. in NYHA II–IV & EF ≤35% *(NEJM* 2011;364:11) 15% ↓ mort. in HF post-MI, EF ≤40% (EPHESUS, *NEJM* 2003;348:1309)
Cardiac resynch therapy (CRT, qv)	*Consider if EF ≤35%, LBBB (QRS >130 ms) and symptomatic HF* 36% ↓ mort. & ↑ EF in NYHA III–IV (CARE-HF, *NEJM* 2005;352:1539) 41% ↓ mort. if EF ≤30%, LBBB and NYHA I/II *(NEJM* 2014;370:1694)
ICD (see "Cardiac Rhythm Mgmt Devices")	*For 1° prevention if EF ≤30–35% or 2° prevention; not if NYHA IV* ↓ mort. in ischemic & non-isch CMP; no Δ mort. early post-MI *(NEJM* 2004;351:2481 & 2009;361:1427), ∴ wait ≥40 d
Diuretics	Loop ± thiazides diuretics (sx relief; no mortality benefit)
Digoxin	23% ↓ HF hosp., no Δ mort *(NEJM* 1997;336:525); ? ↑ mort w/ ↑ levels *(NEJM* 2002;347:1403); optimal 0.5–0.8 ng/mL *(JAMA* 2003;289:871)
Ivabradine (I$_f$ blocker w/o ⊖ ino)	*Consider if EF ≤35%, NYHA II or III, HR ≥70, NSR on max βB.* 18% ↓ CV mort or HF hosp *(Lancet* 2010;376:875)
Iron supplementation	? if NYHA II/III, EF ≤40%, Fe-defic (ferritin <100 or ferritin 100–200 & TSAT <20%). ↑ Sx, ↑ 6MWD, independent of Hct *(NEJM* 2009;361:2436).
Anticoagulation	*If AF, VTE, LV thrombus, ± if large akinetic LV segments* In SR w/ EF <35%, ↓ isch stroke, but ↑ bleed *(NEJM* 2012;366:1859)
Heart rhythm	Catheter ablation of AF → ↑ in EF, ↓ sx *(NEJM* 2004;351:2373) No mortality benefit to AF rhythm vs. rate cntl *(NEJM* 2008;358:2667) Pulm vein isolation ↓ sx c/w AVN ablation & CRT *(NEJM* 2008;359:1778)
Meds to avoid	NSAIDs, nondihydropyridine CCB, TZDs
Experimental	Serelaxin ↓ dyspnea & ? ↓ mortality *(Lancet* 2013;381:29) Empagliflozin (SGLT2i) ↓ death/HF hosp in DM *(NEJM* 2015;373:2117) Interatrial shunting ↓ PCWP & sx *(Lancet* 2016;387:1290)

(Circ 2013;128:e240 & 2016 ACC/AHA/HFSA Update; *EHJ* 2016;37:2129)

Heart failure with preserved EF (HFpEF; "Diastolic HF") *(Circ* 2011;124:e540)

- **Epidemiology:** ~½ of Pts w/ HF have normal or only min. impaired systolic fxn (EF ≥40%); risk factors for HFpEF incl ↑ age, ♀, DM, AF. Mortality ≈ to those w/ systolic dysfxn.
- **Etiologies** (impaired relaxation and/or ↑ passive stiffness): ischemia, prior MI, LVH, HCMP, infiltrative CMP, RCMP, aging, hypothyroidism
- **Precipitants of pulmonary edema:** *volume overload* (poor compliance of LV → sensitive to even modest ↑ in volume); *ischemia* (↓ relaxation); *tachycardia* (↓ filling time in diastole), *AF* (loss of atrial boost to LV filling); *HTN* (↑ afterload → ↓ stroke volume)
- **Dx** w/ clinical s/s of HF w/ preserved systolic fxn. Dx supported by evidence of diast dysfxn:
  (1) echo: abnl MV inflow (E/A reversal and Δs in E wave deceleration time) & ↓ myocardial relax. (↑ isovol relax. time & ↓ early diastole tissue Doppler vel)
  (2) exercise-induced ↑ PCWP (± ↓ response chronotropic & vasodilator reserve)
- **Treatment:** diuresis for vol overload, BP control, prevention of tachycardia and ischemia; no benefit to: ACEI/ARB *(NEJM* 2008;359:2456) or PDE5 inhib *(JAMA* 2013;309:1268) spironolactone ? ↓ CV death & HF hosp (at least in Americas) *(NEJM* 2014;370:1383) ARNi *(Lancet* 2012;380:1387) and serelaxin *(Lancet* 2013;381:29) under study

Diseases with mechanical and/or electrical dysfunction of the myocardium

DILATED CARDIOMYOPATHY (DCM)

Definition and epidemiology (*Circ* 2013;128:e240; *JACC* 2013;62:2046)
- Ventricular dilatation and ↓ contractility ± ↓ wall thickness *in the absence of myocardial disease caused by ischemia/infarct, valvular disease or hypertension*
- Incidence 5–8/100,000/y; prevalence: 1/2500. Most common reason for heart transplant.

Etiologies (*JACC* 2011;57:1641; *Circ Res* 2012;111:131)
- **Familial** (~35%): Pt & ≥2 closely related family members w/ otherwise unexplained DCM; ~30 genes identified to date, encoding structural & nuclear proteins
- **Idiopathic** (<20%): ? undiagnosed infectious, alcoholic or genetic cause
- **Infectious myocarditis** (10–15%; *Lancet* 2012;379:738; *JACC* 2012;59:779)
  Viruses (parvoB19 & HHV6 > Coxsackie, adeno, echo, CMV, HCV): from subacute (dilated LV, mild–mod dysfxn) to fulminant (nondil., thick, edematous LV, sev dysfxn)
  Bacterial, fungal, rickettsial, TB, Lyme (mild myocarditis, often with AVB)
  HIV: ~8% of asx HIV ⊕; due to HIV, other virus or antiretrovirals; also premature CAD
  Chagas: apical aneurysm ± thrombus, RBBB, megaesophagus/colon (*NEJM* 2015;373:456)
- **Toxic:** alcohol (~20%) typ. 7–8 drinks/d ×>5 y, but variable; cocaine; XRT (usu RCMP); anthracyclines (risk ↑ >550 mg/m², may manifest late), cyclophosphamide, trastuzumab
- **Infiltrative** (5%): often mix of DCMP + RCMP (qv) with thickened wall amyloidosis, sarcoidosis, hemochromatosis, tumor
- **Autoimmune:** *collagen vasc. dis.* (3%): PM, SLE, scleroderma, PAN, RA, Wegener's; *peripartum* (last month → 5 mo postpartum; *EHJ* 2015;36:1090): ~1:3000 preg. ↑ risk w/ multiparity, ↑ age, Afr Am; stnd HF Rx (if preg, no ACEi or spironolact.); ? bromocriptine to ↓ prolactin; 72% normalize EF (*JACC* 2015;66:905); ~30% recur w/ next preg
  Idiopathic giant cell myocarditis (GCM): avg age 42, fulminant, AVB/VT (*Circ HF* 2013;6:15)
  Eosinophilic (variable peripheral eos): hypersensitivity (mild HF but at risk for SCD) or acute necrotizing eosinophilic myocarditis (ANEM; STE, effusion, severe HF)
- **Stress-induced** (Takotsubo = apical ballooning): Typically postmenopausal ♀; mimics MI (chest pain, ± STE & ↑Tn; deep TWI & ↑QT); mid/apex dyskinesis; ? Rx w/ βB, ACEi; usu. improves over wks (*JAMA* 2011;306:277). In-hosp morb/mort similar to ACS (*NEJM* 2015;373:929).
- **Arrhythmogenic right ventricular cardiomyopathy** (ACM/ARVC): fibrofatty replacement of RV → dilation (dx w/ MRI); ECG: ± RBBB, TWI V_1–V_3, ε wave; risk VT (*Lancet* 2009;373:1289)
- **Tachycardia:** likelihood ∝ rate/duration; often resolves w/ rate cntl (*Circ* 2005;112:1092)
- **LV noncompaction** (*JACC* 2015;66:578): prominent trabeculae, arrhythmias, cardioemboli
- **Metab/other:** hypothyroid, acromegaly, pheo, OSA, Vit B_1, selenium or carnitine defic.

Clinical manifestations
- **Heart failure:** both congestive & poor forward flow sx; signs of L- & R-sided HF diffuse, laterally displaced PMI, S3, ± MR or TR (annular dilat., displaced pap. muscle)
- Embolic events (~10%), supraventricular/ventricular arrhythmias, & palpitations
- Chest pain can be seen w/ some etiologies (eg, myocarditis)

Diagnostic studies and workup (*JACC* 2016;67:2996)
- CXR: moderate to marked cardiomegaly, ± pulmonary edema & pleural effusions
- ECG: may see PRWP, Q waves or BBB; low-voltage; AF (20%); may be normal
- Echocardiogram: LV dilatation, ↓ EF, regional or global LV HK ± RV HK, ± mural thrombi
- Cardiac MRI: up to 76% Se, 96% Sp for myocarditis or infiltrative dis. (*JACC Imaging* 2014;7:254); extent of midwall fibrosis correlated w/ mortality in NICMP (*JAMA* 2013;309:896)
- Labs: TFTs, Fe panel, HIV, SPEP, ANA; viral sero *not* recommended; others per suspicion
- Family hx (20–35% w/ familial dis.), genetic counseling ± genetic testing (*JAMA* 2009;302:2471)
- Stress test: useful to r/o ischemia (low false ⊖ rate), high false ⊕ rate, even w/ imaging
- Coronary angiography to r/o CAD if risk factors, h/o angina, Qw MI on ECG, equivocal ETT; consider CT angiography (*JACC* 2007;49:2044)
- ? Endomyocardial biopsy (*JACC* 2007;50:1914): yield 10%; of these, 75% myocarditis (for which no proven Rx) & 25% systemic disease; 40% false ⊖ rate (patchy dis.) & false ⊕ (necrosis → inflammation); ∴ biopsy if: acute & hemodyn compromise (r/o GCM, ANEM); arrhythmia or RCMP features (r/o infiltrative); or suspect toxic, allergic, tumor

Treatment (see "Heart Failure" for standard HF Rx)
- Possibility of reversibility of CMP may temper implantation of devices
- Immunosuppression: for giant cell myocarditis (prednisone + AZA), collagen vascular disease, peripartum (? IVIg), & eosinophilic; no proven benefit for viral myocarditis
- Prognosis differs per etiology (*NEJM* 2000;342:1077): postpartum (best), ischemic/GCM (worst)

HYPERTROPHIC CARDIOMYOPATHY (HCM)

Definition and epidemiology
- LV (usually ≥15 mm) and/or RV hypertrophy disproportionate to hemodynamic load
- Prevalence: 1/500; 50% sporadic, 50% familial, most asymptomatic
- Ddx: LVH 2° to HTN, AS, elite athletes (wall usually <13 mm & symmetric and nl/↑ rates of tissue Doppler diastolic relaxation; *Circ* 2011;123:2723), Fabry dis. (↑ Cr, skin findings)

Pathology
- Autosomal dominant mutations in cardiac sarcomere genes (eg, β-myosin heavy chain)
- Myocardial fiber disarray with hypertrophy, which creates arrhythmogenic substrate
- Morphologic hypertrophy variants: asymmetric septal; concentric; midcavity; apical

Pathophysiology
- Subaortic outflow obstruction: narrowed tract 2° hypertrophied septum + systolic anterior motion (SAM) of ant. MV leaflet (may be fixed, variable or nonexistent) and papillary muscle displacement. Gradient (∇) worse w/ ↑ contractility (digoxin, β-agonists, exercise, PVCs), ↓ preload (eg, Valsalva maneuver) or ↓ afterload.
- Mitral regurgitation: due to SAM (mid-to-late, post.-directed regurg. jet) and/or abnl mitral leaflets and papillary muscles (pansystolic, ant.-directed regurg. jet)
- Diastolic dysfunction: ↑ chamber stiffness + impaired relaxation
- Ischemia: small vessel dis., perforating artery compression (bridging), ↓ coronary perfusion
- Syncope: Δs in load-dependent CO, arrhythmias

Clinical manifestations (70% are asymptomatic at dx)
- **Dyspnea** (90%): due to ↑ LVEDP, MR, and diastolic dysfunction
- **Angina** (25%) even w/o epicardial CAD; microvasc. dysfxn (*NEJM* 2003;349:1027)
- **Arrhythmias** (AF in 20–25%; VT/VF): palpitations, syncope, sudden cardiac death

Physical exam
- Sustained PMI, S_2 paradoxically split if severe outflow obstruction, ⊕ S_4 (occ. palpable)
- **Systolic murmur:** crescendo-decrescendo; LLSB; ↑ w/ **Valsalva** & standing (↓ preload)
- ± mid-to-late or holosystolic murmur of MR at apex
- Bifid carotid pulse (brisk rise, decline then 2nd rise); JVP w/ prominent *a* wave
- Contrast to AS, which has murmur that ↓ w/ Valsalva and ↓ carotid pulses

Diagnostic studies (*EHJ* 2014;35:2733)
- CXR: cardiomegaly (LV and LA)
- ECG: LVH, anterolateral TWI and inferior pseudo-Qw, ± apical giant TWI (apical variant)
- **Echo:** any LV wall segment ≥15 mm (or ? even ≥13 if ⊕ HFx), often but not necessarily involving septum; other findings include dynamic outflow obstruction, SAM, MR
- MRI: hypertrophy + patchy delayed enhancement (useful for dx & prog) (*Circ* 2015;132:292)
- Cardiac cath: subaortic pressure ∇; *Brockenbrough sign* = ↓ pulse pressure post-PVC (in contrast to AS, in which pulse pressure ↑ post-PVC)
- ? Genotyping for family screening, but pathogenic mutation ID'd in <½ (*Circ* 2011;124:2761)

Treatment (*Circ* 2011;124:e783 & 2012;125:1432; *Lancet* 2013;381:242)
- Heart failure
  ⊖ **inotropes/chronotropes:** β-blockers, CCB (verapamil), disopyramide
  Careful use of diuretics, as may further ↓ preload. Vasodilators only if systolic dysfxn. Avoid digoxin.
  If sx refractory to drug Rx + *obstructive* physiology (∇ >50 mmHg):
  (a) Surgical myectomy: long-term ↓ symptoms in 90% (*Circ* 2014;130:1617)
  (b) Alcohol septal ablation (*JCHF* 2015;3:896): gradient ↓ by ~80%, only 5–20% remain w/ NYHA III–IV sx; 14% require repeat ablation or myectomy. Good alternative for older Pts, multiple comorbidities. Complic: transient (& occ. delayed) 3° AVB w/ 10–20% req. PPM; VT due to scar formation.
  No clear benefit of dual-chamber pacing (*JACC* 1997;29:435; *Circ* 1999;99:2927)
  If refractory to drug therapy and there is *nonobstructive* pathophysiology: transplant
- Acute HF: can be precip. by dehydration or tachycardia; Rx w/ fluids, βB, phenylephrine
- AF: rate control w/ βB, maintain SR w/ disopyramide or amio; low threshold to anticoag
- SCD: ICD (*JACC* 2003;42:1687). Risk factors: h/o VT/VF, ⊕ FHx SCD, unexplained syncope, NSVT, ↓ SBP or rel HoTN (↑ SBP <20 mmHg) w/ exercise, LV wall ≥30 mm, ? extensive MRI delayed enhancement. EPS *not* useful. Risk 4%/y if high-risk (*JAMA* 2007;298:405).
- Counsel to avoid dehydration, extreme exertion
- Endocarditis prophylaxis not recommended (*Circ* 2007;16:1736)
- 1st-degree relatives: periodic screening w/ echo, ECG (as timing of HCMP onset variable). Genetic testing if known mutation.

RESTRICTIVE CARDIOMYOPATHY (RCM)

Definition (*Circ* 2006;113:1807)
- Impaired ventricular filling with ↓ compliance in nonhypertrophied, nondilated ventricles; normal or ↓ diastolic volumes, normal or near-normal EF; must r/o pericardial disease

Etiology (*JACC* 2010;55:1769)
- **Myocardial processes**
  Autoimmune (scleroderma, polymyositis-dermatomyositis)
  Infiltrative diseases (see primary entries for extracardiac manifestations, Dx, Rx)
  Amyloidosis (*Circ* 2011;124:1079): age at presentation ~60 y; ♂:♀ = 3:2
    AL (eg, MM, etc.); familial (transthyretin, ATTR); AA/senile (dep. of TTR, ANP)
    ECG: ↓ QRS amplitude (50%), pseudoinfarction pattern (Qw), AVB (10–20%), hemiblock (20%), BBB (5–20%)
    Echo: biventricular wall thickening (*yet w/ low voltage on ECG*), granular sparkling texture (30%), biatrial enlargement (40%), thickened atrial septum, valve thickening (65%), diastolic dysfxn, small effusions
    Nl voltage/septal thickness has NPV ~90%
    Labs: ✓ SPEP/UPEP, serum free light chain ratio (<0.25 or >1.65 κ-to-λ ratio)
    MRI: distinct late gadolinium enhancement pattern (*JACC* 2008;51:1022)
  Sarcoidosis (can also be DCM): presents at age ~30 y; ↑'d in blacks, N. Europe, ♀
    5% w/ systemic sarcoid have overt cardiac involvement; cardiac w/o systemic in 10%
    ECG: AVB (75%), RBBB (20–60%), VT; PET: ↑ FDG uptake in affected area
    Echo: regional WMA (particularly basal septum) w/ thinning or mild hypertrophy
    Gallium or FDG uptake at areas of inflam.; sestaMIBI w/ non-cor. perfusion defects
    Cardiac MRI: T2 early gad (edema); fibrosis/scar in basal septum; LGE prognostic
    Cardiac bx low yield b/c patchy
  Hemochromatosis: in middle-aged men (espec N. European); 15% p/w cardiac sx
  Diabetes; storage diseases: Gaucher's, Fabry, Hurler's, glycogen storage diseases
- **Endomyocardial processes**
  Chronic eosinophilic: Löffler's endocarditis (temperate climates; ↑ eos; mural thrombi that embolize); endomyocardial fibrosis (tropical climates; var. eos; mural thrombi)
  Toxins: radiation (also p/w constrictive pericarditis, valvular dis, ostial CAD), anthracyclines
  Serotonin: carcinoid, serotonin agonists, ergot alkaloids. Metastatic cancer.

Pathology & pathophysiology
- Path: normal or ↑ wall thickness ± infiltration or abnormal deposition
- ↓ myocardial compliance → nl EDV but ↑ EDP → ↑ systemic & pulm. venous pressures
- ↓ ventricular cavity size → ↓ SV and ↓ CO

Clinical manifestations (*Circ* 2000;101:2490)
- **Right-sided > left-sided heart failure** with peripheral edema > pulmonary edema
- **Diuretic "refractoriness"; thromboembolic events**
- Poorly tolerated tachyarrhythmias; VT → syncope/sudden cardiac death

Physical exam
- ↑ JVP, ± Kussmaul's sign (JVP not ↓ w/ inspir., classically seen in *constrict. pericarditis*)
- Cardiac: ± S₃ and S₄, ± murmurs of MR and TR
- Congestive hepatomegaly, ± ascites and jaundice, peripheral edema

Diagnostic studies
- CXR: normal ventricular chamber size, enlarged atria, ± pulmonary congestion
- ECG: low voltage, pseudoinfarction pattern (Qw), ± arrhythmias
- Echo: ± symmetric wall thickening, biatrial enlarge., ± mural thrombi, ± cavity oblit.
  w/ diast dysfxn: ↑ early diast (E) and ↓ late atrial (A) filling, ↑ E/A ratio, ↓ decel. time
- Cardiac MRI/PET: may reveal inflammation or evidence of infiltration (but nonspecific)
- Cardiac catheterization
  Atria: **M's** or **W's** (prominent *x* and *y* descents)
  Ventricles: **dip & plateau** (rapid ↓ pressure at onset of diastole, rapid ↑ to early plateau)
  Concordance of LV & RV pressure peaks during respiratory cycle (vs. discordance in constrictive pericarditis; *Circ* 1996;93:2007)
- Endomyocardial biopsy if suspect infiltrative process; fat pad bx for amyloid
- Restrictive cardiomyopathy vs. constrictive pericarditis: see "Pericardial Disease"

Treatment (in addition to Rx'ing underlying disease)
- Gentle diuresis. May not tolerate CCB or other vasodilators.
- Control HR (but can ↓ CO); maintain SR (helps filling). Digoxin ↑ arrhythmias in amyloid.
- Anticoagulation (particularly with AF or low CO)
- Transplantation for refractory cases

AORTIC STENOSIS (AS)

Etiology
- **Calcific**: predominant cause in Pts >70 y; risk factors include HTN, ↑ chol., ESRD
- **Congenital** (ie, bicuspid AoV w/ premature calcification): cause in 50% of Pts <70 y
- **Rheumatic heart disease** (AS usually accompanied by AR and MV disease)
- AS mimickers: subvalvular (HCMP, subAo membrane) or supravalvular stenosis

Clinical manifestations (usually indicates AVA <1 cm² or concomitant CAD)
- **Angina**: ↑ O₂ demand (hypertrophy) + ↓ O₂ supply (↓ cor perfusion pressure) ± CAD
- **Syncope** (exertional): peripheral vasodil. w/ fixed CO → ↓ MAP → ↓ cerebral perfusion
- **Heart failure**: outflow obstruct + diastolic dysfxn → pulm. edema, esp. if ↑ HR/AF (↓ LV fill.)
- Acquired vWF disease (~20% of sev. AS): destruction of vWF; GI angiodysplasia
- Natural hx: usually slowly progressive (AVA ↓ ~0.1 cm²/y, but varies; Circ 1997;95:2262), until sx develop; mean survival based on sx: angina = 5 y; syncope = 3 y; CHF = 2 y

Physical exam
- **Midsystolic crescendo-decrescendo** murmur at **RUSB**, harsh, high-pitched, radiates to carotids, apex (holosystolic = Gallavardin effect), ↑ w/ passive leg raise, ↓ w/ standing & Valsalva. Dynamic outflow obstruction (HCM) is the reverse.
- Ejection click after S₁ sometimes heard with bicuspid AoV
- Signs of severity: late-peaking murmur, paradoxically split S₂ or inaudible A₂, small and delayed carotid pulse ("pulsus parvus et tardus"), LV heave, ⊕ S₄ (occasionally palpable)

Pathophys Heart Dis., 6th ed., 2015. for this ed.

Diagnostic studies
- **ECG**: may see LVH, LAE, LBBB, AF (in late disease)
- **CXR**: cardiomegaly, AoV calcification, poststenotic dilation of ascending Ao, pulmonary congestion
- **Echo**: valve morphology, jet velocity, estim pressure gradient (∇) & calculate AVA, LVEF
- **Cardiac cath**: usually to r/o CAD (in ~½ of calcific AS); for hemodyn. if disparity between exam & echo: ✓ pressure gradient (∇) across AoV, calc AVA (underestim. if mod/sev AR)
- **Dobutamine challenge** (echo or cath): if low EF and mean ∇ <30, use to differentiate: *afterload mismatch*: 20% ↑ SV & ∇, no Δ AVA (implies contractile reserve, ↑ EF post-AVR) *pseudostenosis*: 20% ↑ SV, no Δ in ∇, ↑ AVA (implies low AVA artifact of LV dysfxn) *limited contractile reserve*: no Δ SV, ∇ or AVA (implies EF prob. will not improve w/ AVR)

Classification of Aortic Stenosis (Circ 2014;129:e521)

Stage	Sx	Severity	Max Jet Vel (m/s)	Mean Grad (mmHg)	AVA (cm²)[a]	LVEF
n/a	N	Normal	1	0	3–4	nl
A	N	At risk	<2	<10	3–4	nl
B	N	Mild	2–2.9	<20	>1.5	nl
		Moderate	3–3.9	20–39	1–1.5	nl
C1	N	Severe	≥4	≥40	≤1.0	nl
		Very severe	≥5	≥60	≤0.8	nl
C2		Severe + ↓ EF	≥4	≥40	≤1.0	↓
D1		Severe	≥4	≥40	≤1.0	nl
D2	Y	Severe + low flow/∇ + ↓ EF[b]	<4	<40	≤1.0	↓
D3		Severe + low flow/∇ nl EF[c]	<4	<40	≤1.0	nl

[a]AVA indexed to BSA <0.6 cm²/m² also severe; [b]DSE → max jet vel ≥4 & AVA ≤1.0; [c]small LV w/ ↓ stroke vol.

Treatment (Circ 2014;129:e521; NEJM 2014;371:744; Lancet 2016;387:1312)
- Based on **symptoms**: once they develop, AVR needed. If asx, HTN can be cautiously Rx'd.
- **AVR**: indicated in sx (stage D1); asx severe + EF <50% (stage C2); or asx severe (stage C1) and undergoing other cardiac surgery
  Reasonable if:
      Asx severe (stage C1) but either sx or ↓ BP w/ exercise (can *carefully* exercise asx AS to uncover sx, do *not* exercise sx AS) or **very severe.**
      Sx severe w/ low flow/∇ w/ low EF & response to dobuta (stage D2) or normal EF but AS felt to be cause of sx (stage D3)
      Asx moderate AS (stage B) and undergoing cardiac surgery
- Transcatheter AoV replacement (TAVR, see below) indicated if surgical risk prohibitive or as reasonable alternative to surgery if medium (STS predicted 30-d mortality ~4–8%) or high (mortality 8–15%) operative risk

- Medical (if not AVR candidate or to temporize): careful diuresis prn, control HTN, maintain SR; digoxin if ↓ EF & HF or if AF; *avoid* venodilators (nitrates) & ⊖ inotropes (βB/CCB) if severe AS; avoid vigorous physical exertion once AS mod–severe;
  ? nitroprusside in HF w/ sev. AS, EF <35%, CI <2.2, & MAP >60 (*NEJM 2003;348:1756*) or if low flow w/ ↓ EF and HTN (*Circ 2013;128:1349*)
- IABP: stabilization, bridge to surgery
- Balloon AoV valvotomy (BAV): 50% ↑ AVA & ↓ peak *P*, *but* 50% restenosis by 6–12 mo & ↑ risk of peri-PAV stroke/AR (*NEJM 1988;319:125*), ∴ bridge to AVR or palliation

TAVR (transcatheter AoV replacement)

- Valves: balloon-expandable (Edwards SAPIEN) or self-expanding (Medtronic CoreValve)
- Approaches: most commonly retrograde via perc. transfemoral access; also retrograde via axillary art. or ascend. Ao (via small thoracotomy & aortotomy). Rarely antegrade transapical via small thoracotomy & LV puncture (if narrow iliofem art. or calcified Ao).
- Peri- & postprocedural complic.: low CO; annular rupture or coronary occlusion (both rare); local vascular; paravalvular leaks; CHB.
- Lifelong ASA + ? clopidogrel (or OAC) × 6 mo; ? subclinical valve thrombus in ~20%, ↓ w/ anticoag (*NEJM 2015;373:2015*)
- Outcomes w/ TAVR. In *nonoperative* Pts (ie, vs. med Rx): 44% ↓ mortality but still ~20% annual mortality in TAVR group (*NEJM 2012;366:1696; JACC 2014;63:1972*).
  In *high-risk* Pts vs. surg AVR (*NEJM 2012;366:1686 & 2014;370:1790*): mortality ≈ (balloon-expand) or 26% ↓ (self-expand); ↑ vasc complic; ↑ early stroke of stroke/TIA w/ balloon-expand; PPM required for CHB in ~20% w/ self-expand; paravalvular leaks in ~7%.
  In *medium-risk* Pts (*NEJM 2016;374:1609*): death/stroke ≈, ↑ vasc complic but ↓ bleeding, AKI, AF. If transfemoral 21%, ↓ death/stroke, whereas tended to be 21% ↑ if transapical.

AORTIC REGURGITATION (AR)

Etiology (*Circ 2006;114:422*)

- **Valve disease (43%): rheumatic heart disease** (usually mixed AS/AR + MV disease); **bicuspid AoV** (natural hx: $^{1}/_{3}$ → normal, $^{1}/_{3}$ → AS, $^{1}/_{6}$ → AR, $^{1}/_{6}$ → endocarditis → AR); **infective endocarditis**; valvulitis (RA, SLE, certain anorectics & serotonergics, XRT)
- **Root disease (57%): HTN**, aortic aneurysm/dissection, annuloaortic ectasia (ie, Marfan), **aortic inflammation** (GCA, Takayasu's, ankylosing spond., reactive arthritis, syphilis)

Clinical manifestations

- Acute: sudden ↓ forward SV and ↑ LVEDP (noncompliant ventricle) → pulmonary edema ± hypotension and cardiogenic shock
- Chronic: clinically silent while LV dilates (to ↑ compliance to keep LVEDP low) more than it hypertrophies → chronic volume overload → LV decompensation → CHF
- Natural hx: *variable* progression (unlike AS, can be fast or slow); once decompensation begins, prognosis poor w/o AVR (mortality ~10%/y)

Physical exam

- **Early diastolic decrescendo murmur at LUSB** (RUSB if dilated Ao root); ↑ w/ sitting forward, expir, handgrip; severity of AR ∝ duration of murmur (except in acute & severe late); *Austin Flint murmur:* mid-to-late diastolic rumble at apex (AR jet interfering w/ mitral inflow)
- **Wide pulse pressure** due to ↑ stroke volume, hyper-dynamic pulse; pulse pressure narrows in late AR with ↓ LV fxn; bisferiens (twice-beating) arterial pulse
- PMI diffuse and laterally displaced; soft S_1 (early closure of MV); ± S_3 (≠ ↓ EF but rather just volume overload in AR)

Classic Eponymous Signs in Chronic AR (*South Med J 1981;74:459*)	
Sign	**Description**
Corrigan's pulse	"water hammer" pulse (ie, rapid rise/fall or distention/collapse)
Hill's sign	(popliteal SBP – brachial SBP) >60 mmHg
Duroziez's sign	to-and-fro murmur heard over femoral artery w/ light compression
Pistol shot sounds	pistol shot sound heard over femoral artery
Traube's sound	double sound heard over femoral artery when compressed distally
de Musset's sign	head-bobbing with each heartbeat (low Se)
Müller's sign	systolic pulsations of the uvula
Quincke's pulses	subungual capillary pulsations (low Sp)

Diagnostic studies

- ECG: can see LVH, LAD, abnl repol; CXR: cardiomegaly ± ascending Ao dilatation

- **Echo:** severity of AR (severe = regurg jet width ≥65% LVOT, regurg fraction ≥50%, regurg orifice ≥0.3 cm², flow reversal in descend. Ao; moderate = jet width 25–64%, regurg fraction 30–49%, regurg orifice 0.1–0.29 cm²); LV size & fxn

Treatment *(Circ 2014;129:e521; Lancet 1387:1312)*
- Acute decompensation (consider endocarditis as possible acute precipitant):
  surgery usually urgently needed for acute severe AR, which is poorly tolerated by LV
  IV afterload reduction (nitroprusside) and inotropic support (dobutamine)
  ± chronotropic support (↑ HR → ↓ diastole → ↓ time for regurgitation)
  pure vasoconstrictors and IABP contraindicated
- In chronic AR, management decisions based on *LV size and fxn* (and before sx occur)
- **Surgery** (AVR, replacement or repair if possible):
  severe and **sx** (if equivocal, consider stress test)
  asx and either EF ≤50% or LV dilation (LVESD >50 mm) or undergoing cardiac surg
- Transcatheter AoV replacement (TAVR) being explored *(JACC 2013;61:1577 & 2015;66:169)*
- Medical therapy: **vasodilators** (nifedipine, ACEI/ARB, hydralazine) if severe ASx w/ sx or LV dysfxn & not operative candidate or to improve hemodynamics before AVR; no clear benefit in asx severe AR w/ mild LV dilation & nl LV fxn *(NEJM 2005;353:1342)*

MITRAL REGURGITATION (MR)

Etiology *(Lancet 2009;373:1382; NEJM 2010;363:156)*
- **Primary** (degeneration of valve apparatus)
  leaflet abnl: myxomatous (MVP), endocarditis, calcific RHD, valvulitis (collagen-vascular disease), congenital, anorectic drugs (phen-fen), XRT
  chordae tendineae rupture: myxomatous, endocarditis, spontaneous, trauma
  papillary muscle dysfxn b/c of ischemia or rupture during MI [usu. posteromedial papillary m. (supplied predominantly by PDA) vs. anterolateral (suppl. by diags & OMs)]
- **Secondary (functional):** inferoapical papillary muscle displacement due to ischemic LV remodeling or DCM; HCM *(JACC 2015;65:1231)*

Clinical manifestations
- Acute: **pulmonary edema**, hypotension, cardiogenic shock *(NEJM 2004;351:1627)*
- Chronic: typically asx for yrs, then as LV fails → progressive DOE, fatigue, AF, PHT
- Prognosis: 5-y survival w/ medical therapy is 80% if asx, but only 45% if sx

Physical exam
- **High-pitched, blowing, holosystolic murmur at apex;**
  radiates to axilla; ± thrill; ↑ w/ handgrip (Se 68%, Sp 92%),
  ↓ w/ Valsalva (Se 93%) *(NEJM 1988;318:1572)*
  ant. leaflet abnl → post. jet heard at spine
  post. leaflet abnl → ant. jet heard at sternum
- ± diastolic rumble b/c ↑ flow across valve
- Lat. displ. hyperdynamic PMI, obscured S₁, widely split S₂
  (A₂ early b/c ↓ LV afterload, P₂ late if PHT); ± S₃
- Carotid upstroke brisk (vs. diminished and delayed in AS)

Diagnostic studies *(NEJM 2005;352:875)*
- ECG: may see LAE, LVH, ± atrial fibrillation
- CXR: dilated LA, dilated LV, ± pulmonary congestion
- Echo: MV anatomy (ie, etiol); MR severity: jet area, jet width at origin (vena contracta) or effective regurgitant orifice (ERO; predicts survival); LV fxn (EF should be *supranormal* if compensated, ∴ EF <60% w/ sev. MR = LV dysfxn)
- TEE or cardiac MR if TTE not sufficiently informative
- Cardiac cath: prominent PCWP *c-v* waves (not spec. for MR), LVgram for MR severity & EF

Classification of Primary Mitral Regurgitation

Severity	Regurg. fraction	Jet area (% of LA)	Jet width (cm)	ERO (cm²)	Angio*
Mild	<30%	<20	<0.3	<0.2	1+
Moderate	30–49%	20–40	0.3–0.69	0.2–0.39	2+
Severe†	≥50%	>40	≥0.70	≥0.40	3/4+

*1+ = LA clears w/ each beat; 2+ = LA does not clear, faintly opac. after several beats; 3+ = LA & LV opac. equal.
†For secondary MR, because ERO underestimated & likely progressive LV dysfxn, ERO ≥0.20 is severe

Treatment *(Circ 2014;129:e521; Lancet 2016;387:1324)*
- **Acute severe MR:** consider ischemia & endocarditis as precipitants; IV afterload reduction (nitroprusside), relieve congestion (diuresis & NTG), ± inotropes (dobuta), IABP, avoid vasoconstrictors; *surgery* usually needed as prognosis poor w/o *(JAMA 2013;310:609)*

- **Chronic severe primary MR:** surgery (repair [preferred if feasible] vs. replacement) indicated if sx & EF >30% or if asx & either EF 30–60% or LV sys. diam. ≥40 mm
  MV *repair* reasonable if asx & either EF >60% + LVESD <40 mm or new AF or PHT if AF, concomitant surgical ablation ↓ AF recurrence, ∅ Δ stroke; consider for sx cntl or if planning no anticoag (NEJM 2015;372:1399)
- **Severe secondary MR:** consider surgery if NYHA III-IV; replacement results in more durable correction & ↓ HF & ↓ CV admissions than repair (NEJM 2016;374:344)
- In Pts undergoing CABG w/ moderate fxnal MR, annuloplasty ↓ MR but longer surgery, ↑ neurologic events, & no impact on fxnal status or mortality (NEJM 2016;374:1932)
- Percut. MV repair (Circ 2014;130:1712): edge-to-edge clip less effective than surgery but consider for sev. sx nonoperative Pt (NEJM 2011;364:1395); perc valve under study (JACC 2014;64:1814)
- If sx & EF<60% but not operative candidate: HF Rx (βB, ACEI, ± aldo antag); ↓ preload w/ diuretics, NTG (espec. if ischemic MR) for sx relief ± ↓ ERO; maintain SR
- Asymptomatic: ∅ proven benefit of medical therapy; βB ↑ LV fxn (JACC 2012;60:833).

MITRAL VALVE PROLAPSE (MVP)

Definition and Etiology
- Billowing of MV leaflet ≥2 mm above mitral annulus in parasternal long axis echo view
- Primary: sporadic or familial myxomatous proliferation of spongiosa of MV apparatus
- Secondary: trauma, endocarditis, congenital, CTD (eg, Marfan's, OI, Ehlers-Danlos)

Clinical manifestations (usually asymptomatic)
- MR (MVP most common cause), endocarditis, embolic events, arrhythmias (rarely SCD)
- High-pitched, midsystolic click (earlier w/ ↓ preload) ± mid-to-late systolic murmur
- No Rx per se [endocarditis Ppx no longer rec. (Circ 2007;116:1736)]; Rx MR as above

MITRAL STENOSIS (MS)

Etiology (Lancet 2012;379:953)
- **Rheumatic heart disease** (RHD): *fusion of commissures* → "fish-mouth" valve from autoimmune rxn to β strep infxn; seen largely in developing world today
- **Mitral annular calcification:** encroachment upon leaflets → fxnal MS; espec in ESRD
- Congenital, infectious endocarditis w/ large lesion, myxoma near MV, thrombus
- Valvulitis (eg, SLE, amyloid, carcinoid) or infiltration (eg, mucopolysaccharidoses)

Clinical manifestations (Lancet 2009;374:1271)
- **Dyspnea and pulmonary edema** (if due to RHD, sx usually begin in 30s) precipitants: exercise, fever, anemia, volume overload (incl. pregnancy), tachycardia, AF
- **Atrial fibrillation:** onset often precipitates heart failure in Pts w/ MS
- **Embolic events:** commonly cerebral, espec in AF or endocarditis
- Pulmonary: hemoptysis, frequent bronchitis (due to congestion), PHT, RV failure
- Ortner's syndrome: hoarseness from LA compression of recurrent laryngeal nerve

Physical exam
- **Low-pitched mid-diastolic rumble at apex** w/ presystolic accentuation (if not in AF); best heard in L lat decubitus position during expiration, ↑ w/ exercise; severity proportional to *duration* (not intensity) of murmur; loud S_1
- **Opening snap** (high-pitched early diastolic sound at apex) from fused leaflet tips; MVA proportional to S_2–OS interval (tighter valve → ↑ LA pressure → shorter interval)
- Loud S_1 (unless MV calcified and immobile)

Diagnostic studies
- ECG: **LAE** ("P mitrale"), ± AF, ± RVH
- CXR: **dilated LA** (flat L heart border, R double density, displaced L mainstem bronchus)
- **Echo:** estimate pressure gradient (∇), RVSP, valve area, valve echo score (0–16, based on leaflet mobility & thick, subvalvular thick., Ca++); exer. TTE (to assess Δ RVSP and ∇) if sx & severity of MS at rest discrepant; TEE to assess for LA thrombus before PMBC
- **Cardiac cath:** ∇, calculated MVA; LA tall *a* wave & blunted *y* descent; ↑ PA pressures

Classification of Mitral Stenosis				
Stage	Mean ∇ (mmHg)	Pressure ½ time	MVA (cm²)	PA sys (mmHg)
Normal	0		4–6	<25
Mild-Mod	<5	100–149	1.6–2	<30
Severe	5–9	150–219	1.1–1.5	30–50
Very severe	≥10	≥220	≤1	>50

Treatment *(Circ 2014;129:e521; Lancet 2016;387:1324)*

- Medical: Na restriction, cautious diuresis, βB, AF control, sx-limited physical stress
- Antibiotic Ppx indicated if h/o RHD w/ valvular disease for 10 y or until age 40
- Anticoag: AF; prior embolism; LA clot; ? LA >55 mm or Large LA w/ spont contrast
- Mechanical intervention indicated if **heart failure sx w/ MVA ≤1.5**; reasonable if asx but very severe (MVA ≤1) and morphology favorable for PMBC; may consider PMBC if MVA >1.5 but hemodyn signif w/ exercise, or if asx but MVA ≤1.5 and new-onset AF
- **Percutaneous mitral balloon commissurotomy** (PMBC): preferred Rx if RHD; MVA doubles, ∇ ↓ by 50%; ≈ MVR if valve score <8, ∅ if mod-severe MR or LA clot
- Surgical (MV repair if possible, o/w replacement): consider in sx Pts w/ MVA ≤1.5 if PMBC unavailable/failed/contraindicated or valve morphology unsuitable
- Pregnancy: if NYHA class III/IV → PMBC, o/w medical Rx w/ low-dose diuretic & βB

TRICUSPID REGURGITATION

- 1° etiol: rheumatic, CTD, XRT, IE, Ebstein's, carcinoid, tumors, pacemaker leads
- Fxnl etiol (most common): RV and/or PHT (may be 2° to L-sided dis.), RV dilation ± MI
- Holosystolic murmur, 3rd/4th ICS, ↑ w/ insp (Carvallo's sign); S$_3$; prominent *cv* wave in JVP
- Consider repair, annuloplasty or replacement for sx and severe TR (eg, ERO ≥0.40 cm^2); transcatheter system (provides surface for coaptation) under study *(JACC 2015;66:2475)*

PROSTHETIC HEART VALVES

Mechanical (60%)
- Bileaflet (eg, St. Jude Medical); tilting disk; caged-ball
- Very durable (20–30 y), but thrombogenic and ∴ require anticoagulation consider if age <~60 y or if anticoagulation already indicated *(JACC 2010;55:2413)*

Bioprosthetic (40%)
- Bovine pericardial or porcine heterograft (eg, Carpentier-Edwards), homograft
- Less durable, but min. thrombogenic; consider if >~70 y, lifespan <20 y, or ∅ anticoag
- If 50–69 y, 2× reop but ½ bleeding or stroke vs. mech *(JAMA 2014;312:1323 & 2015;313:1435)*

Physical exam
- **Crisp sounds** ± soft murmur during forward flow (normal to have small ∇)

Anticoagulation & antiplatelet therapy *(Circ 2014;129:e521)*
- *High-risk features:* prior thromboembolism, AF, EF <30–35%, hypercoagulable
- **Warfarin (Ø NOACs):** mech MVR or high-risk mech AVR: INR 2.5–3.5. Low-risk mech AVR or high-risk bio MVR/AVR: INR 2–3. Consider in low-risk bio MVR/AVR for 1st 3 mo.
- **+ ASA** (≤100 mg): all prosth. valves unless h/o GIB, uncontrolled HTN, erratic INR, or >80 y
- If thrombosis, ↑ intensity (eg, INR 2–3 → 2.5-3.5; 2.5-3.5 → 3.5-4.5; add ASA if not on)

Periprocedural "Bridging" of Anticoagulation in Pts with Mechanical Valve(s)	
AVR w/o risk factors	d/c warfarin 2–4 d before surg; restart 12–24 h after surg
MVR or AVR w/ risk factors	Preop: d/c warfarin, start UFH (preferred to LMWH) when INR <2 4–6 h preop; d/c UFH; postop: restart UFH & warfarin ASAP

Procedures include noncardiac surgery, invasive procedures, and major dental work

Correction of overanticoagulation *(Circ 2014;129:e521)*
- Risk from major bleeding must be weighed against risk of valve thrombosis
- Not bleeding: if INR 5–10, withhold warfarin; if INR >10 also give vit K 1–2.5 mg PO
- Bleeding: FFP or PCC + low-dose (1 mg) vit K IV

Endocarditis prophylaxis: for all prosthetic valves (see "Endocarditis")

Complications
- Structural failure (r/o endocarditis); mechanical valves: rare except for Bjork-Shiley; bioprosth: up to 30% rate w/in 10–15 y, mitral > aortic; consider TAVR *(JAMA 2014;312:162)*
- Paravalvular leak (r/o endocarditis); small *central* jet of regurg is normal in mech. valves
- Obstruction from thrombosis *(JACC 2013;62:1731)* or pannus: ✓ TTE, TEE, CTA, or fluoro significantly symptomatic *pannus* ingrowth: remove w/ surgery thrombosis: surgery if L-sided valve & either severe sx or lg (? ≥0.8 cm) thrombus; lytic successful in ~70% of L-sided thrombosis, but w/ 14% risk of stroke; consider UFH ± lytic (? low-dose tPA via slow infusion) *(JACC CV Imaging 2013;6:206)* if mild sx & small clot burden or poor surg candidate; lytic reasonable for R-sided
- Infective endocarditis ± valvular abscess and conduction system dis. (see "Endocarditis")
- Embolization (r/o endocarditis); risk highest 1st 90 d, ~1%/y w/ warfarin (vs. 2% w/ ASA, or 4% w/o meds); mech MVR 2× risk of embolic events vs. mech AVR *(Circ 1994;89:635)*
- Bleeding (from anticoag), hemolysis (espec w/ caged-ball valves or paravalvular leak)

GENERAL PRINCIPLES

Anatomy
- Tissue sac surrounding heart & proximal great vessels; 2 layers (parietal & visceral)

Disease states
- Inflammation (w/ or w/o fluid accumulation) → pericarditis
- Fluid accumulation → effusion ± tamponade
- Decrease in compliance (sequela of inflammation) → constrictive pericarditis
- Tamponade and constriction characterized by increased ventricular interdependence

PERICARDITIS AND PERICARDIAL EFFUSION

Etiologies of Acute Pericarditis (JAMA 2015;314:1498)	
Idiopathic (>80%)	Most presumed to be undiagnosed viral etiologies
Infectious (<5% can be confirmed infectious)	Viral: Coxsackie, echo, adeno, EBV, VZV, HIV, influenza Bacterial (from endocarditis, pneumonia or s/p cardiac surgery): S. pneumococcus, N. meningitidis, S. aureus, Borrelia (Lyme); TB Fungal: Histo, Coccidio, Candida; Parasitic: Entamoeba, Echino
Neoplastic (<10%)	Common: metastatic (lung, breast, lymphoma, leukemia, RCC) Rare: primary cardiac & serosal tumors (mesothelioma)
Autoimmune	Connective tissue diseases: SLE, RA, scleroderma, Sjögren's Vasculitides: PAN, eosin GPA (Churg-Strauss), GPA (Wegener's) Drug-induced: procainamide, hydralazine, INH, CsA
Uremia	~5–13% of Pts prior to HD; ~20% occurrence in chronic HD Pts
Cardiovascular	STEMI, late post-MI (Dressler's syndrome); ascending AoD; chest trauma; postpericardiotomy; procedural complic. (ie, PCI, PPM)
Radiation	>40 Gy to mediastinum; acute or delayed; may be transudative
Effusion w/o pericarditis	CHF, cirrhosis, nephrotic syndrome, hypothyroidism, amyloidosis. Transudative.

Clinical manifestations (NEJM 2014;371:2410)
- **Pericarditis:** retrosternal CP, pleuritic, positional (often ↓ by sitting forward), → trapezius; may be absent in TB, neoplastic, XRT, or uremic; ± fever; ± s/s of systemic etiologies
- **Effusion:** present in ~2/3 of Pts w/ pericarditis; ranges from asx to tamponade

Physical exam
- **Pericarditis:** multiphasic **friction rub** best heard at LLSB w/ diaphragm of stethoscope. Notoriously variable and evanescent leathery sound w/ up to 3 components: atrial contraction, ventricular contraction, ventricular relaxation (NEJM 2012;367:e20).
- **Effusion:** distant heart sounds, dullness over left posterior lung field due to compressive atelectasis from pericardial effusion (Ewart's sign)

Diagnostic studies (JAMA 2015;314:1498; EHJ 2015;36:2921)
- Need ≥2 of the following: chest pain (as noted above), friction rub, ECG findings, effusion
- **ECG:** may show diffuse STE (concave up) & PR depression (except in aVR: ST ↓ & PR ↑), TWI; classically and in contrast to STEMI, TWI do not occur until STs normalize
  Stages: (I) STE & PR ↓; (II) ST & PR normalize; (III) diffuse TWI; (IV) Tw normalize
  ECG may show evidence of large effusion w/ low voltage & electrical alternans (beat-to-beat Δ in QRS amplitude and/or axis due to swinging heart)
- **CXR:** if lg effusion (>250 mL) → ↑ cardiac silhouette w/ "water-bottle" heart & epicardial halo
- **Echocardiogram:** presence, size, & location of effusion; presence of tamponade physiology; pericarditis itself w/o spec. abnl (∴ echo can be nl), although can see pericardial stranding (fibrin or tumor); can also detect LV/RV dysfxn (myocarditis?)
- **CT:** will reveal pericardial effusions, but they often appear larger by CT than by echo.
- **MRI:** may reveal pericardial thickening/inflammation, as well as myocardial involvement
- **CK-MB or troponin** (⊕ in ~30%; JACC 2003;42:2144) if myopericarditis. Consider CRP/ESR.

Workup for effusion
- r/o infxn: usually apparent from Hx & CXR; ? value of ✓ acute and convalescent serologies
- r/o noninfectious etiologies: BUN, Cr, ANA, RF, HIV, relevant malignancy evaluation
- Pericardiocentesis if suspect infxn or malignancy or large effusion (>2 cm) or recurrent
  ✓ cell counts, TP, LDH, glc, Gram stain & Cx, AFB, cytology
  ADA, PCR for MTb, and specific tumor markers as indicated by clinical suspicion
  "exudate": TP >3 g/dL, TP_eff/TP_serum >0.5, LDH_eff/LDH_serum >0.6 or glc <60 mg/dL;
  high Se (~90%) but very low Sp (~20%); overall low utility (Chest 1997;111:1213)
- Pericardial bx if suspicion remains for malignancy or TB

Treatment of pericarditis *(JAMA 2015;314:1498; EHJ 2015;36:2921)*

- High-dose **NSAID** (eg, ibuprofen 600–800 mg tid) or ASA (eg, 650–1000 mg tid) × 7–14 d then taper over wks; ASA preferred over NSAID in acute MI; consider PPI to ↓ risk of GIB
- **Add colchicine** 0.5 mg bid (qd if ≤70 kg) × 3 mo; ↓ risk of refractory or recurrent pericarditis by 50% *(NEJM 2013;369:1522)*
- Avoid steroids except for systemic autoimmune disorder, uremic, preg., NSAIDs contra-indicated, or refractory idiopathic dis. Appear to ↑ rate of pericarditis recurrence *(Circ 2008;118:667)*. If due to TB, steroids ↓ risk of constriction *(NEJM 2014;371:1121)*.
- Avoid anticoagulants (although no convincing data that ↑ risk of hemorrhage/tamponade)
- Infectious effusion → pericardial drainage (preferably surgically) + systemic antibiotics
- Acute idiopathic pericarditis self-limited in 70–90% of cases
- Recurrent pericarditis *(Circ 2007;115:2739)*
  - risk factors: subacute, lg effusion/tamponade, T >38°C, lack of NSAID response after 7 d
  - treatment: colchicine 0.5 mg bid × 6 mo *(Annals 2011;155:409 & Lancet 2014;383:2232)*
- Recurrent effusions: consider pericardial window (percutaneous vs. surgical)

PERICARDIAL TAMPONADE

Etiology
- Any cause of pericarditis but espec. **malignancy, infectious,** uremia, ascending AoD, myocardial rupture, periprocedural complication, trauma, post-cardiotomy
- Rapidly accumulating effusions most likely to cause tamponade as no time for pericardium to stretch (eg, to ↑ compliance) and accommodate ↑ intrapericardial fluid volume

Pathophysiology *(NEJM 2003;349:684)*
- ↑ intrapericardial pressure, compression of heart chambers, ↓ venous return → ↓ CO
- Diastolic pressures ↑ & equalize in all cardiac chambers → minimal flow of blood from RA to RV when TV opens → blunted y descent
- ↑ ventricular interdependence → pulsus paradoxus (pathologic exaggeration of nl physio)
  Inspiration → ↑ intrapericardial & RA pressures → ↓ venous return → ↑ RV size → septal shift to left. Also, ↑ pulmonary vascular compliance → ↓ pulm venous return.
  Result is ↓ LV filling → ↓ **LV stroke volume** & blood pressure & pulse pressure.

Clinical manifestations
- **Cardiogenic shock** (hypotension, fatigue) **without pulmonary edema**
- Dyspnea (seen in ~85%) may be due to ↑ respiratory drive to augment venous return

Physical exam *(EHJ 2014;35:2279)*
- **Beck's triad** (present in minority of cases): **distant heart sounds, ↑ JVP, hypotension**
- ↑ JVP (76%) w/ blunted y descent
- Reflex tachycardia (77%), hypotension (26%; occasionally hypertensive), cool extremities
- **Pulsus paradoxus** (Se 82%, Sp 70%) = ↓ SBP ≥10 mmHg during inspiration
  ⊕ LR 3.3 (5.9 if pulsus >12), ⊖ LR 0.03
  Ddx = PE, hypovolemia, severe COPD, constriction (~$^1/_3$), RV infarct
  ? absent if pre-existing ↑ LVEDP, irregular rhythm, severe AI, ASD, regional tamponade
- Distant heart sounds (28%), ± pericardial friction rub (30%)
- Tachypnea and orthopnea but clear lungs

Diagnostic studies
- ECG: ↑ HR, ↓ voltage (seen in 42%), electrical alternans (20%), ± signs of pericarditis
- CXR: ↑ cardiac silhouette (89%)
- **Echocardiogram:** ⊕ **effusion,** IVC plethora, **septal shift** with inspiration
  diastolic collapse of RA (Se 85%, Sp 80%) and/or RV (Se <80%, Sp 90%)
  respirophasic Δ's in transvalvular velocities (↑ across TV & ↓ across MV w/ inspir.)
  postsurgical tamponade may be localized and not easily visible
- Cardiac cath (right heart and pericardial): elevation (15–30 mmHg) and equalization of intrapericardial and diastolic pressures (RA, RV, PCWP), blunted y descent in RA
  ↑ in stroke volume postpericardiocentesis = ultimate proof of tamponade
  if RA pressure remains elevated after drainage, may have effusive-constrictive disease (constriction from visceral pericardium; *NEJM 2004;350:469*) or myocardial dysfxn (eg, from concomitant myocarditis)

Treatment *(EHJ 2014;35:2279)*
- Volume but be careful as overfilling can worsen tamponade) and ⊕ inotropes (avoid βB)
- Avoid vasoconstrictors as will ↓ stroke volume & potentially ↓ HR
- Avoid positive pressure ventilation as it can further impair cardiac filling *(Circ 2006;113:1622)*
- **Pericardiocentesis** (except if due to aortic/myocardial rupture for which emergent surgery treatment of choice; if too unstable, consider small pericardiocentesis to prevent PEA)
- Surgical drainage considered if fluid rapidly reaccumulates, loculated, or hemorrhagic

Etiology (Circ 2011;124:1270)

- Any cause of pericarditis (~1–2% incidence overall after acute pericarditis)
- Highest risk w/ **TB, bacterial, neoplastic, XRT,** connective tissue, postcardiac surgery
- **Viral/idiopathic,** as most common cause of pericarditis, also account for signif proportion

Pathophysiology

- Adhesion of visceral and parietal pericardial layers → rigid pericardium that limits diastolic filling of ventricles → ↑ systemic venous pressures
- Venous return is limited only after early rapid filling phase; ∴ rapid ↓ in RA pressure with atrial relaxation and opening of tricuspid valve and *prominent x and y descents*
- Kussmaul sign: JVP does not decrease with inspiration (↑ venous return with inspiration, but negative intrathoracic pressure not transmitted to heart because of rigid pericardium)

Clinical manifestations (NEJM 2011;364:1350)

- Right-sided > left-sided heart failure (systemic congestion > pulmonary congestion)

Physical exam

- ↑ **JVP** with **prominent y descent,** ⊕ **Kussmaul sign** [Ddx: tricuspid stenosis, acute cor pulmonale, RV dysfxn (CMP, RV MI), SVC syndrome]
- Hepatosplenomegaly, ascites, peripheral edema. Consider in Ddx of idiopathic cirrhosis.
- PMI usually not palpable, **pericardial knock,** usually no pulsus paradoxus

Diagnostic studies

- ECG: nonspecific, AF common (up to 33%) in advanced cases
- CXR: calcification (MTb most common), espec in lateral view (although not specific)
- Echocardiogram: ± thickened pericardium, "**septal bounce**" = abrupt displacement of septum during rapid filling in early diastole
- Cardiac catheterization: atria w/ Ms or Ws (prominent x and y descents)
  ventricles: **dip-and-plateau or square-root sign** (rapid ↓ pressure at onset of diastole, rapid ↑ to early plateau)
  discordance between LV & RV pressure peaks during respiratory cycle (Circ 1996;93:2007)
- CT or **MRI**: thickened pericardium (>4 mm; Se ~80%) w/ tethering (Circ 2011;123:e418)

Treatment

- Diuresis if intravascular volume overload; surgical pericardiectomy if infectious or advanced

Constrictive Pericarditis vs Restrictive Cardiomyopathy		
Evaluation	**Constrictive pericarditis**	**Restrictive cardiomyopathy**
Physical exam	⊕ Kussmaul sign Absent PMI ⊕ Pericardial knock	± Kussmaul sign Powerful PMI, ± S_3 and S_4 ± **Murmurs of MR, TR**
ECG	± Low voltage	Low voltage if infiltrative myopathy ± **Conduction abnormalities**
Echocardiogram	**Respirophasic variation (25–40%):** inspir. → ↑ flow across TV and ↓ flow across MV E′ (tissue velocity) nl/↑ (>12 cm/sec) **Expir.** hepatic vein flow reversal **Septal bounce** in early diastole Normal wall thickness	<10% respirophasic variation Slower peak filling rate Longer time to peak filling rate **E′** ↓ (<8 cm/sec) (Se 95%, Sp 96%; HF Rev 2013;18:255) **Inspir.** hepatic vein flow reversal **Biatrial enlargement** ± ↑ wall thickness
CT/MRI	**Usually w/ thickened pericardium**	Normal pericardium
NT-proBNP	Variable	Typically ↑/↑↑ (JACC 2005;45:1900)
Cardiac catheterization	Prominent x and y descents (more so in constriction)	
	Dip-and-plateau sign (more so in constriction)	
	LVEDP = RVEDP RVSP <55 mmHg (Se 90%, Sp 29%) RVEDP >$^1/_3$ RVSP (Se 93%, Sp 46%) **Discordance** of LV & RV pressure peaks during respiratory cycle **Systolic area index** (ratio of RV to LV pressure–time area in inspir vs. expir) >1.1 (Se 97%, Sp 100%)	**LVEDP > RVEDP** (esp. w/ vol.) RVSP >55 mmHg RVEDP <$^1/_3$ RVSP Concordance of LV & RV pressure peaks during respiratory cycle Systolic area index ≤1.1 (JACC 2008;51:315)
Endomyocardial biopsy	Usually normal	± **Specific etiology of RCMP** (fibrosis, infiltration, hypertrophy)

HYPERTENSION

JNC 8 Classification		
Category	Systolic	Diastolic
Normal	<120	<80
Pre-HTN	120–139	80–89
Stage 1 HTN	140–159	90–99
Stage 2 HTN	≥160	≥100

Ambulatory Thresholds		
Setting	Systolic	Diastolic
24-hr avg	135	85
Day (awake)	140	90
Night (asleep)	125	75

(Circ 2005;111:697)

BP in mmHg. Average ≥2 measurements >1–2 min apart. Confirm stage 1 w/in 1–4 wk; can Rx stage 2 immediately (J Clin HTN 2014;16:14)

Epidemiology (JAMA 2014;311:1424; Circ 2015;131:e29)
- Prevalence ~30% in U.S. adults, ≥44% in African-Americans; M = F
- Of those with HTN, ~3/4 were treated, ~1/2 achieve target BP, ~1/6 were unaware of dx

Etiologies
- **Essential** (95%): onset 25–55 y; ⊕ FHx. Unclear mechanism but ? additive microvasc renal injury over time w/ contribution of hyperactive sympathetics (NEJM 2002;346:913). ↑ Age → ↓ ↑ art compliance → HTN. Genetics + environment involved (Nature 2011;478:103).
- **Secondary:** Consider if Pt <30 y or if sudden onset, severe, refractory HTN

Secondary Causes of Hypertension			
Diseases		Suggestive findings	Initial workup
RENAL	**Renal parenchymal** (2–3%)	h/o DM, polycystic kidney disease, glomerulonephritis	CrCl, albuminuria See "Renal Failure"
	Renovascular (1–2%) Athero (90%) FMD (10%, young women) PAN, scleroderma	ARF induced by ACEI/ARB Recurrent flash pulm edema Renal bruit; hypokalemia (NEJM 2009;361:1972)	MRA (>90% Se & Sp, less for FMD), CTA, duplex U/S, angio, plasma renin (low Sp)
ENDO	**Hyperaldo or Cushing's** (1–5%)	Hypokalemia Metabolic alkalosis	See "Adrenal Disorders"
	Pheochromocytoma (<1%)	Paroxysmal HTN, H/A, palp.	
	Myxedema (<1%)	See "Thyroid Disorders"	TFTs
	Hypercalcemia (<1%)	Polyuria, dehydration, Δ MS	iCa
OTHER	Obstructive sleep apnea (qv); alcohol		
	Medications: OCP, steroids, licorice; NSAIDs (espec COX-2); Epo; cyclosporine		
	Aortic coarctation: ↓ LE pulses, systolic murmur, radial-femoral delay; abnl TTE, CXR		
	Polycythemia vera: ↑ Hct		

Standard workup
- Goals: (1) identify CV risk factors; (2) seek 2° causes; (3) assess for target-organ damage
- History: CAD, HF, TIA/CVA, PAD, DM, renal insufficiency, sleep apnea, preeclampsia; ⊕ FHx for HTN; diet, Na intake, smoking, alcohol, prescription and OTC meds, OCP
- Physical exam: ✓ **BP in both arms;** funduscopic exam, BMI, cardiac (LVH, murmurs), vascular (bruits, radial-femoral delay), abdominal (masses or bruits), neuro exam
- Testing: K, BUN, Cr, Ca, glc, Hct, U/A, lipids, TSH, urinary albumin:creatinine (if ↑ Cr, DM, peripheral edema), ? renin, ECG (for LVH), CXR, TTE (eval for valve abnl, LVH)
- Ambulatory BP monitoring (ABPM): consider for episodic, resistant, or white coat HTN

Complications of HTN
- Neurologic: **TIA/CVA,** ruptured aneurysms, vascular dementia
- Retinopathy: stage I = arteriolar narrowing; II = copper-wiring, AV nicking; III = hemorrhages and exudates; IV = papilledema
- Cardiac: **CAD, LVH, HF, AF**
- Vascular: aortic dissection, aortic aneurysm (HTN = key risk factor for aneurysms)
- Renal: proteinuria, **renal failure**

Treatment (JAMA 2014;311:507; J Clin HTN 2014;16:14; HTN 2015;65:1372; JACC 2015;65:1998)
- Every ↓ 10 mmHg → 20% ↓ MACE, 28% ↓ HF, 13% ↓ mort. (Lancet 2016;387:957)
- Traditional goal: <140/90; if prior MI/stroke: reasonable to consider <130/80
  If high-risk (CV dis., 10-y risk of CV dis.≥15%, CKD, or ≥75 y; non-DM and no h/o stroke) SBP ~120 vs. ~135 (via unattended automated cuff) → ↓ MACE 25%, ↓ death 27%, ↓ HF 38%, but ↑ HoTN, AKI, syncope, electrolyte abnl (NEJM 2015:373:2103)
  If DM: optimal goal disputed b/c lack of clear benefit in one study (NEJM 2010;362: 1575); may consider <130/80 for renal protection if CKD & albuminuria (ASH/ISH)
  If intermed risk (RF for but w/o CV dis.), benefit only if SBP >~140 (NEJM 2016;374:2009)
  In elderly: ? more lenient targets, but benefit to Rx'ing stage 2 HTN in low-risk (NEJM 2008; 358:1887) and targeting SBP ~120 in high-risk (↓ MACE & mortality; JAMA 2016;315:2673)

- **Lifestyle modifications** (each may ↓ SBP −5 mmHg)
    weight loss: goal BMI 18.5–24.9; aerobic exercise: ≥30 min exercise/d, ≥5 d/wk
    diet: rich in fruits & vegetables, low in saturated & total fat (*DASH, NEJM 2001;344:3*)
    limit Na: ≤2.4 g/d (ideally ≤1.5 g/d); maintain K intake (*NEJM 2007;356:1966 & 2010;362:2102*)
    limit alcohol: ≤2 drinks/d in men; ≤1 drink/d in women & lighter-wt Pts; avoid NSAIDs
- **Pharmacologic options**
    Pre-HTN: ARB prevents onset of HTN, no ↓ in clinical events (*NEJM 2006;354:1685*)
    HTN: *choice of therapy controversial, concomitant disease and stage may help guide Rx*
    uncomplicated: CCB, ARB/ACEI, or thiazide (chlorthalidone preferred) are 1ˢᵗ line (*NEJM 2009;361:2153*). βB not 1ˢᵗ line (*Lancet 2005;366:1545*).
    For non-black Pts <60 y: reasonable to start w/ ARB or ACEI, then add CCB or thiazide if needed, and then add remaining class if still needed
    For black, elderly, and ? obese Pts (all of whom more likely to be salt sensitive):
    reasonable to start with CCB or thiazide, then add either the other 1ˢᵗ choice class or ARB or ACEI if needed, and then all 3 classes if still needed
    +CAD (*Circ 2015;131:e435*): ACEI or ARB (*NEJM 2008;358:1547*); ACEI+CCB superior to ACEI+thiazide (*NEJM 2008;359:2417*) or βB+diuretic (*Lancet 2005;366:895*); may require βB and/or nitrates for anginal relief; if h/o MI, βB + ACEI/ARB ± aldo antag (see "ACS")
    +HF: ACEI/ARB/ARNi, βB, diuretics, aldosterone antagonist (see "Heart Failure")
    +2° stroke prevention: ACEI ± thiazide (*NEJM 2001;358:1033*)
    +diabetes mellitus: consider ACEI or ARB; can also consider thiazide or CCB
    +chronic kidney disease: ACEI or ARB (*NEJM 1993;329:1456 & 2001;345:851 & 861*)
- Tailoring therapy: if stage 1, start w/ monoRx; if stage 2, consider starting w/ combo (eg, ACEI + CCB; *NEJM 2008;359:2417*); start at ½ max dose; after 2–3 wk, uptitrate or add drug
- Pregnancy: methyldopa, labetalol, & nifed pref. Hydral OK; avoid diuretics; ∅ ACEI/ARB. Targeting DBP 85 vs. 105 safe and ↓ severe HTN (*NEJM 2015;372:407*).

Resistant HTN (BP > goal on ≥3 drugs incl diuretic; *JAMA 2014;311:2216*)
- Exclude: 2° causes (see table) and *pseudoresistance:* inaccurate measure (cuff size), diet noncomp (↑ Na), poor Rx compliance/dosing, white coat HTN (✓ ABPM)
- Ensure effective diuresis dosing (chlorthalidone > HCTZ, loop > thiazide if eGFR <30)
- Can add aldosterone antagonist (*Lancet 2015;386:2059*), β-blocker (particularly vasodilators like labetalol, carvedilol, or nebivolol), α-blocker, or direct vasodilator

HYPERTENSIVE CRISES

- **Hypertensive emergency:** ↑ BP → acute target-organ ischemia and damage
    neurologic damage: encephalopathy, hemorrhagic or ischemic stroke, papilledema
    cardiac damage: ACS, HF/pulmonary edema, aortic dissection
    renal damage: proteinuria, hematuria, acute renal failure; scleroderma renal crisis
    microangiopathic hemolytic anemia; preeclampsia-eclampsia
- **Hypertensive urgency:** SBP >180 or DBP >120 (?110) w/ min. or ∅ target-organ damage

Precipitants
- Progression of essential HTN ± medical noncompliance (espec clonidine) or Δ in diet
- Progression of renovascular disease; acute glomerulonephritis; scleroderma; preeclampsia
- Endocrine: pheochromocytoma, Cushing's
- Sympathomimetics: cocaine, amphetamines, MAO inhibitors + foods rich in tyramine

Treatment (*Chest 2007;131:1949*)
- Tailor goals to clinical context. Treat Ao dissection aggressively. Do *not* treat HTN in acute ischemic stroke unless lysis planned or extreme BP (>220/120).
- Emergency: ↓ MAP by ~25% in mins to 2 h w/ IV agents (may need arterial line for monitoring); goal DBP <110 w/in 2–6 h, as tolerated
- Urgency: ↓ BP to ≤160/100 in hrs using PO agents; goal normal BP in ~1–2 d
- Watch UOP, Cr, mental status: may indicate a lower BP is not tolerated

Drugs for Hypertensive Crises		
IV	Nitroprusside* 0.25–10 µg/kg/min	Nitroglycerin 5–1000 µg/min
	Labetalol 20–80 mg IVB q10min or 0.5–2 mg/min. *Preferred in pregnancy.*	Esmolol 0.5 mg/kg load → 0.05–0.2 mg/min
	Fenoldopam 0.1–1.6 µg/kg/min	Hydralazine 10–20 mg q20–30min
	Nicardipine 5–15 mg/h	Clevidipine 1–16 mg/h
	Phentolamine 5–15 mg bolus q5–15min	Enalaprilat 1.25 mg
PO	Captopril 12.5–100 mg q8h	Labetalol 200–800 mg, repeat after 2–3 h
	Clonidine 0.2 mg load → 0.1 mg qh	Hydralazine 10–75 mg qid

*Metabolized to cyanide →Δ MS, lactic acidosis, death. Limit use of very high doses (8–10 µg/kg/min) to <10 min. Monitor thiocyanate levels. Hydroxocobalamin or sodium thiosulfate infusion for treatment of cyanide toxicity.

AORTIC ANEURYSMS

Definitions
- **True** aneurysm (≥50% dilation of all 3 layers of aorta) vs. **false** (rupture within adventitia)
- **Location:** root (annuloaortic ectasia), thoracic aortic aneurysm (TAA), thoracoabdominal aortic aneurysm (TAAA), abdominal aortic aneurysm (AAA)
- **Type:** fusiform (circumferential dilation) vs. saccular (localized dilation of aortic wall)

Epidemiology (Circ 2010;121:e266, 2011;124:2020; Nat Rev Cardiol 2011;8:92)
- **TAA:** ♂:♀ 2:1; ~60% root/ascending; 40% desc.
- **AAA:** ~4–8% prev in those >60y; 5× more common in ♂; mostly infrarenal

Pathophysiology & risk factors (NEJM 2009;361:1114; Nat Med 2009;15:649)
- Medial degen and/or ↑ wall stress; wall stress ∝ [(ΔP × r) / (wall thickness)] (Laplace's law)
- **TAA:** medial degeneration (muscle apoptosis, elastin fiber weakening); a/w CTD, aortitis
- **AAA:** long-standing HTN + athero/inflammation → medial weakening
- Classic **clinical risk factors:** HTN, atherosclerosis, smoking, age, ♂
- **CTD** (Marfan, Ehlers-Danlos type IV, Loeys-Dietz); **congenital** (bicuspid AoV, Turner's) **aortitis** (Takayasu's GCA, spondyloarthritis, IgG4, syphilis); trauma

Screening (Circ 2010;121:e266 & 2011;124:2020; Annals 2015;313:1156)
- **TAA:** if bicuspid AoV or 1° relative w/: (a) TAA or bicuspid AoV, (b) CTD as above
- **AAA:** ✓ for pulsatile abd mass; U/S ♂ >60 y w/ FHx of AAA & ♂ 65–75 y w/ prior tobacco

Diagnostic studies (Circ 2010;121:e266 & 2011;124:2020)
- **Contrast CT:** quick, noninvasive, high Se & Sp for all aortic aneurysms
- **TTE/TEE:** TTE most useful for root and proximal Ao; TEE can visualize other sites of TAA
- **MRI:** favored over CT for AoRoot imaging; useful in AAA but time-consuming; noncontrast "black blood" MR to assess aortic wall
- **Abdominal U/S:** screening/surveillance test of choice for infrarenal AAA

Treatment (Circ 2006;113:e463; 2008;117:1883; 2010;121:e266; NEJM 2014;371:2101)
- Goal is to prevent rupture (50% mortality prior to hospital) by modifying risk factors
- **Risk factor modification:** smoking cessation; LDL-C <70 mg/dL
- **BP control:** βB (↓ dP/dt) ↓ aneurysm growth (NEJM 1994;330:1335); **ACEI** a/w ↓ rupture risk (Lancet 2006;368:659); **ARB** may ↓ rate of aortic root growth in Marfan (NEJM 2008;358:2787)
- Mod CV exercise OK, no burst activity requiring Valsalva maneuvers (eg, heavy lifting)
- **Indications for surgery** (individualized based on FHx, body size, gender, anatomy)
  - **TAA:** sxs, ascending Ao >5.5 cm (4–5 cm if Marfan, bi-AoV, L-D, vascular EDS); size may not predict repair benefit; descending Ao >6 cm; ≥4.5 cm and planned AoV surgery
  - **AAA:** sx; infrarenal >5.5 cm; consider ≥5.0 cm in ♀; ↑ >0.5 cm/y; inflam/infxn

Endovascular repair (EVAR) (NEJM 2008;358:494; Circ 2011;124:2020 & 2015;131:1291)
- Requires favorable aortic anatomy
- **TEVAR** (thoracic EVAR) for descending TAA ≥5.5 cm may ↓ periop morbidity and possibly mortality (Circ 2010;121:2780; JACC 2010;55:986; J Thorac CV Surg 2010;140:1001 & 2012;144:604)
- **AAA:** guidelines support open repair or EVAR for infrarenal AAA in good surg candidates ↓ short-term mort., bleeding, LOS; but long-term graft complic. (3–4%/y; endoleak, need for reintervention, rupture) necessitate periodic surveillance, with no proven Δ in overall mortality in trials, except ? in those <70 y (NEJM 2010;362:1863, 1881 & 2012;367:1988)
  In observ. data, EVAR a/w ↑ early survival but ↑ long-term rupture (NEJM 2015;373:328)
  In Pts unfit for surgery or high periop risks: ↓ aneurysm-related mortality but no Δ in overall mortality over med Rx (NEJM 2010;362:1872). EVAR noninferior (? superior) to open repair in ruptured AAA w/ favorable anatomy (Ann Surg 2009;250:818).

Complications (Circ 2010;121:e266; Nat Rev Cardiol 2011;8:92)
- **Pain:** gnawing chest, back or abdominal pain; new or worse pain may signal rupture
- **Rupture:** risk ↑ w/ diameter, ♀, current smoking, HTN
  - **TAA:** ~2.5%/y if <6 cm vs. 7%/y if >6 cm
  - **AAA:** ~1%/y if <5 cm vs. 6.5%/y if 5–5.9 cm; ~80% mortality at 24 h
- **Aortic insufficiency (TAA), CHF, acute aortic syndromes** (qv)
- **Thromboembolic ischemic events** (eg, to CNS, viscera, extremities)
- **Compression of adjacent structures** (eg, SVC, trachea, esophagus, laryngeal nerve)

Follow-up (Circ 2010;121:e266; Nat Rev Cardiol 2011;8:92; JAMA 2013;309:806)
- Expansion rate ~0.1 cm/y for TAA, ~0.3–0.4 cm/y for AAA
- AAA: <4 cm q2–3 y; 4–5.4 cm q6–12 mos; more often if rate of expansion >0.5 cm in 6 mo
- TAA: 6 mo after dx to ensure stable, and if stable, then annually (Circ 2005;111:816)
- Screen for CAD, PAD and aneurysms elsewhere, espec popliteal. About 25% of Pts w/ TAA will also have AAA, and 25% of AAA Pts will have a TAA: consider pan-Ao imaging.

ACUTE AORTIC SYNDROMES

Definitions *(Circ 2010;121:e266; Eur Heart J 2012;33:26)*
- **Aortic dissection:** intimal tear → blood extravasates into Ao media (creates false lumen)
- **Intramural hematoma** (IMH): vasa vasorum rupture → medial hemorrhage that does not communicate with aortic lumen; 6% of aortic syndromes; clinically managed as AoD
- **Penetrating ulcer:** atherosclerotic plaque penetrates elastic lamina → medial hemorrhage

Classification *(proximal twice as common as distal)*
- **Proximal:** involves ascending Ao, regardless of origin (= Stanford A, DeBakey I & II)
- **Distal:** involves descending Ao only, distal to L subclavian art. (= Stanford B, DeBakey III)

Risk factors *(Lancet 2015;385:800)*
- **Classic** (in older Pts): **HTN** (h/o HTN in >70% of dissections); **age** (60s–70s), **sex** (~65% ♂); **smoking**; ↑ **lipids. Acute ↑ BP:** cocaine, Valsalva (eg, weightlifting).
- **Genetic or acquired predisposition:** *CTD* (Marfan, Loeys-Dietz, Ehlers-Danlos type IV); *congenital anomaly* (bicuspid AoV, coarct [eg, Tuner's syndrome], PCKD); *aortitis* (Takayasu's, GCA, Behçet's, syphilis, TB); *pregnancy* (typically 3rd trimester)
- **Trauma:** blunt, decel. injury (eg, MVA); IABP, cardiac or aortic surgery, cardiac cath

Clinical Manifestations and Physical Exam* *(JAMA 2000;283:897)*		
Feature	Proximal	Distal
"Aortic" pain (abrupt, severe, tearing or ripping quality, *maximal at onset* [vs. crescendo for ACS])	94% (chest, back)	98% (back, chest, abd)
Syncope (often due to tamponade)	13%	4%
HF (usually due to acute AI)	9%	3%
CVA	6%	2%
HTN	36%	70%
HoTN or shock (tamponade, AI, MI, rupture)	25%	4%
Pulse deficit (if involves carotid, subclavian, fem)	19%	9%
AI murmur	44%	12%

*S/S correlate w/ affected branch vessels & distal organs; may Δ as dissection progresses

Initial evaluation & diagnostic studies *(Circ 2010;121:e266; JACC CV Img 2014;7:406)*
- H&P, incl. bilat BP & radial pulses for symmetry; ECG w/ STE if propogates to cor
- **CXR:** abnl in 60–90% [↑ mediast. (absence ⊖ LR 0.3), L pl effusion] but *cannot* r/o AoD
- **CT:** quick and available, Se ≥93%, Sp 98%; facilitates "triple rule-out" ACS vs. PE vs. AoD
- **MRI:** Se & Sp >98%, but time-consuming test & not readily available
- **TEE:** Se >95% prox, 80% for distal; can assess cors/peric/AI; "blind spot" behind trachea
- ⊖ Initial imaging but high clinical suspicion → further studies (²/₃ w/ AoD have ≥2 studies)
- **D-dimer:** Se/NPV ~97%, Sp ~47%; ? <500 ng/mL to r/o dissec *(Circ 2009;119:2702)* but not in Pts at high clinical risk *(Annals EM 2015;66:368)*; does not r/o IMH

Treatment *(Circ 2010;121:1544; JACC 2013;61:1661; Lancet 2015;385:800)*
- ↓ **dP/dt** targeting HR <60 & central BP <120 (or lowest that preserves perfusion; r/o pseudohypotension, eg, arm BP ↓ due to subclavian dissection; use highest BP reading)
- *First IV βB* (eg, esmolol, labetalol) to blunt reflex ↑ HR & inotropy in response to vaso-dilators; verap/dilt if βB contraindic; *then* ↓ **SBP w/ IV vasodilators** (eg, nitroprusside)
- **If HoTN:** urgent surgical consult, IVF to achieve euvolemia, pressors to keep (MAP 70 mmHg); r/o complication (eg, tamponade, contained rupture, severe AI)
- **Proximal:** surgery considered in **all acute** and in chronic if c/b progression, AI or aneurysm
- **Distal:** med Rx unless complication (see below), however pre-emptive endovascular intervention may ↓ late complications, mort *(JACC 2013;61:1661; Circ Cardiovasc Int 2013;6:407)*

Complications *(occur in ~20%; Circ 2010;121:e266; Lancet 2015;385:800)*
- Freq assess (sx, BP, UOP), pulses, labs (Hct, lactic acid), imaging (~7 d or sooner if Δs)
- Uncontrolled BP or persistent pain may indicate complication/extension
- **Progression:** propagation of dissection, ↑ aneurysm size, ↑ false lumen size
- **Rupture:** pericardial sac → tamponade (avoid pericardiocentesis unless PEA); blood in pleural space, mediast., retroperitoneum; ↑ in hematoma on imaging portends rupture
- **Malperfusion** (partial or complete obstruction of branch artery) *coronary* → MI (usually RCA → IMI, since dissection often along outer Ao curvature); *innominate/carotid* → CVA, Horner; *intercostal/lumbar* → spinal cord ischemia/paraplegia; *innominate/subclavian* → upper extremity ischemia; *iliac* → lower extremity ischemia; *celiac/mesenteric* → bowel ischemia; *renal* → AKI or gradually ↑ Cr, refractory HTN
- **AI:** due to annular dilatation or disruption or displacement of leaflet by false lumen
- **Mortality:** historically ~1%/h × 48 h for acute prox AoD w/ 10–35% at 30 d
- **Long-term serial imaging** (CT or MRI; latter may be preferred due to lower cumulative radiation exposure) at 1, 3, and 6 mo, and then annually (18 mo, 30 mo, etc.)

ARRHYTHMIAS

Sinus bradycardia (SB) (NEJM 2000;342:703)
- Etiologies: **meds** (incl βB, CCB, amio, Li, dig), ↑ **vagal tone** (incl. athletes, sleep, IMI), **metabolic** (hypoxia, sepsis, myxedema, hypothermia, ↓ glc), OSA, ↑ ICP
- Treatment: if no sx, none; atropine, β₁ agonists (short-term) or pacing if symptomatic
- Most common cause of sinus pause is *blocked premature atrial beat*

Sick sinus syndrome (SSS)
- Features may include: periods of unprovoked SB, SA arrest, paroxysms of SB and atrial tachyarrhythmias ("tachy-brady" syndrome), chronotropic incompetence w/ ETT
- Treatment: meds alone usually fail (adeq. control tachy → unacceptable brady); usually need **combination of meds** (βB, CCB, dig) for tachy and **PPM** for brady

AV Block	
Type	**Features**
1°	Prolonged PR (>200 ms), all atrial impulses conducted (1:1).
2° Mobitz I (Wenckebach)	Progressive ↑ PR until impulse not conducted (→ "grouped beating"). Due to **AV node** abnl: ischemia (IMI), inflammation (myocarditis, endocarditis, MV surgery), high vagal tone (athletes), drug induced. Classically (~50%), absolute ↑ in PR *decreases* over time (→ ↓ RR intervals, duration of pause <2× preceding RR interval); nl QRS. AVB usually worsens w/ carotid sinus massage, improves w/ atropine. Often paroxysmal/nocturnal/asx, no Rx required.
2° Mobitz II	Blocked impulses w/ consistent PR interval, often prolonged QRS. Due to **His-Purkinje** abnl: ischemia (AMI), degeneration of conduction system, infiltrative disease, inflammation/AoV surgery/TAVR. AVB may improve w/ carotid sinus massage, may worsen w/ atropine. May progress to 3° AVB. Pacing pads; transven. pacing wire.
3° (complete)	No AV conduction. Escape, if present, narrow (jxnal) or wide (vent.)

Nb, if 2:1 block, cannot distinguish type I vs. II 2° AVB (no chance to observe PR prolongation); usually categorize based on other ECG & clinical data. High-grade AVB usually refers to block of ≥2 successive impulses.

AV dissociation
- *Default:* slowing of SA node allows subsidiary pacemaker (eg, AV junction) to take over
- *Usurpation:* acceleration of subsidiary pacemaker (eg, AV junctional tach, VT)
- *3° AV block:* atrial pacemaker unable to capture ventricles, subsidiary pacemaker emerges distinguish from *isorhythmic dissociation* (A ≈ V rate, some P waves nonconducting)

Temporary pacing wires
- Consider w/ bradycardia with hemodyn instability or unstable escape rhythm when perm pacer not readily available. Risks: infxn, RV perf, VT, PTX, CHB if existing LBBB, etc.
- Consider instead of PPM for sx brady from reversible cause (βB/CCB O/D, Lyme, SBE, myocarditis, s/p cardiac surgery/trauma/TAVR), TdP, acute MI (sx brady/high-grade AVB)

Arise above the ventricles, ∴ narrow QRS unless aberrant conduction or pre-excitation.

Common Etiologies of SVT (NEJM 2012;367:1438)		
	Type	**Features**
Atrial	Sinus tachycardia (ST)	Caused by pain, fever, hypovolemia, hypoxia, PE, anemia, anxiety, withdrawal, β-agonists, etc.
	Atrial tachycardia (AT)	Originate at site in atria other than SA node. Seen w/ CAD, COPD, ↑ catechols, EtOH, dig.
	Multifocal atrial tachycardia (MAT)	↑ automaticity at multiple sites in the atria; seen with underlying pulmonary disease
	Atrial flutter (AFL)	Clockwise or counterclockwise macroreentry, usually w/in right atrium
	Atrial fibrillation (AF)	Chaotic atrial activation with rapid, irregular AVN bombardment; often from pulmonary veins
AV Jxn	AV nodal reentrant tach (AVNRT)	Reentrant circuit using dual pathways w/in AVN
	Atrioventricular reciprocating tachycardia (AVRT)	Reentry using AVN & access. path. May show preexcitation (WPW) or not (concealed access. path.). Can be ortho or antidromic (see below).
	Nonparoxysmal junctional tachycardia (NPJT)	↑ jxnal automaticity. May see retro. P, AV dissoc. A/w myo/endocarditis, cardiac surg, IMI, dig.

Diagnosis of SVT Type (NEJM 2012;367:1438)

Onset	Abrupt on/off argues against sinus tachycardia
Rate	Not dx as most can range from 140–250 bpm; *but:* ST usually <150; AFL often conducts 2:1 → vent. rate 150; AVNRT & AVRT usually >150
Rhythm	Irregular → AF, AFL w/ variable block, or MAT

P wave morphology	Before QRS → ST, AT (P different from sinus), MAT (≥3 morphologies)
	After QRS & inverted in inf. leads → *retrograde atrial activation via AVN*
	  AVNRT: buried in or distort terminal portion of QRS (pseudo RSR′ in V_1)
	  AVRT: slightly after QRS (RP interval >100 ms favors AVRT vs. AVNRT)
	  NPJT: either no P wave or retrograde P wave similar to AVNRT
	Fibrillation or no P waves → AF
	Saw-toothed "F" waves (best seen in inferior leads & V_1) → AFL

Response to vagal stim. or adenosine	Slowing of HR often seen with ST, AF, AFL, AT, whereas re-entrant rhythms (AVNRT, AVRT) may abruptly terminate (classically w/ P wave after last QRS) or no response. Occ AT may terminate. In AFL & AF, ↑ AV block may unmask "F" waves or fibrillation

Figure 1-4 Approach to SVT (adapted from *NEJM* 2012;367:1438)

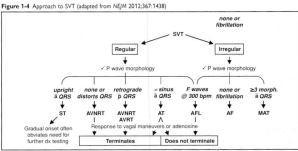

Treatment of SVT (Circ 2016;133:e506)

Rhythm	Acute treatment	Long-term treatment
Unstable	**Cardioversion** per ACLS	n/a
ST	Treat underlying stressor(s)	n/a
AT	βB, CCB or adenosine; ? amiodarone	radiofrequency ablation (RFA); βB or CCB, ± class IC/III antiarrhythmics
AVNRT or AVRT	**Vagal maneuvers** **Adenosine** (caution in AVRT*) **CCB** or βB, DCCV if other Rx fail	*For AVNRT* (see next section for AVRT): **RFA.** CCB, βB, or dig (chronic or prn) ± Class IC/III antiarrhythmics (if nl heart)
NPJT	**CCB, βB,** amiodarone	Rx underlying dis. (eg, dig tox, ischemia)
AF	**βB, CCB,** digoxin, **AAD**	See "Atrial Fibrillation"
AFL	**βB, CCB,** digoxin, **AAD**	RFA; βB or CCB ± class III antiarrhyth.
MAT	CCB or βB if tolerated	Treat underlying disease. CCB or βB. AVN ablation + PPM if refractory to meds

*Avoid adenosine & nodal agents if accessory pathway + pre-excited tachycardia, use below (*JACC* 2003;42:1493)

- *Catheter ablation:* high overall success rate (AFL/AVNRT ~95%, AVRT ~90%, AF ~80%) complications: stroke, MI, bleeding, perforation, conduction block (*JAMA* 2007;290:2768)

ACCESSORY PATHWAYS (WOLFF-PARKINSON-WHITE)

Definitions
- **Accessory pathway** (bypass tract) of conducting myocardium connect-ing atria & ventricles, allowing impulses to bypass normal AVN delay
- **Preexcitation (WPW) pattern:** ↓ PR interval, ↑ QRS width w/ δ wave (slurred onset, *can be subtle*). ST & Tw abnl (can mimic old IMI).
  only seen w/ pathways that conduct antegrade (if pathway only conducts retrograde, then ECG will be normal during SR; "concealed" bypass tract)
  PAC can exaggerate pre-excitation if AV node conduction slowed
- **WPW syndrome:** WPW accessory pathway + paroxysmal tachycardia

Classic tachycardias of WPW accessory pathways
- **Orthodromic AVRT:** narrow-complex SVT (typically), conducting ↓ AVN & ↑ accessory pathway; requires retrograde conduction and ∴ can occur w/ concealed bypass tracts
- **Antidromic AVRT** (rare): wide-complex SVT, conducting ↓ accessory pathway & ↑ AVN; requires antegrade conduction and ∴ should see pre-excitation pattern during SR
- **AF** w/ rapid conduction down accessory pathway ∴ wide-complex irregular SVT; requires antegrade conduction; ∴ should see pre-excitation in SR. Rarely can degenerate into VF.

Treatment (Heart Rhythm 2012;9:1006; Circ 2016;133:e506)
- **AVRT** (orthodromic): vagal, βB, CCB; care w/ adenosine (can precip AF); have defib ready
- **AF/AFL** w/ conduction down accessory pathway: need to Rx arrhythmia and ↑ pathway refractoriness. Use **procainamide, ibutilide,** or DCCV; **avoid** CCB, βB, amio, dig, & adenosine, as can ↑ refractoriness of pathway → ↑ vent. rate → VF (Circ 2016;133:e506).
- **Long term:** RFA if sx; if not candidate for RFA, then antiarrhythmics (IA, III) or CCB/βB. consider RFA if asx but AVRT or AF inducible on EPS (NEJM 2003;349:1803) or if rapid conduction possible (✓ w/ EPS if pre-excitation persists during exercise testing) risk of SCD related to how short RR interval is in AF (eg, ≤250ms) and if SVT inducible

WIDE-COMPLEX TACHYCARDIAS (WCTs)

Etiologies (Lancet 2012;380:1520)
- **Ventricular tachycardia (VT):** accounts for 80% of WCT in unselected population
- **SVT conducted with aberrancy:** either fixed BBB, rate-dependent BBB (usually RBBB), conduction via an accessory pathway or atrially triggered ventricular pacing

Monomorphic ventricular tachycardia (MMVT)
- All beats look similar; predominantly upward in V_1 = RBBB-type vs. downward = LBBB-type
- In structurally abnormal heart: **prior MI** (scar); **CMP; myocarditis; arrhythmogenic RV CMP (ARVC):** incomplete RBBB, ε wave (terminal notch in QRS) & TWI in V_1–V_3 on resting ECG, LBBB-type VT, dx w/ MRI (Lancet 2009;373:1289)
- In structurally normal heart (w/ normal resting ECG):
  RVOT VT: LBBB-type VT w/ inferior axis; typically ablate
  idiopathic LV VT: RBBB-type VT w/ superior axis; responds to verapamil

V_2 — Epsilon

Polymorphic ventricular tachycardia (PMVT)
- QRS morphology changes from beat to beat
- Etiologies: **ischemia; CMP;** catecholaminergic;
  torsades de pointes (TdP = "twisting of the points," PMVT + ↑ QT):↑ QT **acquired** (meds, lytes, stroke, see "ECG") w/ risk ↑ w/ ↓ HR, freq PVCs (pause dependent) or **congenital** (K/Na channelopathies) w/ resting Tw abnl & TdP triggered by sympathetic stimulation (eg, exercise, emotion, sudden loud noises) (Lancet 2008;372:750).
  Brugada syndrome (Na channelopathy): ♂ > ♀; pseudo-RBBB w/ STE in V_1–V_3 (provoked w/ class IA or IC) on resting ECG

V_1

Diagnostic clues that favor VT (assume until proven o/w)
- **Prior MI, CHF** or **LV dysfunction** best predictors that WCT is VT (Am J Med 1998;84:53)
- Hemodynamics and rate do not reliably distinguish VT from SVT
- MMVT is regular, but initially it may be slightly irregular, mimicking AF w/ aberrancy; grossly irregularly irregular rhythm suggests AF w/ aberrancy or pre-excitation
- ECG features that favor VT (Circ 1991;83:1649)
  AV dissociation (independent P waves, capture or fusion beats) proves VT
  very wide QRS (>140 ms in RBBB-type or >160 in LBBB-type); extreme axis deviation
  QRS morphology atypical for BBB
  RBBB-type: absence of tall R' (or presence of monophasic R) in V_1, r/S ratio <1 in V_6
  LBBB-type: onset to nadir >60–100 ms in V_1, q wave in V_6
  concordance (QRS in all precordial leads w/ same pattern/direction)

Long-term management (JACC 2006;48:1064; EHJ 2015;36:2793; Circ 2016;133:1715)
- Workup: **echo** to ✓ LV fxn, **cath** or **stress test** to r/o ischemia, ? MRI and/or RV bx to look for infiltrative CMP or ARVC, ? **EP study** to assess inducibility
- **ICD:** 2° prevention after documented VT/VF arrest (unless due to reversible cause). 1° prev. if high risk, eg, EF <30–35%, ARVC, Brugada, certain LQTS, severe HCMP. See "Cardiac Rhythm Mgmt Devices." Wearable vest if reversible etiology or waiting for ICD? Antitachycardia pacing (ATP = burst pacing faster than VT) can terminate VT w/o shock
- **Meds:** βB, verapamil if idiopathic LV VT, or AAD (eg, amio, mexiletine) to suppress VT
- If med a/w TdP → QT >500 ± VPBs: d/c med, replete K, give Mg, ± pacing (JACC 2010;55:934)
- **RFA** if isolated VT focus or if recurrent VT triggering ICD firing (↓ VT storm by 34%; NEJM 2016;375:111); ablation before ICD implantation ↓ discharge rate by 40% (Lancet 2010;375:31)

Classification (*Circ* 2014;130:e199)
- **Paroxysmal** (self-terminating, usually <48 h, often triggered in pulm veins) vs. **persistent** (>7 d) vs. **long-standing persistent** (>1 y) vs. **permanent** (no plan for SR)
- **Nonvalvular** (AF absent rheumatic MS, prosthetic valve, or mitral valve repair) vs. **valvular**

Epidemiology and etiologies (*Circ* 2011;124:1982)
- 1–2% of pop. has AF (10% of those age ≥80); M > F; lifetime risk ~25%
- Acute (up to 50% w/o identifiable cause)
    Cardiac: HF, new CMP, myo/pericarditis, ischemia/MI, HTN crisis, valve dis., cardiac surg
    Pulmonary: acute pulmonary disease or hypoxemia (eg, COPD flare, PNA), PE, OSA
    Metabolic: high catecholamine states (stress, infection, postop, pheo), thyrotoxicosis
    Drugs: alcohol ("holiday heart"), cocaine, amphetamines, theophylline, caffeine, smoking
    Neurogenic: subarachnoid hemorrhage, ischemic stroke
- Chronic: ↑ age, HTN, ischemia, valve dis. (MV, TV, AoV), CMP, hyperthyroidism, obesity

Evaluation
- H&P, ECG, CXR, TTE (LA size, thrombus, valves, LV fxn, pericardium), K, Mg, Cr, FOBT before anticoag, TFTs; r/o MI not necessary unless other ischemic sx

Figure 1-5 Approach to acute AF (Adapted from *Circ* 2014;130:e199)

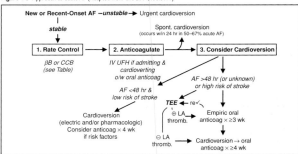

Rate Control (if sx, goal HR <80; if asx & EF >40%, goal HR <110; *Lancet* 2016;388:818)			
Agent	**Acute (IV)**	**Maint. (PO)**	**Comments**
CCB Verapamil	5–10 mg over 2′ may repeat in 30′	120–360 mg/d in divided doses	↓ BP (Rx w/ Ca gluc) Can worsen HF
CCB Diltiazem	0.25 mg/kg over 2′ may repeat after 15′ 5–15 mg/h infusion	120–360 mg/d in divided doses	Preferred if severe COPD Can ↑ dig levels
βB Metoprolol	2.5–5 mg over 2′ may repeat q5′ × 3	25–100 mg bid or tid	↓ BP (Rx w/ glucagon) Preferred if CAD Risks: HF & bronchospas.
Digoxin* (onset >30 min)	0.25 mg q2h up to 1.5 mg/24 h	0.125–0.375 mg qd (adj for CrCl)	Consider in HF or low BP Poor exertional HR ctrl
Amiodarone	300 mg over 1 h → then 10–50 mg/h × 24 h		

Circ 2014;130:e199. IV βB, CCB & dig **contraindicated** if evidence of WPW (ie, pre-excitation or WCT) since may facilitate conduction down accessory pathway leading to VF; ∴ use procainamide, ibutilide or amio.
*Many meds incl. amio, verapamil, quinidine, propafenone, macrolides & azole antifungals ↑ digoxin levels.

Cardioversion
- Consider if: 1st AF, sx, tachycardia-mediated CMP, or difficult to rate control
    if AF >48 h 2–5% risk stroke w/ cardioversion (*pharmacologic or electric*)
    ∴ either TEE to r/o thrombus or ensure therapeutic anticoagulation for ≥3 wk prior if needs to cardiovert urgently, often anticoagulate acutely (eg, IV UFH)
- Likelihood of success ∝ AF duration & atrial size; control precipitants (eg, vol status, thyroid)
- Before electrical cardiovert, consider pre-Rx w/ AAD (eg, ibutilide), esp. if 1st cardiovert failed
- For pharmacologic cardioversion, class III and IC drugs have best proven efficacy
- If SR returns (spont. or w/ Rx), atria may be *mech. stunned;* also, high risk of recurrent AF over next 3 mo. ∴ **Anticoag postcardioversion ≥4 wk** (? unless AF <48 h and low risk).

Rhythm control (Lancet 2016;388:829)
- No ↓ mortality or stroke vs rate control (NEJM 2002;347:1825; 2008;358:2667 & 2016;374:1911)
- Consider if sx w/ rate control (eg, HF), difficult to control rate, or tachycardia-mediated CMP

Antiarrhythmic Drugs (AAD) for AF (EHJ 2012;33:2719; Circ 2014;130:e199)			
Agent	**Conversion**	**Maintenance**	**Comments**
III Amiodarone	5–7 mg/kg IV over 30–60' → 1 mg/min, 10-g load	200–400 mg qd (most effective AAD for SR)	↑ QT, TdP rare. Often delay to convert. Poss. pulm, liver, thyroid tox. ↑ INR w/ warfarin.
III Dronedarone	n/a	400 mg bid	↓ side effects & effic. vs. amio; ∅ if perm AF or ↓ EF; liver tox
III Ibutilide	1 mg IV over 10' may repeat × 1	n/a	Contraindic. if ↓ K or ↑ QT (3–8% risk of TdP): give w/ IV Mg
III Dofetilide	500 mcg PO bid	500 mcg bid	↑ QT, ↑ risk of TdP; renal adj
III Sotalol	n/a	80–160 mg bid	✓ for ↓ HR, ↑ QT; renal adj
IC Flecainide	300 mg PO × 1	100–150 mg qd	PreRx w/ AVN blocker. ø if structural/ischemic heart dis.
IC Propafenone	600 mg PO × 1	150–300 mg tid	
IA Procainamide	10–15 mg/kg IV over 1 h	n/a	↓ BP; ↑ QT ± PreRx w/ AVN blocker
**Underlying disease & maintenance AAD of choice:** _None or minimal (incl HTN w/o LVH):_ class IC ("pill in pocket"), sotalol, dronedarone; **HTN w/ LVH:** amio; **CAD:** sotalol, dofetilide, amio, dronedarone; **HF:** amio, dofetilide			

Nonpharmacologic therapy
- Ablation (pulm vein isolation; radiofreq or cryo): ~80% success; no need to interrupt anticoag. If w/o ↑↑ LA or ↓ EF, superior to AAD. (NEJM 2016;374:2235; JAMA 2014;311:692)
- Surgical "maze" procedure (70–95% success) if undergoing cardiac surgery
- AV node ablation + PPM if other Rx inadequate (NEJM 2001;344:1043; 2002;346:2062)

Oral anticoagulation (Circ 2014;130:e199; JAMA 2015;313:1950; EHRA Practical Guide EHJ 2016:epub)
- _All valvular AF_ (ie, rheum MS, valve prosthesis or repair), as stroke risk very high
- Nonvalvular AF (NVAF): stroke risk ~4.5%/y
- **CHA₂DS₂-VASc** to guide Rx: **C**HF (1); **H**TN (1); **A**ge ≥75 y (2); **D**M (1), **S**troke/TIA (2); **V**ascular disease (eg, MI, PAD, Ao plaque) (1); **A**ge 65–74 (1); ♀ **S**ex **c**ategory (1)
  annual risk of stroke (Lancet 2012;379:648): at low end, ~1% per point: 0 → ~0%, 1 → 1.3%, 2 → 2.2%, 3 → 3.2%, 4 → 4.0%; at higher scores, risk ↑↑ (5 → 6.7%, ≥6 → 9.0%)
  score ≥2 → anticoagulate; score 1 → consider anticoag. or ASA (? latter reasonable if risk factor 65–74 y, vasc dz or ♀) or no Rx; **score 0** → reasonable to not Rx
- **Rx options:** NOAC (NVAF only) or warfarin (INR 2–3); if Pt refuses anticoag, ASA + clopi or, even less effective, ASA alone (NEJM 2009;360:2066)
- AF w/ CAD/ PCI: can combine anticoag + clopi, omit ASA (Lancet 2013;381:1107)
- Periop rate of arterial embolization in NVAF <0.5%; no benefit to bridging anticoag w/ LMWH & ↑ bleeding c/w stopping warfarin 5 d preop (NEJM 2015;373:823)

Non-vit K antag Oral Anticoag (NOACs) for NVAF (Lancet 2014;383:955)		
Anticoag	**Dosing**	**Efficacy & safety vs warfarin**
Dabigatran (Direct thromb inhib)	150 mg bid (110 not avail in U.S.) (75 mg bid if CrCl 15–30)	150 mg: ↓ ischemic stroke & ICH, but ↑ GIB 110 mg: ≈ ischemic stroke & ↓ major bleed/ICH Risks: GI side effects, ↑ MI c/w warfarin
Rivaroxaban (FXa inhib)	20 mg qd (15 mg qd if CrCl 15–50) w/ pm meal	≈ ischemic stroke & major bleeds, but ↓ fatal bleed incl ICH
Apixaban (FXa inhib)	5 mg bid (2.5 mg bid if ≥2 of: ≥80 y, ≤60 kg, Cr ≥1.5 mg/dL)	≈ ischemic stroke & ↓ major bleed incl ICH, 11% ↓ death. In Pts felt not cand for warfarin, apixa 55% ↓ stroke w/o ↑ bleed vs ASA alone.
Edoxaban (FXa inhib)	60 mg qd if CrCl 51–95 (30 mg if CrCl 15–50)	≈ ischemic stroke & ↓ major bleed incl ICH, 14% ↓ CV death. ↑ ischemic CVA if CrCl >95.
No monitoring required. Onset w/in hrs; 1 missed dose may ↓ protection. Specific reversal agents: idarucizumab for dabigatran; adnexanet for FXa (NEJM 2015;373:511 & 373:2413).		

Nonpharmacologic stroke prevent (JACC 2015;66:1497)
- Perc left atrial appendage (LAA) occlusion (Watchman) noninf to anticoag (JACC 2015;65:2614)
- Epicardial snare to ligate LAA. High rate of initial tech success (JACC 2013;62:108).
- Surgical LAA resection reasonable if another indication for cardiac surgery

Atrial flutter
- Macroreentrant atrial loop (typical: counterclockwise w/ flutter waves ⊖ in inf leads)
- Risk of stroke similar to that of AF, ∴ anticoagulate same as would for AF
- Ablation of cavotricuspid isthmus has 95% success rate for typical AFL

Definition
- Symptom of sudden transient loss of consciousness due to global cerebral hypoperfusion
- If CPR or cardioversion required, then SCD and not syncope (different prognosis)
- Presyncope = prodrome of light-headedness without LOC

Etiologies (NEJM 2002;347:878; JACC 2006;47:473; Eur Heart J 2009;30:2631)
- **Neurocardiogenic** (a.k.a. vasovagal, ~25%; NEJM 2005;352:1004): ↑ sympathetic tone → vigorous contraction of LV → mechanoreceptors in LV trigger ↑ vagal tone (hyperactive Bezold-Jarisch reflex) → ↓ HR (cardioinhibitory) and/or ↓ BP (vasodepressor). Cough, deglutition, defecation, & micturition → ↑ vagal tone and thus can be precipitants. Carotid sinus hypersensitivity (exag vagal resp to carotid massage) is related disorder.
- **Orthostatic hypotension** (~10%)
  hypovolemia/diuretics, deconditioning; vasodilat. (esp. if combined w/ ⊖ chronotropes)
  autonomic neuropathy [1° = Parkinson's, MSA/Shy-Drager, Lewy body dementia, POTS (dysautonomia in the young); 2° = DM, EtOH, amyloidosis, CKD] (NEJM 2008;358:615)
- **Cardiovascular** (~20%, more likely in men than women)
  Arrhythmia (15%): challenging to dx as often transient
    Bradyarrhythmias: SSS, high-grade AV block, ⊖ chronotropes, PPM malfunction
    Tachyarrhythmias: VT, SVT (syncope rare unless structural heart disease or WPW)
  Mechanical (5%)
    Endocardial/Valvular: AS, MS, PS, prosthetic valve thrombosis, myxoma
    Myocardial: pump dysfxn from MI or outflow obstruction from HCMP (but usually VT)
    Pericardial: tamponade; Vascular: PE, PHT, AoD, ruptured AAA, subclavian steal
- **Neurologic** (~10%): vertebrobasil insuff, cerebrovasc dissection, SAH, TIA/CVA, migraine
- Misc. causes of LOC (but not syncope): seizure, ↓ glc, hypoxia, narcolepsy, psychogenic

Workup (etiology cannot be determined in ~40% of cases)
- H&P incl. orthostatic VS have highest yield and most cost effective (Archives 2009;169:1299)
- **History** (from Pt and witnesses if available)
  activity and posture before the incident
  precipitating factors: exertion (AS, HCMP, PHT), positional Δ (orthostatic hypotension), stressors such as sight of blood, pain, emotional distress, fatigue, prolonged standing, warm environment, N/V, cough/micturition/defecation/swallowing (neurocardiogenic), head turning or shaving (carotid sinus hypersens.); arm exercise (subclavian steal)
  prodrome (eg, diaphoresis, nausea, blurry vision): cardiac <~5 sec, vasovagal >~5 sec
  associated sx: chest pain, palp., neurologic, postictal, bowel or bladder incontinence (convulsive activity for <10 sec may occur w/ transient cerebral HoTN & mimic seizure)
- **PMH:** prior syncope, previous cardiac or neurologic dis.; no CV disease at baseline → 5% cardiac, 25% vasovagal; CV disease → 20% cardiac, 10% vasovagal (NEJM 2002;347:878)
- **Medications that may act as precipitants**
  vasodilators: α-blockers, nitrates, ACEI/ARB, CCB, hydralazine, phenothiazines, antidep.
  diuretics; ⊖ chronotropes (eg, βB and CCB)
  proarrhythmic or QT prolonging: class IA, IC or III antiarrhythmics (see "ECG")
  psychoactive drugs: antipsychotics, TCA, barbiturates, benzodiazepines, EtOH
- **Family history:** CMP, SCD, syncope (vasovagal may have genetic component)
- **Physical exam**
  VS including **orthostatics** (⊕ if supine → standing results in >20 mmHg ↓ SBP, >10 mmHg ↓ DBP, or >10–20 bpm ↑ HR), BP in both arms
  cardiac: HF (↑ JVP, displ. PMI, S₃), murmurs, LVH (S₄, LV heave), PHT (RV heave, ↑ P₂)
  vascular: ✓ for asymmetric pulses, carotid/vert/subclavian bruits; carotid sinus massage to ✓ for carotid hypersens (if no bruits): ⊕ if asystole >3 sec or ↓ SBP >50 mmHg
  neurologic exam: focal findings, evidence of tongue biting; FOBT
- **ECG** (abnormal in ~50%, but only definitively identifies cause of syncope in <10%)
  Conduction: SB, sinus pauses/sinus arrhythmia, AVB, BBB/IVCD
  Arrhythmia: ectopy, ↑ or ↓ QT, preexcitation (WPW), Brugada, ε wave (ARVC), SVT/VT
  Ischemic changes (new or old): atrial or ventricular hypertrophy
- Lab: glc, Hb, preg test (child-bearing age ♀), ? D-dimer, ? troponin (low yield w/o other s/s)

Other diagnostic studies (consider based on results of H&P and ECG)
- Ambulatory ECG monitoring: if suspect arrhythmogenic syncope
  Holter monitoring (continuous ECG 24–48 h): useful if *frequent* events
    arrhythmia + sx (4%); asx but signif. arrhythmia (13%); sx but no arrhythmia (17%)
  Event recorder (activated by Pt to record rhythm strip): limited role in syncope as only useful if established prodrome (because must be Pt activated)

External loop recorders (continuously saves rhythm, ∴ can be activated *after* an event): useful for episodes (including w/o prodrome) likely to occur w/in 1 mo; can be coupled w/ mobile cardiac telemetry than can be auto-triggered for specific rhythms

Implantable loop recorders (inserted SC; can record >1 y): useful if episodes <1/mo; dx in 55% of cases (*Circ* 2001;104:46); recommended for recurrent syncope w/o prodrome
- Echo: consider to r/o structural heart disease (eg, CMP [incl HCMP & ARVC], valvular disease [incl AS, MS, MVP], myxoma, amyloid, PHT, ± anomalous coronaries)
- ETT/CCTA/Cath: esp. w/ exertional syncope; r/o ischemia or catechol-induced arrhythmia
- Electrophysiologic studies (EPS): consider in high-risk Pts in whom tachy or brady etiology is strongly suspected, but cannot be confirmed;
  50% (inducible VT, conduction abnormalities) if heart disease, but ? significance 3–20% abnl if abnl ECG; <1% abnl if normal heart and normal ECG (*Annals* 1997;127:76)
- ? Tilt table testing: debated utility due to poor Se/Sp/reproducibility; consider only if vasovagal dx suspected but cannot be confirmed by hx
- Cardiac MRI: helpful to dx ARVC if suggestive ECG, echo (RV dysfxn) or ⊕ FHx of SCD
- Neurologic studies (cerebrovascular studies, CT, MRI, EEG): if H&P suggestive; low yield

Figure 1-6 Approach to syncope

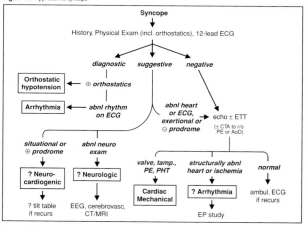

(Adapted from *JACC* 2006;47:473)

High-risk features (usually admit w/ telemetry & testing; *J Emerg Med* 2012:42:345)
- Age >60 y, h/o CAD, HF/CMP, valvular or congenital heart dis., arrhythmias, FHx SCD
- Syncope c/w cardiac cause (lack of prodrome, exertional, resultant trauma) or recurrent
- Complaint of chest pain or dyspnea; abnl VS, cardiac, pulm, or neuro exam
- ECG suggesting conduction abnormality, arrhythmia, or ischemia; Pt w/ PPM/ICD

Treatment
- Arrhythmia, cardiac mechanical or neurologic syncope: treat underlying disorder
- Vasovagal syncope: ? benefit of fludrocortisone, midodrine or SSRI (*Int J Cardiol* 2013;167:1906; *JACC* 2016;68:1); no proven benefit for disopyramide or βB (*Circ* 2006;113:1164)
  ? 16 oz of H₂O before at-risk situations (*Circ* 2003;108:2660)
  ? benefit w/ PPM if ≥3 episodes/2y & loop recorder w/ asystole >3 sec (*Circ* 2012;125:2566); PPM likely ineffective if positive tilt-test and no arrhythmia (*EHJ* 2014;35:2211)
- If orthostatic: vol replete (eg, 500 mL PO a.m.); if chronic → rise from supine to standing *slowly*, stockings, midodrine, ? atomoxetine (*HTN* 2014;64:1235), fludrocort, ↑ Na diet

Prognosis (*Ann Emerg Med* 1997;29:459; *NEJM* 2002;347:878)
- 22% overall recurrence rate if idiopathic, else 3% recurrence
- Cardiac syncope: 2-fold ↑ in mort., 20–40% 1-y SCD rate, median survival ~6 y
- Unexplained syncope w/ 1.3-fold ↑ in mort., but noncardiac or unexplained syncope w/ nl ECG, no h/o VT, no HF, age <45 → low recurrence rate and <5% 1-y SCD rate
- Vasovagal syncope: Pts not at increased risk for death, MI, or stroke
- ✓ state driving laws and MD reporting requirements. Consider appropriateness of Pt involvement in exercise/sport, operating machinery, high-risk occupation (eg, pilot).

CARDIAC RHYTHM MANAGEMENT DEVICES

Pacemaker Code

A, atrial; V, vent; O, none; I, inhibition; D, dual; R, rate-adaptive	1st letter	2nd letter	3rd letter	4th letter
	Chamber paced	Chamber sensed	Response to sensed beat	Program features

Common Pacing Modes

VVI	Ventricular pacing on demand w/ single lead in RV. Sensed ventricular beat inhibits V pacing. Used in chronic AF with symptomatic bradycardia.
DDD	A & V sensing/pacing (RA & RV leads). Native A beat inhib A pacing & *triggers V pacing* → tracking of intrinsic atrial activity. Maintains AV synchrony, ↓ AF.
Mode Switch	In atrial tachyarrhythmia (eg, AF), PPM Δs from DDD to nontracking mode (eg, VVI). Prevents PPM from pacing at max V rate in response to rapid atrial rate.
Magnet over generator	PPM: fixed rate pacing (VOO/DOO). ICD: no shock, pacing preserved. Indic: ✓ capture; surgery; inapprop PPM inhib/ICD shock, PM-mediated tachy
Leadless intracardiac PPM with emerging indications (NEJM 2015;373:1125 & 2016;374:53)

Indications for Permanent Pacing (Circ 2008;117:350 & 2012;126:1784)

AV block	3° or type II 2° AVB a/w sx or w/ either HR <40 or asystole ≥3 sec (≥5 if in AF) while awake; ? asx 3° or type II 2° AVB; bifasc or alter. L & R BBB
Sinus node	SB, pauses (SSS), chronotrop incompet a/w sx or ? if sx w/o clear assoc
Tachy-arrhythmia	AF w/ SSS; sx recurrent SVT term. by pacing after failing drugs/ablation; Sustained pause-dependent VT; ? high-risk congenital long QT
Syncope	Carotid sinus hypersensitivity with asystole >3 sec ? Neurocardiogenic syncope w/ prominent cardioinhib. response ? Syncope with bi- or trifascicular block and not likely 2° to other causes

Pacemaker Complications

Issue	Manifestation	Description & etiologies
Perforation	Effusion/tamp/pain	Typically acute, consider if HoTN
Failure to pace	Bradycardia	↓ Battery, lead fx/dislodgment, ↑ pacing threshold due to tissue rxn/injury; oversense → inapprop inhib
Failure to sense	Inapprop. pacing	Lead dislodgment or sensing threshold too high
PM-mediated tachycardia	WCT at device upper rate	Seen w/ DDD. V → A retrograde conduction; sensed by A lead → triggers V pacing → etc.
PM syndrome	Palpit, HF	Seen w/ VVI, due to loss of AV synchrony

Cardiac resynch therapy (CRT)/Biventricular (BiV) pacing (JACC 2013;61:e6)
- 3-lead pacemaker (RA, RV, coronary sinus to LV); R > S in V1 suggests approp LV capture
- Synchronize & enhance LV fxn (↑ CO, ↓ adverse remodeling)
- **Indications:** LVEF ≤35% + NYHA II–IV despite med Rx + SR + LBBB ≥150 (? ≥120) ms; mort. benefit w/ CRT-D only if LBBB (& QRS ≥130ms) (NEJM 2014;370:1694) ? benefit in NYHA I–III, EF ≤50% w/ PPM indication for AVB (NEJM 2013;368:1585) consider in AF: need rate control or AVN ablation; more pacing → greater CRT effect
- **Benefits:** ↓ HF sx, ↓ HF hosp., ↑ survival (NEJM 2005;352:1539 & 2010;363:2385)

Implantable cardiac defibrillator (ICD) (JACC 2013;61:e6; Circ 2015;132:1613)
- RV lead: defib & pacing (± antitachycardia pacing [ATP] = burst pacing ↑ ↑ VT rate to stop VT); ± RA lead for dual chamber PPM. Wearable defib & subcut-ICD, but ∅ pace/ATP.
- **Pt selection** (NEJM 2004;350:2151 & 351:2481; 2005;352:225; 2009;361:1427; Circ 2012;126:1784)
  2° prevention: survivors of VF arrest, unstable VT w/o reversible cause; structural heart disease & spontaneous sustained VT (even if asx)
  1° prevention: LVEF ≤30% & post-MI *or* LVEF ≤35% & NYHA II–III (wait: ≥40 d if post-MI, ≥90 d for NICMP) *or* LVEF ≤40% & inducible VT/VF; *life expectancy must be > 1 y*; consider if unexplained syncope + DCM, or if HCM, ARVC, Brugada, sarcoid, LQTS, Chagas or congenital heart disease if at risk for SCD; ? wearable vest as bridge to ICD
- **Risks:** inapprop shock in ~15–20% at 3 y (commonly d/t misclassified SVT); infxn; lead fx
- **ICD discharge:** ✓ device to see if approp; r/o ischemia; 6-mo driving ban (✓ state law); if recurrent VT, ? drug Rx (eg, amio + βB; NEJM 2006;295:165) or VT ablation (NEJM 2007;357:2657); ablation at time of ICD ↓ risk of VT by 40% (Lancet 2010;375:31)

Device infection (Circ 2010;121:458; JAMA 2012;307:1727; NEJM 2012;367:842)
- Presents as *pocket infection* (warmth, erythema, tenderness) and/or *sepsis w/ bacteremia*
- Incidence ~2% over 5 y; if *S. aureus* bacteremia, infxn in ≥35%
- TTE/TEE used to help visualize complic. (eg, vegetation), but even ⊖ TEE does not r/o
- Rx: abx; system removal if pocket infxn or GPC bacteremia; ∅ routine abx prior to inv. proc.

Goal: characterize risk of Pt & procedure → appropriate testing (ie, results will Δ management) and interventions (ie, reasonable probability of ↓ risk of MACE)

Preoperative evaluation (NEJM 2015;373:2258)

Figure 1-7 Approach to preop CV eval for non-CV surgery (modified from Circ 2014;130:e278)

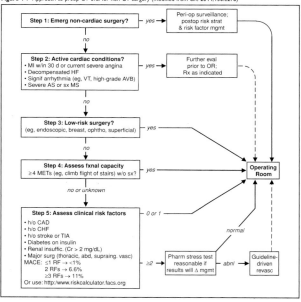

Noninvasive Testing Result		
High risk	**Intermediate risk**	**Low risk**
Ischemia at <4 METs manifested by ≥1 of:	*Ischemia at 4–6 METs* manifested by ≥1 of:	*No ischemia or at >7 METs w/*
• Horiz/down ST ↓ ≥1 mm or STE	• Horiz/down ST ↓ ≥1 mm	• ST ↓ ≥1 mm or
• ≥5 abnl leads or ischemic ECG Δs lasting >3 min after exertion	• 3–4 abnl leads	• 1–2 abnl leads
• SBP ↓ 10 mmHg or typical angina	• 1–3 min after exertion	

Additional preoperative testing (Circ 2014;130:e278)
- ECG if known cardiac disease and possibly reasonable in all, except if low-risk surgery
- TTE if any of following & prior TTE >12 mo ago or prior to Δ in sx: dyspnea of unknown origin; hx of HF w/ ↑ dyspnea; suspect (eg, murmur) or known ≥ moderate valvular dis.

Coronary artery disease
- If possible, wait ~60 d after MI in the absence of revascularization before elective surgery
- Coronary revasc guided by standard indications. Has not been shown to Δ risk of death or postop MI when done prior to elective vasc. surgery (NEJM 2004;351:2795).

Heart failure (JACC 2014;64:e77)
- Decompensated HF should be optimally Rx'd prior to elective surgery
- 30-d CV event rate: symptomatic HF > asx HFrEF > asx HFpEF > no HF

Valvular heart disease
- If meet criteria for valve intervention, do so before elective surgery (postpone if necessary)
- If severe valve disease and surgery urgent, intra- & postoperative hemodynamic monitoring reasonable (espec for AS, since at ↑ risk even if sx not severe; be careful to maintain preload, avoid hypotension, and watch for atrial fibrillation)

- If severe symptomatic AS and surg AVR not an option, balloon aortic valvuloplasty (BAV) or transcatheter aortic valve replacement (TAVR) can be considered (JACC 2014;64:e77)

Cardiac implantable electronic devices
- Discuss w/ surgical team need for device (eg, complete heart block) & consequences if interference w/ fxn, and likelihood of electromagnetic interference
- Consider reprogramming, magnet use, etc. as needed

Pre- & perioperative pharmacologic management
- **ASA:** continue in Pts w/ existing indication. Initiation prior to surgery does not ↓ 30-d ischemic events and ↑ bleeding (NEJM 2014;370:1494), but Pts w/ recent stents excluded.
- **Dual antiplatelet therapy:** delay elective surg 14 d after balloon angioplasty, 30 d after BMS and ideally 6 mos (min 3 mos) after DES implantation (2016 ACC/AHA Update) unless risk of bleeding > risk of stent thrombosis or ACS. If must discontinue $P2Y_{12}$ inhibitor, continue ASA and restart $P2Y_{12}$ inhibitor ASAP.
- **β-blockers** (Circ 2009;120:2123; JAMA 2010;303:551; Am J Med 2012;125:953)
    Continue βB in Pts on them chronically. Do not stop βB abruptly postop (may cause reflex sympathetic activation). Use IV if Pt unable to take PO.
    In terms of initiating, conflicting evidence; may depend on how done. Some studies show ↓ death/MI, another ↓ MI, but ↑ death & stroke and ↑ brady/HoTN (Lancet 2008;371;1839).
    Reasonable to initiate if intermed- or high-risk ⊕ stress test, or RCRI ≥3, espec if vasc surgery. Initiate ≥1 wk prior to surgery (not day of), use low-dose, short-acting βB, and titrate to achieve HR and BP goal (? HR ~55–65). Avoid bradycardia and HoTN.
- **Statins:** ↓ ischemia & CV events in Pts undergoing vascular surg (NEJM 2009;361:980). Consider if risk factors & non–low-risk surgery and in all Pts undergoing vascular surgery.
- ACEI/ARB: may cause HoTN if held before surgery, restart ASAP.
- Amiodarone: ↓ incidence of postop AF if started prior to surgery (Circ 1997;337:1785)

Postoperative monitoring
- ECG if known CAD or high-risk surgery. Consider if >1 risk factor for CAD.
- Routine troponin prognostic (JAMA 2012;307:2295) but ✓ only if sx/ECG Δs suggestive of ACS

PERIPHERAL ARTERY DISEASE (PAD)

Clinical features (NEJM 2016;374:861)
- Prev. ↑ w/ age: <1% if <40 y, ~15% if ≥70 y; risk factors incl. **smoking, DM,** HTN, chol
- **Claudication** (dull ache, often in calves) precip by walking and relieved by stopping (vs. spinal stenosis, qv); Leriche synd = claudication, ↓ or ∅ femoral pulses, & erectile dysfxn
- **Critical limb ischemia (CLI):** rest pain (↑ w/ elevation b/c ↓ perfusion), **ulcer** (typically at pressure foci, often dry; in contrast, venous ulcers are more often at medial malleolus, wet, and with hemosiderin deposition) or **gangrene,** due to PAD, and >2-wk duration (implies chronicity vs. acute limb ischemia; see below)

Diagnosis
- ↓ peripheral pulses; other signs of chronic PAD: hair loss, skin atrophy, nail hypertrophy
- Ankle:brachial index (ABI): nl 1–1.4; borderline 0.91–0.99; abnl ≤0.90; if >1.4, non-dx possibly due to calcified noncompressible vessel → ✓ PVR. If ABI abnl → segmental ABI w/ PVR to localize disease. If ⊕ sx but nl ABI, ✓ for ↓ lower extrem BP after exercise.
- Duplex arterial U/S; CTA w/ distal run-off; MRA or angio if dx in ? or possible intervention

Treatment (JACC 2013;61:1555; JAMA 2013;309:453 & 2015;314:1936)
- Risk factor modification. Screen for CAD. Structured exercise program (JAMA 2013;310:57).
- If sx, ASA or clopi to ↓ D/MI/stroke. More intensive Rx (eg, adding ticagrelor or vorapaxar) ↓ both MACE and limb ischemic events (Circ 2013;112:679 & JACC 2016;67:2719).
- Cilostazol (if no HF) & ? ACEI & statins to ↓ sx (Circ 2003;108:1481)
- Endovascular (angioplasty vs. stent) or surgical revasc if limiting/refractory sx or CLI

Acute limb ischemia (ALI)
- Sudden decrement in limb perfusion that threatens viability;
    viable (no immed threat of tissue loss): audible art. Doppler signals, sensory, & motor OK
    threatened (salvage requires prompt Rx): loss of arterial Doppler signal, sensory, or motor
- Etiologies: embolism > acute thrombosis (eg, athero, APS, HITT), trauma to artery
- Clinical manifestations (**6 Ps**): pain (distal to proximal, ↑ in severity), poikilothermia, pallor, pulselessness, paresthesias, paralysis
- Testing: thorough pulse & neuro exam; arterial Doppler; angiography, either CT w/ bilateral run-off through feet or arteriography
- Urgent consultation w/ vascular medicine and/or vascular surgery
- Treatment: immediate anticoagulation ± intra-arterial lytic; angioplasty or surgery

DYSPNEA

Pathophysiology	Etiologies
Airway obstruction (↑ resistance to airflow)	**Asthma, COPD,** bronchiectasis, cystic fibrosis, tumor, foreign body, **anaphylaxis**
Alveolar / Parenchymal disease	**Pulmonary edema:** *cardiogenic* or *noncardiogenic* **ILD;** pneumonia; atelectasis
Vascular (V/Q mismatch)	Large vessel: **PE,** tumor emboli Small vessel: **PHT,** vasculitis, ILD, emphysema, PNA
Chest wall (↑ resistance to expansion; weakness of respir. muscles)	**Pleural disease:** large effusion, fibrosis; pneumothorax **Chest wall/diaphragm:** kyphoscoliosis, ↑ abd girth **Neuromuscular disorders** (ALS, GBS, MG) **Hyperinflation** (COPD, asthma)
Stimulation of receptors	Chemoreceptors: **hypoxemia,** metabolic acidosis Mechanoreceptors: **ILD,** pulmonary edema, PHT, PE
↓ O_2 **carrying cap.** (but nl P_aO_2)	**Anemia,** methemoglobinemia, CO poisoning
Psychological	Anxiety, panic attack, depression, somatization

Evaluation
- History: quality of sensation, tempo, positional dependence, exac./allev. factors, exertion
- Cardiopulmonary exam, S_aO_2, CXR (see Appendix & Radiology inserts), ECG, ABG, U/S predictors of CHF: h/o CHF, PND, S_3, CXR w/ venous congestion, AF (*JAMA* 2005;294:1944) dyspnea w/ nl CXR → CAD, asthma, PE, early ILD, anemia, acidosis, NM disease
- Based on results of initial evaluation: PFT, chest CT, TTE, cardiopulmonary testing
- **BNP & NT-proBNP** ↑ in CHF (also ↑ in AF, RV strain from PE, COPD flare, PHT, ARDS) BNP <100 pg/mL to r/o CHF (90% Se), >400 to r/i (*NEJM* 2002;347:161) NT-proBNP <300 pg/mL to r/o CHF (99% Se); age-related cut points to r/i: >450 pg/mL (<50 y), >900 (50–75 y), >1800 (>75 y) (*EHJ* 2006;27:330) in chronic heart failure, ∴ need to compare to known "dry BNP"

PULMONARY FUNCTION TESTS (PFTs)

- **Spirometry:** evaluate for obstructive disease
  Flow-volume loops: diagnose and/or localize obstruction
  Bronchodilator: indicated if obstruction at baseline or asthma clinically suspected
  Methacholine challenge: helps dx asthma if spirometry nl, >20% ↓ FEV_1 → asthma
- **Lung volumes:** evaluate for hyperinflation or restrictive disease including NM causes
- **D_LCO:** evaluates functional surface area for gas exchange; helps differentiate causes of obstructive and restrictive diseases and screens for vascular disease & early ILD

Figure 2-1 Approach to abnormal PFTs

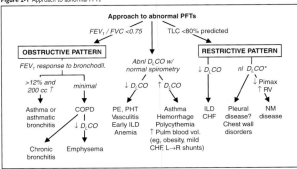

*D_LCO can be diminished due to secondary atelectasis

ASTHMA

Definition and epidemiology (Lancet 2013;382:1360)
- Chronic inflam. disorder w/ **airway hyperresponsiveness + variable airflow obstruction**
- Affects 5–10% population; ~85% of cases by age 40 y

Clinical manifestations (NEJM 2013;369:549)
- Classic triad = **wheezing, cough and dyspnea;** others include chest tightness, sputum; symptoms typically *chronic* with *episodic exacerbation*
- Precipitants (**triggers**)
  respiratory irritants (smoke, perfume, etc.) & *allergens* (pets, dust mites, pollen, etc.)
  infections (URI, bronchitis, sinusitis)
  drugs (eg, ASA & NSAIDs via leukotrienes, βB via bronchospasm, MSO_4 via histamine)
  emotional stress, cold air, exercise (increase in ventilation dries out airways)

Physical examination
- Wheezing and prolonged expiratory phase
- Presence of nasal polyps, rhinitis, rash → *allergic component*
- Exacerbation → ↑ RR, ↑ HR, accessory muscle use, diaphoresis, pulsus paradoxus

Diagnostic studies
- **Peak exp flow (PEF):** ≥60 L/min ↑ after bronchodil or ≥20% diurnal variation c/w asthma. <80% personal best c/w poor control, <50% c/w severe exacerbation.
- **Spirometry:** ↓ FEV_1, ↓ FEV_1/FVC, coved flow-volume loop; lung volumes: ± ↑ RV & TLC ⊕ bronchodilator response (↑ FEV_1 ≥12% & ≥200 mL) c/w asthma; methacholine challenge (↓ FEV_1 ≥20%) if PFTs nl: Se >90% (AJRCCM 2000;161:309)
- Allergy suspected → consider ✓ serum IgE, eos, skin testing/RAST

Ddx ("all that wheezes is not asthma...")
- Hyperventilation & panic attacks
- Upper airway obstruction or inh foreign body; laryngeal/vocal cord dysfxn (eg, 2° to GERD)
- CHF ("cardiac asthma"); COPD; bronchiectasis; ILD (including sarcoidosis); vasculitis; PE

"Asthma plus" syndromes (Lancet 2002;360:1313)
- Atopy = asthma + allergic rhinitis + atopic dermatitis
- ASA-sensitive asthma (Samter's syndrome) = asthma + ASA sensitivity + nasal polyps
- ABPA = asthma + pulmonary infiltrates + allergic rxn to *Aspergillus*
  Dx: ↑ IgE to *Asperg.* & total (>1000), ↑ *Asperg.* IgG levels, ↑ eos, central bronchiect.
  Rx: steroids ± itra-/voriconazole for refractory cases (NEJM 2000;342:756)
- Churg-Strauss = asthma + eosinophilia + granulomatous vasculitis

CHRONIC MANAGEMENT

"Reliever" medications (used prn to quickly relieve sx)
- *Short-acting* inh **β₂-agonists** (SABA): albuterol Rx of choice
- *Short-acting* inh **anticholinergics** (ipratropium) ↑ β₂-agonist delivery → ↑ bronchodilation

"Controller" meds (taken daily to keep control) (NEJM 2009;360:1002)
- Inh **corticosteroids** (ICS): Rx of choice (JAMA 2001;285:2583). PO steroids may be needed for severely uncontrolled asthma, but avoid if possible b/c systemic side effects.
- *Long-acting* inh **β₂-agonists** (LABA; eg, salmeterol): safe & ↓ exacerbations when added to ICS (NEJM 2016;374:1822). Except for exercise-induced asthma, should *not* be used w/o ICS (may ↑ mortality, esp. in African-Americans) (Chest 2006;129:15; Annals 2006;144:904).
- *Long-acting* inh **antimuscarinics** (LAMA; eg, tiotropium): add if sx despite ICS (super. to ↑ ICS, ≈ to adding LABA; NEJM 2010;363:1715) or if sx despite ICS+LABA (NEJM 2012;367:1198)
- **Nedocromil/cromolyn:** limited use in adults. Useful in young Pts, exercise-induced bronchospasm; ineffective unless used before trigger or exercise exposure.
- **Theophylline:** useful if hard to control sx; PO convenient, but high side-effect profile
- **Leukotriene receptor antagonists** (LTRA): some Pts very responsive, esp. ASA-sens (AJRCCM 2002;165:9) and exercise-induced (Annals 2000;132:97). May be noninf to ICS initial Rx and LABA add-on Rx (NEJM 2011;364:1695).
- **Anti-IgE:** for uncontrolled mod-to-severe allergic asthma (↑ IgE) on ICS ± LABA (NEJM 2006;354:2689; Annals 2011;154:573); not cost-effective for most Pts (JACI 2007;120:1146)

Other (Lancet 2015;386:1086)
- Behavior modification: identify and avoid triggers; PPI w/o benefit (NEJM 2009;360:1487)
- ImmunoRx may be useful if significant allergic component (JAMA 2016;315:1715)
- TNF antagonists may be helpful in refractory asthma (NEJM 2006;354:697)
- Anti-IL5 (mepolizumab, reslizumab) ↓ exac. in sev asthma (NEJM 2014;371:1189 & 1198)
- Anti-IL13 (lebrikizumab) ↑ FEV_1 (NEJM 2011;365:1088), not yet FDA approved
- Anti-IL4 (dupilumab): ↓ exac. in sev asthma (NEJM 2013;368:2455; Lancet 2016;388:31)

- Bronchial thermoplasty (exp'tal): radiofrequency destruction of airway smooth muscle no Δ in FEV_1, but ↓ in sx and # of exacerbations (NEJM 2007;356:1327)

Principles of treatment
- Education and avoidance of environmental triggers (Lancet 2015;386:1075); yearly flu shot
- Use quick-relief rescue medication as needed for all Pts
- Goal to achieve **complete control** = daily sx ≤2/wk, Ø nocturnal sx or limitation of activity, reliever med ≤2/wk, nl PEF or FEV_1; partly controlled = 1–2 of the above present in a wk; uncontrolled = ≥3 of the above present in a wk
- Step up treatment as needed to gain control, step down as tolerated
- If PEF ↓ 15% × 2 d or ↓ 30%, 4× ICS dose ↓ need for PO steroids (AJRCCM 2009;180:598)

Asthma Stepwise Therapy (Adapted from Global Initiative for Asthma [GINA] 2015 update)				
Step 1	Step 2	Step 3	Step 4	Step 5
		Rapid-acting β_2-agonists prn		
	Select one	*Select one*	*Do one or more*	*Add one or both*
Controller options	**Low-dose ICS**	**Low-dose ICS + LABA**	↑ **ICS dose** (w/ LABA)	Oral steroids (lowest dose)
	LTRA	Low-dose ICS + LAMA	**Add LAMA**	Anti-IgE Rx
		Med-dose ICS	Add LTRA	
		Low-dose ICS + LTRA	Add Theo	
		Low-dose ICS + Theo		

EXACERBATION

Evaluation
- History: baseline PEF, steroid requirement, ED visits, hospital admissions, prior intubation
  Current exacerbation: duration, severity, potential precipitants, meds used
  Risk factors for life-threatening: prior intubation, h/o near-fatal asthma, ED visit/hosp for asthma w/in 1 y, current/recent PO steroids, not using ICS, overdependent on SABA, Ψ, h/o noncompliance
- Physical exam: VS, pulm, accessory muscle use, pulsus paradoxus, abdominal paradox
  Assess for barotrauma: asymmetric breath sounds, tracheal deviation, subcutaneous air → pneumothorax, precordial (Hamman's) crunch → pneumomediastinum
- Diagnostic studies: **PEF** (used to follow clinical course); S_aO_2; **CXR** to r/o PNA or PTX
  ABG if severe: low P_aCO_2 initially; nl or high P_aCO_2 *may signify tiring*

Severity of Asthma Exacerbation			
Feature	**Mild**	**Moderate**	**Severe**
Breathless w/...	Walking	Talking	At rest
Talking in ...	Sentences	Phrases	Words
Mental status	± Agitated	Agitated	Agitated
RR	↑	↑	>30
Accessory muscles	Ø	⊕	⊕
Wheeze	Moderate, end-expir	Loud	Usually loud
HR	<100	100–120	>120
Pulsus paradoxus	Normal (<10)	10–25	>25
PEF	>80%	60–80%	<60%
S_aO_2	>95%	91–95%	<90%
P_aO_2	Normal	>60	<60
P_aCO_2	<45	<45	>45

Resp arrest imminent: drowsy, abdominal paradox, wheezes inaudible (b/c Ø air movement), bradycardia, loss of abdominal paradox (respiratory muscle fatigue). Presence of several parameters (not necessarily all) indicates classification (adapted from Chest 2003;123:1018; GINA 2015 update).

Initial treatment (NEJM 2010;363:755)
- **Oxygen** to keep S_aO_2 ≥90%
- **Inhaled SABA** (eg, albuterol) by MDI (4–8 puffs) or nebulizer (2.5–5 mg) q20min
- **Corticosteroids**: prednisone 0.5–1 mg/kg PO; IV if impending resp arrest
- **Ipratropium** MDI (4–6 puffs) or nebulizer (0.5 mg) q20min if severe (Chest 2002;121:1977)
- Epinephrine (0.3–0.5 mL SC of 1:1000 dilution) no advantage over inh SABA
- Montelukast IV ↑ FEV_1 but did not Δ rate of hosp (J Allergy Clin Immunol 2010;125:374)
- *Reassess after 60–90 min of Rx*
  Mild-mod exacerbation: cont SABA q1h
  Severe exacerbation: SABA & ipratropium q1h or continuously; ± Mg 2 g IV over 20 min (Lancet 2003;361:2114); ± heliox (60–80%)
- *Decide disposition within 4 h of presentation and after 1–3 h of Rx*

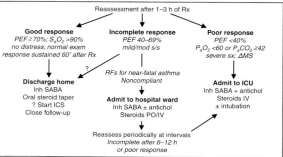

Figure 2-2 Disposition of patients after initial treatment of asthma exacerbation

Reassessment after 1–3 h of Rx

Good response
PEF ≥70%; S_aO_2 >90%
no distress; normal exam
response sustained 60' after Rx

Incomplete response
PEF 40–69%
mild/mod s/s

Poor response
PEF <40%
P_aO_2 <60 or P_aCO_2 ≥42
severe sx; ΔMS

Discharge home
Inh SABA
Oral steroid taper
? Start ICS
Close follow-up

RFs for near-fatal asthma
Noncompliant

Admit to hospital ward
Inh SABA ± antichol
Steroids PO/IV

Admit to ICU
Inh SABA + antichol
Steroids IV
± intubation

Reassess periodically at intervals
Incomplete after 6–12 h
or poor response

ICU-level care
- **High-dose steroids:** methylprednisolone 125 mg IV q6h (*Archives* 1983;143:1324)
- **Invasive ventilation:**
  large ET tube, P_{plat} <30 cm H_2O (predicts barotrauma better than PIP), max exp time
  PEEP individualized to Pt physiology
  paralysis, inhalational anesthetics, bronchoalveolar lavage w/ mucolytic, heliox
  (60–80% helium) and ECMO have been used with success
- NPPV likely improves obstruction (*Chest* 2003;123:1018), but controversial and rarely used

ANAPHYLAXIS

Definition and pathophysiology (*Ann Emerg Med* 2006;47:373)
- Severe, rapid-onset (mins to hrs), potentially life-threatening systemic allergic response
- IgE-mediated mast cell degranulation with release of histamine, tryptase and TNF
- Precipitates systemic reactions (bronchospasm, tissue swelling, fluid shifts, vasodilation)
- Common triggers: penicillins, cephalosporins, shellfish, nuts, insect stings, IV contrast (not truly an IgE-mediated mechanism, but clinically similar)

Diagnosis: any of the three following criteria
1) Acute illness with skin ± mucosal involvement (rash, flushing, hives), AND at least one of:
   - Respiratory compromise (wheeze, stridor, dyspnea, hypoxemia)
   - Hypotension or hypoperfusion (syncope, incontinence)
2) Two or more of the following after exposure to a **likely** allergen: skin/mucosal involvement, respiratory compromise, ↓ BP or hypoperfusion, GI symptoms
3) Hypotension after exposure to **known** allergen for that Pt

Treatment
- **Epi:** IM/SC 0.3–0.5 mL of 1:1000 dilution q5–20min; if HoTN 1 mg IVB q5min ± gtt
- **Airway:** suppl O_2 ± intubation or cricothyroidotomy (if laryngeal edema); β₂-agonists
- Fluid resuscitation w/ lg volume of crystalloid (may extravasate up to 35% of blood volume)
- Antihistamines relieve hives & itching, *no effect on airway or hemodynamics*
  H1RA (diphenhydramine 50 mg IV/IM) ± H2RA (eg, ranitidine 50 mg IV)
- Corticosteroids have no immediate effect but may help prevent relapse:
  methylprednisolone 125 mg IV q6h if severe or prednisone 50 mg PO
- Avoid unopposed α-adrenergic vasopressors

Disposition
- Mild rxn limited to urticaria or mild bronchospasm can be observed for ≥6 h; admit all others
- Watch for **biphasic reaction;** occurs in 23%, typically w/in 8–10 h but up to 72 h
- At time of d/c: education re: allergen avoidance, instruction and Rx for EpiPen, allergist f/u

Angioedema (*Ann Allergy Asthma Immunol* 2000;85:521; *J Allergy Clin Immunol* 2013;131:1491)
- Localized swelling of skin/mucosa; involves face, lips, tongue, uvula, larynx, and bowels
- Etiologies: mast cell-mediated (eg, NSAIDs); bradykinin-mediated (eg, **ACEi**, ARNi, hereditary angioedema, acquired C1 inhibitor deficiency); idiopathic
- Diagnosis: C4 and C1 inhibitor level, tryptase (if suspect anaphylaxis)
- Rx: intubation if risk of airway compromise; allergic angioedema: H1/H2 antihist., steroids
  if 2° ACEi: d/c ACEi, antihist., **icatibant** (bradykinin-receptor antag) *NEJM* 2015;372:418)
  Hereditary angioedema: synthetic C1 inhibitor cinryze (*NEJM* 2010;363:513)

Definition and epidemiology (Lancet 2014;385:1778)
• Progressive airflow limitation caused by airway and parenchymal inflammation

Emphysema vs. Chronic Bronchitis		
	Emphysema	**Chronic Bronchitis**
Definition	Dilation/destruction of parenchyma (path definition)	Productive cough >3 mo/y × ≥2 y (clinical definition)
Pathophysiology	Tissue destruction V/Q: ↑ dead space fraction → hypercarbia, but only mild hypoxemia	Small airways affected V/Q: ↑ shunt fraction → severe hypoxemia, hypercapnia PHT, cor pulmonale
Clinical manifestations	Severe, constant dyspnea Mild cough	Intermittent dyspnea Copious sputum production
Physical exam	"Pink puffer" Tachypneic, noncyanotic, thin Diminished breath sounds	"Blue bloater" Cyanotic, obese, edematous Rhonchi & wheezes

Pathogenesis (Lancet 2003;362:1053)
• **Cigarette smoke** (centrilobular emphysema, affects 15–20% of smokers)
• Recurrent airway infections
• α_1-antitrypsin defic.: early-onset panacinar emphysema, 1–3% of COPD cases. Suspect if age <45, lower lungs affected, extrathoracic manifestations (liver disease [not if MZ subtype], FMD, pancreatitis). ✓ serum AAT level (nb, acute phase reactant).
• Low FEV_1 in early adulthood important in genesis of COPD (NEJM 2015;373:111)
• Misc: biomass (eg, cooking fuels in enclosed space), chronic asthma (Lancet 2009;374:733)

Clinical manifestations
• Chronic cough, sputum production, dyspnea; later stages → freq exac., a.m. HA, wt loss
• Exacerbation triggers: infxn, other cardiopulmonary disease, incl. PE (Annals 2006;144:390)
Infxn: overt tracheobronchitis/pneumonia from viruses, S. pneumoniae, H. influenzae, M. catarrhalis or triggered by changes in strain of colonizers (NEJM 2008;359:2355)
• Physical exam: ↑ AP diameter of chest ("barrel-chest"), hyperresonance, ↓ diaphragmatic excursion, ↓ breath sounds, ↑ expiratory phase, rhonchi, wheezes during exacerbation: tachypnea, accessory muscle use, pulsus paradoxus, cyanosis
• Asthma-COPD overlap syndrome (ACOS; NEJM 2015;373:1241): features of both present. For example: reversibility of airway obstruction w/ bronchodilator in COPD; neutrophilic inflammation in asthma (more classic in COPD); eos in COPD.

Diagnostic studies
• CXR (see Radiology inserts): hyperinflation, flat diaphragms, ± interstitial markings & bullae
• PFTs: **obstruction:** ↓↓ FEV_1, ↓ FVC, **FEV_1/FVC <0.7 (no sig Δ post bronchodilator)**, expiratory scooping of flow-volume loop; **hyperinflation:** ↑↑ RV, ↑ TLC, ↑ RV/TLC; **abnormal gas exchange:** ↓ D_LCO (in emphysema)
• ABG: ↓ P_aO_2, ± ↑ P_aCO_2 (in chronic bronchitis, usually only if FEV_1 <1.5 L) and ↓ pH
• ECG: PRWP, S1S2S3, R-sided strain, RVH, ↑ P waves in lead II ("P pulmonale")

Chronic treatment (Lancet 2015;1789)
• **Bronchodilators** (first-line therapy): **anticholinergics**, β_2-agonists (BA), theophylline Long-acting (LA) antimuscarinic (LAMA; eg, tiotropium): ↓ exac., ↓ admit, ↓ resp failure (NEJM 2008;359:1543), better than ipratropium or LABA as mono Rx (NEJM 2011;364:1093)
LABA: ~11% ↓ in exacerbations, no ↑ in CV events (Lancet 2016;387:1817)
LABA + inh steroid: ? ↓ mort. vs. either alone (NEJM 2007;356:775)
LAMA + LABA: ↑ FEV_1, ↓ sx vs. either alone (Chest 2014;145:981) and superior to LABA + inh steroid (NEJM 2016;374:2222)
• **Corticosteroids** (inhaled, ICS): ~11% ↓ in exacerb & slow ↓ FEV_1; no Δ in risk of PNA or in mortality (Lancet 2016;387:1817)
• Roflumilast (PDE-4 inhibitor): ↑ FEV_1 & ↓ exacerbations when added to bronchodilator (Lancet 2009;374:685, 695 & 2015;385:857)
• Antibiotics: daily azithro ↓ exacerb, but not yet routine (JAMA 2014;311:2225)
• Mucolytics: no Δ FEV_1, but ? ↓ exacerbation rate (Lancet 2008;371:2013)
• **Oxygen:** if P_aO_2 ≤55 mmHg or S_aO_2 ≤89% (during rest, exercise, or sleep) to prevent cor pulmonale; only Rx proven to ↓ mortality (Annals 1980;93:391; Lancet 1981;i:681)
• **Prevention:** Flu/Pneumovax; smoking cessation (eg, varenicline, bupropion) → 50% ↓ in lung function decline (AJRCCM 2002;166:675) and ↓ long-term mortality (Annals 2005;142:223)
• Rehabilitation: ↓ dyspnea and fatigue, ↑ exercise tolerance, ↓ QoL (NEJM 2009;360:1329)

- **Experimental**
  - Lung volume reduction surgery: ↑ exer. capacity, ↓ mort. *if* FEV$_1$ >20%, upper-lobe, low exer. capacity (*NEJM* 2003;348:2059)
  - Bronchoscopic lung reduction w/ endobronchial valves or coils: ↑ lung fxn but significant complications (PTX, PNA) (*NEJM* 2015;373:2325; *Lancet* 2015;386:1066; *JAMA* 2016;315:175)
  - Nocturnal BiPAP: may improve survival, ? decrease QoL (*Thorax* 2009;64:561)
- **Lung transplant**: ↑ QoL and ↓ sx (*Lancet* 1998;351:24), ? survival benefit (*Am J Transplant* 2009;9:1640)

Staging and prognosis
- **COPD assessment test (CAT)**: 8 question tool assessing cough, sputum, exercise capacity & energy, with score ranging 0–40 (http://www.catestonline.org)
- **mMRC score**: ≥2 defined as walking slowly b/c breathlessness or having to stop to catch breath walking level
- Ratio of diam PA/aorta >1 associated with ~3× ↑ risk of exacerbations (*NEJM* 2012;367:913)

COPD Staging and Recommended Therapies by GOLD Criteria

Stage	FEV$_1$	3-y mort	Exac. in past yr	CAT <10 or mMRC 0-1	CAT ≥10 or mMRC ≥2
I: Mild	≥80%	?	≤1 (and 0 hosp)	**A** Short-acting inh dilator prn	**B** Standing inh dilator (LAMA > LABA)
II: Mod	50–80%	~11%			
III: Severe	30–50%	~15%	≥2 or ≥1 hosp	**C** [ICS + LABA] or LAMA	**D** ICS + [LAMA and/or LABA] + Experimental as indicated
IV: Very severe	<30%	~24%			
					Consider adding PDE-4 inhib to bronchodilator

Smoking cessation & vaccinations in all. Pulm rehab in groups B–D. Consider theophylline as alternative. O$_2$ as indicated per S$_a$O$_2$. (Adapted from Global Initiative for Chronic Obstructive Pulmonary Disease, 2016)

EXACERBATION

COPD Exacerbation Treatment (*NEJM* 2002;346:988)

Agent	Dose	Comments
Ipratropium	MDI 4–8 puffs q1–2h *or* Nebulizer 0.5 mg q1–2h	First-line therapy (*NEJM* 2011; 364:1093)
Albuterol	MDI 4–8 puffs q1–2h *or* Nebulizer 2.5–5 mg q1–2h	Benefit if component of reversible bronchoconstriction
Corticosteroids	No consensus for optimal dose & duration (*Cochrane* 2009:CD001288) Consider: Prednisolone 30–40 mg/d × 10–14 d or even 5 d (*JAMA* 2013;309:2223) Methylprednisolone 125 mg IV q6h × 72 h for more severe exacerbations	↓ treatment failure, ↓ hospital stay, ↑ FEV$_1$ but no mortality benefit, ↑ complications (*Cochrane* 2009:CD001288) OutPt Rx after ED visit ↓ relapse (*NEJM* 2003;348:2618) ? use periph eos >2% to trigger use (*AJRCCM* 2012;186:48)
Antibiotics	Amox, TMP-SMX, doxy, clarithro, antipneumococcal FQ, etc., all reasonable (no single abx proven superior). Consider local flora and avoid repeat courses of same abx. ≤5d course likely enough for mild-mod exacerbation (*JAMA* 2010;303:2035).	*H. flu, M. catarrhalis, S. pneumo* freq. precipitants. ↑ PEF, ↓ Rx failure, ? ↓ short-term mort, ↓ subseq exacerb (*Chest* 2008;133:756 & 2013;143:82) Consider if ↑ sputum purulence or CRP >40 (*Chest* 2013;144:1571)
Oxygenation	↑ F$_i$O$_2$ to achieve P$_a$O$_2$ ≥55–60 or S$_a$O$_2$ 90–93%	**Watch for CO$_2$ retention** (due to ↑ V/Q mismatch, loss of hypoxemic resp drive, Haldane effect) *but must maintain oxygenation!*
Noninvasive positive-pressure ventilation	Initiate *early* if mod/severe dyspnea, ↓ pH / ↑ P$_a$CO$_2$, RR >25 Results in 58% ↓ intubation, ↓ LOS by 3.2 d, 59% ↓ mortality Contraindications: Δ MS, inability to cooperate or clear secretions, hemodynamic instability, UGIB (*NEJM* 1995;333:817; *Annals* 2003;138:861; *Cochrane* 2004:CD004104; *ERJ* 2005;25:348)	
Endotracheal intubation	Consider if P$_a$O$_2$ <55–60, ↑ing P$_a$CO$_2$, ↓ing pH, ↑ RR, respiratory fatigue, Δ MS or hemodynamic instability	
Other measures	Mucolytics overall not supported by data (*Chest* 2001;119:1190) Monitor for cardiac arrhythmias	

HEMOPTYSIS

Definition and pathophysiology
- Expectoration of blood or blood-streaked sputum
- **Massive hemoptysis:** ->600 mL/24–48 h; gas exchange more important than blood loss
- Massive hemoptysis usually from tortuous or invaded **bronchial arteries**

	Etiologies (Crit Care Med 2000;28:1642)
Infection/ Inflammation	**Bronchitis** (most common cause of trivial hemoptysis) **Bronchiectasis** incl. **CF** (common cause of massive hemoptysis) TB or aspergilloma (can be massive); pneumonia or lung abscess
Neoplasm	Usually primary **lung cancer**, sometimes metastasis (can be massive)
Cardiovasc.	**PE** (can be massive), pulmonary artery rupture (2° to instrumentation), CHF, mitral stenosis, trauma/foreign body, bronchovascular fistula
Other	**Vasc** (GPA, Goodpasture's, Behçet's; can be massive), AVM, anticoag (w/ underlying lung dis), coagulopathy, cocaine, pulm hemosiderosis

Diagnostic workup
- Localize bleeding site (r/o GI or ENT source by H&P ± endo); determine whether **unilateral or bilateral, localized or diffuse, parenchymal or airway** by CXR/ chest CT ± bronch
- PT, PTT, CBC to rule out **coagulopathy**
- Sputum culture/stain for bacteria, fungi and AFB; cytology to **r/o malignancy**
- ANCA, anti-GBM, urinalysis to ✓ for **vasculitis** or **pulmonary-renal syndrome**

Treatment
- Mechanism of death is asphyxiation not exsanguination; maintain gas exchange, reverse coagulation and treat underlying condition; cough supp. may ↑ risk of asphyxiation
- Massive hemoptysis: **put bleeding side dependent**; selectively intubate nl lung if needed
  Angiography: Dx & Rx (vascular occlusion balloons or **selective embol of bronchial art**)
  Rigid bronch: allows more options (electrocautery, laser) than flex. *Surgical resection.*

BRONCHIECTASIS

Definition and epidemiology (NEJM 2002;346:1383)
- Obstructive airways disease of bronchi and bronchioles, chronic transmural inflamm w/ airway dilatation and thickening, collapsibility, mucus plugging w/ impaired clearance

Initial workup
- H&P: cough, dyspnea, copious sputum production, ± hemoptysis, inspiratory "squeaks"
- CXR: scattered or focal; rings of bronchial cuffing; "tram track" of dilated, thick airways
- PFTs: obstructive; chest CT: airway dilation & thickening ± cystic Δs, infiltrates, adenopathy

Etiology	Other Features	Diagnostic Testing
Chronic infxns (eg, MTb, ABPA)	Chronic cough, freq/persist infiltrate, refract asthma (ABPA)	Sputum cx (incl myobact, fungal), ± bronch/BAL, IgE & eos (ABPA)
1° ciliary dyskin	Sinusitis, infertility, otitis	Dynein mutations
Immunodefic.	Recurrent infxns often as child	IgA, IgG, IgM, IgG subclasses
RA, SLE	Resp sx may precede joint sx	RF, ANA
IBD	Not relieved by bowel resection	Colonoscopy, biopsy
α_1-AT deficiency	Lower lobe emphysema	α_1-AT level
Anatomic	R middle lobe synd. from sharp takeoff, foreign body aspir.	Bronchoscopy

Treatment
- Treat underlying condition; mucolytics & bronchodilators
- Prophylactic azithro shown to ↓ exacerb. in non-CF bronchiectasis (JAMA 2013:1251)
- Antibiotics: at time of acute exacerbation directed against suspected or prior pathogens

Cystic fibrosis (NEJM 2015;372:351)
- Autosomal recessive genetic disorder due to mutations in chloride channel (CFTR gene)
- ↑ mucus thickness, ↓ mucociliary clearance, ↑ infections → bronchiectasis
- Clinical: recurrent PNA, weight loss, sinus infxns, infertility, pancreatic insuffic (fatty stools)
- Rx: airway clearance (chest PT, inh hypertonic saline, DNAse), abx for exacerb. for drug-resistant org. (eg, *Pseudomonas, Burkholderia*), gene targeted with CFTR potentiator (ivakaftor) & corrector (lumakaftor) (NEJM 2011;365:1663 & 2015;373:220), lung transplant

Non-tuberculous mycobacterium (NTM; ubiquitous hydrophilic bacteria)
- Chronic cough, ↓ wt; Lady Windermere synd.: R middle lobe bronchiectasis in elderly ♀ who suppress expectoration; in HIV ⊕ disseminated disease (see HIV/AIDS)
- Dx: CT scan (tree-in-bud, nodules, cavities, bronchiect.), sputum ×3 or BAL, AFB stain + cx
- Treatment: [clarithro or azithro] + rifamycin & ethambutol for ≥12 mo (Chest 2004;126:566)

SOLITARY PULMONARY NODULE

Principles
- Definition: single, <3 cm, surrounded by normal lung, no LAN or pleural effusion
- Often "incidentalomas," esp with ↑ CT use, but may still be early, curable malignancy

Etiologies	
Benign (70%)	**Malignant (30%)**
Granuloma (80%): TB, histo, coccidio	**Bronchogenic carcinoma** (75%):
Hamartoma (10%)	adeno & large cell (peripheral)
Bronchogenic cyst, AVM, pulm infarct	squamous & small cell (central)
Echinococcosis, ascariasis, aspergilloma	**Metastatic** (20%): breast, head & neck, colon,
Wegener's, rheumatoid nodule	testicular, renal, sarcoma, melanoma
Lipoma, fibroma, amyloidoma, pneumonitis	Carcinoid, primary sarcoma

Initial evaluation
- **History:** h/o cancer, smoking, age (<30 y = 2% malignant, +15% each decade >30)
- **CT:** size/shape, Ca^{2+}, LAN, effusions, bony destruction, **compare w/ old studies**
  Ø Ca → ↑ likelihood malignant; laminated → granuloma; "popcorn" → hamartoma
- High-risk features for malig: size (eg, ≥2.3 cm diameter), spiculated, upper lobe, ♀, >60 yo, >1 ppd current smoker, no prior smoking cessation (NEJM 2003;348:2535 & 2013;369:910)

Diagnostic studies
- **PET:** detects metab. activity of tumors, 97% Se & 78% Sp for malig. (esp. if >8 mm)
  also useful for surgical staging b/c may detect unsuspected mets (JAMA 2001;285:914)
  useful in deciding which lesions to bx vs. follow w/ serial CT (J Thor Oncol 2006;1:71)
- **Transthoracic needle biopsy** (TTNB): if tech. feasible, 97% will obtain definitive tissue dx
  (AJR 2005;185:1294); if noninformative or malignant → resect
- **Video-assisted thoracoscopic surgery** (VATS): for percutaneously inaccessible lesions;
  highly sensitive and allows resection; has replaced thoracotomy
- Transbronchial bx (TBB): most lesions too small to reliably sample w/o endobronchial
  U/S (Chest 2003;123:604); bronch w/ brushings low-yield unless invading bronchus;
  navigational bronchoscopy w/ 70% yield, ↑ sens w/ larger nodules (Chest 2012;142:385)
- PPD, fungal serologies, ANCA

Management (for solid SPN >8 mm; if ≤8 mm, serial CT) (Chest 2013;143:840)
- **Low risk** (<5%, see ref): serial CT (freq depending on risk); shared decision w/ Pt re: bx
- **Intermediate risk** (5–60%): PET, if ⊖ → follow low-risk protocol; if ⊕ → high-risk protocol
- **High risk** (and surgical candidate): TBB, TTNB, or VATS → lobectomy if malignant
- **Ground-glass nodules:** longer f/u b/c if malignant can be slow-growing & PET ⊖

SLEEP APNEA

Definition and pathophysiology
- **Obstructive:** pharyngeal collapse → apnea (≥10 s) or hypopnea (↓ airflow) ± desaturation;
  risk factors: obesity (present in 70%), large neck, male sex, ↓ muscle tone, ↑ age, alcohol
- **Central:** ↓ neurologic feedback w/ oscillating drive. Apneas w/o resp effort ± subsequent
  ↑ resp rate. Associated with CHF & atrial fibrillation; worsened by sedatives.
- **Complex:** obstructive + central (nb, untreated obstructive → complex)
- Proposed mech: Apnea/arousals → sympathetic nervous system activation, negative
  intrathoracic pressure → ↑ preload, ↑ afterload. Consequently → HTN, pulm HTN.

Clinical manifestations (Lancet 2002;360:237; Lancet Resp Med 2013;1:61)
- Snoring, witnessed apneas/gasping, daytime sleepiness
- **Cardiovascular:** HTN (JAMA 2012;307:2169); a/w ↑ risk of stroke and death (NEJM
  2005;353:2034) & possibly CAD & endothelial dysfxn (AJRCCM 2001;163:19; Circ 2008;117:2270)
- **Neurocognitive:** ↓ cognitive performance, ↓ QoL, ↑ motor vehicle and work accidents
  (NEJM 1999;340:847; AJRCCM 2001;164:2031)

Diagnosis and treatment (JAMA 2013;310:731 & Lancet 2014;383:736)
- **Polysomnography** (sleep study); can do home-testing
- **Obstructive: CPAP** ↓↓ apnea/hypopnea, ↓ BP (JAMA 2013;310:2407 & NEJM 2014;370:2276),
  ↓ sleepiness, ↑ performance (AJRCCM 2012;186:677), ↑ EF in Pts with CHF (NEJM 2003;348:1233),
  ↓ metab syndrome (NEJM 2011;365:2277), ↓ mortality after stroke (AJRCCM 2009;180:36)
- Oral appliances if refusing CPAP; upper-airway stimulator under study (NEJM 2014;370:139)
- **Central:** adaptive servoventilation (ASV) if w/o CHF (nb, ↑ mortality if CHF; NEJM 2015;373:1095)
- Avoid alcohol and sedatives
- Surgery (eg, uvulopalatopharyngoplasty, UPPP) of limited benefit (Chest 1997;111:265)

WORKUP OF ILD (Thorax 2008;63:v1)

Broad categories
- **Sarcoid; exposure-related** (eg, drugs, toxins, hypersens. pneumonitis, pneumoconiosis); **collagen vasc. dis.** (eg, scleroderma, GPA); **idiopathic PNAs** (eg, IPF, COP); **misc.**

Rule out mimickers of ILD
- **Congestive heart failure** (✓ BNP, trial of diuresis)
- **Infection:** viral, atypical bacterial, fungal, mycobacterial, parasitic
- **Malignancy:** lymphangitic carcinomatosis, bronchoalveolar, leukemia, lymphoma

History and physical exam
- Occupational, travel, exposure (including tobacco), meds, FHx, precipitating event
- Tempo (acute → infxn, CHF, hypersens pneumonitis, eos PNA, AIP, COP, drug-induced)
- Extrapulmonary signs/sx (skin Δs, arthralgias/arthritis, clubbing, neuropathies, etc.)

Diagnostic studies (see Appendix & Radiology inserts)
- CXR and **high-resolution chest CT:** reticular, nodular or ground-glass pattern
  - Upper lobe-predominant → coal, silica, hypersens, sarcoid, TB, RA
  - Lower lobe-predominant → IPF, asbestos, scleroderma
  - Adenopathy → sarcoidosis, berylliosis, silicosis, malignancy, fungal infections
  - Pleural disease → collagen-vascular diseases, asbestosis, infections, XRT
- PFTs: ↓ D_LCO (early sign), restrictive pattern (↓ volumes), ↓ P_aO_2 (esp. w/ exercise); if also obstructive, consider sarcoid, LAM, silicosis
- Serologies: ✓ ACE, ANA, RF, ANCA, anti-GBM, HIV, ± myositis panel & other serologies
- Bronchoalveolar lavage: dx infxn, hemorrhage, eosinophilic syndromes, PAP
- Biopsy (transbronch, CT-guided, VATS, open) if no clear precipitant and w/u unrevealing

SPECIFIC ETIOLOGIES OF ILD

Sarcoidosis (Lancet 2014;383:1155)
- Prevalence: African-Americans, northern Europeans, and females; onset in 3rd–4th decade
- Pathophysiology: depression of cellular immune system peripherally, activation centrally

Clinical Manifestations of Sarcoidosis	
Organ system	**Manifestations**
Pulmonary	Hilar LAN; fibrosis; pulm hypertension. Stages: I = bilat hilar LAN; II = LAN + ILD; III = ILD only; IV = diffuse fibrosis.
Cutaneous (~15%)	Waxy skin plaques; lupus pernio (violaceous facial lesions) Erythema nodosum = red tender nodules due to panniculitis, typically on shins; Ddx: idiopathic (34%), infxn (33%, strep, TB), sarcoid (22%), drugs (OCP, PCNs), vasculitis (Behçet's), IBD, lymphoma.
Ocular (10–30%)	Anterior > posterior uveitis; ↑ lacrimal gland
Endo & renal (10%)	Nephrolithiasis, hypercalcemia (10%), hypercalciuria (40%) Due to vitamin D hydroxylation by macrophages
Neuro (10% clin, 25% path)	CN VII palsy, periph neuropathies, CNS lesions, seizures
Cardiac (5% clin, 25% path)	Conduction block, VT, CMP
Liver, spleen, BM	Granulomatous hepatitis (25%), splenic & BM gran. (50%)
Constitutional	Fever, night sweats, anorexia & wt loss (a/w hepatic path)
Musculoskeletal	Arthralgias, periarticular swelling, bone cysts

- Löfgren's syndrome: erythema nodosum + hilar adenopathy + arthritis (good prognosis)
- Diagnostic studies: LN bx → **noncaseating granulomas** + multinucleated giant cells endobronchial ultrasonography superior to conventional bronch (JAMA 2013;309:2457)
  ^{18}FDG PET can be used to identify extent and potentially targets for dx bx
  ↑ **ACE** (Se 60%, 90% w/ active dis., Sp 80%, false ⊕ in granulomatous diseases)
- To assess extent: CXR, PFTs, full ophtho exam, ECG, CBC (lymphopenia, ↑ eos), Ca, 24-h urine for Ca, LFTs; ± Holter, echo, cardiac MRI, brain MRI, etc., based on s/s
- Rx: **steroids** if sx or extrathoracic organ dysfxn (eg, prednisone 20–40 mg/d), improves sx, but doesn't Δ long-term course; hydroxychloroquine for extensive skin disease; anti-TNF, MTX, AZA, mycophenolate or cyclophosphamide for chronic/refractory disease
- Prognosis: ~$^2/_3$ spontaneously remit w/in 10 y (60–80% of stage I, 50–60% stage II, 30% stage III), w/ relapses uncommon; ~$^1/_3$ have progressive disease

Exposure
- **Drugs/Iatrogenic**

Amio (dose & duration depend.): chronic interstitial PNA ↔ ARDS; Rx: d/c amio; steroids
Other drugs: nitrofurantoin, sulfonamides, thiazides, INH, hydralazine, gold
Chemo: **bleomycin** (triggered by hyperoxia), busulfan, cyclophosphamide, MTX, etc.
XRT: COP/BOOP w/ sharply linear, nonanatomic boundaries; DAH
- **Pneumoconioses** (inorganic dusts) (NEJM 2000;342:406; Clin Chest Med 2004:467)
    Coal worker's: upper lobe coal macules; may progress to massive fibrosis
    Silicosis: upper lobe opacities ± eggshell calcification of lymph nodes; ↑ risk of TB
    Asbestosis: lower lobe fibrosis, calcified pleural plaques, DOE, dry cough, rales on
    exam. Asbestos exposure also → pleural plaques, benign pleural effusion, diffuse
    pleural thickening, rounded atelectasis, mesothelioma, lung Ca (esp. in smokers).
    Berylliosis: multisystemic granulomatous disease that mimics sarcoidosis
- **Hypersensitivity pneumonitides** (organic dusts): loose, noncaseating *granulomas*
    Antigens: farmer's lung (spores of thermophilic actinomyces); pigeon fancier's lung
    (proteins from feathers and excreta of birds); humidifier lung (thermophilic bacteria)

Collagen vascular diseases (Chest 2013;143:814)
- **Rheumatologic disease**
    Scleroderma: fibrosis in ~67%; PHT seen in ~10% of CREST Pts
    PM-DM: ILD & weakness of respiratory muscles; MCTD: PHT & fibrosis
    SLE & RA: pleuritis and pleural effusions more often than ILD; SLE can cause DAH
- **Vasculitis** (can p/w *DAH*)
    GPA (Wegener's granulomatosis) (⊕ c-ANCA) w/ necrotizing granulomas
    EGPA (Churg-Strauss) (⊕ c- or p-ANCA) w/ eosinophilia & necrotizing granulomas
    Microscopic polyangiitis (⊕ p-ANCA) w/o granulomas
- **Goodpasture's syndrome** = DAH + RPGN; typically in smokers; ⊕ anti-GBM in 90%
- **Lymphangioleiomyomatosis** (LAM): cystic, ↑ in ♀, Rx w/ sirolimus (NEJM 2011;364:1595)

Idiopathic interstitial pneumonias (IIPs) (AJRCCM 2013;188:733; NEJM 2014;370:1820)
- Definition: **ILD of unknown cause**; dx by radiographic, histologic, and clinical features

IIPs		
Type	**Imaging/Histology**	**Clinical**
UIP/IPF	Reticular opacities, honeycombing, traction bronchiectasis; periph, subpl., & basal	Sx >12 mo 5-y mort. ~80%
NSIP	Homogenous ground-glass opacities or consolid., reticular irreg lines; symmetric, periph, basal, subpl. Mimics CTD ILD. Cellular and fibrotic subtypes, latter similar to UIP but homogenous.	Sx mos–y 5-y mort. 10% (fibrotic = UIP)
COP/BOOP	Patchy bilat consolid., nodules; subpl. & peribronchial. Prolif of granulation tissue in small bronchioles & inflam of surrounding alveoli.	Can be post-infxn, HSCT, XRT, rxn to drugs. 5-y mort <5%.
AIP	Diffuse ground-glass opacities, consolid. w/ lobular sparing. Path similar to DAD.	Sx <3 wk 6-mo mort. 60%
DIP	Diffuse ground-glass opacities, reticular lines; lower zones, periph. Mφ in alveoli.	30–50 yo *smokers* Sx wks–mos
RB-ILD	Bronchial thickening, centrilobular nodules, patchy ground-glass opacities. Mφ in alveoli.	Death rare

UIP, usual interstitial PNA (NEJM 2012;366:1968); IPF, idiopathic pulm fibrosis (Lancet 2011;378:1949); NSIP, nonspecific IP; COP, cryptogenic organizing PNA; BOOP, bronchiolis obliterans w/ organizing PNA; AIP, acute IP (Hamman-Rich syndrome); DIP, desquamative IP; RB-ILD, resp bronchiolitis-assoc ILD.

- Rx for UIP/IPF: suppl O₂, pulm rehab, Rx for GERD, lung transplant referral
    Pirfenidone (antifibrotic) or **nintedanib** (tyrosine kin. inhib mediating fibrogenic growth
    factors) ↓ rate of FVC decline (NEJM 2014;370:2071 & 2083; AJRCCM 2015;192:3)
    High-dose steroids may be used for acute exacerbations
- Steroids for other IIPs: NSIP (esp. cellular type) and COP (AJRCCM 2000;162:571); ?
    benefit for AIP and DIP/RB-ILD (for which Pts should stop smoking)

Pulmonary infiltrates w/ eosinophilia (PIE) = eos on BAL ± periph. blood
- **Allergic bronchopulmonary aspergillosis (ABPA)**
- Löffler's syndrome: parasites/drugs → transient pulm infilt + cough, fever, dyspnea, eos
- Acute eosinophilic PNA (AEP): acute hypox febrile illness; Rx: steroids, tobacco cessation
- Chronic eosinophilic pneumonia (CEP): "photonegative" of CHF, typically in women

Miscellaneous
- Pulm alveolar proteinosis (PAP): accum of surfactant-like phospholipids; ♂ smokers; white
    & gummy sputum; BAL milky fluid (NEJM 2003;349:2527); Rx w/ lung lavage & GMCSF
- Langerhans cell granulomatosis (LCG): young ♂ smokers; apical cysts; PTX (25%)
- Lymphocytic interstitial PNA: polyclonal B-cell infiltration (? lymphoma); Rx: steroids

PLEURAL EFFUSION

Pathophysiology
- **Systemic factors** (eg, ↑ PCWP, ↓ oncotic pressure) → *transudative* effusion
- **Local factors** (ie, Δ pleural surface permeability) → *exudative* effusion

Transudates
- **Congestive heart failure (40%):** 80% bilateral, ± cardiomegaly on CXR occasionally exudative (esp. after aggressive diuresis or if chronic), but ~75% of exudative effusions in CHF Pts found to have non-CHF cause *(Chest 2002;122:1518)*
- **Constrictive pericarditis** (knock on exam, calcification or thickening on imaging)
- **Cirrhosis** ("hepatic hydrothorax"): diaphragmatic pores allow passage of ascitic fluid often right-sided (²/₃) & massive (even w/o marked ascites)
- Nephrotic syndrome: usually small, bilateral, asymptomatic (r/o PE b/c hypercoag)
- Other: PE (usually exudate), malignancy (lymphatic obstruction), myxedema, CAPD

Exudates
- **Lung parenchymal infection (25%)**
  bacterial (parapneumonic): can evolve along spectrum of *exudative* (but sterile) → *fibropurulent* (infected fluid) → *organization* (fibrosis & formation of rigid pleural peel). Common causes: Strep pneumo, Staph aureus, Strep milleri, Klebsiella, Pseudomonas, Haemophilus, Bacteroides, Peptostreptococcus, mixed flora in aspiration pneumonia.
  mycobacterial: >50% lymphs 80% of the time, ADA >40, pleural bx ~70% Se
  fungal, viral (usually small), parasitic (eg, amebiasis, echinococcosis, paragonimiasis)
- **Malignancy (15%):** primary lung cancer most common, metastases (eg. breast, lymphoma, etc.), mesothelioma (✓ serum osteopontin levels; *NEJM 2005;353:15*)
- **Pulmonary embolism (10%):** effusions in ~40% of PEs; exudate (75%) > transudate (25%); hemorrhagic—must have high suspicion b/c presentation highly variable
- **Collagen vascular disease:** RA (large), SLE (small), Wegener's, Churg-Strauss
- **Gastrointestinal diseases:** pancreatitis, esophageal rupture, abdominal abscess
- **Hemothorax** (Hct_eff/Hct_blood >50%): trauma, PE, malignancy, coagulopathy, leaking aortic aneurysm, aortic dissection, pulmonary vascular malformation
- **Chylothorax** (triglycerides >110): thoracic duct damage due to trauma, malignancy, LAM
- Other:
  post-CABG: left-sided; initially bloody, clears after several wks
  Dressler's syndrome (pericarditis & pleuritis post-MI), uremia, postradiation therapy
  Asbestos exposure: benign; ⊕ eosinophils
  Drug-induced (eg, nitrofurantoin, methysergide, bromocriptine, amiodarone): ⊕ eos
  Uremia; post-XRT; sarcoidosis
  Meigs' syndrome = benign ovarian tumor → ascites & pleural effusion
  Yellow-nail syndrome: yellow nails, lymphedema, pleural effusion, bronchiectasis

Diagnostic studies
- **Thoracentesis** *(NEJM 2006;355:e16)*
  Indications: **all effusions >1 cm in decubitus view**
    if suspect due to CHF, can diurese and see if effusions resolve (75% do so in 48 h)
    asymmetry, fever, chest pain or failure to resolve → thoracentesis
    parapneumonics should be tapped ASAP (cannot exclude infxn clinically)
  Diagnostic studies: ✓ total protein, LDH, glucose, cell count w/ differential, Gram stain & culture, pH; remaining fluid for additional studies as dictated by clinical scenario
  Complications: PTX (5–10%), hemothorax (~1%), re-expansion pulm edema (if >1.5 L removed), spleen/liver lac.; post-tap CXR not routinely needed *(Annals 1996;124:816)*
  ↓ PTX w/ U/S and experienced supervisor; even with INR ~1.9, risk of bleed low w/ U/S & experienced operator *(Chest 2009;135:1315 & 2013;144:456; Archives 2010;170:332)*
- **Transudate vs. exudate** *(JAMA 2014;311:2422)*
  Light's criteria: exudate = TP_eff/TP_serum >0.5 or LDH_eff/LDH_serum >0.6 or LDH_eff >²/₃ ULN of LDH_serum; 97% Se, 85% Sp; best Se of all methods; however, will misidentify 25% of transudates as exudates; ∴ if clinically suspect transudate but meets criterion for exudate, confirm w/ test w/ higher Sp
  exudative criteria w/ better Sp: chol_eff >55 mg/dL (95–99% Sp); chol_eff >45 mg/dL and LDH_eff >200 (98% Sp); chol_eff/chol_serum >0.3 (94% Sp); serum-effusion alb gradient ≤1.2 (92% Sp); serum-effusion TP gradient ≤3.1 (91% Sp)
  CHF effusions: TP may ↑ with diuresis or chronicity → "pseudoexudate"; alb gradient ≤1.2, chol_eff >60 mg/dL (Se 54%, Sp 92%) or clin judgment to distinguish *(Chest 2002;122:1524)*
- **Complicated vs. uncomplicated parapneumonic** *(Chest 1995;108:299)*
  complicated = ⊕ Gram stain or culture or pH <7.2 or glucose <60
  complicated parapneumonic effusions usually require *drainage* to achieve resolution
  empyema = frank pus, also needs drainage to achieve resolution

- Additional pleural fluid studies (NEJM 2002;346:1971)
    - NT-proBNP ≥1500 pg/mL has 91% Se & 93% Sp for CHF (Am J Med 2004;116:417)
    - WBC & diff.: exudates tend to have ↑ WBC vs. transudates but nonspecific
        - neutrophils → parapneumonic, PE, pancreatitis
        - lymphocytes (>50%) → cancer, TB, rheumatologic
        - eos (>10%) → blood, air, drug rxn, asbestos, paragonimiasis, Churg-Strauss, PE
    - RBC: Hct$_{eff}$ 1–20% → cancer, PE, trauma; Hct$_{eff}$/Hct$_{blood}$ >50% → hemothorax
    - AFB: yield in TB 0–10% w/ stain, 11–50% w/ culture, ~70% w/ pleural bx
    - adenosine deaminase (ADA): seen w/ granulomas, >70 suggests TB, <40 excludes TB
    - cytology: ideally ≥150 mL and at least 60 mL should be obtained (Chest 2010;137:68)
    - glucose: <60 mg/dL → malignancy, infection, RA
    - amylase: seen in pancreatic disease and esophageal rupture (salivary amylase)
    - rheumatoid factor, C$_H$50, ANA: limited utility in dx collagen vascular disease
    - triglycerides: >110 → chylothorax, 50–110 → ✓ lipoprotein analysis for chylomicrons
    - cholesterol: >60; seen in chronic effusions (eg, CHF, RA, old TB)
    - creatinine: effusion/serum ratio >1 → urinothorax
    - fibulin-3: ↑ plasma and/or effusion levels → mesothelioma (NEJM 2012;367:1417)
- Chest CT; pleural biopsy; VATS
- Undiagnosed persistent pleural effusions (Clin Chest Med 2006;27:309)
    - Transudative: most commonly CHF or hepatic hydrothorax. ✓ s/s CHF or cirrhosis, NT-proBNP$_{eff}$; consider intraperitoneal injection of technetium-99m sulfur colloid
    - Exudative (ensure using Sp test listed above): most commonly malig, empyema, TB, PE. ✓ s/s malig, chest CT (I⁺), ADA or IFN-γ release assay; consider thoracoscopy.

Characteristics of Pleural Fluid (not diagnostic criteria)						
Etiology	Appear	WBC diff	RBC	pH	Glc	Comments
CHF	clear, straw	<1000 lymphs	<5000	normal	≈ serum	bilateral, cardiomegaly
Cirrhosis	clear, straw	<1000	<5000	normal	≈ serum	right-sided
Uncomplicated parapneumonic	turbid	5–40,000 polys	<5000	normal to ↓	≈ serum (>40)	
Complicated parapneumonic	turbid to purulent	5–40,000 polys	<5000	↓↓	↓↓ (<40)	need drainage
Empyema	purulent	25–100,000 polys	<5000	↓↓↓	↓↓	need drainage
Tuberculosis	serosang.	5–10,000 lymphs	<10,000	normal to ↓	normal to ↓	⊕ AFB ⊕ ADA
Malignancy	turbid to bloody	1–100,000 lymphs	<100,000	normal to ↓	normal to ↓	⊕ cytology
Pulmonary embolism	sometimes bloody	1–50,000	<100,000	normal	≈ serum	no infarct → transudate
Rheumatoid arthritis/SLE	turbid	1–20,000 variable	<1000	↓	RA ↓↓↓ SLE nl	↑ RF, ↓ C$_H$50 ↑ imm. complex
Pancreatitis	serosang. to turbid	1–50,000 polys	<10,000	normal	≈ serum	left-sided, ↑ amylase
Esophageal rupture	turbid to purulent	<5000 >50,000	<10,000	↓↓↓	↓↓	left-sided, ↑ amylase

Treatment

- Symptomatic effusion: therapeutic thoracentesis, treat underlying disease process
- Parapneumonic effusion (Chest 2000;118:1158)
    - uncomplicated → antibiotics for pneumonia
    - >½ hemithorax or complicated or empyema → tube thoracostomy
        (otherwise risk of organization and subsequent need for surgical decortication)
    - loculated→ tube thoracostomy or VATS; intrapleural t-PA + DNase ↓ need for surgical referral (NEJM 2011;365:518)
- Malignant effusion: serial thoracenteses vs. tube thoracostomy + pleurodesis (success rate ~80–90%) vs. indwelling pleural catheter (JAMA 2012;307:2383); systemic steroids & pH <7.2 a/w ↑ pleurodesis failure rate
- TB effusions: effusion will often resolve spontaneously; however, treat Pt for active TB
- Hepatic hydrothorax
    - Rx: Δ pressure gradient (ie, ↓ ascitic fluid volume, NIPPV)
    - avoid chest tubes; prn thoracenteses, pleurodesis, TIPS or VATS closure of diaphragmatic defects if medical Rx fails; NIPPV for acute short-term management
    - spontaneous bacterial empyema (SBEM) can occur (even w/o SBP being present), ∴ thoracentesis if suspect infection
    - transplant is definitive treatment and workup should begin immediately

Definitions
- Superficial thrombophlebitis: pain, tenderness, erythema along superficial vein
- Deep venous thrombosis (DVT): **Proximal** = thrombosis of iliac, femoral, or popliteal veins (nb, "superficial" femoral vein part of deep venous system). **Distal** = calf veins below knee; lower risk of PE/death than proximal (Thromb Haem 2009;102:493).
- Pulmonary embolism (PE): thrombosis originating in venous system and embolizing to pulmonary arterial circulation; 1 case/1000 person y; 250,000/y (Archives 2003;163:1711)

Risk factors
- Virchow's triad for thrombogenesis
  - **stasis:** bed rest, inactivity, CHF, CVA w/in 3 mo, air travel >6 h (NEJM 2001:779)
  - **injury to endothelium:** trauma, surgery, prior DVT, inflamm., central catheter
  - **thrombophilia:** genetic disorders (qv), HIT, OCP, HRT, tamoxifen, raloxifene
- Malignancy (12% of "idiopathic" DVT/PE; Circ 2013;128:2614)
- History of thrombosis (greater risk of recurrent VTE than genetic thrombophilia)
- Obesity, smoking, acute infection, postpartum (JAMA 1997;277:642; Circ 2012;125:2092)

Thromboprophylaxis (Chest 2012;141:e195S, 227S, 278S)	
Patient & situation	**Prophylaxis**
Low-risk med; same-day surg & <40 y	Early, aggressive ambulation
Minor surgery in mobile Pt	Mechanical Ppx
High-risk med (immobile, h/o VTE, thrombophilia or cancer) & most surgery Pts	UFH 5000 U SC bid or tid, or **LMWH**, or fonda (if HIT ⊕), or mech Ppx (esp. if high bleed risk); ? extended Ppx w/ NOAC (NEJM 2016;375:534)
High-risk surg (trauma, stroke, spinal cord injury, h/o VTE/thrombophilia)	[LMWH or UFH SC] + mech Ppx
Orthopedic surgery	LMWH [or fonda, direct oral anticoag (qv) or warfarin (INR 2–3)] + mech Ppx; NOACs overall appear favorable vs LMWH

For enoxaparin, 30 mg bid for highest risk or 40 mg qd for moderate risk or spinal/epidural anesth. Dose adjust: qd in CrCl <30 mL/min, ↑ 30% if BMI >40 (Ann Pharmacother 2009;43:1064).

Clinical manifestations—DVT
- Calf pain, swelling (>3 cm c/w unaffected side), venous distention, erythema, warmth, tenderness, palpable cord, ⊕ Homan's sign (calf pain on dorsiflexion, seen in <5%)
- *Phlegmasia cerulea dolens:* massive prox DVT w/ edema, *cyanosis*, pain, compart. synd.
- 50% of Pts with sx DVT have asx PE
- Popliteal (Baker's) cyst: may lead to DVT due to compression of popliteal vein

"Simplified Wells" Pretest Probability Scoring of DVT (JAMA 2006;295:199)
+1 point each for: active cancer (Rx ongoing or w/in 6 mo or palliative); paralysis, paresis, or recent immobilization of lower extremities; recently bedridden for ≥3 d or major surgery w/in 12 wk; localized tenderness along distribution of deep venous system; entire leg swelling; calf ≥3 cm larger than asx calf (at 10 cm below tibial tuberosity); pitting edema confined to sx leg; collateral superficial veins (nonvaricose); previous DVT −2 points if alternative dx at least as likely as DVT

Pretest Probability Assessment (useful if outPt, less so if inPt; JAMA IM 2015;175:1112)		
Score ≤0	Score 1 or 2	Score ≥3
Low probability (5%)	Moderate probability (17%)	High probability (53%)

- For UE DVT, +1 point each for venous cath, local pain, & unilateral edema, −1 if alternative dx. ≤1 = unlikely; ≥2 = likely. U/S if likely or if unlikely but abnl D-dimer (Annals 2014;160:451)

Diagnostic studies—DVT
- D-dimer: <500 helps r/o; ? use 1000 as threshold if low risk (Annals 2013;158:93)
- Compression U/S >95% Se & Sp for sx DVT (lower if asx); survey whole leg if ≥mod prob

Figure 2-3 Approach to suspected DVT (Chest 2012;141:e351S)

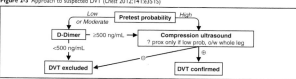

Clinical manifestations—PE
- Dyspnea (~50%), pleuritic chest pain (~40%), cough (~23%), hemoptysis (~8%)
- ↑ RR (>70%), crackles (51%), ↑ HR (30%), fever, cyanosis, pleural friction rub, loud P_2
- *Massive:* syncope, HoTN, PEA; ↑ JVP, R-sided S_3, Graham Steell (PR) murmur

Simplified Wells Pretest Probability Scoring for PE (Annals 2011;154:709)	
• Prior PE or DVT	• Clinical signs of DVT
• Active cancer	• HR >100 bpm
• Immobilization (bed rest ≥3 d) or surgery w/in 4 wk	• Hemoptysis
• Alternative dx less likely than PE	
Dichotomized Wells Probability Assessment	
≤1 Variable = "Unlikely" (13% probability)	≥2 Variables = "Likely" (39% probability)

Diagnostic studies—PE (EHJ 2014;35:3033)
- CXR (limited Se & Sp): 12% nl, atelectasis, effusion, ↑ hemidiaphragm, Hampton hump (wedge-shaped density abutting pleura); Westermark sign (avascularity distal to PE)
- ECG (limited Se & Sp): sinus tachycardia, AF; signs of RV strain → RAD, P pulmonale, RBBB, $S_I Q_{III} T_{III}$ & TWI V_1-V_4 (McGinn-White sign) (Chest 1997;111:537)
- ABG: hypoxemia, hypocapnia, respiratory alkalosis, ↑ A-a gradient (Chest 1996;109:78) 18% w/ room air P_aO_2 85–105 mmHg, 6% w/ nl A-a gradient (Chest 1991;100:598)
- D-dimer (JAMA 2015;313:1668): high Se, poor Sp (~25%); ⊖ ELISA has >99% NPV ∴ use to r/o PE if "unlikely" pretest prob. (JAMA 2006;295:172) consider age-specific cut point: 500 if <50 y, 10× age if ≥50 y (JAMA 2014;311:1117)
- Echocardiography: useful for risk stratification (RV dysfxn), but not dx (Se <50%)
- V/Q scan: high Se (~98%), low Sp (~10%). Sp improves to 97% for high prob VQ. Use if pretest prob of PE high and CT not available or contraindicated. Can also exclude PE if low pretest prob, low prob VQ, but 4% false ⊖ (JAMA 1990;263:2753).
- **CT angiography** (CTA; see Radiology inserts; JAMA 2015;314:74): Se ~90% & Sp ~95%; PPV & NPV >95% if imaging concordant w/ clinical suspicion, ≤80% if discordant (∴ need to consider both); ~1/4 of single & subseg may be false ⊕; CT may also provide other dx
- Lower extremity compression U/S shows DVT in ~9%, sparing CTA, but when added to CTA, does not Δ outcomes (Lancet 2008;371:1343)

Figure 2-4 Approach to suspected PE (Annals 2015;163:701)

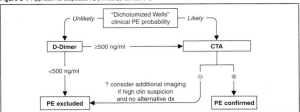

Workup for idiopathic VTE (NEJM 2015;373:697)
- **Thrombophilia workup:** ✓ if ⊕ FH, may be helpful but consider timing as thrombus, heparin and warfarin Δ results. Not helpful for Pt if will not Δ management (eg, plan for long-term anticoagulation regardless), although could be of use to relatives.
- **Malignancy workup:** 12% Pts w/ "idiopathic" DVT/PE will have malignancy; age-appropriate screening adequate; avoid extensive w/u

Risk stratification for Pts with PE
- **Clinical:** hypotension and/or tachycardia (~30% mortality), hypoxemia
- **CTA:** RV/LV dimension ratio >0.9 (Circ 2004;110:3276)
- **Biomarkers:** ↑ troponin & ↑ BNP a/w ↑ mortality; w/ ⊖ Tn, decomp extremely unlikely (Circ 2002;106:1263 & 2003;107:1576; Chest 2015;147:685)
- **Echocardiogram:** RV dysfxn (even if normal troponin) (Chest 2013;144:1539)

Whom to treat (Lancet 2012;379:1835; Chest 2012;141:e419S)
- **Superficial venous thrombosis:** elevate extremity, warm compresses, compression stockings, NSAIDs for sx. *Anticoag* if high risk for DVT (eg, ≥5 cm, proximity to deep vein ≤5 cm, other risk factors) for 4 wk as ~10% have VTE w/in 3 mo (Annals 2010;152:218)
- **LE DVT:** proximal → anticoag. If distal: anticoag if severe sx, o/w consider serial imaging over 2 wk and anticoag if extends (although if bleeding risk low, many would anticoag).

- **UE DVT:** anticoagulate (same guidelines as LE; *NEJM* 2011;364:861). If catheter-associated, need not remove if catheter functional and ongoing need for catheter.
- **PE:** anticoagulate

Anticoagulation options (*Chest* 2012;141:e419S & 2016;149:315; *JAMA* 2014;311:717)

- *Initiate parenteral Rx immediately if high or intermed suspicion while dx testing underway*
- **Non-vitamin K antag oral anticoag** (*NEJM* 2010;363:2499; 2012;366:1287; 2013;369:799 & 1406)
  Preferred b/c as good/better than warfarin in preventing recurrent VTE w/ less bleeding
  Can give as sole anticoag w/ initial loading dose (riva or apixa) or initiate after ≥5 d *of parenteral anticoag* (edox or dabi); 1st dose when d/c IV UFH or w/in 2 h before when next LMWH dose would have been due)
- **LMWH** (eg, enoxaparin 1 mg/kg SC bid *or* dalteparin 200 IU/kg SC qd)
  Preferred over UFH (espec in *cancer*): renal failure (CrCl <25), extreme obesity, hemodynamic instability or bleeding risk (*Cochrane* 2004;CD001100)
  Can use as outpatient bridge to long-term oral anticoagulation
- If cancer, LMWH ↓ recurrence and mortality c/w UFH & warfarin (*NEJM* 2003;349:146; *Lancet Oncol* 2008;9:577); ✓ head CT for brain mets if melanoma, renal cell, thyroid, chorioCA
- **Fondaparinux:** 5–10 mg SC qd (*NEJM* 2003;349:1695); use if HIT ⊕; avoid if renal failure
- **IV UFH:** 80 U/kg bolus → 18 U/kg/h → titrate to PTT 1.5–2.3 × cntl (eg, 60–85 sec); preferred option when contemplating thrombolysis or catheter-based Rx (qv)
- IV Direct thrombin inhibitors (eg, argatroban, lepirudin) used in HIT ⊕ Pts
- **Warfarin** (goal INR 2–3): start same day as parenteral anticoag unless instability and ? need for lytic, catheter-based Rx or surgery; overlap ≥5 d w/ parenteral anticoag & until INR ≥2 × ≥24 h

Systemic thrombolysis (*Chest* 2012;141:e419S & 2016;149:315)

- Typically TPA 100 mg over 2 h *or* wt-adjusted TNK bolus; risk of ICH ~1.5%, ↑ w/ age
- **Massive PE** (hemodynamic compromise): ↓ death and recurrent PE each by ~50% (*JAMA* 2014;311:2414; *EHJ* 2015;36:605) & lower PVR long term (*JACC* 1990;15:65)
- **Submassive PE** (hemodyn. stable but RV dysfxn on echo or enlargement on CTA, or ? marked dyspnea or severe hypoxemia): ↓ hemodyn. decompensation, ↑ ICH, ↓ mortality; consider if <75 y and/or low bleed risk (*NEJM* 2014;370:1402; *JAMA* 2014;311:2414). Some centers prefer catheter-directed therapy.
- **Moderate PE w/ large clot burden** (≥2 lobar arteries or main artery on CT or high-prob VQ w/ ≥2 lobes w/ mismatch): *low-dose lytic* (50 mg if ≥50 kg or 0.5 mg/kg if <50 kg; for both 10-mg bolus → remainder over 2 h) ↓ pulm HTN w/ ≈ bleeding vs. heparin alone
- **DVT:** consider if (a) acute (<14 d) & extensive (eg, iliofemoral), (b) severe sx swelling or ischemia, (c) catheter-directed Rx not available, and (d) low bleed risk

Mechanical intervention

- **Catheter-directed** (fibrinolytic & thrombus fragmentation/aspiration; *Circ* 2012;126:1917)
  Consider if extensive DVT (see above) and to ↓ postthrombotic synd (*Lancet* 2012;379:31)
  Consider if PE w/ hemodyn. compromise or high risk & not candidate for systemic lysis or surgical thrombectomy (*Circ* 2011;124:2139). Preferred to systemic lytic by some centers.
  U/S-assisted improves hemodynamics & RV fxn vs. anticoag alone (*EHJ* 2015;36:597)
- **Thrombectomy:** if large, proximal PE + hemodynamic compromise + contra. to lysis; consider in experienced ctr if large prox. PE + RV dysfxn (*J Thorac CV Surg* 2005;129:1018)
- **IVC filter:** use instead of anticoagulation if latter contraindicated
  No benefit to adding to anticoag (including in submassive) (*JAMA* 2015;313:1627)
  Consider removable filter for temporary indications
  Complications: migration, acute DVT, ↑ risk of recurrent DVT & IVC obstruction (5–18%)

Duration of full-intensity anticoagulation

- Superficial venous thrombosis: 4 wk
- 1st prox DVT *or* PE 2° reversible/time-limited risk factor *or* distal DVT: 3–6 mo
- 1st *unprovoked* prox DVT/PE: ≥3 mo, then reassess; benefit to prolonged Rx
  Consider clot, bleed risk, Pt preference, and intensity of Rx when crafting strategy:
  full-dose NOAC: 80–90% ↓ recurrent VTE, 2–5× bleeding, but no signif excess in major bleeding (*NEJM* 2010;363:2499; 2013;368:699 & 709)
    ½ dose apixa (2.5 mg bid): 80% ↓ recur. VTE, w/o signif ↑ bleeding (*NEJM* 2013;368:699)
    warfarin, either regular (*JAMA* 2015;314:31) or low-intensity (*NEJM* 2003;348:1425)
    aspirin: 32% ↓ recurrent VTE (*NEJM* 2012;366:1959 & 367:1979)
- 2nd VTE event or cancer: indefinite (or until cancer cured) (*NEJM* 2003;348:1425)

Complications & prognosis

- Postthrombotic syndrome (23–60%): pain, edema, venous ulcers
- Recurrent VTE: 1%/y (after 1st VTE) to 5%/y (after recurrent VTE)
- Chronic thromboembolic PHT after acute PE ~3.8%, consider thromboendarterectomy
- Mortality: ~10% for DVT and ~10–15% for PE at 3–6 mo (*Circ* 2008;117:1711)

PHT defined as PA mean pressure ≥25 mmHg at rest
$PA\ mean = CO \times PVR + PA\ wedge\ pressure.\ Trans\ pulm\ gradient = PA\ mean - PA\ wedge.$

Etiologies (Revised WHO Classification) (Circ 2009;119:2250)

Primary Pulmonary arterial HTN (PAH) (group 1) Precapillary PHT PCWP ≤15 mmHg ↑ transpulm grad ↑ PVR	• Idiopathic (IPAH): yearly incidence 1–2 per million; mean age of onset 36 y (♂ older than ♀); ♂:♀ = ~2:1, usually mild ↑ in PAP
	• Familial (FPAH)
	• Associated conditions (APAH)
	  Connective tissue dis.: CREST, SLE, MCTD, RA, PM, Sjögren
	  Congenital L→R shunts: ASD,VSD, PDA
	  Portopulmonary HTN (? 2° vasoactive substances not filtered in ESLD; ≠ hepatopulmonary syndrome)
	  HIV; drugs & toxins: anorexic agents, L-tryptophan
	• Pulmonary veno-occlusive disease: ? 2° chemo; BMT; orthopnea, pl eff, CHF, nl PCWP; art vasodil. worsen CHF (AJRCCM 2000;162:1964)
	• Pulmonary capillary hemangiomatosis

Left heart disease (group 2). ↑ PCWP	• Left atrial or ventricular (diastolic or systolic) dysfunction • Left-sided valvular heart disease (eg, MS/MR)
Lung diseases and/ or chronic hypoxemia (group 3)	• COPD • Alveolar hypoventilation (eg, NM disease) • ILD • Chronic hypoxemia (eg, high altitude) • Sleep apnea • Developmental abnormalities
Chronic thrombo-embolic dis (group 4)	• Prox or distal PEs; ~½ w/o clinical h/o PE (NEJM 2011;364:351) • Nonthrombotic emboli (tumor, foreign body, parasites)
Miscellaneous (group 5)	• Sarcoidosis, histiocytosis X, LAM, schistosomiasis, ESRD • Compression of pulm vessels (adenopathy, tumor, fibrosing mediastinitis, histoplasmosis, XRT) • Other: thyroid dis., glycogen storage dis., Gaucher dis., HHT, sickle cell etc, chronic myeloprolif d/o, splenectomy

Clinical manifestations
• Dyspnea, exertional syncope (hypoxia, ↓ CO), exertional chest pain (RV ischemia)
• Symptoms of R-sided CHF (eg, peripheral edema, RUQ fullness, abdominal distention)
• WHO class: I = asx w/ ordinary activity; II= sx w/ ord. activ; III = sx w/ min activ; IV = sx at rest

Physical exam
• PHT: prominent P_2, R-sided S_4, RV heave, PA tap & flow murmur, PR (Graham Steell), TR
• ± RV failure: ↑ JVP, hepatomegaly, peripheral edema

Diagnostic studies & workup (JACC 2013;62:D40; Circ 2014;130:1820)
• High-res chest CT: dil. & pruning of pulm arteries, ↑ RA & RV; r/o parenchymal lung dis.
• ECG: RAD, RBBB, RAE ("P pulmonale"), RVH (Se 55%, Sp 70%)
• PFTs: disproportionate ↓ D_Lco, mild restrictive pattern; r/o obstructive & restrict. lung dis.
• ABG & polysomnography: ↓ P_aO_2 and S_aO_2 (espec w/ exertion), ↓ P_aCO_2, ↑ A-a gradient; r/o hypoventilation and OSA
• TTE: ↑ RVSP (but estimate over/under by ≥10 mmHg in ½ of PHT Pts; Chest 2011;139:988) ↑ RA, RV, & PA; ↑ pressure → interventricular septum systolic flattening ("D" shape) ↓ RV systolic fxn (TAPSE <1.6 cm);TR, PR; r/o LV dysfxn, MV,AoV, congenital disease
• RHC: ↑ RA, RV, & PA pressures; ✓ L-sided pressures and for shunt
   if PAH: nl PCWP, ↑ transpulm gradient (mean PAP-PCWP >12–15), ↑ PVR, ± ↓ CO
   if 2° to L-heart disease: PCWP (or LVEDP) >15; if PVR nl → "passive PHT"; PVR >240 suggests mixed picture: if ↓ PCWP → ↓ PVR, then "reactive" PHT; if no Δ, then "fixed"
• CTA (large/med vessel),V/Q scan (small vessel to r/o CTEPH), ± pulm angio if still concern
• Vasculitis labs: ANA (~40% ⊕ in PAH), RF, anti-Scl-70, anticentromere, ESR
• LFTs & HIV: r/o portopulmonary and HIV-associated PAH
• 6-min walk test (6MWT) or cardiopulmonary exercise testing to establish fxnl capacity

Treatment (JACC 2013;62:25S & 2015;65:1976; EHJ 2016;37:67)
• Principles: 1) prevent & reverse vasoactive substance imbalance and vascular remodeling
   2) prevent RV failure: ↓ wall stress (↓ PVR, PAP, RV diam); ensure adeq. systemic DBP
• **Supportive**
   Oxygen: maintain S_aO_2 >90–92% (reduces vasoconstriction)
   Diuretics: ↓ RV wall stress and relieve RHF sx; gentle b/c RV is preload dependent
   Digoxin: control AF, ? counteract neg. inotropic effects CCB
   Dobutamine and inhaled NO or prostacyclin for decompensated PHT
   Anticoag: not routinely used; ↓ VTE risk of RHF; ? prevention of in situ microthrombi; ? mort. benefit even if in NSR, no RCTs (Circ 1984;70:580; Chest 2006;130:545)
   Supervised exercise training; aggressive apnea/hypoventilatory Rx w/ CPAP/BiPAP

- **Vasodilators** (ideally right heart catheterization prior to initiation; *NEJM* 2004;351:1425) *acute vasoreactivity test:* use inh NO, adenosine or prostacyclin to identify Pts likely to have long-term response to CCB (⊕ response = ↓ PAP ≥10 mmHg to <40 mmHg w/ ↑ or stable CO); ~10% Pts acute responders; no response → still candidate for other vasodil.

Vasoactive agents	Comments (data primarily in Group 1; little evidence in 2° PHT)
PDE-5 Inhibitor Sildenafil, tadalafil, vardenafil	↑ cGMP → vasodilation, ↓ smooth muscle proliferation, ↓ sx, ↑ 6MWT, no data on clinical outcomes. Often first-line b/c minimal side-effect profile: HA, vision Δ's, sinus congestion (*NEJM* 2009;361:1864).
Endothelin receptor antagonists (ERAs) Bosentan, ambrisentan, macitentan	↓ Smooth muscle remodeling, vasodilation, ↓ fibrosis, ↓ sx, ↑ 6MWT, ↓ worsening PAH or need for prostanoids w/ trend for ↓ PAH mort. (w/ macitentan). Side effects: ↑ LFTs, HA, anemia, edema, teratogen (*NEJM* 2002;346:896; *Circ* 2008;117:3010; *NEJM* 2013;369:809).
IV Prostacyclin Epoprostenol (Flolan)	Vasodilation, ↓ plt agg, ↓ smooth muscle proliferation; benefits ↑ w/ time (? vascular remodeling). ↑ 6MWT, ↑ QoL, ↓ **mortality.** Side effects: HA, flushing, jaw/leg pain, abd cramps, nausea, diarrhea, catheter infxn (*NEJM* 1996;334:296 & 1998;338:273; *Annals* 2000;132:425).
Prostacyclin analogues [Iloprost (inh) Treprostinil (IV, inh, SC)] & **receptor agonist** selexipag (PO)	Same mechanism as prostacyclin but easier to take, ↓ side effects, and w/o risk of catheter infxn, ↓ sx, ↑ 6MWT; trend to ↓ clinical events w/ iloprost but not treprostinil. Inh Rx with improved V/Q matching. Selexipag ↓ disease prog & hosp by ~40% (*NEJM* 2015;373:2522).
Soluble guanylate cyclase (sGC) stim. Riociguat	NO-independent ↑ cGMP → vasodilation, ↓ smooth muscle proliferation, ↓ sx, ↑ 6MWT in PAH; ↓ sx, ↓ PVR, ↑ 6MWT in CTEPH (*NEJM* 2013;369:319 & 330).
Oral CCB Nifedipine, diltiazem	Consider if ⊕ acute vasoreactive response; <½ long-term responder (NYHA I/II & near-full hemodynamics) have ↓ mortality. Not 1st line b/c side effects: HoTN, lower limb edema (*Circ* 2005;111:3105).

- Upfront combination Rx (tadalafil + ambrisentan vs. monotherapy): ↓ sx, ↓ NT-BNP, ↑ 6MWT, ↓ hospitalizations (*NEJM* 2015;373:834)
- Treat underlying causes of 2° PHT; can use vasodilators, although little evidence
- CTEPH: Rx as above. Pulm endarterectomy potentially curative (*AJRCCM* 2011;183:1605).
- Refractory PHT:
  balloon atrial septostomy: R→L shunt causes ↑ CO, ↓ S$_a$O$_2$, net ↑ tissue O$_2$ delivery
  lung transplant (single or bilateral); heart-lung needed if Eisenmenger physiology

Figure 2-5 Treatment of PAH (modified from *JACC* 2013;62:D60 & *EHJ* 2016;37:67)

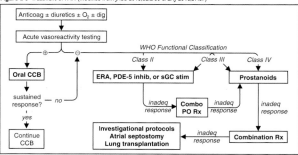

Management of ICU patient
- Avoid tachyarrhythmias & overly aggressive volume resuscitation
- Caution w/ vasodilators if any L-sided dysfxn. *Intubation can cause hemodynamic collapse.*
- May benefit from inotropes/chronotropes
- Consider fibrinolysis if acute, refractory decompensation (eg, TPA 100 mg over 2 h)

Prognosis
- Median survival after dx ~2.8 y; PAH (all etiologies): 2-y 66%, 5-y 48% (*Chest* 2004;126:78-S)
- Poor prognostic factors: clinical evidence of RV failure, rapidly progressive sx, WHO (modified NYHA) class IV, 6MWT <300 m, peak VO$_2$ <10.4 mL/kg/min, ↑ RA or RV or RV dysfxn, RA >20 or CI <2.0, ↑ BNP (*Chest* 2006;129:1313)
- Lung transplant: 1-y survival 66–75%; 5-y survival 45–55% (*Chest* 2004;126:63-S)

$$\text{Hypoxemia} \rightarrow P_AO_2 = F_iO_2 \times (760 - 47) - \frac{P_aCO_2}{R}$$

- **A-a gradient** = $P_AO_2 - P_aO_2$: normal (*on room air*) = "4 + age/4" or "2.5 + (0.2 × age)"
- Hypoxemia + nl A-a gradient: problem is ↓ P_iO_2/F_iO_2 or ↑ P_aCO_2 (ie, hypoventilation)
- Hypoxemia + ↑ A-a gradient: problem is either
  - R → L shunt, anatomic (congen. heart dis.) or severe pathophys. (alveoli filled w/ fluid; eg, PNA, pulm edema); cannot overcome w/ 100% O_2 b/c of sigmoidal Hb-O_2 curve
  - V/Q mismatch where "shunt-like" areas (↓ V & nl Q) cause unoxygenated blood to mix with oxygenated blood; can be overcome w/ ↑ O_2 delivery
  - Diffusion limitation: generally seen with exercise/↑CO

Figure 2-6 Workup of acute hypoxemia

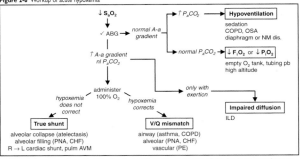

- **Cyanosis:** seen when >4 g/dL of reduced Hb in blood vessels of skin/mucous membranes
  - central: ↓ S_aO_2 (pulm disease, shunt); abnl Hb [metHb, sulfHb, COHb (not true cyanosis)]
  - peripheral: ↓ blood flow → ↑ O_2 extraction (eg, ↓ CO, cold, arterial or venous obstruction)

Chemical Causes of Cellular Hypoxia

Condition	Causes	Classic features	P_aO_2	Pulse Ox sat	CO-Ox sat	Treatment (+ 100% O_2)
Carbon monoxide	Fires, portable heaters, auto exhaust	Cherry-red skin (COHb color)	nl	nl	↓	Hyperbaric O_2
Methemoglobinemia	Nitrates, sulfonamide, benzocaine, dapsone	Chocolate brown blood	nl	mild ↓	↓	Methylene blue
Cyanide	Nitroprusside, fires, industrial	Bitter almond odor; pink skin	nl	nl (↑ S_vO_2)	nl	Hydroxycobalamin

CO binds to Hb more avidly than does O_2. Pulse oximeter (Ox) misreads COHb as HbO_2 → falsely nl sat.
Oxidizing drugs Δ Hb (ferrous) to MetHb (ferric), which cannot carry O_2. Pulse ox misreads MetHb as HbO_2.
Cyanide inhibits mitochondrial O_2 use → cellular hypoxia but pink skin and ↑ venous O_2 sat.

$$\text{Hypercapnia} \rightarrow P_aCO_2 = k \times \frac{V_{CO_2}}{RR \times V_T \times \left(1 - \frac{V_D}{V_T}\right)}$$

Etiologies of High ↑ P_aCO_2

"Won't Breathe"	"Can't Breathe"		
↓ RR	↓ V_T		↑ V_D and/or ↓ V_T
Respiratory Drive	**NM System**	**CW/Pleura**	**Lung/Airways**
Voluntary hypervent. Nl PI_{max} & A-a grad.	↓ PI_{max} ↓ PE_{max}	Abnl PEx Abnl CT	Abnl PFTs ↓ End Tidal CO_2
Metabolic alkalosis **1° neurologic:** brainstem stroke, tumor, 1° alveolar hypovent	**Neuropathies:** cervical spine, phrenic nerve, GBS, ALS, polio	**Chest wall:** obesity, kyphosis, scoliosis	**Lung parench.:** emphysema, ILD/fibrosis, CHF, PNA
2° neurologic: sedatives, CNS infxn, hypothyroidism	**NMJ:** MG, LE **Myopathies:** diaphragm PM/DM; ↓ PO_4 musc dystrophies	**Pleura:** fibrosis effusion	**Airways:** asthma, COPD, OSA, bronchiect., CF

↑VCO_2 typically transient cause of ↑ P_aCO_2; Ddx: exercise, fever, hyperthyroidism, ↑ work of breathing, ↑ carbs.

Indications

- Improve gas exchange: ↑ oxygenation, ↑ alveolar vent. and/or reverse acute resp. acidosis
- Relieve respiratory distress: ↓ work of breathing (can account for up to 50% of total O_2 consumption), ↓ respiratory muscle fatigue
- Apnea, airway protection, pulmonary toilet

SUPPORTIVE STRATEGIES PRIOR TO INTUB. OR AFTER EXTUB.

Oxygen Delivery Systems (Lancet 2016;387:1867)		
System or Device	**O_2 Flow[a]**	**F_iO_2 range & Comments**
Low-flow nasal cannula	1–6	24–40%, 1L adds approx 3% F_iO_2
Standard face mask	5–10	35–50%, minimum 5 L/min
Partial rebreather mask	>10	40–70%
Nonrebreather mask	>10	60–80% (not 100% b/c air leaks)
Air-entrainment mask (Venturi or Vmask)	10–15[b]	24–50%, F_iO_2 stays constant
High-flow nasal O_2 (NEJM 2015;372:2185 JAMA 2015;313:2331 & 2016;315:1354)	≤40	21–100%. In nonhypercapnic acute hypoxemic resp failure, ± ↓ intub. (espec if P_aO_2/F_iO_2 <200) & ↓ 90-d mort vs. stnd O_2 or NPPV. Routine use after extub. ↓ need for reintub.

[a]L/min. [b]Total airflow >60L/min. (Adapted from Marino P. The ICU Book, 4th ed, Philadelphia: LWW, 2014:431)

Noninvasive Positive Pressure Ventilation (NPPV) (NEJM 2015;372:e30)	
Indications Lancet 2009;374:250	*Clinical:* mod–severe dyspnea, RR >24–30, signs of ↑ work of breathing, accessory muscle use, abd paradox *Gas exchange:* P_aCO_2 >45 mmHg (& significantly worse than baseline), hypoxemia, P_aO_2/F_iO_2 <200
Contraindications Crit Care Med 2007;35:2402	Claustrophobia, poor mask fit, Δ**MS**, vomiting, **cannot protect airway**, extrapulm organ failure, HD instab, sev UGIB, ↑ secretions
Continuous positive airway pressure (CPAP)	≈ PEEP. Pt breathes spont. at own rate while vent maintains constant positive airway pressure throughout respiratory cycle. No limit on O_2 delivered (ie, can give hi-flow → F_iO_2 ~1.0) Used if primary problem *hypoxemia* (eg, CHF)
Bilevel positive airway pressure (BiPAP)	≈ PSV + PEEP. Able to set both inspiratory (usually 8–10 cm H_2O) and expiratory pressures (usually <5 cm H_2O). Used if primary problem *hypoventilation*; F_iO_2 delivery limited
Mask ventilation (? helmet better; JAMA 2016;315:2435)	Tight-fitting mask connecting patient to a standard ventilator Can receive PS ~20–30 cm H_2O, PEEP ~10 cm H_2O, F_iO_2 ~1.0 Used for short-term support (<24 h) for a reversible process
Conditions w/ strong evidence Lancet 2000;355:1931 AJRCCM 2006;173:164 JAMA 2016;315:1345 NEJM 2001;344:481	**Cardiogenic pulmonary edema:** may ↓ intub. & mortality (JAMA 2005;294:3124; Lancet 2006;367:1155) although recent trial (w/ high crossover) did not show any mortality benefit (NEJM 2008;359:142) **COPD exac.** w/ ↑ P_aCO_2: ↓ intub. & mort., but if pH <7.3 → intubate High-risk extub. (age >65, CHF, APACHE II >12): NPPV × 24 h directly after extub. → ↓ reintub. and, if P_aCO_2 >45 mmHg during SBT, ↓ mortality Hypoxemic resp failure after abdominal surgery: ↓ reintubation **Immunosupp.** w/ infiltrates: ↓ complications & mortality

VENTILATOR MANAGEMENT

Ventilator Modes and Principles (NEJM 2001;344:1986, CHEST 2015;148:340–355)	
Cont. mandatory ventilation (CMV), aka Assist control (AC)	Vent delivers a minimum number of supported breaths Additional Pt-initiated breaths trigger *fully assisted* vent breaths ∴ Vent-triggered breaths identical to Pt-triggered breaths Tachypnea → ↑ resp. alkalosis, breath-stacking, & auto-PEEP May be pressure targeted or volume targeted (qv)
Pressure support vent (PSV)	Support Pt-initiated breaths w/ a set inspiratory pressure & PEEP A mode of *partial* vent support because no set rate
Other	Synch intermittent mand. vent: deliver min. # supported breaths; V_T of additional Pt-initiated breaths determined by Pt's effort Proportional assist ventilation (PAV): delivers variable pressure to achieve targeted % of work of breathing

Volume or Pressure Targeted	
Volume targeted	Vent delivers a set V_T; pressures depend on airway resist. & lung/CW compl. **Benefit:** ↑ control over ventilation (ideal initial ventilator setting); benefit in ALI/ARDS; easy to measure mechanics (PIP, P_{plat}, airway resist., compl.) Volume control (VC) ⊕: vent delivers variable pressure (depending on real-time lung compliance) to achieve V_T.
Pressure targeted	Vent delivers a fixed inspiratory pressure regardless of V_T V_T depends on airway resistance and lung/chest wall compliance **Benefit:** May ↑ patient comfort (PSV) requiring less sedation
General principles	**Institutional/practitioner preference** and **patient comfort** usually dictate ventilator strategy; no strategy has proven superior **Alarms** can be set for ↑ volumes and ↑ airway pressures in pressure-targeted and volume-targeted strategies, respectively **Risks:** volutrauma (ie, overdistention, if set volume too high; *NEJM 2013;369:2126*), barotrauma [can happen w/ relatively high set volumes (espec if stiff lungs) or if pressure target set too high; key is to monitor transpulmonary pressure (difference between P_{plat} and esophageal ≈ intrapleural), not just airway pressure]; can result in PTX, pneumomediastinum **Hypo-/hyperventilation:** need to ✓ minute vent & pH/P_aCO_2

Variables on the Ventilator	
F_iO_2	Fraction of inspired air that is oxygen
V_T (tidal vol)	Volume of breath delivered; Lung protective ventilation: goal ≤6 cc/kg IBW
f (resp. rate)	Rate set by ventilator, f may be lower than RR if Pt triggering breaths. Adjust to achieve desired P_aCO_2.
Positive end-expiratory pressure (PEEP)	Positive pressure applied during exhalation via resistor in exhalation port Benefits: prevents alveolar collapse, ↓ shunt, ↑ O_2 via alveolar recruitment and improved compliance, allows severely obstructed Pt to initiate breath Cardiac effects: ↓ preload by ↑ intrathoracic pressure → ↓ venous return; ↓ afterload by ↓ cardiac transmural pressure; may ↑ or ↓ CO and may ↑ or ↓ oxygen delivery based on the above Auto-PEEP or intrinsic PEEP: inadequate exhalation time → lungs unable to completely empty before the next breath (ie, "breath stacking"); if flow at end-expiration, there must be pressure = auto-PEEP Will ↓ preload and may ↓ CO, espec if hypovolemic Will ↑ work of breathing as must be overcome by Pt to trigger breaths; can prevent Pt from triggering ventilator, extrinsic PEEP helps Can be detected if end-expiratory flow ≠ 0 before next breath Can measure by occluding expiratory port of vent at end-expiration Can ↓ by: ↑ exp time, ↓ RR, ↓ V_T, Rx bronchospasm and secretions
Inspiratory time	Normally I:E ratio is ~1:2; however, can alter I time (and consequently flow rate, see later); use in pressure-control mode
Inspiratory flow rates	↑ flow rate → ↓ I time → ↑ E time → ∴ may improve ventilation in obstructive disease, but may affect resp rate and bronchodilation/constriction
Peak inspiratory pressure (PIP)	Dynamic measurement during inspiration; set in pressure-targeted mode Determined by airway resistance and lung/chest wall compliance ↑ PIP w/o ↑ P_{plat} → ↑ airway resist (eg, bronchospasm, plugging) ↓ PIP → ↓ airway resistance or air leak in the system
Plateau pressure (P_{plat})	Static measurement at the end of inspiration when there is no flow Determined by resp system compliance (resist. not a factor since Ø flow) ↑ P_{plat} → ↓ lung or chest wall compliance (eg, PTX, pulmonary edema, pneumonia, atelectasis), ↑ PEEP or auto-PEEP P_{plat} <30 cm H_2O ↓ barotrauma (↓V_T, ↓ PEEP or ↑ compl [eg, by diuresis])

Tailoring the ventilator settings
- To improve oxygenation: options include ↑ F_iO_2, ↑ PEEP
  S_aO_2 88–92% acceptable (*AJRCCM 2016;193:43*)
  First, ↑ F_iO_2. If >0.6 and oxygenation remains suboptimal, then try ↑ PEEP: If ↑ P_aO_2/F_iO_2 and P_{plat} stable, suggests recruitable lung (ie, atelectasis). Continue to ↑ PEEP until either can ↓ F_iO_2 to <0.6 or P_{plat} ≥30 cm H_2O. If PEEP 20 & F_iO_2 1.0 and oxygenation remains suboptimal, consider rescue/expt strategies (see "ARDS").

If ↑ PEEP yields no Δ or ↓ P_aO_2/F_iO_2 or ↑ P_aCO_2, suggests additional lung *not* recruitable and instead overdistending lung → ↑ shunt & dead space; ∴ ↓ PEEP
- To improve ventilation: ↑ V_T or inspiratory pressure, ↑ RR (may need to ↓ I time). Nb, tolerate ↑ P_aCO_2 (permissive hypercapnia) in ALI/ARDS (qv) as long as pH >7.15.

Acute ventilatory deterioration (usually ↑ PIP)
- Response to ↑ PIP: disconnect Pt from vent., bag, auscultate, suction, ✓ CXR & ABG

Figure 2-7 Approach to acute ventilatory deterioration

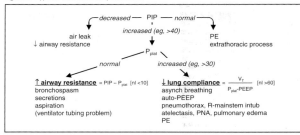

(Adapted from Marino PL. *The ICU Book*, 3rd ed., Philadelphia: Lippincott Williams & Wilkins, 2007:467)

Weaning from the ventilator (NEJM 2012;367:2233; Lancet 2016;387:1856)
- Perform daily assessment of readiness for spontaneous breathing trial (SBT)
- Clinical screening criteria: VS stable, minimal secretions, adequate cough, cause of respiratory failure or previously failed SBT reversed
- Vent parameters: P_aO_2/F_iO_2 >200, PEEP ≤5, f/V_T <105, V_E <12 L/min, VC >10 mL/kg; rapid shallow breathing index (f/V_T) >105 predicts failure, NPV 0.95 (NEJM 1991;324:1445)
- Daily awakening trial (d/c all sedation; Lancet 2008;371:126): open eyes & w/o: agitation, RR >35, S_aO_2 <88%, resp distress or arrhythmias (if fail, restart sedation at ½ prior dose)
- SBT = CPAP or T piece × 30–120 min
  failure if: deteriorating ABGs, ↑ RR, ↑ or ↓ HR, ↑ or ↓ BP, diaphoresis, anxiety
- Tolerate SBT → extubation. Fail SBT → ? cause → work to correct → retry SBT qd
- ? acetazolamide in Pts w/ COPD & metabolic alkalosis (JAMA 2016;315:480)

Complications
- Oxygen toxicity (theoretical); proportional to duration + degree of ↑ oxygen (F_iO_2 >0.6)
- Ventilator-induced lung injury (see "ARDS")
- Ventilator-associated pneumonia (~1%/day, mortality rate ~30%)
  typical pathogens: MRSA, *Pseudomonas*, *Acinetobacter* and *Enterobacter* species
  preventive strategies (AJRCCM 2005;171:388): wash hands, HOB elevated, non-nasal intub., enteral nutrition rather than TPN, routine suction of subglottic secretions, avoid unnecessary abx & transfusions, routine oral antiseptic, stress-ulcer prophylaxis w/ ? sucralfate (↓ VAP, ↑ GIB) vs. H_2RA/PPI, ? silver-coated tubes (JAMA 2008;300:805)
- Laryngeal
  edema: for Pts vent >36 h; ? predicted by ⊕ cuff leak test. Methylprednisolone 20 mg IV q4h starting 12 h pre-extub. → ↓↓ edema and 50% ↓ in reintubation (Lancet 2007;369:1003).
  ulceration: consider *tracheostomy* for patients in whom expect >14 d of mech vent → ↓ duration mech vent, ↓ # ICU days (BMJ 2005;330:1243); no benefit to performing at ~1 wk vs. waiting until ~2 wk (JAMA 2010;303:1483)
- Malnutrition (for all critically ill Pts): enteral nutrition initiated early is safe but not necessary (JAMA 2012;307:795), but bolus may ↑ risk of VAP & *C diff.* (JPEN 2002;26:174); no clear benefit to ✓ing gastric residuals (JAMA 2013;309:249); permissive enteral underfeeding (~½ of calculated caloric req) & standard enteral feeding w/ similar outcomes (NEJM 2015;372:2398); *parenteral* nutrition should be delayed until after day 8 to ↓ risk of infections, cholestasis, RRT, ventilator days (NEJM 2011;365:506)
- Oversedation/delirium: BDZs and polypharmacy are risk factors
  propofol: HoTN in ~25%; *propofol infusion syndrome* (PRIS) ? espec w/ high (>5 mg/kg/h) & prolonged (>48 h) infusions ↓ cardiac vasopressors → ↑ AG, cardiac dysfxn, rhabdomyolysis, ↑ triglycerides, & renal failure (Crit Care 2009;13:R169)
  dexmedetomidine: ↑ vent-free days, but brady & HoTN c/w BDZ (JAMA 2012;307:1151 & 2016;315:1460)

ACUTE RESPIRATORY DISTRESS SYNDROME

Berlin definition (*JAMA 2012;307:2526*)
- **Acute onset** within 1 wk of clinical insult or worsening respiratory status
- **Bilateral infiltrates** without alternative explanation (eg, effusion, atelectasis, nodules)
- **Edema not fully explained** by fluid overload or congestive heart failure
- **Hypoxemia:** P_aO_2/F_iO_2 determined with 5 cm H_2O of PEEP
  P_aO_2/F_iO_2 200–300 = mild ARDS (may be on NPPV), 100–200 = mod, <100 = severe
- Chest CT: heterogeneous lung with densities greater in dependent areas
- Lung bx: diffuse alveolar damage (DAD); Ø req, may give useful dx info (*Chest 2004;125:197*)

Pathophysiology
- ↑ intrapulmonary shunt → hypoxemia (∴ Rx w/ PEEP to prevent derecruitment)
- ↑ increased dead space fraction (see Appendix), predicts ↑ mort. (*NEJM 2002;346:1281*)
- ↓ compliance: $V_T/(P_{plat} - PEEP) <50$ mL/cm H_2O

Etiologies			
Direct injury		**Indirect injury**	
• Pneumonia (~40%)	• Inhalation injury	• Sepsis (~25%)	• Pancreatitis
• Aspiration (~15%)	• Lung contusion	• Shock	• Trauma/multiple fractures
• Near drowning		• DIC	• Transfusion (TRALI)

Treatment (primarily supportive) (*Lancet 2007;369:1553; NEJM 2007;357:1113*)
- Goal is to maintain gas exchange, sustain life, & avoid ventilator-induced lung injury (VILI)

Mechanisms of VILI	Ventilator Strategies (see ARDSnet.org)
Barotrauma/volutrauma: alveolar dist → mech damage	V_T ≤6 mL/kg, P_{plat} ≤30 cm H_2O, tolerate ↑ P_aCO_2 (but keep pH >7.15), ↓ mortality (*NEJM 2000;342:1301*)
Biotrauma → SIRS	Low V_T, open lung strategy w/ high PEEP
Atelectrauma: repetitive alveoli recruit & derecruit	**Titrate PEEP to prevent tidal alveolar collapse** See below for options
Hyperoxia: ? injury; worsened V/Q matching	↑ **PEEP** rather than F_iO_2 (keep <0.60) O_2-induced injury only theoretical in humans

PEEP titration methods (best method unclear)
- No benefit at given V_T if titrated to P_aO_2 alone (*NEJM 2004;351:327; JAMA 2008;299:637*)
- Best PEEP trial: incremental PEEP titration using compliance, O_2, hemodynamics
  If able to ↑ PEEP w/o ↑ P_{plat}, suggests "recruitability"
  ∴ ↑ PEEP if → ↑ S_aO_2 (target ≥88–90%) & P_{plat} ≤30 cm H_2O → ↓ time on vent, better lung mechanics (*JAMA 2008;299:646*), ? ↓ mortality (*JAMA 2010;303:865*)
- ARDSnet "high" PEEP table for optimal F_iO_2/PEEP combo for goal S_aO_2 (ARDSnet.org)
- Esophageal balloon: used to determine true transpulmonary pressure, adjust PEEP according to esoph pressure (≈pleural pressure) to maintain positive transpulm pressure and optimal PEEP; improves oxygenation and lung compliance but no effect on mortality (*NEJM 2008;359:2095*); helpful in obese Pts or w/ ↑ abdominal pressure

Other treatment considerations
- **Fluid balance:** target CVP 4–6 cm H_2O (if nonoliguric & normotensive) → ↑ vent/ICU-free days, but no Δ mortality (*NEJM 2006;354:2564*); PA catheter unproven (*NEJM 2006;354:2213*); consider using BNP >200 to trigger diuresis (UOP goal 4.5–9 mL/kg/h × 3 h)
- **Steroids:** debate continues. Adverse effects include neuromuscular weakness, poor glc control, ? infection. Benefit may vary by time since ARDS onset:
  <72 h: older studies w/o benefit (*NEJM 1987;317:1565*); ? ↓ mortality, ↑ vent/ICU-free days in more recent, controversial study (*Chest 2007;131:954*)
  7–13 d: ? benefit → ↑ vent/ICU-free days, no mortality difference (*NEJM 2006;354:1671*)
  ≥14 d: ↑ mortality (*NEJM 2006;354:1671*)
- **Paralysis:** if P_aO_2/F_iO_2 <150, cisatracurium × 48 h ↓ mortality by 32% (*NEJM 2010;363:1107*)
- **Proning:** if P_aO_2/F_iO_2 <150, prone-positioning ≥16 h ↓ mort. by ~50% (*NEJM 2013;368:2159*)
- **Experimental** (*JAMA 2010;304:2521*)
  Inhaled NO or prostacyclins: ↑ P_aO_2/F_iO_2, no ↓ mort. or vent-free days (*BMJ 2007;334:779*)
  Lung recruitment: apply CPAP 40–45 cm H_2O × 2 min to recruit lung and then ↑ PEEP to maintain; sicker Pts had ↑ recruitable lung (*NEJM 2006;354:1775 & 1839*)
  Driving pressure (ΔP = $P_{plateau}$–PEEP): ↓ ΔP a/w ↑ survival; target <15 (*NEJM 2015;372:747*)
  V-V ECMO: may be useful in refractory ARDS, but no good trial data (*NEJM 2011;365:1905*)

Prognosis (*JAMA 2016;315:788*)
- Mortality ~40% overall in clinical trials; 9–15% resp. causes, 85–91% extrapulm (MODS)
- Survivors: PFTs ~normal, ↓ D_LCO, muscle wasting, weakness persists (*NEJM 2003;348:683*), ↓ exercise tolerance, ↓ QoL, ↑ psych morbidity (*NEJM 2011;364:1293*)

SEPSIS AND SHOCK

Definitions	*(JAMA 2016;315:801)*
Systemic inflammatory response synd. (SIRS)	≥2 of the following: (1) Temp >38 or <36°C; (2) HR >90; (3) RR >20 or P_aCO_2 <32; (4) WBC >12k or <4k or >10% bands
Sepsis	Life-threatening organ dysfxn (SOFA Δ ≥2) due to infxn qSOFA ≥2 useful in triage of potentially septic pts
Septic shock	Sepsis-induced circulatory abnl: pressor required for MAP ≥65 and lactate >2 despite adequate fluid resuscitation

Sequential [Sepsis-Related] Organ Failure Assessment (SOFA, 0-24 points)					
Points	**0**	**1**	**2**	**3**	**4**
Resp: P_aO_2/F_iO_2	≥400	<400	<300	<200[a]	<100[a]
Coag: plt ($10^3/\mu L$)	≥150	<150	<100	<50	<20
Liver: bili (mg/dL)	<1.2	1.2–1.9	2.0–5.9	6.0–11.9	≥12
CV: MAP[b]	≥70	<70	dopa ≤5 or any DBA	dopa 5.1–15 or norepi/epi ≤0.1	dopa >15 or norepi/epi >0.1
Neuro: GCG	15	13–14	10-12	6-9	<6
Renal: Cr or UOP	<1.2	1.2–1.9	2.0–3.4	3.5–4.9 <500	>5 <200

Quick SOFA (qSOFA): ≥2 of following: RR ≥22, ΔMS, SBP ≤110 mmHg

[a]w/ respiratory support; [b]catechols (in μg/kg/min) for ≥1 h *(JAMA 2016;315:762;775; & 801)*

Shock (see "PA Catheter & Tailored Therapy" for subtypes; *NEJM 2013;369:1726*)
- Tissue hypoxia due to ↓ tissue perfusion and hence ↓ tissue O_2 delivery and/or ↑ O_2 consumption or inadequate O_2 utilization
- Typical signs include HoTN (SBP <90 mmHg or drop in SBP >40 mmHg), tachycardia, oliguria (UOP <0.5 cc/kg/h), Δ mentation, metabolic acidosis ± ↑ lactate
- Hard to dx as ↑ SVR can maintain SBP, but tissue perfusion poor; shock index (HR/SBP) >0.9 and pulse pressure [(SBP − DBP)/SBP] <25% clues to significant shock

Fluids & Early Goal-Directed Therapy in Septic Shock *(JAMA 2015;314:708)*
- EGDT uses IVF & pressors to target MAP ≥65 mmHg, CVP 8–12 mmHg and UOP ≥0.5 mL/kg/h, and inotropes & PRBCs to achieve $S_{cv}O_2$ ≥70% in first 6 h *(NEJM 2001;345:1368)*
- Did not ↓ mortality c/w usual care in recent trials *(NEJM 2014;371:1496, 2014;370:1683, & 2015;372:1301)*; however Pts had already rcvd >2 L fluid & abx, underscoring importance of these interventions (see below), and avg $S_{cv}O_2$ was >70%, ∴ no need for inotropes
- Lactate clearance (≥20%/2 h) as effective as $S_{cv}O_2$ to guide resusc. *(JAMA 2010;303:739)*
- Crystalloid as good as colloid for resuscitation *(JAMA 2013;310:1809; NEJM 2014;370:1412)*
- Predictors of fluid responsiveness: pulse pressure variation >13% w/ respiration *(Chest 2008;133:252)*; resp. variation in IVC diam, & passive leg raise. Static CVP poor surrogate.
- Hb >7 g/dL as good as >9, except perhaps if coronary insuffic. *(NEJM 2014;371:1381)*
- After early resuscitation, if ALI/ARDS, target CVP 4–6 mmHg as additional fluids may be harmful → ↑ ventilator/ICU days *(NEJM 2006;354:2564; Chest 2008;133:252)*

Pressors (also see "ICU Medications")
- MAP target 65–70 mmHg as good as 80–85 and ↓ AF *(NEJM 2014;370:1583)*
- Norepinephrine: ↓ arrhythmia & mortality c/w dopamine *(NEJM 2010;362:779; Crit Care Med 2012;40:725)* and ∴ is pressor of choice in septic shock
- Vasopressin: added to low-dose norepi not superior to high-dose norepi but ? benefit in less severe shock (norepi 5–14) *(NEJM 2008;358:877)*; consider if HoTN catechol refractory

Antibiotics
- Start empiric IV abx w/in 1 h of recognition of severe sepsis or septic shock; every hour delay in abx admin a/w 8% ↑ in mortality *(Crit Care Med 2006;34:1589)*
- If possible, obtain 2 sets of BCx before urgently starting abx (but do not delay abx)
- Broad gram-positive (incl MRSA) & gram-neg (incl highly resistant) coverage, ± anaerobes

Steroids *(NEJM 2003;348:727 & 2008;358:111; JAMA 2002;288:1038 & 2009:301:2362)*
- Cortisol secretion helps predict mortality, but treatment of adrenal insufficiency is unproven
- *Possible* mortality benefit w/in 8 h of severe septic shock (SBP <90 for >1 h despite fluids & pressors) if post ACTH stim cortisol Δ ≤ 9 μg/dL *(NEJM 2002;288:862)*
- No mortality benefit to early (<72 h) empiric corticosteroids in all Pts w/ septic shock, regardless of ACTH stim; faster resolution of shock, more superinfxn *(NEJM 2008;358:111)*
- Hydrocortisone 50–100 q6–8h ± fludrocortisone 50 μg daily in septic shock refractory to fluids & pressors, regardless of ACTH stim *(Crit Care Med 2008;36:296)*

Intensive glycemic control *(NEJM 2010;363:2540)*
- No clear benefit; reasonable to keep glc <150 mg/dL using validated protocol

Drug/toxin	Signs/Sx and Diagnostics	Management options
Acetaminophen	Vomiting, ↑ AG & nl OG metabolic acidosis, hepatitis & hepatic failure, renal failure	N-acetylcysteine (NAC) infusion Hemodialysis if massive O/D See "Acute liver failure"
Salicylates	Tinnitus, hyperventilation, abd. pain, vomiting, ∆MS, mixed ↑ AG & nl OG metabolic acidosis + respiratory alkalosis	IVF resuscitation Alkalinization w/ NaHCO₃ Maintain respiratory alkalosis Consider hemodialysis
Opioids	↓ mentation, ↓ RR, miosis	IV naloxone
Benzodiazepines	↓ mentation, ataxia, ↓ RR	Flumazenil *not* rec (can precipitate withdrawal/seizures)
Calcium channel blockers	Bradycardia, AV block, hypotension, HF, hyperglycemia	IVF, vasopressors, Ca infusion, hyperinsulinemic euglycemia, ? intralipid emulsion, pacing
Beta-blockers	Bradycardia, AV block, hypotension, HF, hypoglycemia	Glucagon, vasopressors, pacing
Digoxin	N/V, bradycardia, AV block, delirium, xanthopsia. ✓ serum dig level (but may be inaccurate if <6 h since last dose), renal function	Correct hypokalemia Digibind if hyperkalemia, life-threatening dysrhythmia Consider hemodialysis Lidocaine for arrhythmias
Tricyclic antide-pressants	Hypotension, seizures, arrhythmia, ↑ QRS, ↑ QT	IVF resuscitation, IV sodium bicarbonate, vasopressors
Lithium	N/V/D, tremor, hyperreflexia, clonus, drowsiness, seizure, ↑ QT, AV block, bradycardia	IVF (NS), maintain UOP Consider hemodialysis
Ethylene glycol	CNS depression, ↑ AG & OG metabolic acidosis	Ethanol or fomepizole, NaHCO₃ Consider hemodialysis
Methanol	CNS depression, blindness ↑ AG & OG met. acidosis	Ethanol or fomepizole, NaHCO₃ Consider hemodialysis
Isopropanol	CNS depression, gastritis	Supportive care
Carbon monoxide	HA, dizziness, nausea, ∆MS, carboxyHb level, CO-oximetry (pulse ox. invalid)	100% normobaric oxygen, hyperbaric O₂ in severe cases
Organophosphate	Salivation, lacrimation, diaphoresis, miosis, emesis, bronchospasm, ∆MS	Endotracheal intubation for respiratory failure, atropine, pralidoxime, benzodiazepines
Cyanide	Coma, seizure, metabolic acidosis, hypotension	IV Na nitrite and Na thiosulfate IV hydroxocobalamin

(Chest 2011;140:1072)

LUNG TRANSPLANT

Overview
- Indications: end stage, progressive decline despite max medical Rx, <2-y life expectancy; COPD, ILD (IPF), pulmonary HTN, cystic fibrosis, alpha 1-antitrypsin
- Contraindic: age >65 (relative), uncontrolled/unRx'd infxn, malig in prior 2 y, severe non-pulm dis., BMI ≥35, active smoking, drug dependence, med noncompliance, psychosocial

Posttransplant care
- Immunosuppression: center dependent; no single best regimen. Tacro > cyclosporine (↓ acute rejection) + steroids + MMF/azathioprine
- Serial PFTs, chest X-ray, clinic visits, bronchoscopy w/ transbronchial biopsy

Complications
- Anastomotic: vascular (stenosis, thrombosis) and airway (infection, necrosis, dehiscence, granulation tissue, tracheobronchomalacia, stenosis, fistula)
- Acute rejection: ↓ lung fxn, cough, SOB, fever. Dx w/ trans-bronch bx. Rx immunosupp.
- Chronic rejection: bronchiolitis obliterans w/ obstruction. Dx w/ PFTs, trans-bronch bx. Rx limited (azithromycin, montelukast, ∆ immunosuppressives).
- Infection: ↑ bacterial, fungal, viral pneumonia, systemic infections, CMV, OI
- Malignancy: 2× ↑ risk overall. 5.5× ↑ risk lung cancer. PTLD (assoc w/ EBV) common.
- Misc: GVHD, CKD, DM, CAD, CHF, stroke, encephalopathy, drug toxicity

DYSPHAGIA

Definitions
- Oropharyngeal: inability to propel food from mouth through UES into esophagus
- Esophageal: difficulty swallowing & passing food from esophagus into stomach

Figure 3-1 Etiologies of and approach to dysphagia (*NCP Gastrohep* 2008;5:393; *Neurogastro* 2012;24:57)

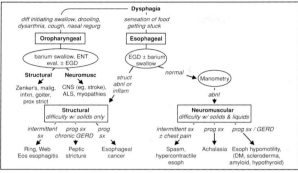

Structural dysphagia (*JAMA* 2015;313:18; *Gastro* 2014;147:1238)
- Caused by inflammatory or malignant changes in oropharynx/esophagus; *solids > liquids*
- Oropharyngeal
  Zenker's diverticulum (post pharyngeal pouch): in elderly, a/w aspiration, dx w/ video fluoroscopy, Rx w/ endo/surg
  malignancy, radiation injury, infection, goiter, osteophytes, proximal strictures/rings/webs
- Esophageal
  rings (concentric obstructing tissue, eg, Schatzki ring): near GE jxn, a/w food impaction, linked to GERD; Rx w/ PPI, dilation
  webs (nonconcentric): usually prox, can be a/w Fe defic. (Plummer-Vinson synd.)
  peptic or XRT strictures, foreign body, tumor, vascular compression (dysphagia lusoria)
- Infxn esophagitis: odynophagia > dysphagia; often immunosupp w/ *Candida*, HSV, CMV
- Pill esophagitis: odynophagia > dysphagia; NSAID, KCl, bisphosp., doxy & tetracycline
- Eosinophilic esophagitis: predominantly young or middle-aged ♂. Dx:>15 eos/hpf on bx, esoph dysfxn (ie, dysphagia, food impaction) & exclude GERD (empiric PPI trial).
  Rx: 3**D**s: 1st modify **D**iet (Ø milk, soy, eggs, wheat, nuts, fish); if no Δ, Rx w/ **D**rugs (swallow inh steroids); if ongoing sx & stricturing, **D**ilation.

Neuromuscular dysphagia
- Caused by aberrant motility or innervation of oropharynx/esophagus; *solids & liquids*
- Oropharyngeal: consider CNS disorders (eg, stroke, ALS, myopathies, CNS tumors)
- Esophageal: motility disorder a/w dysphagia, CP, GERD; dx via manometry or high-res esophageal pressure topography. Entities include:
  Distal spasm: uncoordinated peristalsis w/ simultaneous contractions
  Hypercontractile: high amp contractions; Rx w/PPI, nitrates/CCB/PDEi,TCA/SSRI
  Hypomotility: ↓ amp of distal esoph contractions; seen in scleroderma, DM, hypothyroidism; Rx w/ PPI & Rx underlying disorder
  Achalasia: simult. ↓ amp contractions & ↓ LES relaxation; barium swallow w/ dilated esophagus & distal "bird's beak" narrowing; mostly idiopathic, although can be a/w Chagas; Rx: pneumatic dilation as effective as Heller myotomy (*NEJM* 2011;364:1868); per oral endoscopic myotomy; CCB/nitrates/PDEi; Botox inj if not candidate for surgery

GASTROESOPHAGEAL REFLUX DISEASE (GERD)

Pathophysiology
- ↑ acid exposure in esophagus, caused by ↑ transient LES relaxations. Worsened by ↑ intrabd pressure (eg, obesity, pregnancy), ↓ esophagogastric motility, hiatal hernia. Rarely caused by ↑ acid production except in ↑ secretory states (eg, Zollinger-Ellison).
- Precipitants: supine position, fatty foods, caffeine, alcohol, cigarettes, CCB, pregnancy

Clinical manifestations
- Esophageal: **heartburn**, atypical chest pain, regurgitation, water brash, dysphagia
- Extraesophageal: **cough**, asthma (often poorly controlled), laryngitis, dental erosions

Diagnosis (Annals 2015;163:ITC1)
- Clinical diagnosis based on sx and response to empiric trial of PPI ("PPI test")
- EGD: if (1) Ø response to PPI; or if (2) *alarm features:* dysphagia, vomiting, ↓ wt, anemia
- If dx uncertain & EGD nl → esoph manometry w/ 24-h esoph pH monitoring ± impedance

Treatment (Lancet 2013;381:1933)
- Lifestyle: avoid precipitants, lose weight, avoid large & late meals, elevate head of bed
- Medical: PPI achieve relief in 80–90% of Pts; H2 blockers for intermittent sx
- Refractory: confirm w/ pH testing (on PPI to assess need for ↑ Rx, or off PPI to verify dx).
   If acidic or sx correlate w/ reflux episodes: surgical fundoplication (emerging Rx: LES
      sphincter augmentation w/ radiofrequency, implantable magnetic or electrical devices)
   If nl pH or no sx correlation: Dx esoph hypersensitivity. Rx w/ TCA, SSRI or baclofen.

Complications (NEJM 2014;371:836; Gastro 2011;140:1084.e18 & 2015;149:1599)
- Reflux esophagitis (erosions/ulcers above GE jxn), strictures (caused by chronic inflamm)
- Barrett's esophagus (BE; NEJM 2014;371:836): metaplastic columnar mucosa above GE jxn
   replaces squam esoph epithelium (dx via EGD/bx)
   Screen if GERD w/ ≥1 risk factor for esophageal adeno.: >50 y, ♂, white, hiatal hernia,
      central adiposity, smoking. 0.1–0.3%/y risk of esoph adenocarcinoma, ↑ if ↑ dysplasia.
   Management: PPI. W/o dysplasia: surveillance EGD no sooner than q3–5y (limited data
      on utility of EGD screening in nondysplastic BE). Low-grade dysplasia: EGD q6–12mo;
      potential benefit of endoscopic eradication, eg RFA (JAMA 2014;311:1209).
   High-grade dysplasia: endoscopic eradication (resection or ablation treatment).

PEPTIC ULCER DISEASE (PUD)

Definition & etiologies (Lancet 2009;374:1449)
- Ulcers (break in mucosal lining >5 mm) & erosions (<5 mm) in stomach and duodenum
- Principal risk factors: H. pylori infection > NSAID/ASA use
- **H. pylori infection:** causes ~80% of duodenal ulcers (DU) & ~60% of gastric ulcers (GU).
   ~50% of world colonized w/ H. pylori, but only 5–10% will develop PUD.
- **ASA & NSAIDs:** damage to mucosa caused by ↓ prostaglandin synthesis. Cause majority
   of non–H. pylori–related DU & GU. Regular use a/w 5–6× ↑ odds of GIB.
- Other: smoking, stress, excessive EtOH, gastric cancer/lymphoma, Crohn's, viral infxn (eg,
   CMV/HSV in immunosupp), bisphosphonates, steroids (in combo w/ NSAIDs, but not risk
   factor alone); rarely gastrinoma (Zollinger-Ellison synd.), mastocytosis, idiopathic
- Stress ulcer: risk factors = ICU & coagulopathic, mech vent, h/o GIB, steroid use; Rx w/ PPI

Clinical manifestations
- **Epigastric abdominal pain:** relieved with food (DU) or worsened by food (GU)
- Complications: UGIB, perforation & penetration, gastric outlet obstruction

Diagnostic studies
- Testing for H. pylori: stool antigen or EGD + rapid urease test. False ⊖ if on abx, bismuth,
   PPI, so stop prior to testing if possible. Serology: ↓ utility, useful only to exclude infection
   in low prevalence areas (most of U.S.).
- EGD (definitive dx): if fail empiric Rx or alarm features (see above); bx GU to r/o malig & H.
   pylori; relook in 6–12 wk if >2 cm, malig features, risk factors for gastric cancer (ie, ⊕ FHx,
   ⊕ H. pylori, atrophic gastritis, dysplasia/ metaplasia on bx, > 50 y.o.), or sx persist

Treatment (NEJM 2010;362:1597; Gut 2012;61:646; BMJ 2013;347:f4587)
- **If H. pylori ⊕, eradicate** ("test and treat") (Gastro 2016;151:51):
   Triple Rx: clarith + [amox, MNZ or levoflox] + PPI bid × 10–14 d (if clarith resist rate <20%)
   Quadruple Rx: MNZ + TCN + bismuth + PPI (if clarith resist rate >15% or amox allergy)
      erad vs. triple 93 vs. 70%, clarith sens 95 vs. 85%, resist 91 vs. 8% (Lancet 2011;377:905)
   Sequential Rx: PPI + amox × 7 d → PPI + clarith + MNZ × 7 d (Lancet 2013;381:205)
   Besides PUD, test & Rx if: gastric MALT lymphoma, atrophic gastritis, FHx gastric ca
- If H. pylori ⊖: gastric acid suppression w/ PPI
- Lifestyle changes: d/c smoking and probably EtOH; diet does not seem to play a role
- Surgery: if refractory to med Rx (↑↑ r/o NSAID use) or for complications (see above)

Prophylaxis if ASA/NSAID required (JACC 2016;67:1661; Aliment PharmRx 2016;43:1262)
- PPI if (a) h/o PUD/UGIB; (b) also on clopidogrel (although ? ↓ antiplt effect); (c) ≥2 of
   the following: age >60, steroids or dyspepsia; prior to start test & Rx H. pylori
- Consider misoprostol; consider H2RA if ASA monotherapy (Lancet 2009;374:119)
- Consider Δ to COX-2 inhibit (↓ PUD & UGIB but ↑ CV events) if low CV risk & not on ASA

GASTROINTESTINAL BLEEDING

Definition
- Intraluminal blood loss anywhere from the oropharynx to the anus
- Classification: **upper** = above the ligament of Treitz; **lower** = below the ligament of Treitz
- "Severe" GIB: defined as having associated shock, orthostatic hypotension, ↓ Hct by 6% (or ↓ Hb by 2 g/dL), or requiring transfusion ≥2U PRBCs. Requires hospitalization.

Clinical manifestations
- **Hematemesis** = blood in vomitus (UGIB)
- **Coffee-ground emesis** = blood exposed to gastric acid (UGIB)
- **Melena** = black, tarry stools from digested blood (usually UGIB, but can be from R colon)
- **Hematochezia** = bloody or maroon-colored stools (LGIB or rapid UGIB)

Initial management
- **Assess severity:** VS including orthostatic Δs, JVP. Tachycardia (can be masked by βB use) suggests 10% volume loss, orthostatic hypotension 20% loss, shock >30% loss
- **History:** prior GIB, tempo of current bleed, specific bleeding manifestations (see above), other GI s/s (eg, abd pain, Δ in bowel habits, weight loss, N/V), NSAID/ASA or EtOH use, anticoag/antiplt drugs, h/o or risk factors for cirrhosis, radiation, prior GI or aortic surgery.
- **Physical exam:** localizable abd tenderness, peritoneal signs, masses, LAN, prior surgery signs of liver disease (hepatosplenomegaly, ascites, jaundice, telangiectasias) rectal exam: masses, hemorrhoids, anal fissures, stool appearance, color, occult blood
- **Resuscitation:** placement of 2 large-bore (18-gauge or larger) intravenous lines Volume replacement: NS or LR to achieve normal VS, UOP, & mental status
- **Lab studies: Hct** (may be normal in first 24 h of acute GIB before equilibration) 2–3% → 500 mL blood loss; low MCV → Fe deficient and chronic blood loss; **plt, PT, PTT;** BUN/Cr (ratio >36 in UGIB b/c GI resorption of blood ± prerenal azotemia); LFTs
- **Transfuse:** BB sample for type & cross; use O-neg if emerg; for UGIB (esp. w/ portal HTN) transfuse w/ more restrictive Hb goal (eg, 7 g/dL) or >8 g/dL if CAD (NEJM 2013;368:11)
- **Reverse coagulopathy:** FFP & vit K to normalize PT; plts to keep count >50,000
- **Triage:** alert endoscopist. Consider ICU if unstable VS or poor end organ perfusion. Intubation for emergent EGD, if ongoing hematemesis, shock, poor resp status, Δ MS ? OutPt management if SBP ≥110, HR <100, Hb ≥13 (♂) or ≥12 (♀), BUN <18, Ø melena, syncope, heart failure, liver disease (Lancet 2009;373:42)

Diagnostic studies
- **Nasogastric tube** can aid localization: fresh blood or coffee grounds → active or recent UGIB; nonbloody → does not exclude UGIB (~15% missed). ⊕ occult blood test no value.
- UGIB: **EGD** w/in 24 h. If severe bleed, ↑ Dx/Rx yield by gastric lavage and **erythro 250 mg IV 30 min prior to endoscopy** to clear stomach contents (Am J Gastro 2006;101:1211).
- LGIB: **colonoscopy** (identifies cause in >70%); if severe, colo w/in 12 h → consider rapid purge w/ PEG solution (6–8 L over 4–6 h). If hematochezia a/w orthostasis, concern for brisk UGIB → **exclude UGIB w/ EGD first.** Push enteroscopy, anoscopy, capsule endoscopy in combo w/ urgent colo results in dx >95% of cases (GI Endo 2015;81:889).
- Imaging: if too unstable for endo or recurrent bleeding, can then → IR procedure or surgery **tagged RBC scan:** can identify general luminal location ≥0.04 mL/min **arteriography:** can localize exact vessel if bleeding rates ≥0.5 mL/min, allows for IR Rx
- Emergent exploratory laparotomy (last resort) if no localization and life-threatening bleed

Etiology UGIB	Comment & Treatment
PUD (20–67%) (NEJM 2016;374:2367) See "PUD"	Treatment: **PPI:** 80 mg IV bolus + 8 mg/h drip ≈ 40 mg IV BID boluses **Endoscopic therapy:** epi inj + bipolar cautery or hemoclip. Biopsies for ? H. pylori and treat if ⊕. High-risk (for rebleeding) ulcer: arterial spurting, adherent clot, visible vessel. Endo Rx, IV PPI × 72 h post EGD, then Δ to high-dose oral PPI. Arteriography w/ embolization; surgery (last resort). Intermediate-risk ulcer: oozing, in o/w stable Pt. Endo Rx, can Δ to oral PPI after EGD and observe 24–48 h. Low-risk ulcer: clean-based or flat. Oral PPI and ? discharge. Hold anticoag & antiplatelet Rx until hemostasis; can resume after hemostasis & PPI on board (BMJ 2012;344:e3412).
Erosive gastropathy (4–31%)	Precipitants: NSAIDs, ASA, EtOH, cocaine, gut ischemia, XRT Stress-related mucosal injury in ICU Pts. Risk factors include severe coagulopathy, mech vent >48 h, high dose glucocorticoids Treatment: high-dose PPI
Erosive esophagitis (5–18%)	Risk factors: cirrhosis, anticoagulation, critical illness. Rx offending cause + high dose PPI; repeat EGD later to r/o underling Barrett's.

Esophageal or gastric varices (4–20%) *(Hep 2007;46:922; NEJM 2010;362:823)* See "Cirrhosis"			2° to portal HTN. If isolated gastric → r/o splenic vein thrombosis. <u>Pharmacologic</u> **Octreotide** 50 μg IV bolus → 50 μg/h infusion (84% success). Usually × 5 d, but most benefit w/in 24–48 h. Abx: 20% cirrhotics p/w UGIB have infxn, & ~50% develop infxn during hospitalization; Ppx w/ IV CTX, cipro, or levoflox × 7 d <u>Nonpharmacologic</u> **Endoscopic band ligation** (>90% success) or sclerotherapy Arteriography w/ coiling, or if available, endoscopic injection of cyanoacrylate (glue) for gastric varices Covered esophageal stent placement or balloon tamponade used for bleeding refractory to ligation as bridge to TIPS (consider early if persistent bleed on EGD or Child-Pugh C; NEJM 2010;362:2370) For persistent gastric variceal bleed: TIPS or balloon-retrograde transvenous obliteration
Portal HTN gastropathy			↑ portal venous pressure → ectatic vessels, hyperemia in prox. gastric body. No endoscopic option; Rx portal HTN (octreotide), βB.
Vascular (2–8%)	Angioectasia AVMs, HHT (see below)		AVMs congenital. Angioectasia (ectatic submucosal vessels) a/w ↑ age, CKD, cirrhosis, CTD, severe CV dis. **Heyde syndrome:** GIB d/t angioectasias + aortic stenosis. Endo Rx.
	Dieulafoy's lesion		Large (1–3 mm) submucosal artery protruding through fundal mucosa → sudden, massive UGIB. Difficult to identify. Endo Rx.
	Gastric antral vasc. ectasia (GAVE)		"Watermelon stomach"; ectatic gastric vessels, often a/w cirrhosis, CTD, typically older ♀. Rx w/ thermal hemostasis, repeat q4–8wk to eradicate lesions. TIPS does *not* improve outcomes.
	Aortoenteric fistula		AAA or aortic graft erodes into 3rd portion of duodenum. P/w "herald bleed"; if suspected, diagnose by endoscopy or CT.
Malignancy (2–8%)			Endoscopic hemostasis of mass temporizing measure till cancer Rx
Mallory-Weiss tear (4–12%)			GE jxn lacerations due to vomiting → ↑ intraabd pressure & shearing effect. Can self-resolve w/o endo Rx. Rx w/ antiemetics, PPI.
Cameron's lesions			Linear erosions in hiatal hernia due to mech trauma of diaphragm
Post-sphincterotomy bleeding			Occurs in ~2% of cases, ↑ risk w/ more complicated procedure. Bleeding into duodenum. Rx w/ endo hemostasis.

(GI Endosc Clin N Gastro 2015;25:415)

Etiology LGIB	Comment & Treatment *(Am J Gastro 2015;110:1265 & 2016;111:755)*
Diverticular bleed (30%)	*Pathophysiology:* Intimal thickening and medial thinning of vasa recta as they course over dome of diverticulum → weakening of vascular wall → arterial rupture. Diverticula more common in left colon; but *bleeding diverticula more often in right colon*. *Clinical:* older, ASA/NSAIDs, painless hematochezia, ± abd cramping *Treatment:* Usually stops spont. (~75%) but may take hrs–days; ~20% recur. Can perform endo hemostasis w/ epi injections ± electrocautery *(NEJM 2000;342:78)*, hemoclip, banding. Intra-arterial vasopressin or embo. Surgery (partial colectomy) last resort.
Polyp/Tumor (20%)	Typically slow ooze, p/w fatigue, weight loss, iron deficiency anemia
Colitis (20%)	Infectious (see "Acute Diarrhea"), IBD, ischemic colitis, XRT
Anorectal disorders (20%)	Internal, external hemorrhoids; anal fissures, rectal ulcers, rectal varices (Rx by ↓ portal venous pressure in cirrhotics), XRT
Vascular (<10%)	Angioectasia & AVMs (see above). *Hereditary Hemorrhagic Telangiectasia* (Weber-Osler-Rendu): diffuse AVMs, telangiectasias throughout GI mucosa (also involve lips, oral mucosa, fingertips).
Meckel's diverticulum	Congenital blind intestinal pouch due to incomplete obliteration of vitelline duct. 2% of pop, w/in 2′ of IC valve, 2′ long, ♂:♀ 2:1, often present age 2 (but can cause obscure GIB in adults). Dx w/ 99mTc-pertechnetate scintigraphy. Rx w/ angioembo, surgical resection.

Obscure GIB *(Gastro 2007;133:1694; GIE 2010;72:471)*
- **Definition:** continued bleeding (melena, hematochezia) despite ⊖ EGD & colo; 5% of GIB
- **Etiologies:** Dieulafoy's lesion, GAVE, small bowel angiodysplasia, ulcer or cancer, Crohn's disease, aortoenteric fistula, Meckel's diverticulum, hemobilia
- **Diagnosis:** repeat EGD w/ push enteroscopy/colonoscopy when bleeding is active
  If ⊖, video capsule to evaluate small intestine *(Gastro 2009;137:1197)*
  If still ⊖, consider 99mTc-pertechnetate scan ("Meckel's scan"), enteroscopy (single-balloon, double-balloon or spiral), tagged RBC scan and arteriography

ACUTE DIARRHEA (<4 WEEKS' DURATION)

Acute Infectious Etiologies (NEJM 2014;370:1532; JAMA 2015;313:71)		
Pathogen	**Epidemiology & Clinical Sx**	
Noninflammatory	Predom. disruption small intestine absorp. & secretion. Voluminous diarrhea, N/V. ⊖ fecal WBC & FOB.	
Preformed toxin	"Food poisoning," <24 h dur. *S. aureus* (meats & dairy), *B. cereus* (fried rice), *C. perfringens* (rewarmed meats).	
Viral	Rotavirus	Outbreak person to person (PTP), daycare; lasts 4–8 d.
	Norovirus	~50% of all diarrhea. Winter outbreaks; PTP & food/water; no immunity. Lasts 1–3 d. Vomiting prominent.
Bacterial	*E. coli* (toxigenic)	>50% of traveler's diarrhea; cholera-like toxin; <7 d.
	Vibrio cholerae (Lancet 2012;379:2466)	Contam H$_2$O, fish, shellfish; 50 cases/y in U.S. Gulf Coast. Severe dehydration & electrolyte depletion.
Parasitic	*Giardia*	Streams/outdoor sports, travel, outbreaks. Bloating. Acute (profuse, watery) → chronic (greasy, malodorous).
(± malab for mos after Rx)	*Cryptosporidia* (NEJM 2002;346:1723)	Water-borne outbreak; typically self-limited, can cause chronic infxn if immunosupp. Abd pain (80%), fever (40%).
	Cyclospora	Contaminated produce
Inflammatory		Predom. colonic invasion. Small vol diarrhea. LLQ cramps, tenesmus, fever, typically ⊕ fecal WBC or FOB.
Bacterial	*Campylobacter*	Undercooked poultry, unpasteurized milk, travel to Asia; carried by puppies & kittens. Prodrome; abd pain → "pseudoappendicitis"; c/b GBS, reactive arthritis.
	Salmonella (nontyphoidal)	Eggs, poultry, milk. Bacteremia in 5–10%. 10–33% of bacteremic Pts >50 y may develop aortitis.
	Shigella	Abrupt onset; gross blood & pus in stool; ↑↑ WBC.
	E. coli (O157:H7 & inv/hemorrhagic non-O157:H7)	Undercooked beef, unpasteurized milk, raw produce; PTP. O157 & non-O157 sp. (40%) produce *Shiga* toxin → HUS (typically in children). Gross blood in stool.
	C. difficile	See later
	Vibrio parahaem.	Undercooked seafood
	Salmonella typhi	Travel to Asia. Systemic toxicity, relative bradycardia, rose spot rash, ileus → pea-soup diarrhea, bacteremia.
	Other	*Yersinia*: undercooked pork; unpasteurized milk, abd pain → "pseudoappendicitis" (aka mesenteric adenitis) *Aeromonas, Plesiomonas, Listeria* (meats & cheeses)
Parasitic	*E. histolytica*	Contaminated food/water, travel (rare in U.S.); liver abscess
Viral	CMV	Immunosuppressed; dx by shell vial cx of colon bx

Evaluation (NEJM 2014;370:1532)
- **History:** stool freq, bloody, abd pain, duration of sxs [~1 wk for viral & bacterial (except *C. diff*), >1 wk for parasitic], travel, food, recent abx, immunocompromise
- **PEx:** vol depletion (VS, UOP, axillae, skin turgor, MS), fever, abd tenderness, ileus, rash
- **Laboratory:** ✓ fecal WBC (high false ⊕ & ⊖) or stool lactoferrin & calprotectin (PMN products; Se/Sp >90%), stool cx, BCx, lytes, *C. diff* (if recent hosp/abx), stool O&P (if >10 d, travel to endemic area, exposure to unpurified H$_2$O, community outbreak, daycare, HIV ⊕ or MSM); ± stool ELISAs (viruses, *Crypto, Giardia*), serologies (*E. histolytica*)
- **Imaging/endoscopy** warranted if **warning signs**: fever, signific abd pain, blood or pus in stools, >6 stools/d, severe dehydration, immunosupp, elderly, duration >7 d, hosp-acquired. CT/KUB if ? toxic megacolon; sig/colo if immunosupp or cx ⊖

Treatment (Am J Gastro 2016;111:602)
- If none of the above warning signs *and* Pt able to take POs → supportive Rx only: oral hydration, loperamide, bismuth subsalicylate (avoid anticholinergics)
- If moderate dehydration: 50–200 mL/kg/d of oral solution (½ tsp salt, 1 tsp baking soda, 8 tsp sugar, & 8 oz OJ diluted to 1 L w/ H$_2$O) or Gatorade, etc. If severe: IV fluids.
- Fluoroquinolone or rifaximin if high suspicion for traveler's diarrhea
- If high suspicion for protozoal infection can consider metronidazole or nitazoxanide
- *Empiric* abx for non–hospital-acquired *inflammatory* diarrhea reasonable: FQ × 5–7 d abx rec for *Shigella*, cholera, *Giardia*, amebiasis, *Salmonella* if Pt >50 y or immunosupp or hospitalized, ? *Campylobacter* (if w/in 4 d of sx onset)
  avoid abx if suspect *E. coli* O157:H7 as may ↑ risk of HUS

CLOSTRIDIUM DIFFICILE-ASSOCIATED DIARRHEA (CDAD)

Pathogenesis & epidemiology (NEJM 2015;372:825)
- Ingestion of *C. diff* spores → colonization when colonic flora Δd by abx or chemo → release of toxin A/B → colonic mucosal necrosis & inflammation → pseudomembranes
- Most frequently reported nosocomial infxn; community-acquired infxn may account for up to 1/3 of new cases. Associated w/ all abx (esp. β-lactams, clinda, quinolones).
- Additional risk factors: elderly, nursing home residents, IBD, PPI (CID 2011;53:1173)

Clinical manifestations (a spectrum of disease)
- Asx colonization: <3% healthy adults; ~20% in hospitalized patients on antibiotics
- Acute watery diarrhea (occ bloody) ± mucus, often w/ lower abd pain, fever, ↑↑↑ WBC
- Pseudomembranous colitis: above sx + pseudomembranes + bowel wall thickening
- Fulminant colitis (2–3%): **toxic megacolon** (colon dilatation ≥6 cm on KUB, colonic atony, systemic toxicity) and/or bowel perforation

Diagnosis
- Only test if *symptomatic* (diarrhea, s/s of colitis); test *liquid* stool (unless concern for ileus)
- **Stool EIA:** detects toxin B and/or A (1–2% strains make A); fast (2–6 h); ⊕ result highly Sp
- **Stool PCR:** has ↑ Se, but ⊕ if colonized in absence of active CDAD; should not necessarily Rx if ⊕ PCR w/ ⊖ neg toxin assay (JAMA IM 2015;175;1792)
- Consider flex sig if dx uncertain and/or evidence of no improvement w/ standard Rx

Treatment (NEJM 2015;372:1539; JAMA 2015;313:398)
- If possible d/c abx ASAP; stop antimotility agents
- **Non-severe:** vanco 125 mg PO q6h or MNZ 500 mg PO q8h × 10–14 d; equal cure rates, but MNZ less well tolerated
- **Severe** (any of the following: >12 BM/d, Temp >103°F, WBC >25, HoTN, ICU care required, ileus): vanco 125 mg PO q6h + MNZ 500 mg IV q8h
- If worsening (ileus, ↑ WBC, ↑ lactate, shock, toxic megacolon, peritonitis): abd CT & urgent surgical consult re: subtotal colectomy (? possible role for diverting loop ileostomy or colonic lavage); may also consider vanco PR
- If Pt needs to continue on abx, continue *C. diff* Rx for ≥7 d post-abx cessation
- Stool carriage may persist 3–6 wk postcessation of sx & should not trigger further Rx (retesting for *C. diff* of limited utility during this time)
- **Recurrent infection:** 15–30% risk after d/c of abx, most w/in 2 wk of stopping abx
  1st recurrence: vanco 125 mg PO q6h × 10–14 d or fidaxomicin 200 mg PO bid × 10 d
  Subsequent recurrences: vanco PO pulse → taper. Consult ID physician. Consider fecal microbial transplant (NEJM 2013;368:407 & JAMA 2016;315:142) or fidaxomicin (200 mg bid × 10 d). Pilot data for oral admin of nontoxigenic *C. diff* strain spores (JAMA 2015;313:1719).
- Probiotics w/o clear benefit (Lancet 2013;382:1249)

CHRONIC DIARRHEA (>4 wk; JAMA 2016;315:2712)

General evaluation
- Clinically can be organized into *watery, fatty,* or *inflammatory* stools
- Additional hx: timing (freq, relation to meals; *nocturnal diarrhea* a/w organic causes like IBD rather than IBS), abd pain, wt loss, prior surg, chemo/XRT, diet (incl caffeine or poorly absorbed carbs/sugars), infectious sxs, immunocompromise, travel, laxative use, etc.
- Hx offending meds: PPI, colchicine, abx, H2RA, SSRIs, ARBs, NSAIDs, chemo, caffeine
- PEx: appearance (BMI), signs of systemic disease, surgical scars, rectal tone/DRE
- Lab testing: CBC, metabolic profile, alb, TSH, Fe studies, ESR; *see under each category*
- Imaging/endoscopy: colonoscopy for chronic diarrhea of unknown cause. Abd CT/MRI usually warranted if systemic problem suspected.

Osmotic (watery; ⊖ fecal fat, ↑ osmotic gap, ↓ diarrhea with fasting)
- Caused by ingestion of poorly absorbed cations/anions (Mg, sulfate, phos; found in laxatives) or poorly absorbed sugars (eg, mannitol, sorbitol; found in chewing gum; or lactose if lactose intolerant). *Diarrhea resolves w/ cessation of offending substance.*
- Dx: ↑ **stool osmotic gap** (see Figure); stool pH <6 if unabsorbed carbohydrates
- **Lactose intolerance** (75% nonwhites & 25% whites lactase-deficient): can be acquired after gastroenteritis, med illness, GI surg. Clin: bloating, flatulence, discomfort, diarrhea. Dx: H+ breath test or empiric lactose-free diet. Rx: lactose-free diet & lactase tablets.

Secretory (watery; normal osmotic gap, no Δ diarrhea w/ fasting, often nocturnal diarrhea)
- Caused by secretion of anions or K+ into lumen or inhib of Na absorption → ↑ H₂O in stool. Most commonly caused by bacterial toxins from **infxn** (see above). Other causes:
- **Endocrine:** Addison's, VIPoma, carcinoid, Zollinger-Ellison, mastocytosis, hyperthyroid (↑ motility). ✓ serum peptide levels (eg, gastrin, calcitonin, VIP) & urinary histamine.
- **GI neoplasm:** carcinoma, lymphoma, villous adenoma

- **Microscopic colitis:** common cause of chronic diarrhea w/ obscure origin. Often seen in middle-aged women w/ autoimmune disorders. NSAIDs, SSRIs, PPIs notable triggers. Grossly nl on colo but bx shows lymphocytic & plasmacytic infiltration of mucosa ± thickened submucosal collagen. Rx: antidiarrheals, cholestyramine, bismuth, budesonide; consider anti-TNFs if refractory.
- **Bile acid-induced diarrhea:** ileal resection or disease (eg Crohn's), etc. → bile acids in colon → electrolyte & H_2O secretion. Rx w/ empiric bile-acid binders (eg, cholestyramine).

Fxnal/IBS (watery; normal osmotic gap, ↓ diarrhea with fasting): see Dysmotility

Malabsorption (fatty; ↑ fecal fat, ↑ osmotic gap, ↓ diarrhea w/ fasting)
- Defective mucosal absorption of nutrients b/c Δs in: mucosal surface (surgical resection) or gen. mucosal dis. (celiac, IBD). Bloating, foul-smelling, floating stools (steatorrhea).
- **Celiac disease** (NEJM 2012;367:2419; Gastro 2015;148:1175)
  Immune rxn in genetically predisposed Pts (~1% pop) to gliadin, a component of gluten (wheat protein) → small bowel inflammatory infiltrate → impaired absorption
  Other s/s: Fe/folate defic anemia; osteoporosis; dermatitis herpetiformis; ↑ AST/ALT
  Dx: IgA anti-tissue transglutaminase Ab (most Se), IgA anti-deaminated gliadin peptide Ab; IgA α-endomysial Ab. Duodenal bx to confirm dx (blunted villi, crypt hyperplasia, inflamm infiltrate) but may not be necessary if serology ⊕ and Pt sx. HLA-DQ2/Q8 testing useful for high ⊖ predictive value if ⊖ serologies already on gluten-free diet.
  Rx: gluten-free diet; 7–30% do not respond to diet → ? wrong dx or noncompliant
  Complic: ~5% refractory sx, risk of T-cell lymphoma and small bowel adenocarcinoma
- **Whipple's disease:** infxn w/ *T. whipplei* (NEJM 2007;365:55)
  Other s/s: fever, LAN, edema, arthritis, CNS Δs, gray-brown skin pigmentation, AI & MS, oculomasticatory myorhythmia (eye oscillations + mastication muscle contract)
  Rx: (PCN + streptomycin) or 3rd-gen ceph × 10–14 d → Bactrim for ≥1 y
- **Small intestinal bacterial overgrowth** (SIBO): colonic bacteria in SI → steatorrhea, B12/Fe defic, protein-losing enteropathy. A/w dysmotility (DM neuropathy, scleroderma), Δ'd anatomy (Crohn's, surgery, fistulae), immune deficiency, celiac, CF. Dx w/ H^+ or ^{14}C-xylose breath testing or empiric abx. Rx w/ 7–10 d abx (eg, rifaximin, MNZ, FQ).
- Other: s/p short bowel resection (short bowel syndrome), chronic mesenteric ischemia, eosinophilic gastroenteritis, intestinal lymphoma, tropical sprue, *Giardia* infection

Maldigestion (fatty; ↑ fecal fat, ↑ osmotic gap, ↓ diarrhea w/ fasting)
- Defective intraluminal hydrolysis of nutrients, typ. 2/2 pancreatic/hepatobiliary pathology
- **Pancreatic insufficiency:** most commonly from chronic pancreatitis or pancreatic cancer. Test w/ stool elastase, chymotrypsin levels, or empiric pancreatic enzyme replacement.
- ↓ **bile acids** due to ↓ synthesis (cirrhosis), cholestasis (PBC), or s/p ileal resection. Test w/ empiric bile acid replacement therapy.

Inflammatory (⊕ fecal WBC or lactoferrin or calprotectin, ⊕ FOB, fever, abd pain)
- **Infections:** chronic *C. diff*, *Entamoeba histolytica*, *Yersinia*, CMV, TB especially in immunocompromised hosts. CMV, *C. diff* notorious for causing exacerbations of IBD.
- **Inflammatory bowel disease** (Crohn's, UC)
- Radiation enteritis, ischemic colitis, neoplasia (colon cancer, lymphoma)

Figure 3-2 Workup of chronic diarrhea

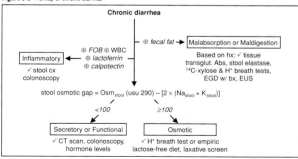

Functional GI Disease
- Functional GI sx caused by abnl gut–brain interactions rather than structural cause
- >20 types of FGIDs per Rome III criteria; now Rome IV (Gastro 2016;150:1257)
- **Irritable Bowel Syndrome (IBS)** (JAMA 2015;313:949)
  Abd discomfort a/w ≥2 of following: improve w/ defecation, Δ stool frequency, Δ stool form
  IBS-C (constipation predominant) vs. **IBS-D** (diarrhea predominant) vs. IBS-M (mixed) vs.
  IBS-U (unclassified). Sx may be related to stress, diet, lifestyle, possibly microbiome.
  Treatment: exercise, cognitive behavioral Rx, Δ diet, probiotics, ? peppermint oil
  IBS-C: laxatives (eg, lubiprostone, linaclotide, PEG), biofeedback
  IBS-D: rifaximin or loperamide; eluxadoline, μ & κ agonist, δ antag (NEJM 2016;374:242)
- **Cyclical Vomiting Syndrome:** stereotypic episodes of acute recurrent vomiting;
  a/w marijuana use, family hx of migraine
  acute Rx: antiemetics, IVF, sumatriptan, BZDs; prevention: TCAs/AEDs; avoid marijuana

Gastroparesis (Gastro Clinics of NA 2015;44:1; World J Gastro 2015;21:6842)
- Delayed gastric emptying w/o obstruction, typically p/w nausea (>90%), vomiting (>80%),
  early satiety (60%), postprandial fullness/pain
- Etiol: DM, post-surg, thyroid disease, critical illness, Parkinson's, opiates, CCB, anti-cholin
- Dx: gastric emptying scintigraphy
- **Treatment:** prokinetic agents (metoclopramide or erythromycin), antiemetics for sx; feeding
  tube if refractory; intrapyloric botox & gastric stimulation experimental

Acute colonic pseudo-obstruction (Ogilvie's syndrome) (ANZ J Surg 2015;85:728)
- Definition: loss of intestinal peristalsis in absence of mechanical obstruction
- Abd discomfort & distention, ↓ / absent bowel sounds, ± N/V, hiccups
- Typically in elderly, hospitalized, ill Pts, precipitated by: intra-abd process (surgery,
  pancreatitis, peritonitis, intestinal ischemia), severe medical illness (eg, sepsis), meds
  (opiates, CCB, anticholinergics), metab/endo abnl (thyroid, DM, kidney failure, liver
  failure), spinal cord compression/trauma, neurologic d/o (Parkinson's, Alzheimer's, MS)
- KUB or CT w/ colonic dilatation w/o mech obstruction; cecal diam >14 cm a/w high risk perf
- **Treatment:** conservative measures (NPO, avoid offending meds) usually effective;
  IV **neostigmine** (monitor for bradycardia), methylnaltrexone; bowel decompression w/
  NGT, rectal tube, colonoscopy; if refractory, colostomy or colectomy

Constipation (Annals 2015;162:ITC1)
- Defined as dissatisfaction w/ defecation or (per Rome III): ≥2 of following during last 3 mo
  ≥25% of the time: straining, lumpy/hard stools, incomplete evacuation, sensation of
  anorectal obstruction, manual maneuvers to facilitate defecation, stool frequency <3/wk
- **Secondary etiologies (4 M's)**
  Mech obstruction: malignancy, compression, rectocele, strictures
  Meds: opioids, TCAs, anticholinergics, CCB, NSAIDs, diuretics, Ca^{2+}, Fe
  Metabolic/endo: DM, hypothyroid, uremia, preg, panhypopit, porphyria, ↑ Ca, ↓ K, ↓ Mg
  Myopathy/Neuro: Parkinson's, Hirschsprung's, amyloid, MS, spinal injury, dysautonomia
- **Dx:** H&P w/ DRE. Labs: consider CBC, electrolytes, TSH. Colonoscopy if alarm sx.
  Anorectal manometry/balloon expulsion test; colonic transit study; defecography.
- **Treatment:** diet change w/ ↑ fluid intake, fiber supplementation
  Bulk laxatives (psyllium, methylcellulose, polycarbophil): ↑ colonic residue, ↑ peristalsis
  Osmotic laxatives (Mg, sodium phosphate [avoid if CKD], lactulose): ↑ water in colon
  Stimulant laxatives (senna, castor oil, bisacodyl, docusate sodium): ↑ motility & secretion
  Enema/suppository (phosphate, mineral oil, tap water, soapsuds, bisacodyl)
  Lubiprostone (↑ secretion); methylnaltrexone and alvimopan for opioid-induced
  Linaclotide ↑ stool freq, ↓ straining/bloating (NEJM 2011;365:6:527)

Nutrition in critical illness (see "Mech Ventilation" as well) (NEJM 2014;370:1227)
- In theory, enteral superior to parenteral as maintains integrity and function of GI tract,
  however, both routes with similar outcomes (NEJM 2014;371:1673)
- **Enteral (EN):** start w/in 24–48 hr of ICU admission tends to ↓ infxn & mort. Contraindic. if
  obstruction, major GIB. Complications: ischemic bowel injury due to ↑ demand for
  splanchnic blood flow, esp. if hemodynamically unstable; aspiration PNA (possibly ↓ risk if
  jejunal feeds but conflicting data), nasopharyngeal ulceration/bleeding due to tube.
- **Parenteral (PN):** start after 7 d if unable to tolerate enteral feeds, or ? sooner (JAMA
  2013;309:2130); late (>day 8 of ICU stay) initiation of PN to supplement insufficient EN ↓
  infxn & time on vent (NEJM 2011;365:506). Contraindic: hyperosmolality, severe electrolyte
  disturbances, severe hyperglycemia; sepsis is *relative* contraindication. Complications:
  hyperglycemia (due to dextrose), catheter sepsis/thrombus, refeeding syndrome, LFT
  abnl (steatosis, cholestasis, gallbladder sludge due to lack of enteric stimulation.

DISORDERS OF THE COLON

DIVERTICULOSIS

Definition & pathophysiology (*Lancet* 2004;363:631)
- Acquired herniations of colonic mucosa & submucosa in areas where vasa recta penetrate
- Thought to occur in setting of abnormal motility and ↑ intraluminal pressure

Epidemiology
- Risk factors: ↓ fiber, ↑ red meat, obesity, smoking, physical inactivity, EtOH, NSAIDs
- Prevalence higher w/ ↑ age (10% if <40 y; 50–66% if >80 y); "Westernized" societies
- **Left side** (90%, mostly sigmoid) > R side of colon (except in Asia where 75–85% R-sided)

Clinical manifestations
- Usually asx, but 5–15% develop diverticular hemorrhage (see "GIB") and <5% diverticulitis
- For asx diverticulosis, limited data for ↑ fiber diet or avoiding nuts/seeds (*JAMA* 2008;300:907)

DIVERTICULITIS

Pathophysiology (*NEJM* 2007;357:2057; *Gastroenterol* 2015;147:1944)
- Retention of undigested food and bacteria in diverticulum → fecalith formation → obstruction → compromise of diverticulum's blood supply, infection, perforation
- **Uncomplicated:** microperforation → localized infection
- **Complicated** (15%): macroperf → abscess, peritonitis, fistula (65% w/ bladder), obstrxn

Clinical manifestations
- **LLQ abdominal pain, fever,** nausea, vomiting, constipation or diarrhea
- PEx ranges from LLQ tenderness ± palpable mass to peritoneal signs & septic shock
- Ddx includes IBD, infectious colitis, PID, tubal pregnancy, cystitis, colorectal cancer

Diagnostic studies
- Plain abdominal radiographs to r/o free air, ileus or obstruction
- **Abdominal CT** (I⁺O⁺): >95% Se & Sp; assess complicated disease (abscess, fistula)
- Colonoscopy *contraindicated* acutely ↑ risk of perforation; do 6 wk after to r/o neoplasm

Treatment (*JAMA* 2014;311:287; *Dis Colon Rectum* 2014;57:284)
- Mild: outPt Rx indicated if Pt has few comorbidities and can tolerate POs
  PO abx: (MNZ + FQ) or amox/clav for 7–10 d; liquid diet until clinical improvement
  Possible that abx not be needed for uncomplicated diverticulitis (*Cochrane* CD009092)
- Severe: inPt Rx if cannot take POs, narcotics needed for pain, or complications
  NPO, IVF, NGT (if ileus)
  IV abx (GNR & anaerobic coverage; eg, CTX/MNZ or pip-tazo)
- Abscesses >4 cm should be drained percutaneously or surgically
- Surgery: if progression despite med Rx, undrainable abscess, free perforation
  Resection superior to laparoscopic lavage (*JAMA* 2015;314:1364)
  After source control, 4 d abx may be sufficient (*NEJM* 2015;372:1996)
  Resection for recurrent bouts of diverticulitis on a case by case basis
  Consider lower threshold for urgent & elective surgery for immunocompromised Pts

Prevention
- Mesalamine ± rifaximin may provide sx relief in chronic/recurrent dis. (*Dig Sci* 2007;52:2934)
- Risk of recurrence 10–30% w/in 10 y of 1ˢᵗ episode; more likely 2ⁿᵈ episode complicated

POLYPS & ADENOMAS

Pathophysiology & Epidemiology (*NEJM* 2016;374:1065)
- Accumulation of mutations in colonic epithelial cell DNA affecting oncogenes & tumor suppressor genes → *tumor initiation* (formation of adenoma; *APC* loss of fxn) → *tumor progression* (adenoma → carcinoma; *K-ras* gain of fxn, *DCC*, *p53* loss of fxn).
- Risk factors: ↑ age, FHx (sporadic in 1° relatives, Lynch, FAP), IBD, ↑ dietary fat, central adiposity, ↑ EtOH, ↓ fiber, ↑ red meat, ? smoking, DM
- Protective factors: ↑ physical activity, ASA/NSAIDs, Ca²⁺ intake, HRT, ↓ BMI; possibly ↑ fiber, vitamin D, fish oil, statins, selenium
- Neoplastic polyps: adenomas (tubular, villous, tubulovillous dysplasia), sessile serrated adenomas/polyps (concern for interval CRC), carcinomas.
- Nonneoplastic polyps: hyperplastic, juvenile, Peutz-Jeghers, inflammatory

Detection
- *Colonoscopy* is gold standard
- Recommended in all Pts starting at age 50 and then typically q10y unless pathology found
- If ⊕ FHx, start age 40, or 10 y before age of dx in youngest family member, repeat q5y

INFLAMMATORY BOWEL DISEASE

Definition
- **Ulcerative colitis (UC):** inflammation of the colonic *mucosa*; *contiguous*, starting at rectum
- **Crohn's disease (CD):** *transmural* inflammation occurring anywhere in GI tract, *skip areas*

Epidem & pathophys (NEJM 2009;361:2066; Gastro 2011;140:1785; Lancet 2016;387:156)
- 1.4 million people in U.S.; prev 1:1000 UC & 1:3000 CD; ↑ incidence in Caucasians, Jews
- Age of onset 15–30 y in UC and CD; CD is bimodal and has second peak at 50–70 y
- Smokers at ↑ risk for CD, whereas nonsmokers & former smokers at ↑ risk for UC
- Genetic predisposition + environmental risk factors → T cell dysregulation → inflammation

ULCERATIVE COLITIS (NEJM 2011;365:1713; Lancet 2012;380:1606)

Clinical manifestations
- **Grossly bloody diarrhea,** lower abdominal cramps, urgency, tenesmus
- Extracolonic (>25%): erythema nodosum, pyoderma gangrenosum, aphthous ulcers, uveitis, episcleritis, thromboembolic events (esp. during a flare; Lancet 2010;375:657), AIHA, seroneg arthritis, chronic hepatitis, cirrhosis, PSC (↑ risk cholangio CA, CRC)

Diagnosis
- **Colonoscopy:** involves rectum (95%) & extends proximally and *contiguously within colon*
- Classify by location: proctitis (25–55%), left-sided colitis (50–70%) and pancolitis (20%)
- Appearance: granular, friable mucosa with diffuse ulceration; *pseudopolyps*
- Histology: superficial chronic inflammation; crypt abscesses & architectural distortion
- Barium enema with featureless and tubular appearance of colon (*leadpipe appearance*)
- Flares: ↑ ESR & CRP (not Se or Sp); ⊕ fecal calprotectin (Se 77%, Sp 71%)

Complications
- **Toxic megacolon** (5%): colon dilatation (≥6 cm on KUB), colonic atony, systemic toxicity, & ↑ risk of perf. Rx w/ IV steroids & broad-spectrum abx; surgery if needed.
- Stricture (5%): occurs in rectosigmoid after repeated episodes of inflammation
- CRC and dysplasia (see below)
- For patients s/p surgery w/ ileal pouch, may develop *pouchitis* (inflammation of ileal pouch, up to ½ of pts), Rx w/ abx (MNZ, cipro), probiotics

Prognosis
- 50% of Pts in remission at any given time; intermittent exacerbations in 90%; continual active disease in ~18%. Rate of colectomy at 10 y is 24%.
- Mortality rate of severe UC flare is <2%, & overall life expectancy in UC = non-UC Pts

CROHN'S DISEASE (Lancet 2012;380:1590)

Clinical manifestations
- **Abdominal pain,** loose/frequent stools (up to 50% ⊕ FOBT), fever, malaise, wt loss
- Mucus-containing, **nongrossly bloody diarrhea**
- N/V, bloating, obstipation if presence of obstruction; extracolonic manifestations as in UC

Diagnosis
- **Ileocolonoscopy + bx** is gold standard; **small bowel imaging** (eg MR-enterography – 91% accuracy in identifying Crohn's compared to endoscopy); capsule endoscopy
- Classify by location: small bowel (47%), ileocolonic (21%), colonic (28%); upper tract rare
- Montreal classification: age at dx, disease location & behavior (stricturing vs. nonstricturing, penetrating vs. nonpenetrating), plus modifiers for upper tract & perianal disease
- Appearance: nonfriable mucosa, cobblestoning, aphthous ulcers, deep & long **fissures**
- Histology: **transmural inflammation** with mononuclear cell infiltrate, **noncaseating granulomas** (seen in <25% of mucosal biopsies), fibrosis, ulcers, fissures
- Track disease severity w/ Crohn's Disease Activity Index (CDAI) questionnaire

Complications
- **Perianal disease:** fissures, fistulas, skin tags, perirectal abscesses (in 24% of Pts; perianal disease *precedes* intestinal symptomatology)
- **Stricture:** small bowel, postprandial abd pain; can lead to complete SBO & require surgery
- **Fistulas:** perianal, enteroenteric, rectovaginal, enterovesicular, enterocutaneous
- **Abscess:** fever, tender abd mass, ↑WBC; *steroids mask sx*, ∴ need high-level suspicion
- **Malabsorption:** ileal disease/resection: ↓ bile acids abs → gallstones; ↓ fatty acid abs → Ca oxalate kidney stones; ↓ fat soluble vitamin abs → vit D deficiency → osteopenia

Prognosis
- Variable at 1 y: ~50% in remission, ~20% flare, ~20% low activity, ~10% chronic active
- At 20 y, majority will have required some surgery; overall life expectancy is slightly ↓

Initial evaluation

- **H&P** (✓ for intestinal & extraintestinal manifestations) and **diagnostic studies** as above
- **Lab:** consider CBC/diff, LFTs, iron studies, B12, folate, vit D. Fecal calprotectin & lactoferrin have higher Se & Sp than ESR & CRP.
- **Exclude other etiologies:** infectious/ischemic colitis, intestinal lymphoma/carcinoma, CRC, IBS, vasculitis, Behçet's, celiac disease, small intestinal bacterial overgrowth
- **Rule out infection** (esp. CMV) before treating with immunosuppressants and biologics

Goals of treatment

- Induce remission of acute flare → maintain remission; mucosal healing 1° goal
- Convention is step up Rx (least → most toxic). Early combined immunosuppression Rx not yet widely adopted; consider if severe disease (Lancet 2015;386:1825).

Medical Therapy for IBD (in stepwise sequence)	
Ulcerative colitis	
Mild	**5-ASA:** many formulations (sulfasalazine, mesalamine, olsalazine, balsalazide) depending on disease location. Used to induce remission & for maintenance. Complications: diarrhea, abd pain, pancreatitis.
Mild-Moderate	**MMX-budesonide:** oral formulation of budesonide released throughout entire colon for flare. 1ˢᵗ pass metab ↓ systemic adverse effects of steroid.
Moderate-Severe	**PO prednisone:** 40–60 mg w/ taper over several wks to induce remission. **AZA/6-MP:** 0.5–1 mg/kg and uptitrate over several wks for maintenance. Complic: BM suppression, lymphoma, pancreatitis, hepatitis; ✓ TPMT levels prior to dosing to ↓ risk of generation of toxic metabolites. In selected cases can add allopurinol to boost activity in non-responders.
Severe or refractory disease	**IV steroids:** eg, 100 mg hydrocort q8h or 16–20 mg methylprednisolone q8h to induce remission w/ plan to taper & switch to non-steroid maintenance. **Cyclosporine:** for severe flares refractory to steroids, 2–4 mg/kg infusion × 7 d w/ goal to Δ to maintenance medication (eg, AZA/6-MP) **Anti-TNF** (infliximab, adalimumab & golimumab): 15–20% remission rates (Gastro 2012;142:257). For steroid-refractory flares or to maintain remission. Complic: reactivation TB (✓ PPD prior to Rx); exclude viral hepatitis; small ↑'d risk NHL; infusion & lupus-like rxn, psoriasis, MS, CHF. **Vedolizumab** (see below) Investigational: tofacitinib (janus kinase inhib; NEJM 2012;367:616), fecal transplant (Gastro 2015;149:102)
Crohn's disease	
Mild	**5-ASA:** Sulfasalazine 4–6 g/d may be useful in inducing remission **Abx:** FQ/MNZ or amox/clav for pyogenic complic (fistulas, perineal dis.)
Mild-mod	**Budesonide:** oral formulation able to reach ileum
Moderate-severe	**PO prednisone:** same as UC, for inducing remission, not maintenance **AZA/6-MP:** same as UC, for maintenance **MTX:** 15–25 mg IM/SC or PO qwk for maintenance; 1–2 mo to take effect
Severe or refractory disease	**Anti-TNF:** infliximab, adalimumab or certolizumab (pegylated) If flare on infliximab, ✓ trough & presence of anti-infliximab Ab. Low & ⊖ Ab → ↑ dose/freq. If ⊕ Ab → Δ to other biologic (Am J Gastro 2011;106:685). **Vedolizumab** (anti-α4β7 integrin) and **ustekinumab** (anti-IL 12/23) if refractory to anti-TNFs SMAD7 anti-sense oligonucleotide (NEJM 2015;372:1104) under study

Surgery

- **UC:** colectomy if sx refractory to or intolerable side effects from meds, CRC, perforation, toxic megacolon, uncontrolled hemorrhage. Often *ileal pouch-anal anastomosis* (IPAA).
- **CD:** resection if refractory disease; endoscopic dilation or surgery for strictures; diverting ileostomy for perineal disease

Cancer screening (NEJM 2015;372:1441)

- **Colon cancer:** risk in UC ~2% at 10 y, ~8% at 20 y, ~18% at 30 y. Similar for colonic CD, plus risk of small bowel cancer as well. Dysplasia best marker for risk. Other risk factors include: PSC, ⊕ FHx, greater extent of disease, stricture, & pseudopolyps.
- **Surveillance:** *colonoscopy* w/ random bx 8 y after dx to eval for dysplasia, q1–3y thereafter based on risk factors. *Chromoendoscopy* using dye to stain high-risk lesions for targeted biopsy is emerging technique. If high-grade dysplasia or dysplasia assoc. lesion/mass → colectomy. Chemoprophylaxis: 5-ASA & ursodeoxycholic acid (if PSC) ? beneficial (AJG 2011;106:731; Aliment Pharmacol Ther 2012;35:451).

ACUTE MESENTERIC ISCHEMIA

Definition and Causes
- Reduced or absent blood flow to small intestine, typically caused by *arterial* (ie, SMA or its branches) occlusion or transient hypoperfusion or less often by *venous* occlusion
- **SMA thrombosis** (~60%): typically due to atherosclerosis at origin of SMA; other risk factors incl. vascular injury from abd trauma, infl'y, or mesenteric dissections/aneurysms
- **SMA embolism** (~30%): embolic occlusion to SMA (has narrow take-off angle), often in setting of AF, valvular disease incl. endocarditis, atherosclerotic plaque in aorta
- **Nonocclusive mesenteric ischemia** (~10%): transient intestinal hypoperfusion due to ↓ CO, athero, sepsis, drugs that ↓ gut perfusion (pressors, cocaine, amphetamines)
- Mesenteric **venous thrombosis** (MVT, ~5%): a/w hypercoag. states, portal hypertension, IBD, malignancy, inflammation (pancreatitis, peritonitis), pregnancy, trauma, surgery
- **Focal segmental ischemia of the small bowel** (<5%): vascular occlusion to small segments of the small bowel (vasculitis, atheromatous emboli, strangulated hernias, XRT)

Clinical manifestations
- Total arterial or venous occlusion: **sudden abd pain out of proportion to abdominal tenderness on exam,** progressing to frank infarction w/ peritoneal signs if untreated
- Nonocclusive: abd distention & pain, N/V, **lower GI bleeding** due to mucosal sloughing; often occurring after episode of hypoperfusion (e.g. cardiac event or shock)

Physical Exam
- From unremarkable ± abd distention to peritoneal signs (bowel infarction); ⊕ **FOBT ~75%**

Diagnostic Studies
- Dx relies on high level of suspicion; rapid dx essential to avoid infarction (occurs w/in hrs)
- Mortality 20 to >70% if bowel infarcted; dx prior to infarction strongest predictor of survival
- Laboratory: often nl; ~75% ↑ WBC; ↑ amylase, LDH, PO₄, D-dimer; ~50% ↑ lactate (late)
- KUB: nl early before infarct; "thumbprinting," ileus, pneumatosis in later stages
- **CT angiography** (arterial phase): noninvasive test of choice; *venous* phase for dx MVT
- **Angiography**: gold standard; potentially therapeutic; indicated if vasc occlusion suspected

Treatment (NEJM 2016;374:959)
- IVF, NPO, **optimize hemodynamics** (minimize pressors), **broad-spectrum abx, anticoagulation** w/ heparin ± tPA (for occlusive disease), **IV papaverine** (vasodilator; for all)
- If evidence of peritonitis: to OR for surgical endovascular therapies & bowel resection
- **SMA thrombosis:** percutaneous (stenting) or surgical revascularization
- **SMA embolism:** embolectomy (catheter-based aspiration vs. surgical)
- **Nonocclusive:** correct underlying cause (esp. cardiac)
- **Mesenteric venous thrombosis:** 3–6 mo. warfarin after initial heparinization. Fibrinolysis or thrombectomy typically reserved for Pts w/ hemodynamic instability or refractory sx.
- **Focal segmental ischemia:** typically surgical resection

CHRONIC MESENTERIC ISCHEMIA
- Definition and causes: ↓ blood flow to gut typically because of mesenteric atherosclerosis
- Sx: "intestinal angina" = **postprandial abd pain,** early satiety, & ↓ wt due to fear of eating. If pain becomes constant → could represent acute thrombosis (see above).
- Dx: angiography (gold std) ≈ gastric tonometry exercise testing + duplex U/S (if available)
- Treatment: surgical revascularization (1st line); could also consider angioplasty ± stenting

ISCHEMIC COLITIS

Definition & pathophysiology
- Nonocclusive disease 2° to Δs in systemic circulation or anatomic/fxnal Δs in local mesenteric vasculature; often underlying etiology unknown, frequently seen in elderly
- **"Watershed"** areas (splenic flexure & rectosigmoid) most susceptible, 25% involve R side

Clinical manifestations, diagnosis, & treatment
- Disease spectrum: reversible colopathy (35%), transient colitis (15%), chronic ulcerating colitis (20%), resulting stricture (10%), gangrene (15%), fulminant colitis (<5%)
- Usually p/w **cramping LLQ pain w/ overtly bloody stool;** fever and peritoneal signs should raise clinical suspicion for infarction
- Dx: **flex sig/colonoscopy** or **CT abd/pelvis** to make diagnosis; r/o IBD, infectious colitis
- Treatment: bowel rest, IV fluids, **broad-spectrum abx,** serial abd exams; **surgery** for infarction, fulminant colitis, hemorrhage, failure of med Rx, recurrent sepsis, stricture
- Resolution w/in 48 h w/ conservative measures occurs in >50% of cases

ACUTE PANCREATITIS (AP)

Pathogenesis

- Pancreatic duct and acinar injury via direct or indirect toxicity → impaired secretion and premature activation of digestive enzymes → autodigestion and acute inflammation

Etiologies *(Lancet 2015;386:85)*

- **Gallstones (40%):** ♀ > ♂, usually small stones (<5 mm) or microlithiasis/sludge
- **Alcohol (30%):** ♂ > ♀, 1st attack after ~10 y heavy use; usually chronic w/ acute flares
- Anatomic: divisum, annular pancreas, duodenal duplication cysts, Sphincter of Oddi dysfxn
- Autoimmune: can p/w chronic disease, panc mass or panc duct strictures, ↑ IgG4, ⊕ ANA
- Drugs: 5-ASA, 6-MP/AZA, ACEI, cytosine, didanosine, dapsone, estrogen, furosemide, isoniazid, metronidazole, pentamidine, statins, sulfa, thiazides, tetracycline, valproate
- Familial: a/w mutations in *PRSS1, CFTR, SPINK1*; suspect if early onset (age <20 y)
- Infections: ascariasis, clonorchiasis, coxsackie, CMV, HIV, mumps, mycoplasma, TB, toxo
- Ischemia: vasculitis, cholesterol emboli, hypovolemic shock, cardiopulmonary bypass
- Metabolic: hypertriglyceridemia (TG >1000; type I and V familial hyperlipemia), hyperCa
- Neoplastic: panc/ampullary tumors, mets (RCC most common, breast, lung, melanoma)
- Post ERCP (5%): Ppx w/ PR indomethacin *(NEJM 2012;366:1414)*, panc duct stent if high risk
- Post trauma: blunt abdominal trauma, pancreatic/biliary surgery
- Toxins: organophosphates, scorpion toxin, methanol

Clinical manifestations

- **Epigastric abdominal pain (90%),** only 50% p/w classic bandlike pain radiating to back
- 10% pain-free (due to analgesic/steroid use, immunosuppressed, ∆MS, ICU, post-op), ∴ ✓ amylase/lipase in Pts w/ unexplained shock *(Am J Gastro 1991;86:322)*.
- **Nausea and vomiting (90%)**
- Abdominal tenderness/guarding, ↓ bowel sounds (ileus), jaundice if biliary obstruction
- Signs of retroperitoneal hemorrhage (Cullen's = periumbilical; Grey Turner's = flank) rare
- Ddx: acute cholecystitis, perforated viscus, SBO, mesenteric ischemia, IMI, AAA leak, distal aortic dissection, ruptured ectopic pregnancy

Diagnostic studies

- **Dx requires 2 of 3:** characteristic abd pain; lipase or amylase >3× ULN; ⊕ imaging
- Laboratory *(Am J Gastro 2013;108:1400)*
    levels of both amylase and lipase do *not* correlate w/ severity of disease
    ↑ **amylase:** >3× ULN >90% sensitive, >70% specific for acute pancreatitis
        false ⊖: acute on chronic (eg, alcoholic); hypertriglyceridemia (↓ amylase activity)
        false ⊕: other abd or salivary gland process, acidemia, renal failure, macroamylasemia
    ↑ **lipase:** >3× ULN 99% sensitive, 99% specific for acute pancreatitis
        false ⊕: renal failure, other abd process, diabetic ketoacidosis, HIV, macrolipasemia
        longer half-life than amylase: useful in Pts w/ delayed presentation after onset of sx
    lipase >10,000 has 80% PPV for biliary dx, 99% NPV for EtOH *(Dig Dis Sci 2011;56: 3376)*
    ALT >3× ULN has 95% PPV for gallstone pancreatitis *(Am J Gastro 1994;89:1863)*
- Imaging studies *(Am J Gastro 2013;108:1400)*
    Abd U/S: typically not useful to visualize pancreas (obscured by bowel gas) but *should be ordered for all pts with AP to r/o biliary etiology* (ie, gallstones, BD dilatation)
    Abd CT: not rec for initial eval unless dx unclear (local complic. not yet visible & concern for AKI w/ IV contrast). However, if persistent pain and/or clinical deterioration after 48– 72 h, CT(I⁺) useful to r/o local complications (necrosis, fluid collections).
    MRI/MRCP: Can detect necrosis; also used to assess for stones & ductal disruption
    Endoscopic U/S (EUS): limited role; useful for occult biliary disease (microlithiasis)

Severity *(Am J Gastro 2009;104:710)*

- Severity defined by presence of organ failure (AKI, resp failure, GIB, shock) & local or systemic complic. (panc necrosis, fluid collections, gastric outlet obstrxn, splenic & PVT).
    Mild: 80% of cases. No organ failure or local/systemic complications, low mortality.
    Moderate: transient (<48 h) organ failure ± local/systemic complications, high morbidity.
    Severe: persistent (>48 h) organ failure, very high mortality

Prognosis

- Scoring systems *(Crit Care Med 1999;27:2272; Am J Gastro 2009;104:966)*
    Ranson's/APACHE II: earliest scoring systems predicting severity at 48 h using multiple physiological criteria; may have poor PPV for severe AP
    BISAP: simple 5-point scoring system (BUN >25, impaired MS, SIRS, age >60, pleural effusion) used w/in first 24 h; score ≥3 predicts ↑ risk of organ failure, mortality
    CTSI: uses CT findings at 48–72h (fluid collections, necrosis) to predict mortality
- Other criteria: SIRS >48 h, rising BUN/Hct, obesity, comorbid disease predict ↑ mortality

Treatment (Clin Gastro Hepatol 2011;9:710; Am J Gastro 2012;107:1146; NEJM 2014;370:150)

- **Fluid resuscitation:** early aggressive IVF, titrate to UOP ≥0.5 mL/kg/h, goal to ↓ BUN & Hct over first 12–24 h. LR may be superior to NS (↓ SIRS, CRP at 24 h; avoid if ↑ Ca)
- **Nutrition** (Clin Gastro Hepatol 2007;5:946; Intern Med 2012;51:523; Crit Care 2013;17:R118)
    Early enteral feeding encouraged (maintains gut barrier, ↓ bacterial translocation) though new data suggest may not be superior to oral feeding at 72 h (NEJM 2014;317:1983)
    Mild: Start feeding once pain-free w/o ileus. Low-fat low-residue diet as safe as liquid diet.
    Severe: early (w/in 48–72 h) enteral nutrition indicated and preferred over TPN b/c ↓ infectious complications, organ failure, surgical interventions, and mortality.
    Nasogastric feeding shown to be non-inferior to nasojejunal feeding
- **Analgesia:** IV opioids (monitor respiratory status, adjust dosing if ↑ renal impairment)
- **Gallstone pancreatitis:** urgent (w/in 24 h) ERCP w/ sphincterotomy if cholangitis, sepsis, or Tbili ≥5. For mild disease, CCY during initial hosp to ↓ risk of recurrence (Lancet 2015;386:1261); defer surgery if necrotizing AP until improvement in inflam., fluid collections.
- **Hypertriglyceridemia:** insulin gtt (activates lipoprotein lipase), fibrates, ± apheresis
- No role for ppx abx in absence of infectious complications (World J Gastroenterol 2012;18:279)

Complications
- Systemic: ARDS, abdominal compartment syndrome, AKI, GIB (pseudoaneurysm), DIC
- Metabolic: hypocalcemia, hyperglycemia, hypertriglyceridemia
- Fluid collections:
    Acute fluid collection: seen early, not encapsulated, most resolve w/in 1–2 wk w/o Rx
    Pseudocyst: ~4 wk after initial attack, encapsulated. No need for Rx if asx (regardless of size/location). If sx → endoscopic (Gastro 2013;145:583) vs. perc/surg drainage.
- Pancreatic necrosis: Nonviable pancreatic tissue. CT-guided FNA if infection suspected
    Sterile necrosis: if asx, can be managed expectantly, no role for ppx antibiotics
    Infected necrosis (5% of all cases, 30% of severe): high mortality. Rx w/ carbapenem or MDZ+FQ. "Step-up" Rx w/ perc drainage and minimally invasive surg debridement or endoscopic necrosectomy superior to open necrosectomy (NEJM 2010;362:1491)
    Pancreatic abscess: circumscribed collection of pus (usually w/o pancreatic tissue), usually seen ≥4 wk into course. Rx with abx + drainage (CT-guided if possible).

CHRONIC PANCREATITIS

Pathogenesis & Etiology
- Often, but not always, recurrent acute attacks → inflammatory infiltrate → fibrosis → pancreatic insufficiency (need to lose 90% of panc fxn to develop DM, fat/protein malabs.)
- Toxins (60–80% due to EtOH; smoking also important risk factor), idiopathic, genetic, autoimmune, relapsing AP, obstruction

Clinical manifestations
- Sxs include epigastric pain, N/V; over time will be painless and p/w steatorrhea and wt loss

Diagnostic studies
- Labs: amylase/lipase ↑ early, may be nl later. ⊕ fecal fat, ↓ stool elastase & A1AT.
    ✓ A1c, consider IgG4/ANA & genetic testing (CFTR, SPINK1, PRSS1) if young or ⊕ FHx.
- Imaging: Ca²⁺ on KUB/CT. ERCP/MRCP/EUS high Sens for dx: stricture, dilated ducts

Treatment (Lancet 2016;387:1957)
- Pancreatic enzyme replacement (may ↓ pain by reducing CCK)
- Pain control: smoking & EtOH cessation, analgesics, ESWL for duct stones, celiac nerve plexus block, thoracoscopic splanchnicectomy, resection.

Complications
- Pseudocysts, pseudoaneurysms, pancreatic ascites or pleural effusion, ↑ **risk of panc Ca**

AUTOIMMUNE PANCREATITIS

Pathogenesis
- Lymphoplasmacytic sclerosing pancreatitis w/ dense fibrosis and ↑ IgG4 (type 1), or granulocytic epithelial lesions with minimal IgG4 cells (type 2)

Clinical Manifestations
- **Abdominal pain,** can p/w obstructive jaundice and panc mass mimicking panc Ca.
- Extrapancreatic: Sjögren's, interstitial nephritis, autoimmune thyroiditis, UC/PSC, RA

Diagnosis
- Labs: cholestatic LFTs (↑ Aφ > AST/ALT), ↑ γ-globulins and IgG4, ⊕ ANA, RF
- HISORt criteria: Histology, Imaging ("sausage pancreas", bile duct stricture), Serology, other Organ involvement, Response to therapy

Treatment
- Corticosteroids 1ˢᵗ-line, immunomodulators (AZA, MMF, cyclophosphamide) if relapse

ABNORMAL LIVER TESTS

Tests of hepatocellular injury or cholestasis

- **Aminotransferases** (AST, ALT): intracellular enzymes released 2° necrosis/inflammation
  ALT more specific for liver than is AST (heart, skeletal muscle, kidney, brain, RBC/WBC)
  ↑ levels seen w/ most types of hepatocellular injury; skeletal musc. injury, MI (AST > ALT)
- **Alkaline phosphatase** (Aφ): enzyme bound in hepatic canalicular membrane.
  ↑ levels seen w/ biliary obstrxn or intrahepatic cholestasis
  also found in bone, intestines, kidney, placenta; confirm from liver w/: ↑ GGT (or ↑ 5'-NT)
- **Bilirubin:** product of heme metab (unconjugated, "indirect") carried by alb to liver
  where taken up for conjugation ("direct") to make soluble, then excreted into bile.
  ↑ direct hyperbili seen w/ cholestasis, enzymatic disorders (eg, Dubin-Johnson, Rotor's)
  ↑ indirect hyperbili seen with hemolysis, enzymatic disorders (eg, Crigler-Najjar, Gilbert's)
  jaundice seen when bili >2.5 mg/dL (esp. in sclera or under tongue);
  if hyperbili conjugated then ↑ urine bilirubin

Tests of hepatic function

- **Albumin:** marker for liver protein synthesis, ↓ slowly in liver failure (t½ ~15–18 d)
- **Prothrombin time** (PT): depends on synthesis of coag factors by liver (except FVIII);
  b/c t½ of some factors (eg, V, VII) is short, ↑ PT can occur w/in hrs of liver dysfxn

Patterns of LFTs

Pattern	ALT	AST	Aφ	Bilirubin
Hepatocellular	↑↑	↑↑	±↑	±↑ (direct)
Viral hepatitis, NASH	Often ALT > AST		±↑	±↑ (direct)
Alcoholic hepatitis	AST:ALT ≥ 2:1		±↑	±↑ (direct)
Ischemic injury	↑↑↑	↑↑↑	↑↑	↑↑ (direct)
Wilson's disease	↑	↑	Aφ:Tbili < 4	
Cholestatic	±↑	±↑	↑↑	↑↑ **(direct)**
Infiltrative	near nl	near nl	↑↑	±↑
Nonhepatic				
Skeletal muscle injury	AST >> ALT		nl	nl
Bone disease	nl	nl	↑ (w/ nl GGT)	nl
Hemolysis	nl	nl	nl	↑ (indirect)

- **R-value** = ratio of ALT:Aφ normalized to ULN for each = (ALT/ULN) ÷ (Aφ/ULN)
  R >5 suggests hepatocellular injury, <2 suggests cholestatic injury, 2–5 suggests mixed

Figure 3-3 Approach to abnormal liver tests with hepatocellular pattern

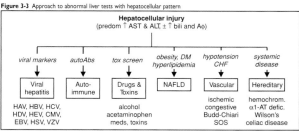

- **Workup for *acute* enzyme elevation** (often symptomatic)
  Severe ALT & AST elevation (>1000):
    toxins (usu. acetaminophen) → ✓ tox screen, EtOH, acet. levels. Other toxins: INH,
      disulfiram, pyrazinamide, OTC/herbal, fenofibrate, niacin, amiodarone, MDMA.
    ischemia (eg, sepsis, hypotension, Budd Chiari) → ✓ liver U/S w/ Doppler. Etiologies
      usually lead to ↑ LDH, ∴ usually ratio ALT:LDH <1.5 (vs. >1.5 w/ toxins, viruses).
    viruses (Hep A-E; HSV, CMV, VZV) → ✓ viral serologies
    other (AIH, acute Wilson Disease, acute biliary obstrxn) → see ALF & cirrhosis sections
  Acute mild-moderate ALT & AST elevation: as above, think meds/toxins (*see list at end of
    section*), viruses, ischemia/vascular issues in hospitalized Pts, obstruction (if mixed
    picture), systemic disease (see "Workup for chronic enzyme elevation," below)
- **Workup for *chronic* enzyme elevation** (often asymptomatic)
  Screen for common causes: hep serologies, EtOH, liver U/S (? NAFLD, cirrhosis), meds

If suspect underlying systemic disease: iron studies (HFE); ANA, ASMA, Ig levels (AIH); ceruloplasmin, urinary copper (Wilson); α1-AT (can cause liver dis even w/o lung involvement); celiac screening (rare cause of liver dis); thyroid studies; see "Cirrhosis"

If ⊖ evaluation → lifestyle modification (wt loss, DM control) & repeat testing 3–6 mo

If evidence of chronic liver disease or persistent lab abnl, consider liver bx

Figure 3-4 Approach to abnormal liver tests with cholestatic pattern

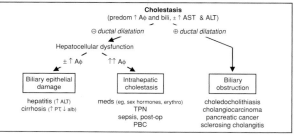

- **Workup for cholestatic pattern:** ✓ RUQ U/S to assess for ductal dilatation.
  If ⊕ (extrahepatic obstruction) → Pt may need ERCP ± imaging (MRCP, CT) for dx/Rx
  If no dilatation on U/S → ✓ AMA (for PBC), viral serologies (Hep A-E, EBV, CMV); if work-up negative, consider MRCP and liver bx. See offending med list below.

Figure 3-5 Approach to abnormal liver tests with infiltrative pattern

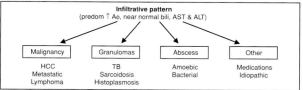

- **Workup for infiltrative pattern:** ✓ GGT level to ensure GI source of Aφ elevation.
  If ⊕ (↑ GGT & ↑ Aφ) → often imaging first step (RUQ U/S or CT; consider MRCP if these studies negative); ✓ SPEP (for amyloid), often need liver bx for definitive diagnosis.

Common medications that cause abnormal liver tests (http://livertox.nlm.nih.gov)

Hepatocellular		Cholestatic		Mixed
Acarbose	Prednisone	ACE inhibitors	6-MP	Amox-Clav
Acetaminophen	Protease	Anabolic	OCP	Azathioprine
Allopurinol	Inhibitors	Steroids	Penicillins	Carbamazepine
Amiodarone	Pyrazinamide	Azathioprine	Protease	Clindamycin
Azathioprine	Risperidone	Chlorpromazine	Inhibitors	Mirtazapine
Clindamycin	Statins	Estrogens	Sulfonamides	Nitrofurantoin
Fibrates	Sulfonamides	Macrolides	Terbinafine	Penicillins
Hydralazine	Tamoxifen	Methimazole	Tricyclics	Phenobarbital
Isoniazid	Tetracyclines			Phenytoin
Ketoconazole	TNF-alpha			Protease
Methotrexate	inhibitors			Inhibitors
Mirtazapine	Trazodone			Sulfonamides
Nitrofurantoin	Tricyclics			Trazodone
(Some) NSAIDs	Valproic Acid			Tricyclics
Phenytoin				Valproic acid
				Verapamil

VIRAL

Hepatitis A (ssRNA; 30–45% of acute viral hepatitis in U.S.)
- Transmission: fecal–oral route; contaminated food, water, shellfish; daycare center outbreaks
- Incubation: 2–6 wk; no chronic carrier state
- Sx: ↓ appetite, malaise, fever, N/V, RUQ pain, jaundice; rarely fulminant (↑ w/ chronic HCV)
- Diagnosis: acute hepatitis → ⊕ IgM anti-HAV; past exposure → ⊕ IgG anti-HAV (⊖ IgM)
- Rx for acute HAV: supportive care; refer to liver txplnt center if fulminant hepatitis
- Postexposure ppx: age 1–40 y → vaccine; age <1 y or >40 y, immunosupp, liver dis. → Ig

Hepatitis B (dsDNA; ~45% of acute viral hepatitis in U.S.; *Lancet* 2014;384:2053)
- Transmission: blood (IVDU, transfusion), sexual, perinatal
- Incubation: 6 wk–6 mo (mean 12–14 wk)
- Acute infxn: 70% subclinical, 30% jaundice, <1% fulminant hepatitis (up to 60% mortality)
- Chronic infxn: HBsAg ⊕ >6 mo in <5% of adult-acquired (↑ if immunosupp), >90% of perinatal; ~40% chronic HBV → cirrhosis (↑ risk w/ HCV, HDV, or HIV coinfxn, EtOH)
- HCC: ↑ risk if cirrhotic, FHx HCC, African >20 y old, Asian ♂ >50 y old or ♀ >40 y old or ↑ ALT ± HBV DNA >2000. Screen w/ AFP & U/S q6mo.
- Extrahepatic syndromes: PAN (<1%), membranous nephropathy, MPGN, arthritis
- Serologic and virologic tests (see *Annals* 2014;161:58 for screening guidelines)
  HBsAg: appears before sx; used to screen blood donors; persists >6 mo = chronic HBV
  HBeAg: evidence of viral replication and ↑ infectivity
  IgM anti-HBc: 1st Ab to appear; indicates acute infection
   window period = HBsAg becomes ⊖, anti-HBs not yet ⊕, anti-HBc only clue to infxn
  IgG anti-HBc: indicates previous (HBsAg ⊖) or ongoing (HBsAg ⊕) HBV infection
  anti-HBe: indicates waning viral replication & ↓ infectivity
  anti-HBs: indicates resolution of acute disease & immunity (sole marker after vaccination)
  HBV DNA: presence in serum correlates w/ active viral replication in liver

Diagnosis	HbsAg	anti-HBs	anti-HBc	HBeAg	anti-HBe	HBV DNA
Acute hepatitis	⊕	⊖	IgM	⊕	⊖	⊕
Window period	⊖	⊖	IgM	±	±	⊕
Recovery	⊖	⊕	IgG	⊖	±	⊖
Immunization	⊖	⊕	⊖	⊖	⊖	⊖
Chronic hepatitis *HBeAg* ⊕	⊕	⊖	IgG	⊕	⊖	⊕
Chronic hepatitis *HBeAg* ⊖	⊕	⊖	IgG	⊖	⊕	±*

*Precore mutant: HBeAg not made, but anti-HBe can develop due to x-reactivity w/ HBcAg; a/w ↑ HBV DNA

- Rx for acute HBV: supportive; hospitalize for Δ MS or ↑ INR (liver transplant center); consider antiviral therapy if severe

Phases of Chronic HBV					
Phase	ALT (ULN*)	HBV DNA (IU/mL)	HBeAg	Liver Histology (inflammation/fibrosis)	Progression to cirrhosis
Immune-tolerant	Nl	≥10⁶	⊕	Minimal	<0.5%/y
Immune-active *HBeAg* ⊕	≥2×	≥20k	⊕	Moderate-to-severe	2–5.5%/y
Inactive	Nl	≤2k	⊖	Min necroinflam.; variable fibrosis	0.05%/y
Immune React- ivation; *HBeAg* ⊖ precore mutant	≥2×	≥2k	⊖	Moderate-to-severe	8–10%/y

*ALT ULN <30 U/Ll for ♂, <19 U/L for ♀. Adapted from *Hepatology* 2016;63:261.

- Rx of chronic HBV: Rx in immune-active or immune reactivation phases or cirrhotics w/ elevated HBV DNA or decomp. Consider bx if ALT 1–2× ULN or in immune-tolerant phase if age >40 y; Rx if mod-to-severe inflammation or fibrosis on bx.
- **Entecavir** or **tenofovir**: nucleo(s/t)ide analogs, well tolerated, low resistance; at 5 y, HBeAg seroconversion is 30–40% & loss of HBsAg is 5–10% (*Gastro* 2012;142:1360; *Lancet* 2013;381:468). Tenofovir preferred if h/o lamivudine resistance.
- **PEG IFN-α2a**: At 2 y, HBeAg seroconversion is 27%; contraindicated if autoimmune disease, uncontrolled psych disorder, seizures, decompensated cirrhosis

- Rx duration: (1) HBeAg ⊕ immune-active w/o cirrhosis: if seroconversion (HBeAg ⊖, anti-HBe ⊕), can stop after 1 y if ALT nl & HBV DNA suppressed or until HBsAg clears; (2) HBeAg ⊖ immune reactivation: indefinite; (3) cirrhotic: indefinite
- If undergo liver transplant: HBIG + nucleo(s/t)ide analogue effective in preventing reinfection
- HIV/HBV coinfection: Rx w/ 2 drugs active against both HBV & HIV (NEJM 2007;356:1445)
- Immunosuppression: prior to initiating chemoRx, anti-TNF, steroids (>20 mg/d > 1 mo), screen Pts for HBV; Rx if moderate to high risk of reactivation (Gastro 2015;148:215)
- Postexposure (risk infxn ~30%) ppx: HBIG → vaccine (if unvac or known nonresponder)

Hepatitis C (ssRNA; ~10% of acute viral hepatitis in U.S.; Lancet 2015;385:1124)
- Transmission: blood (IVDU, transfusion rare cause) > sexual; 20–30% w/o clear precipitant
- Incubation: 1–5 mo; mean 6–7 wk
- Acute infxn: 80% subclinical; 10–20% sx hepatitis w/ jaundice; fulminant hepatitis rare; prob of spont clearance a/w IL28B & HLA class II genotypes (Annals 2013;158:235)
- Chronic: up to 85% → chronic hepatitis, 20–30% of whom develop cirrhosis (after ~20 y ↑ risk of cirrhosis in men, EtOH, HIV; HCC in 1–4% of cirrhotics/y
- Extrahepatic syndromes: mixed cryoglobulinemia, porphyria cutanea tarda, lichen planus, leukocytoclastic vasculitis, thyroiditis, MPGN, IPF, NHL and monoclonal gammopathies
- Serologic, virologic, & genetic tests
  anti-HCV (ELISA): ⊕ in 6 wk, does *not* = recovery or immunity; can be ⊖ after recovery
  HCV RNA: ⊕ w/in 2 wk, marker of active infection
  HCV genotype (1–6): guides duration & predicts response to Rx; geno. 3 a/w ↑ risk HCC
- Dx: *acute hepatitis* = ⊕ HCV RNA, ± anti-HCV; *resolved* = ⊖ HCV RNA, ± anti-HCV; *chronic* = ⊕ HCV RNA, ⊕ anti-HCV
- Treatment indications (www.hcvguidelines.org)
  Acute: if no spont. clearance at 12–16 wk, can Rx w/ same regimens for chronic HCV
  Chronic: Rx recommended for all except those with ↓ life expectancy
- Rx: NS3/4A protease inhibitors ("…previr"; PI), NS5a inhibitors ("…asvir"; NS5ai), RNA polymerase inhibitors ("…buvir"; RNAPi), ribavirin (RBV), pegylated-interferon (PEG-IFN)

Approved HCV Regimens for Treatment-Naïve Patients						
PI	**NS5ai**	**RNAPi**	**RBV**	**PEG-IFN**	**Genotypes**
	Daclatasvir	Sofosbuvir	±		1a, 1b, 2, 3
	Ledipasvir	Sofosbuvir			1a, 1b, 4, 5, 6
	Velpatasvir	Sofosbuvir			1, 2, 3, 4, 5, 6
Paritaprevir*	Ombitasvir	Dasabuvir	±		1a, 1b
Paritaprevir*	Ombitasvir		±		4
Simeprevir		Sofosbuvir	±		1a, 1b
		Sofosbuvir	⊕		2, 3, 4, 5, 6
Grazoprevir	Elbasvir		±		1, 4

*Boost with ritonavir. www.hcvguidelines.org. NEJM 2014;370:211, 220, 1483, 1574, 1879, 1889, 1973, 1983, 1993 & 2015;373:2608 & 2618; Lancet 2014;384:1756.

- Monitoring on Rx: CBC, INR, LFTs, GFR, HCV VL, and TSH (if IFN is used) prior to starting Rx. PIs contraind. if decomp. liver dx (ascites, encephalopathy) or CTP score ≥7. D/c Rx if jaundice, N/V, weakness, 10x ↑ in ALT, or significant ↑ in bili, A⊕, INR after 4 wk.
- Goal is sustained virologic response (SVR) = ∅ viremia 12 wk after completion of Rx. Success depends on genotype but SVR rates >90% with current regimens
- Special populations (HCV/HIV coinfection, decompensated cirrhosis, s/p liver transplant, renal impairment): www.hcvguidelines.com for updated recs on mgmt
- Vaccinate all chronic HCV patients against HBV and HAV if not immune
- Postexposure (needlestick risk ~3%) ppx: none; if HCV RNA → ⊕, consider Rx w/in 3 mo

Hepatitis D (RNA)
- Transmission: blood or sexual; endemic in Africa & E. Europe. Generally requires host to already have HBV infxn in order to cause co-infection or superinfection; in rare cases (immunosupp s/p liver txplt) can replicate autonomously.
- Natural hx: acute HBV-HDV coinfection resolves in >80% of cases; however acute HDV superinfection leads to chronic HBV-HDV in most cases (↑ progression to cirrhosis, HCC)

Hepatitis E (ssRNA; NEJM 2012;367:1237; Lancet 2012;379:2477)
- Most common cause of acute viral hepatitis in endemic areas
- Transmission: fecal–oral; travelers to central & SE Asia, Africa and Mexico, exp. to swine
- Natural hx: acute hepatitis w/ ↑ mort. (10–20%) if pregnant; rare chronic in transplant Pts
- Dx: IgM anti-HEV (through CDC), HEV RNA
- Extrahepatic sx: arthritis, pancreatitis, anemia, neuro (GBS, meningoencephalitis)

Other viruses (human pegivirus, CMV, EBV, HSV, VZV)

AUTOIMMUNE HEPATITIS (AIH)

Classification (J Hep 2011;55:171; Hep 2010;51:2193)
- Type 1: antismooth muscle Ab (ASMA), ANA; antisoluble liver antigen (anti-SLA), a/w more severe disease and relapsing disease
- Type 2: anti-liver/kidney microsome 1 (anti-LKM1); anti-liver cytosol type 1 (ALC-1);
- Overlap syndrome: AIH + PBC (suspect if ⊕ antimitochondrial Ab or ⊕ histology → "autoimmune cholangitis") or PSC (suspect if ⊕ IBD, pruritus, or radiology/histology)
- Drug-induced: minocycline, nitrofurantoin, infliximab, hydralazine, α-methyl DOPA, statins

Diagnosis and treatment (Lancet 2013;382:1433)
- 70% female; 40% present w/ severe AIH (3% fulminant) w/ ALT >10 × ULN; 34–45% asx
- Extrahepatic syndromes: thyroiditis, arthritis, UC, Sjögren's, Coombs' ⊕ hemolytic anemia
- Dx: scoring system combining serologies, ↑ IgG, Ø viral hepatitis, & liver bx (interface hepatitis & lymphoplasmacytic infiltrate) has high Sp & mod Se (Hep 2008;48:169)
- Rx: (1) ALT 10× ULN; (2) ALT 5× ULN & IgG 2× ULN; or (3) bridging/multiacinar necrosis
- Induction Rx: (1) prednisone monoRx; (2) prednisone + AZA, or (3) budesonide (if non-cirrhotic) + AZA → 65–80% remission (asx, nl LFTs, bili, & IgG, none to minimal interface hepatitis); taper steroids as able; relapse rate of 50–80% (J Hep 2015;62:S100)
- Nonresponders or AZA intolerant: cyclosporine, tacrolimus, MMF, rituximab, infliximab
- HCC screening and liver transplant referral for ESLD

OTHER CAUSES OF HEPATITIS OR HEPATOTOXICITY

Alcoholic hepatitis (J Hep 2012;57:399; Hep 2010;51:307)
- Sx: progressive jaundice, tender hepatomegaly, fever, ascites, GIB, encephalopathy
- Labs: ALT usually <300–500 w/ AST:ALT > 2:1, ↓ plt, ↑ Tbili & INR indicate severe hepatitis
- Prognosis: scoring systems include Maddrey's discriminant fxn (MDF), Lille model, MELD
  MDF (4.6 × [PT − control] + Tb) >32 w/ 30–50% 1-mo mortality if un Rx'd (Gastro 1996;110:1847)
  Lille model: predicts nonresponse to steroids after 1st week of Rx; score > 0.45 predicts poor response to further steroid Rx and a/w ↓ in 6-mo survival (Hep 2007;45:1348)
  Combination of Lille + MELD scores best predictor of mortality (Gastro 2015;149:398)
- Rx: consider if MDF >32, MELD >18, or presence of encephalopathy
  Steroids (eg, methylprednisolone 32 mg/d or prednisolone 40 mg/d × 4 wk → 4–6 wk taper) ↓ death but ↑ rate of infections (NEJM 1992;326:507 & 2015;372:1619)
  Contraindications: active GIB, pancreatitis, untreated HBV, uncontrolled infections
  Pentoxifylline of no benefit alone or when added to steroids (NEJM 2015;372:1619)
  Addition of NAC to steroids ↓ 1-mo but not 6-mo mortality (NEJM 2011;365:1781)

Acetaminophen hepatotoxicity (NEJM 2008;359:285; BMJ 2011;342:2218)
- Pathophysiology: >90% of acetaminophen (N-acetyl-p-aminophenol, APAP) metab into nontoxic metab, but ~5% metab by CYP2E1 into NAPQI, a hepatotoxic metab detoxified by glutathione conjugation; APAP overdose (>10 g) depletes glutathione stores → injury
- CYP2E1 induced by fasting, alcohol, and certain anticonvulsants and anti-TB drugs, resulting in a "therapeutic misadventure" with even low doses (2–6 g) of acetaminophen
- Liver dysfunction may not be apparent for 2–6 d
- Rx: NG lavage, activated charcoal if w/in 4 h. Consider early transfer to transplant ctr.
  N-acetylcysteine: administer up to 72 h after ingestion, if time of ingestion unknown or chronic ingestion >4g/d; low threshold to start NAC w/ low or undetectable APAP levels
  PO NAC (preferred): 140 mg/kg loading dose → 70 mg/kg q4h × 17 additional doses
  IV NAC: 150 mg/kg × 1 h → 50 mg/kg × 4 h → 100 mg/kg × 16 h; risk of anaphylaxis (↓ w/ 12-h regimen; Lancet 2014;383:697); use if unable to take POs, GIB, pregnancy, ALF

Ischemic hepatitis
- "Shock liver" w/ AST & ALT >1000 + ↑↑ LDH; delayed ↑↑ Tbili
- Seen in HoTN & CHF; often requires ↑ venous + ↓ portal/arterial pressure + hypoxia

Nonalcoholic fatty liver disease (Hep 2012;55:2005)
- Definition: fatty infiltration of liver and absence of EtOH or other cause of steatosis
  NAFL = steatosis, Ø inflam; **NASH** = steatosis + inflam ± fibrosis on bx
- NAFLD: 10–30% of U.S. pop. & over 60% in T2DM & obesity
- NASH: 2–5% of NAFLD & risk of cirrhosis in NASH w/ fibrosis on bx is 30% at 10 y
- Clinical: 80% asx, ↑ ALT > AST, but nl ALT/AST does not exclude poss. of NASH on bx
- Dx: liver bx remains gold standard. NAFLD fibrosis score = clinical variables to predict NASH w/ advanced fibrosis with PPV >80% (www.nafldscore.com)
- Rx: wt loss (ideally ≥10%, Gastro 2015;149:367), exercise, DM control (liraglutide, Lancet 2016;387:679 or pioglitazone), statins (Lancet 2010;376:1916); vit E ↓ steatosis but not fibrosis in Pts w/o DM (NEJM 2010;362:1675). HCC is a complication of NAFLD that has progressed to NASH cirrhosis but can occur in absence of advanced liver disease.

Definition

- Acute insult to liver + coagulopathy + encephalopathy; most w/o known preexisting liver dis.
- *Fulminant* if encephalopathy w/in 8 wk from jaundice onset; *subfulminant* if 8 wk to 6 mo
- Acute on chronic liver failure: acute insult to liver in Pt w/ underlying chronic liver disease

Etiology *(Lancet 2010;376:190)*

- **Drugs/toxins** (nearly 80% of cases in U.S.; *Hepatology 2010;52:2065*)
  Drugs: acetaminophen (most common cause; >40% of all cases in U.S., typically unintentional overdose); anti-TB drugs (INH, rifampin, pyrazinamide); AEDs (phenytoin, valproate, carbamazepine); NSAIDs (idiosyncratic, not dose-related); abx (eg, fluoroquinolones, macrolides); MDMA (ecstasy)
  Toxins: *Amanita phalloides* (mushroom spp. in West Coast), certain herbal preparations
- **Viral** (12% of cases in the US): HAV, HBV, HCV (rare), HDV + HBV, HEV (esp. if pregnant). In immunosupp: HSV (50% have skin lesions), EBV, VZV, CMV, HHV6
- **Vascular:** Budd-Chiari, ischemic hepatitis, hepatic sinusoidal obstruction syndrome
- **Other:** Wilson's disease, pregnancy-related ALF (acute fatty liver, preeclampsia, HELLP), initial presentation of autoimmune hepatitis; idiopathic

Clinical manifestations

- Initial presentation usually nonspecific: n/v, malaise; then jaundice & multiorgan failure
- Neurologic: **encephalopathy:** grade 1 = attn deficit, tremor; grade 2 = *asterixis*, lethargy, confusion, ataxia; grade 3 = somnolence, rigidity, clonus, hyperreflexia; grade 4 = coma
  cerebral edema: astrocyte swelling likely related to ↑ ammonia levels
- Cardiovascular: **hypotension** with low SVR, shock
- Pulmonary: **respiratory alkalosis,** impaired peripheral O_2 uptake, pulm edema, ARDS
- GI: bleeding (due to bleeding diathesis), pancreatitis (? due to ischemia, drugs, infxn)
- Renal: ATN, **hepatorenal syndrome,** hyponatremia, hypokalemia, hypophosphatemia
- Hematology: thrombocytopenia, ↑ PT/PTT, ↓ fibrinogen, **bleeding diathesis** (↓ synthesis of coag factors balanced by ↓ protein C/S; bleeding mostly due to low platelet count), DIC
- **Infection** (~90% of Pts): esp. with *Staph, Strep,* GNRs and fungi (↓ immune fxn, invasive procedures); SBP in 32% of Pts; *fever and ↑ WBC may be absent*
- Endocrine: **hypoglycemia** (↓ glc synthesis), metabolic acidosis (↑ lactate), adrenal insuf.

Workup *(Hepatology 2012;55:965)*

- CBC, PT/PTT, LFTs, lytes, BUN/Cr, pH, lactate, NH_3, acetaminophen level, viral serologies (qv) in all Pts, with additional labs as below if suspected
- Autoimmune hep serologies & IgG levels, ceruloplasmin & serum/urine copper, preg test
- Imaging studies (RUQ U/S or abd CT, Doppler studies of portal and hepatic veins)
- Liver biopsy if underlying etiology remains elusive after initial testing

Management *(NEJM 2013;369:2525)*

- **ICU care at liver transplant center** for hemodynamic & ventilatory support; CVVH for AKI
- Early listing for liver transplantation in selected Pts (see below)
- Cerebral edema: consider ICP monitoring if grade 3/4 enceph; if ↑ ICP → mannitol 0.5–1.0 mg/kg; if arterial NH_3 >150, grade 3/4 enceph, AKI or hernia vasopressors → prophylactic 3% saline for goal Na 145–155 mEq/L; barbiturates & hypothermia if refractory ↑ ICP
- Encephalopathy: intubate for grade 3 or 4; lactulose is of little benefit
- Coagulopathy: vit K, FFP/plts/cryo if active bleeding or before invasive procedure; PPI ppx
- Infection: low threshold for abx (broad spectrum, eg, vancomycin & 3rd-gen ceph.) if suspect infection; anti-fungal coverage in high-risk Pts. Daily blood cultures.
- Rx of specific causes: NAC if acetaminophen-related; antiviral (eg, entecavir) for HBV; plasma exchange can be temporizing measure for Wilson's; IV acyclovir for HSV; PCN-G for *A. phalloides;* delivery of child for pregnancy-related; TIPS, anticoag for Budd-Chiari. Lack of data for use of steroids in autoimmune, but often given *(Hepatology 2014;59:612).*
- NAC may benefit pts w/ non-APAP ALF but data inconclusive *(Gastro 2009;137:856)*
- **Liver transplantation** if poor prognosis but could survive surgery

Prognosis

- Non-acetaminophen ALF mortality ~80%, acetaminophen-induced ALF mortality ~30%
- Predictors of poor outcome (King's College Hospital, UK):
  Acetaminophen-induced: pH <7.25, INR >6.5 or PT>100, Cr >3.4, or grade 3/4 enceph.
  Non-acetamin.-induced: INR >6.5 or PT>100; *or* ≥3 of the following: unfavorable etiology (seronegative hepatitis or drug reaction); age <10 or >40 y; INR >3.5 or PT >50; Tbili >17.5; duration of jaundice >7 d prior to onset of encephalopathy
- ~25–30% of Pts undergo liver transplantation w/ 5-y survival rate of 70%
- BMI >30, Cr >2, age >50 y, need for pressors/vent support a/w poorer acute transplant outcome

CIRRHOSIS

Definition (Hep 2011;54:1864 & 2012;56:1983; J Hep 2012;56:S13)
- Definition: **fibrosis and regenerative nodules** resulting from hepatocellular injury
- **Decompensated** = jaundice, variceal bleed, encephalopathy, ascites; worse prognosis

Etiologies
- **Alcohol** (~60–70%) and other toxins (eg, arsenic)
- **Viral hepatitis** (~10%): chronic HBV, HCV, HDV infection
- **Autoimmune hepatitis:** ♀, ↑ IgG, ⊕ ANA, antismooth muscle Ab, anti-LKM-1, anti-LC1
- **Metabolic diseases** (~5%): hemochromatosis, Wilson's disease, α_1-AT deficiency
- **Biliary tract disease** (~5%): primary biliary cholangitis, secondary biliary cirrhosis (calculus, neoplasm, stricture, biliary atresia), primary sclerosing cholangitis
- **Vascular diseases:** Budd-Chiari syndrome, R-sided CHF, constrictive pericarditis, SOS
- **Nonalcoholic fatty liver dis. (NAFLD,** 10–15%) cause of most "cryptogenic cirrhosis"
- **Medications:** amiodarone, methotrexate, vitamin A, valproate acid

Clinical manifestations
- Nonspecific sx (anorexia, fatigue) or jaundice, encephalopathy, ascites, variceal bleeding

Physical exam
- Liver: *initially* enlarged, palpable (L lobe predom), firm; *eventually* shrunken, nodular
- Signs of liver failure: jaundice (bili >2.5), spider angiomata & palmar erythema (↑ estradiol), Dupuytren's contractures, white nail lines (Muehrcke's lines) & proximal nail beds (Terry's nails), ↑ parotid & lacrimal glands, gynecomastia, testicular atrophy, asterixis, encephalopathy, fetor hepaticus, clubbing, hypertrophic osteoarthropathy
- Signs of portal hypertension: splenomegaly, ascites, dilated superficial abdominal veins (caput medusae), epigastric Cruveilhier-Baumgarten venous hum

Laboratory studies
- LFTs: ↑ **bili,** ↑ **PT/INR** (poor correlation w/ bleeding; factor VIII nl as not synthesized by liver), ↓ **alb,** ± ↑ aminotransferases (AST > ALT if late) and ↑ Aϕ (variable)
- Hematologic tests: anemia (marrow suppress., hypersplenism, Fe ± folate defic.), neutropenia (hypersplenism), thrombocytopenia (hypersplenism, ↓ Tpo production, EtOH tox)
- Chem: ↓ Na (↑ ADH due to ↓ EAV); ↑ Fe/TIBC, ↑ ferritin (released from hepatocytes)
- Lab predictors of cirrhosis: AST/plt >2; Lok index; Bonacini score (JAMA 2012;307:832)

Workup (Lancet 2014;383:1749)
- Abd **U/S w/ Doppler:** liver size & echotexture, r/o HCC, ascites, ✓ patency of vasculature
- Determine etiology: hepatitis serologies (HBsAg, anti-HBs, anti-HCV), autoimmune hepatitis studies (IgG, ANA, anti–smooth muscle Ab), Fe and Cu studies, α_1-AT, AMA
- Assess fibrosis: biomarkers (FibroSURE = panel of 5 markers validated in HCV, ↑ score predictive of fibrosis); elastography (U/S or MR-based; measurement of liver stiffness)
- Liver bx (gold standard): percutaneous or transjugular (consider if ascites or coagulopathy), used to confirm presence of cirrhosis & dx etiology.

Prognosis

Modified Child-Turcotte-Pugh (CPS) Scoring System

	Points scored		
	1	**2**	**3**
Ascites	None	Easily controlled	Poorly controlled
Encephalopathy	None	Grade 1 or 2	Grade 3 or 4
Bilirubin (mg/dL)	<2	2–3	>3
Albumin (g/dL)	>3.5	2.8–3.5	<2.8
PT (sec > control)	<4	4–6	>6
or INR	<1.7	1.8–2.3	>2.3
	Classification		
	A	**B**	**C**
Total points	5–6	7–9	10–15
1-y survival	100%	80%	45%

- **MELD (M**odel for **E**nd-**S**tage **L**iver **D**isease): used to stratify Pts on liver tx list & to predict 3-mo survival in Pts w/ cirrhosis and some acute forms of liver disease. Based on Cr, INR, & total bili. Calculator: www.mayoclinic.org/meld/mayomodel6.html (Gastro 2011;14:1952). If MELD <21 additional predictors of mortality include Na <130 (NEJM 2008;359:1018; Clin Gastroenterol Hepatol 2009;7:1236), refractory ascites, ↑ HVPG and low QoL.

Ascites (see "Ascites" for details on dx evaluation; Am J Gastro 2009;104:1802)
- Due to portal HTN (defined as hepatic venous pressure gradient [HVPG] >5 mmHg)
- Develops in 60% w/in 10 y; ~50% mortality at 5 y

- Treatment: ↓ **Na intake** (1–2 g/d); restrict intake of free water if Na <125
  Diuretics: goal diurese ~1 L/d. Use spironolactone ± furosemide in 5:2 ratio (eg, 100 & 40 mg daily); urine Na/K >1 implies effective natriuresis if Pt compliant w/ low-Na diet
  Avoid NSAIDs in cirrhotic Pts as interfere w/ diuretic action and are nephrotoxic
- **Refractory ascites:** seen in 5–10% of Pts; 2-y survival 25%
  Diuretic-resistant on 2 g Na diet, minimal weight loss on maximal diuretic doses, or diuretic-induced complications (AKI, Na <125, ↑ K, encephalopathy)
  Med mgmt: conflicting evidence for d/c'ing βB (Hep 2016;63:1968); if limited by HoTN, add midodrine
  Large-volume paracenteses (LVP; >5 L removal): give 6–8 g albumin per L fluid removed (above 5 L) as colloid replacement a/w ↓ risk of post-para circulatory dysfxn & possibly ↓ mortality (Hep 2012;55:1172). Avoid LVP if SBP present as ↑ risk of AKI.
  Transjugular intrahepatic portosystemic shunt (TIPS) (Clin Gas Hep 2011;9:936)
  ↓ ascites in 75%; ↑ CrCl, ↑ enceph, survival benefit over LVP remains controversial
  Contraindic: grade II enceph, CHF or pulm HTN, active infxn or biliary obstruction
  Complications: bleeding, fistula; stent thrombosis (1-y patency w/ coated stents ~80%); infxn ("endotipsitis"); new or ↑ enceph in 20–30%, hemolysis (Hep 2010;51:306)
  Consider for liver transplant if above fail
- **Hepatic hydrothorax:** 2° diaphragmatic defect; often unilateral, R > L, ± ascites
  Treatment: avoid chest tube (↑ complications); Rx same as ascites (TIPS if refractory)
  Spontaneous *empyema* can occur (even w/o SBP); dx thoracentesis; Rx abx

(SBP; see "Ascites" for details; J Hep 2010;53:397)
- Develops in ~20%; 20% mortality; risk factors: ascitic TP <1 g/dL, hx of SBP, current GIB
- Can p/w encephalopathy, abd pain, fever, *but often* (25%) *asx*; perform paracentesis in all hospitalized cirrhotics w/ ascites
- Micro: GNRs (E. coli, Klebs) > GPCs (S. pneumo, enterococcus) (see "Ascites")
- Rx: 3°-gen. ceph or amox/clav × 5 d. If uncomplicated (no encephalopathy or AKI) can use FQ but avoid if already on for ppx or if in ↑ FQ resistance area. (NEJM 1999;341:403)
  IV albumin 1.5 g/kg at time of dx & 1 g/kg on day 3 → ↑ survival (NEJM 1999;341:403)
  If not improving, repeat paracentesis at 48 h: expect 25% ↓ in PMNs if Rx working
- Indefinite Ppx if (1) h/o SBP or (2) ascitic TP <1.5 plus: Na ≤130 or Cr ≥1.2 or BUN ≥25 or [CPS ≥9 + Tbili ≥3] (Am J Gastro 2009;4:993) → cipro 500 mg qd or Bactrim DS qd.
  Short-term Ppx: CTX 1 g IV × 7 d if GIB; cipro 500 mg PO qd × 1 y if ascitic fluid TP <1.5

(see also "GIB"; Lancet 2014;383:1749)
- Presence of varices correlates w/ severity of liver dis (40% of Child A Pts → 85% Child C)
- ↑ varix size, Child B/C, & red wale marks assoc w/ ↑ risk of bleeding
- UGIB 1° prevention: screen at time of dx w/ EGD; data best for Pts w/ med-large varices
  nonselective β-blockers: ~50% ↓ risk of bleeding & ↓ mortality if med-large varices.
  Nadolol or propranolol typically used, titrate to max tolerated dose; carvedilol can be considered in nonresponders or if systemic HTN (α1 blockade → ↓ intrahepatic vasc resistance, Gut 2013;62:1634). EGD not req. to document improvement.
  endoscopic variceal ligation (EVL): superior to βB in ↓ risk of 1st bleed but no diff in mortality (Ann Hep 2012;11:369); risk of serious complications (esoph perf, ulcers).
  Repeat q1–2wk until varices gone, then w/ f/u EGD at 3 mo then q6–12mo
  βB vs. EVL: choice based on Pt/physician preference, βB often 1st (Hepatol 2008;47:1764); using both βB and EVL for primary prevention currently not recommended
- 2° prevention: for all Pts after 1st bleed, given ~50% risk of rebleed & ~30% mortality
  βB + EVL → either alone (Annals 2008;149:109); TIPS if refractory, or consider in Child B or C w/in 72 h of admission for esoph variceal bleed (↑ 1-y survival; NEJM 2010;362:2370)

(Clin Gas Hep 2012;10:1208)
- Pathogenesis: failure of liver to detoxify NH3 + other substances (eg, ADMA; J Hepatol 2013;58:38) that cause cerebral edema, ↓ O2 consumption, ↑ ROS → brain dysfxn
- Precipitants: bleeding, infxn, med nonadherence, ↓ K, ↓ Na, dehydration, hypoxia, portosystemic shunt (eg, TIPS), meds (eg, sedatives), acute insult to liver (eg, PVT)
- Stages: see section in "Acute Liver Failure"
- Dx: NH3 levels have poor Se for dx & monitoring Rx; remains a *clinical dx*
- Rx: identify/correct precipitants; **lactulose** (acidification of colon: NH3 → NH4+) w/ goal 2–4 stools/d (PEG may be more effective; JAMA IM 2014;174:1727); alternatively, **rifaximin** 550 mg bid (↓ gut bacteria → ↓ NH3 prod); rifaximin + lactulose may be more effective than lactulose alone; Am J Gastro 2013;108:1458); acarbose & probiotics may benefit
- 2° prevention: lactulose or rifaximin 550 bid (Gastro 2009;137:885; NEJM 2010;362:1071)

(NEJM 2009;361:1279; Crit Care 2012;16:R23(1))
- Pathophys: splanchnic vasodilation and renal vasoconstriction w/ ↓ renal blood flow
- Criteria: (1) cirrhosis w/ ascites; (2) **acute kidney injury** (serum Cr ↑ ≥0.3 mg/dL w/in 48 h or ≥50% ↑ in serum Cr from baseline; Gut 2015;64:531); (3) Ø improvement in Cr after d/c

diuretic & volume expansion (1 g/kg/d of albumin × 2 d); (4) Ø shock (prerenal azotemia/ATN); (5) Ø nephrotoxic meds; (6) Ø intrinsic kidney disease

Type I: development in <2 wk; usually occurs in severe liver failure, often following precipitating event (see later); median survival 2 wk

Type II: more indolent course, median survival 6 mo; liver failure present < in type I

- Precipitants: GIB, overdiuresis, infection, serial LVP, drugs (aminoglycosides, NSAIDs)
- Rx: *if critically ill* → vasopressor (eg, norepinephrine or vasopressin) + albumin (1 g/kg, max 100 g, bolus daily) to ↑ MAP 10 mmHg. *If not critically ill* → octreotide (100–200 mcg SC tid) + midodrine (max 15 mg PO tid) + 1 g/kg (max 100 g) albumin on day of presentation followed by 20–60 g albumin qd to ↑ MAP (Hep 2010;51:576). May need dialysis or TIPS as bridge to liver transplant.

Hepatocellular carcinoma (HCC) (Hep 2011;53:1020; Lancet 2012;379:1245)
- Epi: worldwide, 6th most prevalent cancer, 3rd most frequent cancer-related death, 80% of cases due to HCV/HBV. Increased risk of HCC is ~3–8% (Gastro 2012;142:1264). ↑'d risk w/ cirrhosis of any type but esp. w/ viral, HFE, PBC, ? α1-AT.
- Clinical: asx vs. hepatic decompensation (eg, ascites, PSE), PVT w/ tumor thrombus
- Dx: screen cirrhotics q6mo w/ U/S ± AFP, though many centers choose dual phase CT/MRI (if arterial enhancing & venous phase or delayed washout, no bx req for dx)
- Rx: *radiofrequency ablation* (RFA) for HCCs <3 cm in size; consider *resection* if single lesion <2 cm and Child-Pugh A w/o portal HTN; *transarterial chemoembolization* (TACE) preferred for large cancers (not curative) or if not amenable to RFA (near IVC/lung); consider *liver transplant* if up to 3 HCCs ≤3 cm or 1 HCC ≤5 cm (Milan criteria)

Other Complications
- **Hepatopulmonary syndrome** (HPS) (Dig Dis Sci 2015;60:1914)
  Abnl gas exchange (A-a gradient ≥15 or P_aO_2 <80) caused by intrapulmonary vascular dilatations leading to intrapulmonary shunting
  S/S: platypnea-orthodeoxia, clubbing, cyanosis
  Dx w/ contrast echo showing "late" A-V shunting (contrast in LA 3–6 cycles after RA)
  Rx: O_2; potential embolization if large vessel on CT, ? TIPS, liver tx only definitive Rx
- **Portopulmonary hypertension** (POPH) (Expert Rev Gastro Hepatol 2015;9:983)
  Pulm HTN in Pt w/ portal HTN w/o other cause. ESLD→ ↑ endothelin → pulm vasoconst.
  Rx w/ same therapies as for idiopathic PAH, incl prostacyclin analogs, endothelin receptor antagonists, sildenafil; liver transplant is often curative.
- **Cirrhotic cardiomyopathy:** ↓ inotropic & chronotropic response, ↓ systolic and diastolic fxn, prolonged QT, hyperkinetic circulation; ↑ troponin, BNP (Circulation 2016;56:539)
- **Infxns:** unless already immune, vaccinate for HAV, HBV, PCV13 & PPSV23; flu yearly. Cellulitis in ~20% of Pts hospitalized w/ cirrhosis, often in abd wall or LE a/w skin edema.
- Endocrine: diabetes (15–30%), ↑ frequency of adrenal insufficiency (Hep 2015;1282)
- Coagulopathy: balanced defects w/ ↓ synth of coag factors, hyperfibrinolysis, ↓ plt balanced by ↓ synthesis anticoag factors (protein C/S), defic. of profibrinolytic factors, ↑ levels of vWF. No support for routine administration of FFP, plt, cryo unless in DIC.
- Nutrition: monitor and supplement fat soluble vitamins, zinc
- Meds: acetaminophen can be used up to 2 g/d; avoid ASA/NSAIDs; aminoglycosides contraindicated; oral hypoglycemics if compensated but insulin if decompensated

Liver transplantation
- Undertake evaluation when MELD ≥15. Exception points added if HCC as above
- Indic: recurrent/severe enceph, refractory ascites, recurrent variceal bleeng, HPS, PPH, HCC (if no single lesion is >5 cm or ≤3 lesions with largest ≤3 cm), acute liver failure
- Contraindic: inadequate social support, active substance abuse (EtOH w/in 6 mo), sepsis, advanced cardiopulm dis., extrahepatic Ca, cholangio Ca, hemangiosarcoma, persistent noncompliance, AIDS, fulminant LF w/ sustained ICP >50 mmHg or CPP <40 mmHg
- Survival: 1-y up to 90%, 5-y up to 80%, though lower with HCV; autoimmune liver disease, such as AIH/PBC/PSC may recur in 10–30% (or more) of allografts

OTHER ETIOLOGIES OF CIRRHOSIS

Hemochromatosis & Iron Overload Syndromes (Lancet 2016;388:706)
- Recessive disorder of iron sensing or transport leading to tissue **iron deposition**
- **HFE** mutations (85% of cases): typically C282Y homozyg. (~0.5% of N. Europeans), rarely C282Y/H63D compound heterozyg. C282Y homozygotes: 28% of ♂ & 1% of ♀ develop sx (delayed since menses ↓ Fe load). C282Y/H63D: only 1.5% manifest sx.
- Non-HFE mutations: hemojuvelin, hepcidin, transferrin receptor 2, & ferroportin
- 2° causes of iron overload: iron-loading anemias (eg, thalassemia major, sideroblastic anemia, aplastic anemia), parenteral iron-overload (RBC transfusions, long-term HD), chronic liver disease (due to ETOH, HBV, HCV, NASH, etc), dietary iron overload

- Sx: fatigue & arthralgias, loss of libido in ♂. In *advanced disease* (rare): bronze skin (melanin + iron), hypogonadism (esp. in juvenile onset), DM, arthropathy (MCP), CHF, infxns (↑ risk *Vibrio, Listeria, Yersinia*), cirrhosis (↑ risk if EtOH/fatty liver disease; 15% risk of HCC). Disease also a/w ALS (H63D homozygotes) & porphyria.
- Dx: iron sat >45% (iron/TIBC × 100%); ↑ ferritin (acute phase reactant, so poor Sp; often nl in young Pts). If ↑ iron sat. → ✓ HFE to confirm dx, imaging by MRI (black liver). If HFE ⊕ & ferritin >1000 ng/mL or ↑ LFTs → liver bx for quant Fe index & to stage fibrosis
- Treatment: phlebotomy (250 mL = 1 unit, ~250 mg of Fe) qwk until Fe sat <50% & ferritin 50–100 μg/L, then q3–4mo; PPI ↓ intestinal Fe absorption & may ↓ need for phlebotomy; avoid vit C & uncooked seafood; deferoxamine if phleb. contraindic.; genetic counseling

Wilson's disease (J Hep 2012;56:671)

- Recessive disorder of copper transport (mutation in *ATP7B*) → **copper overload;** primarily affects liver, but also other tissues (brain, eye)
- Epidemiology: 1 in 30,000, majority present b/t 5 & 35 y/o, only 3% of Pts present >40 y/o
- Extrahepatic s/s: neuro ψ disease, parkinsonism & movement disorder (hepatolenticular disease), Kayser-Fleischer rings in 99% w/ neuro ψ but in <50% w/ hepatic disease), Coombs ⊖ hemolytic anemia, renal disease
- Dx: ↑ 24-h urine Cu, ↓ serum ceruloplasmin (Se 90%), rarely penicillamine challenge w/ ↑ urine Cu excretion, liver bx w/ hepatic Cu content. In *acute liver failure*, Aφ/bili <4 + AST/ALT >2.2 better Se & Sp than urine Cu or ceruloplasmin (Hepatology 2008;4:1167).
- Treatment: chelation w/ D-penicillamine (supplement B6 as d-pen inactivates); 2ⁿᵈ-line trientine (↓ toxicity w/ ≈ efficacy, but $$). Zinc: ↓ intestinal Cu transport & can help delay disease; best used in conjunction w/ chelation (must give 4–5 h apart from chelators). Elim. Cu-rich foods. Transplant for fulminant LF or for chronic dis. unresponsive to Rx.

α₁-antitrypsin deficiency (α₁-AT) (J Hepatol 2016;65:413)

- Abnl α_1-AT → polymerization in liver (cirrhosis) & uninhibited protease activity in lung (emphysema). Affects 1/3000 of European ancestry. Varied presentations: neonatal hepatitis; cholestatic jaundice in children; ↑ AST/ALT or cirrhosis in children/adults.
- Extrahepatic disease includes: emphysema, necrotizing panniculitis, ANCA vasculitis
- Dx: serum α_1-AT level (acute phase reactant), level <50% of nl typically diagnostic; gold standard = phenotyping of protease inhibitor (Pi). Alleles most a/w hepatic dis.: Z (63% of ZZ adults found to have chronic liver dis) & M (malton) (Am J Respir Crit Care Med 2013;137:502). Liver bx shows characteristic PAS ⊕ cytoplasmic inclusion bodies.
- Treatment: standard Rx for cirrhosis/chronic liver dis., including liver transplantation

Primary biliary cholangitis (PBC) (Lancet 2015;386:1565)

- Autoimmune destruction of *intrahepatic* bile ducts (previously "primary biliary cirrhosis")
- Epi: ♀ 40–60 y/o; a/w Sjögren's, Raynaud's, scleroderma, celiac & thyroid disease; may be triggered by certain infxns or toxins; a/w X monosomy, variants in IL12α & IL12R genes
- Sx (late): fatigue/sleep disturbance, pruritus, steatorrhea, xanthelasma, jaundice, cirrhosis
- Ddx: PSC, AIH, hepatic sarcoidosis, meds, idiopathic adult ductopenia, biliary stricture/Ca
- Dx: ↑ Aφ, ↑ bili, ↑ IgM, ↑ chol, ⊕ antimitochondrial Ab (AMA) in 95%. If ⊕ AMA, liver bx not needed due to high Se & Sp. 0.5% gen pop ⊕ AMA & nl LFTs → 10% develop PBC at 6 y. If AMA ⊖, liver bx (Pts often ⊕ ANA, smooth muscle Ab; same prognosis as ⊕ AMA).
- Rx: **ursodeoxycholic acid** (13–15 mg/kg/d) regardless of stage
  ~25% complete response, ↑ survival & ↓ histologic stage & complications (eg, varices) (Gastro 2005;128:297). Budesonide may benefit in short term.
  Pruritus: cholestyramine (give 2–4 h after UDCA); if refractory sx: naltrexone, rifampin
  Fat-soluble vitamins; screen/Rx osteoporosis (risk independent of vit D deficiency)
  If ESLD: liver tx: ~20% recur but no impact on long-term survival

Primary sclerosing cholangitis (PSC) (Lancet 2013;382:1587; World J Hepatol 2016:8:265)

- Diffuse inflammation of *intrahepatic and extrahepatic* bile ducts leading to fibrosis & stricturing of biliary system. A/w HLA-B8 and -DR3 or DR4, frequent ⊕ autoantibodies.
- Epi: ♂ > ♀ (20–50y) ~70% Pts w/ PSC have IBD (usually UC); only 1–4% w/ UC have PSC.
- Clinical: fatigue, pruritus, jaundice, fevers, RUQ pain, concomitant IBD, ESLD
- Ddx: extrahepatic obstruction, PBC, may also have overlap w/ AIH and similar presentation to IgG4 autoimmune cholangitis (steroid responsive) (Gastro 2008;134:706)
- Dx: MRCP ± ERCP → *multifocal beaded bile duct strictures*, but may miss dx if confined to small intrahepatic ducts (~2% "small duct PSC": better prognosis, ? different disease). Liver bx may show "onion-skin" fibrosis around bile ducts but not necessary for dx.
- Treatment: supportive care, fat-soluble vitamins; no meds have improved survival
  Ursodeoxycholic acid may ↓ colon CA risk in Pts w/ UC & improve LFTs in Pts w/o UC
  Dominant stricture: endoscopic dilation, short-term stenting or surgical resection
  Cholangiocarcinoma (20%): ? biannual surveillance w/ MRCP/RUQ U/S and CA19-9
  Liver transplantation: ~30% recurrence, though if UC, colectomy may ↓ recurrence

Portal vein thrombosis (PVT) (Hepatology 2009;49:1729 & 2015;61:660)

- **Definition:** thrombosis, constriction or invasion of portal vein → portal HTN → varices. Isolated splenic vein thrombosis (eg, 2° to pancreatitis) → isolated gastric varices.
- **Etiologies:** cirrhosis, neoplasm (pancreas, HCC), abdominal infxn, hypercoag states, pancreatitis, collagen vascular diseases, Behçet's, IBD, surgery, trauma, OCPs, preg
- **Clinical manifestations**
    acute: can p/w abd or lumbar pain; often asx w/ incidental finding on U/S or CT. If mesenteric vein involved may p/w intestinal infarct; if fever consider pylephlebitis.
    chronic: asx/incidental finding; may p/w s/s of **portal HTN** → hematemesis 2° variceal bleeding, splenomegaly, encephalopathy; ascites uncommon unless cirrhosis
- **Diagnostic studies:** LFTs usually normal; U/S w/ Doppler, MRA, CT (I⁺), angiography; "portal cavernoma" network of hepatopetal collaterals in chronic PVT—can rarely cause biliary obstruction and cholestatic LFTs → portal cholangiopathy (may require surgery)
- **Treatment:**
    Acute: If noncirrhotic, LMWH → warfarin × 6 mo, or indefinitely if irreversible cause. If cirrhotic, preliminary studies support anticoag if no contraindications; should screen for high-risk varices prior to initiation (Nat Rev Gastroenterol Hepatol 2014;11:435).
    Chronic: Anticoag if noncirrhotic or hypercoag state; screen for varices prior to anticoag. Esophageal varices: 1° Ppx recommended; if bleed, endoscopic Rx and βB. If refractory bleed consider TIPS, shunt.
    Isolated gastric varices 2° splenic vein thrombosis: splenectomy is curative

Budd-Chiari syndrome (Hepatology 2009;49:1729)

- Occlusion of hepatic vein(s) or IVC → sinusoidal congestion and portal HTN
- **Etiologies:** ~50% due to myeloproliferative d/o a/w JAK2 mutations (esp. P. vera), other hypercoag state, tumor invasion (HCC, renal, adrenal), IVC webs, trauma, 25% idiopathic
- **Symptoms:** hepatomegaly, RUQ pain, ascites, dilated venous collaterals, acute liver failure
- **Dx:** ± ↑ aminotransferases & Aφ; Doppler U/S of hepatic veins (85% Se & Sp); CT (I⁺) or MRI/MRV → vein occlusion or ↑ caudate lobe (separate venous drainage); "spider-web" pattern on hepatic venography; liver bx showing congestion (r/o right-sided CHF)
- **Treatment:** Rx underlying condition, anticoag (LMWH → warfarin); consider thrombolysis acutely; if short stenosis, stent may be possible; consider TIPS (↑ occlusion risk c/w side-to-side portocaval shunt); liver transplant if ALF or failed shunt (J Gastro Surg 2012;16:286)

Sinusoidal obstruction syndrome (SOS) (Hepatology 2009;49:1729)

- Occlusion of hepatic venules and sinusoids (formerly **veno-occlusive disease**)
- **Etiologies:** HSCT, chemo (esp. cyclophosphamide), XRT, Jamaican bush tea
- **Clinical manifestations:** hepatomegaly, RUQ pain, ascites, weight gain, ↑ bilirubin
- **Dx:** U/S w/ reversal of portal flow, but often not helpful; dx made clinically (↑ bili, wt gain/ascites and RUQ pain) or, if necessary, by liver bx or HVPG (>10 mmHg)
- **Treatment** (20% mortality): supportive; ? defibrotide (adenosine agonist ↑ TPA levels)
- **Ppx:** defibrotide; ursodeoxycholic acid for high-risk HSCT pop; ? use of low-dose heparin

Figure 3-6 Hepatic vasculature

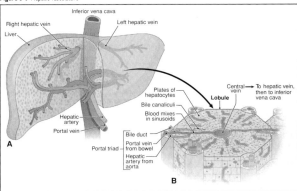

Modified from *The Nature of Disease Pathology for the Health Professions*, 2007. *Hepatology* 2009;49:1729.

Pathophysiology
- Portal hypertension → systemic vasodilatation (? due to release of NO) → ↓ effective arterial volume → renal Na retention → volume overload and ascites
- In malignant or inflammatory ascites, pathophysiology related to leaking of proteinaceous material from tumor or from inflamed/infected/ruptured intraabdominal structures

Etiologies

Portal HTN related (SAAG ≥1.1)	Non-portal HTN related (SAAG <1.1)
Presinusoidal obstruction portal or splenic vein thrombosis, schistosomiasis, sarcoidosis *Sinusoidal* obstruction: **cirrhosis** (81%), including SBP, acute hepatitis, malignancy (HCC or mets) *Postsinusoidal* obstruction right-sided CHF incl constriction & TR Budd-Chiari syndrome, SOS	**Malig:** peritoneal carcinomatosis; chylous ascites from malignant lymphoma; Meigs' syndrome (ovarian tumor) **Infection:** TB, chlamydia/gonorrhea (ie, Fitz-Hugh-Curtis syndrome) **Inflam:** pancreatitis, ruptured pancreatic/biliary/lymph duct; bowel obstrxn Hypoalbuminemic states: **nephrotic syndrome,** protein-losing enteropathy

Symptoms
- ↑ abd girth, wt gain, new abd hernia, abd pain, dyspnea, nausea, early satiety

Evaluation (JAMA 2008;299:1166; Hepatology 2009;29:2087)
- Physical exam: flank dullness (NPV ~90%; >1500 mL needed), shifting dullness (Se ~83%)
- Radiologic: **U/S** detects >100 mL; MRI/CT (also help with Ddx)
- Paracentesis (Hep 2013;57:1651): perform in all Pts w/ new ascites, consider in all hosp. cirrhotics w/ ascites. Low complic. rate (~1% hematoma formation). Prophylactic FFP or plts does *not* ↓ bleeding complic. Most useful tests: cell count, alb, total protein, culture.
- **Serum-ascites albumin gradient (SAAG)** – serum alb (g/dL) – ascites alb (in g/dL)
  If ≥1.1 g/dL → cause of ascites likely portal HTN (~95% accuracy; Annals 1992;117:215)
  If <1.1 g/dL → non–portal hypertension related
  If portal HTN + another cause (~5% of cases) SAAG still ≥1.1
- Ascites fluid total protein (**AFTP**): useful when SAAG ≥1.1 to distinguish cirrhosis (AFTP <2.5 g/dL) from cardiac ascites (AFTP ≥2.5 g/dL). Low AFTP (<1 g/dL) assoc. w/ ↑ risk of SBP (see "Cirrhosis" for guidelines on SBP Ppx based on AFTP).
- **Cell count:** normal limit of PMNs in ascitic fluid up to 250 PMNs/mm³. Bloody tap (typically from traumatic para) can skew cell count; subtract 1 PMN for every 250 RBCs to correct PMN count. Ascites PMNs ≥250 suggest infection (see below).
- Other tests: amylase (pancreatitis, gut perforation); bilirubin (test in dark brown fluid, suggests bile leak or proximal intestinal perf); TG (chylous ascites); BNP (HF); cytology (peritoneal carcinomatosis, ~95% Se w/ 3 samples). SBP a/w ↓ glc & ↑ LDH is fluid.

Treatment (see "Cirrhosis" for details)
- If 2° to portal HTN: ↓ **Na intake + diuretics**; if refractory → LVP or TIPS
- If non–portal HTN related: depends on underlying cause (TB, malignancy, etc.)

Bacterial peritonitis (Gut 2012;61:297)

Type	Ascites cell count/mm³ & cx
Spontaneous bacterial peritonitis (SBP): spontaneous bacterial translocation from gut to ascitic fluid. Ascitic fluid in cirrhosis has ↓ opsonins (esp. if low AFTP), leading to ↑ risk of infxn.	≥250 polys; Cx ⊕ (1 org.) *E. coli* (37%), *Klebs* (17%), *S. pneumo* (12%), misc. GPC (14%), misc. GNR (10%)
Culture-⊖ neutrocytic ascites (CNNA): cell counts suggest infxn but cx ⊖. No recent abx, w/o other explanation for counts. Rare when sens cx methods.	≥250 polys; Cx ⊖
Nonneutrocytic bacterascites (NNBA): ⊕ cx w/o ↑PMNs. Natural course may resolve w/o tx or may progress to SBP.	<250 polys; Cx ⊕ (1 org.) Misc. GPC (30%), *E. coli* (27%), *Klebs* (11%), misc. GNR (14%)
2° bacterial peritonitis: caused by intraabd abscess or perf. AFTP >1 g/dL, glc <50 mg/dL plus LDH >225 U. Rx 3ʳᵈ-gen ceph. + MNZ; urgent abd imaging ± ex lap.	≥250 polys; Cx ⊕ (polymicro)
Peritoneal dialysis-associated: cloudy fluid, abd pain, fever, nausea. Rx: vanc + gent (IV load, then administer in PD).	≥100, poly predom. Cx ⊕ (typ. 1 org.). Misc. GPC (50%), misc. GNR (15%).

CHOLELITHIASIS (GALLSTONES)

Epidemiology & pathogenesis (*J Hep* 2008:48:S124)
- >10% adults in the U.S. have gallstones; a/w ↑ overall mortality (*Gastro* 2011:140:508)
- Bile = bile salts, phospholipids, cholesterol; ↑ cholesterol saturation in bile + accelerated nucleation + gallbladder hypomotility → gallstones
- Risk factors: ♀; South, Central, Native American; ↑ age (>40 y), obesity, pregnancy, TPN, rapid ↓ wt; drugs (OCPs, estrogen, clofibrate, octreotide, ceftriaxone); ileal disease
- ? statin use >1 y ↓ risk of sx gallstones & cholecystectomy (*JAMA* 2009:302:2001)

Types of gallstones
- Cholesterol (90%): 2 subtypes
    mixed: contain >50% cholesterol; typically smaller, multiple stones
    pure: 100% cholesterol; larger, yellow, white appearance
- Pigment (10%)
    Black: unconjugated bili & calcium; seen w/ chronic hemolysis, cirrhosis, CF, Gilbert synd
    Brown: stasis & infection in bile ducts → bacteria deconjugate bilirubin → precipitates w/ calcium; seen w/ duodenal diverticula, biliary strictures, parasites

Clinical manifestations
- Asx in 80% of cases; biliary pain in ~2%/y; once sx, rate of complications ~2%/y
- **Biliary pain ("colic") = episodic RUQ or epigastric abd pain** that begins abruptly, is continuous, resolves slowly and lasts for 30 min–3 h; ± radiation to scapula; **nausea**
- May be precipitated by **fatty foods**
- Physical exam: afebrile, ± RUQ tenderness or epigastric pain

Diagnostic studies
- RUQ U/S: Se & Sp >95% for stones >5 mm; can show complications (cholecystitis); should be performed only after fasting ≥8 h to ensure distended, bile-filled gallbladder

Treatment (*J Hepatol* 2016:65:146)
- Cholecystectomy (CCY), usually laparoscopic, if symptomatic
- CCY in asx Pts w/: GB calcification (~7% risk of ca) (*Surgery* 2001:129:699), GB polyps >10 mm, Native American, stones >3 cm or bariatric surgery or cardiac transplant candidates
- Ursodeoxycholic acid (rare) for cholesterol stones w/ uncomplicated biliary pain or if poor surgical candidate; also reduces risk of gallstone formation with rapid wt loss
- Biliary pain: NSAIDs (eg, diclofenac 50 mg IM) drug of choice, efficacy ≈ opiates & ↓ complications (*Aliment Pharmacol Ther* 2012:35:1370)

Complications
- Cholecystitis: 20% of sx biliary pain → cholecystitis w/in 2 y
- Choledocholithiasis → cholangitis or gallstone pancreatitis
- Mirizzi syndrome: common hepatic duct compression by cystic duct stone → jaundice, biliary obstruction
- Cholecystenteric fistula: stone erodes through gallbladder into bowel
- Gallstone ileus: SBO (usually at term ileum) due to stone in intestine that passed thru fistula
- Gallbladder carcinoma: ~1% in U.S.

CHOLECYSTITIS (*NEJM* 2008:358:2804)

Pathogenesis
- Acute cholecystitis: stone impaction in cystic duct → inflammation behind obstruction → GB swelling ± secondary infection (50%) of biliary fluid
- Acalculous cholecystitis: gallbladder stasis and ischemia → inflammatory response; occurs mainly in critically ill, hosp. Pts (postop major surgery, TPN, sepsis, trauma, burns, opiates, immunosuppression, infxn [eg, CMV, *Crypto*, *Campylobacter*, typhoid fever])

Clinical manifestations
- History: RUQ/epigastric pain ± radiation to R shoulder/back, nausea, vomiting, fever
- Physical exam: **RUQ tenderness, Murphy's sign** = ↑ RUQ pain and inspiratory arrest with deep breath during palpation of R subcostal region, ± palpable gallbladder
- Laboratory evaluation: ↑ WBC, ± mild ↑ bilirubin, AΦ, ALT/AST and amylase; AST/ALT >500 U/L, bili >4 mg/dL or amylase >1000 U/L → choledocholithiasis

Diagnostic studies
- **RUQ U/S**: high Se & Sp for stones, but need *specific signs of cholecystitis*: GB wall thickening >4 mm, pericholecystic fluid and a sonographic Murphy's sign

- **HIDA scan:** most Se test (80–90%) for acute cholecystitis. IV inj of HIDA (selectively secreted into biliary tree). In acute cholecystitis, HIDA enters BD but not GB. 10–20% false ⊕ (cystic duct obstructed from chronic cholecystitis, lengthy fasting, liver disease).

Treatment
- NPO, IV fluids, nasogastric tube if intractable vomiting, analgesia
- **Antibiotics** (*E. coli, Klebsiella* and *Enterobacter* sp. are usual pathogens) ([2nd- or 3rd-generation cephalosporin or FQ] + MNZ) or piperacillin-tazobactam
- **CCY** (typically laparoscopic) w/in 24 h ↓ morbidity vs. waiting 7–45 d (*Ann Surg* 2013:258:385)
- If unstable for surgery, EUS-guided transmural, ERCP-guided transcystic duct drainage, or percutaneous cholecystotomy (if w/o ascites or coagulopathy) are alternatives to CCY (*NEJM* 2015:373:357)
- Intraoperative cholangiogram or ERCP to r/o choledocholithiasis in Pts w/ jaundice, cholangitis or stone in BD on U/S

Complications
- Gangrenous cholecystitis: necrosis w/ risk of empyema and perforation
- Emphysematous cholecystitis: infection by gas-forming organisms (air in GB wall)
- Post CCY: bile duct leak, BD injury or retained stones, cystic duct remnant, sphincter of Oddi dysfxn

---

CHOLEDOCHOLITHIASIS

Definition
- Gallstone lodged in common bile duct (CBD)

Epidemiology
- Occurs in 15% of Pts w/ gallbladder stones; can form de novo in CBD

Clinical manifestations
- Asymptomatic (50%)
- RUQ/epigastric pain 2° obstrxn of bile flow → ↑ CBD pressure, jaundice, pruritus, nausea

Diagnostic studies
- Labs: ↑ bilirubin, Aφ; transient spike in ALT or amylase suggests passage of stone
- RUQ U/S: BD stones seen ~50% of cases; usually inferred from dilated CBD (>6 mm)
- ERCP preferred dx modality when likelihood high; cholangiogram (percutaneous, operative) when ERCP unavailable or unsuccessful; EUS/MRCP to exclude BD stones when suspicion low

Treatment
- ERCP & papillotomy w/ stone extraction (± lithotripsy)
- CCY typically w/in 6 wk unless contraindication (>15% Pts will develop indication for CCY if left unRx'd)

Complications
- Cholangitis, cholecystitis, pancreatitis, stricture

CHOLANGITIS

Definition & etiologies
- BD obstruction → infection proximal to the obstruction
- Etiologies: **BD stone** (~85%)
  Malignant (biliary, pancreatic) or benign stricture
  Infection w/ fluke (*Clonorchis sinensis, Opisthorchis viverrini*)

Clinical manifestations
- Charcot's triad: RUQ pain, jaundice, fever/chills; present in ~70% of Pts
- Reynolds' pentad: Charcot's triad + shock and Δ MS; present in ~15% of Pts

Diagnostic studies
- RUQ U/S
- Labs: ↑ WBC, bilirubin, Aφ, amylase; ⊕ BCx
- ERCP; percutaneous transhepatic cholangiogram if ERCP unsuccessful

Treatment
- **Antibiotics** (broad-spectrum) to cover common bile pathogens (see above) ampicillin + gentamicin (or levofloxacin) ± MNZ (if severe); carbapenems; pip/tazo
- ~80% respond to conservative Rx and abx → biliary drainage on elective basis
- ~20% require **urgent biliary decompression** via ERCP (papillotomy, stone extraction and/or stent insertion). If sphincterotomy cannot be performed (larger stones), decompression by biliary stent or nasobiliary catheter can be done; otherwise, percutaneous transhepatic biliary drainage or surgery.

GENERAL

Definitions
- **Acidemia** → pH <7.36, **alkalemia** → pH >7.44
- **Acidosis** → process that increases [H$^+$]; **alkalosis** → process that decreases [H$^+$]
- Primary disorders: metabolic acidosis or alkalosis, respiratory acidosis or alkalosis
- Compensation
  respiratory: hyper- or hypoventilation alters P_aCO_2 to counteract 1° metabolic process
  renal: excretion/retention of H$^+$/HCO$_3^-$ to counteract 1° respiratory process
  respiratory compensation occurs in minutes; renal compensation takes hours to days
  compensation usually never fully corrects pH; if pH normal, consider mixed disorder

Consequences of Severe Acid-Base Disturbances (NEJM 1998;338:26 & 107)		
Organ system	**Acidemia (pH <7.20)**	**Alkalemia (pH >7.60)**
Cardiovascular	↓ contractility, arteriolar vasodilation ↓ MAP & CO; ↓ response to catecholamines ↑ risk of arrhythmias	Arteriolar vasoconstriction ↓ coronary blood flow ↑ risk of arrhythmias
Respiratory	Hyperventilation, ↓ resp. muscle strength	Hypoventilation
Metabolic	↑ K (resp. > metab.), insulin resistance	↓ K, ICa, Mg, PO$_4$
Neurologic	Δ MS	Δ MS, seizures, tetany

Workup (NEJM 2014;371:1434)
- **Traditional or physiologic approach** (Brønsted-Lowry definition of acids & bases)
  Determine **primary disorder**: ✓ pH, P_aCO_2, HCO$_3$
  Determine if **degree of compensation** is appropriate

Primary Disorders				
Primary disorder	**Problem**	**pH**	**HCO$_3$**	**P_aCO_2**
Metabolic acidosis	gain of H$^+$ or loss of HCO$_3$	↓	⇓	↓
Metabolic alkalosis	gain of HCO$_3$ or loss of H$^+$	↑	⇑	↑
Respiratory acidosis	hypoventilation	↓	↑	⇑
Respiratory alkalosis	hyperventilation	↑	↓	⇓

Compensation for Acid/Base Disorders (JASN 2010;21:920)	
Primary disorder	**Expected compensation**
Metabolic acidosis	↓ P_aCO_2 = 1.2 × ΔHCO$_3$ or P_aCO_2 = (1.5 × HCO$_3$) + 8 ± 2 (Winters' formula) (also, P_aCO_2 ≈ last 2 digits of pH)
Metabolic alkalosis	↑ P_aCO_2 = 0.7 × ΔHCO$_3$
Acute respiratory acidosis	↑ HCO$_3$ = 0.1 × ΔP_aCO_2 (also, ↓ pH = 0.008 × ΔP_aCO_2)
Chronic respiratory acidosis	↑ HCO$_3$ = 0.35 × ΔP_aCO_2 (also, ↓ pH = 0.003 × ΔP_aCO_2)
Acute respiratory alkalosis	↓ HCO$_3$ = 0.2 × ΔP_aCO_2 (also, ↑ pH = 0.008 × ΔP_aCO_2)
Chronic respiratory alkalosis	↓ HCO$_3$ = 0.4 × ΔP_aCO_2

- **Alternative approaches**
  Base excess/deficit (Curr Opin Crit Care 2006;12:569; Am J Emerg Med 2016;34:626)
  Strong Ion Difference or "Stewart Method" (NEJM 2014;371:1821)

Mixed disorders (more than 1 primary disorder at the same time)
- If compensation less or greater than predicted, may be 2 disorders:
  P_aCO_2 too low → concomitant 1° resp. alk.
  P_aCO_2 too high → concomitant 1° resp. acid.
  HCO$_3$ too low → concomitant 1° met. acid.
  HCO$_3$ too high → concomitant 1° met. alk.
- Normal pH, *but* ...
  ↑ P_aCO_2 + ↑ HCO$_3$ → resp. acid. + met. alk.
  ↓ P_aCO_2 + ↓ HCO$_3$ → resp. alk. + met. acid.
  normal P_aCO_2 & HCO$_3$, but ↑ AG → AG met. acid. + met. alk.
  normal P_aCO_2, HCO$_3$, & AG → no disturbance *or* non-AG met. acid. + met. alk.
- *Cannot* have resp. acid. (hypoventilation) and resp. alk. (hyperventilation) simultaneously

Figure 4-1 Acid-base nomogram

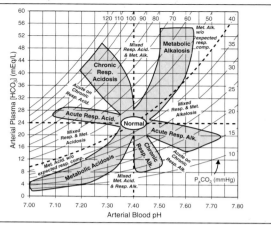

(Adapted from Brenner BM, ed., *Brenner & Rector's The Kidney*, 8th ed., 2007; Ferri F. ed. *Practical Guide to the Care of the Medical Patient*, 7th ed., 2007)

- **ABG vs.VBG:** concordant for pH (–0.04), HCO_3 (~2 mEq) but **not** PCO_2 (–8±17 mmHg) VBG can be used to *screen* for hypercarbia w/ PCO_2 cutoff ≥45 mmHg (100% Se), **but** may not accurately assess *degree* of hypercarbia (*Am J Emerg Med* 2012;30:896).

METABOLIC ACIDOSIS

Initial workup (*NEJM* 2014;371:1434)

- √ **anion gap** (AG) = $Na^+ - (Cl^- + HCO_3^-)$ = unmeasured anions – unmeasured cations if ↑ glc, use measured *not* corrected Na
  expected AG is [albumin] × 2.5 (ie, 10 if albumin is 4 g/dL, 7.5 if albumin is 3 g/dL)
  ↑ AG → ↑ unmeasured anions such as organic acids, phosphates, sulfates
  ↓ AG → ↓ alb or ↑ unmeasured cations (Ca, Mg, K, Li, bromide, iodide, immunoglobulin)]
- If ↑AG, √ **delta-delta** (ΔΔ = ΔAG/ΔHCO₃) to assess if there is an additional metabolic acid-base disturbance; ΔAG = (calculated AG – expected AG), ΔHCO₃ = (24 – HCO₃)
  ΔΔ = 1–2 → pure AG metabolic acidosis
  ΔΔ < 1 → AG metabolic acidosis *and* simultaneous non-AG acidosis
  ΔΔ > 2 → AG metabolic acidosis *and* simultaneous metabolic alkalosis

Etiologies of AG Metabolic Acidosis	
Ketoacidosis	**Diabetes mellitus,** alcoholism, starvation (*NEJM* 2014;372:546)
Lactic acidosis (*NEJM* 2014; 371:2309)	**Type A:** impairment in tissue oxygenation eg, **circulatory or respiratory failure**, sepsis, ischemic bowel, carbon monoxide, cyanide **Type B:** no impairment in tissue oxygenation. ↓ clearance (eg, hepatic dysfxn) or ↑ generation [eg, malig, EtOH, thiamine def., meds (metformin, NRTIs, salicylates, propylene glycol, isoniazid, linezolid)] **D-lactic acidosis:** short bowel syndrome → precip by glc ingest → metab by colonic bacteria to D-lactate; not detected by standard lactate assay
Renal failure	Accumulation of organic anions such as phosphates, sulfates, urate, etc.
Ingestions	**Methanol** (windshield fluid, antifreeze, solvents, fuel): metab to formic acid **Ethylene glycol** (antifreeze): metab to glycolic and oxalic acids **Propylene glycol** (pharmaceutical solvent, eg, IV diazepam, lorazepam, and phenobarbital; antifreeze): lactic acidosis **Salicylates:** metabolic acidosis (from lactate, ketones) + respiratory alkalosis due to stimulation of CNS respiratory center **Glutathione depletion:** acetaminophen → ↑ endogenous organic acid 5-oxoproline in susceptible hosts (malnourished, female, renal failure)

- ✓ for **ketonuria** (dipstick acetoacetate) or plasma β-hydroxybutyrate (βOHB)
  nb, urine acetoacetate often not present in early ketoacidosis due to shunting to βOHB; ∴ acetoacetate may later turn ⊕ but does not signify worsening disease
- If ⊖ ketones, ✓ **renal function, lactate, toxin screen,** and **osmolal gap**
- **Osmolal gap** (OG) = measured osmoles − calculated osmoles
  calculated osmoles = $(2 \times Na) + (glucose/18) + (BUN/2.8)$
  (can + [EtOH/4.6] if have EtOH level and want to test if other ingestions)
  OG >10 → suggests ingestion (see below) but lacks specificity (can be elevated in lactic acidosis, DKA, and alcoholic ketoacidosis)
  for methanol/ethylene glycol: early on, OG precedes AG; later OG may be nl with ⊕ AG

AG	OG	Ingestion	Other manifestations
↑	nl	Acetaminophen	Hepatitis
		Salicylates	Fever, tachycardia, tinnitus; met. acid. + resp. alkalosis
↑	↑	Ethanol	Alcoholic fetor, ∆MS, hepatitis; keto + lactic acidosis ± met. alk. (vomiting)
		Methanol	∆MS, blurred vision, pupillary dilation, papilledema
		Ethylene glycol	∆MS, cardiopulm. failure, hypoCa. **Ca oxalate crystals →** AKI. Urine fluoresces under UV light.
		Propylene glycol	AKI
nl/↑	↑	Isopropyl alcohol	∆MS, fruity breath (acetone)

Table title: **Ingestions**

Etiologies of Non-AG Metabolic Acidosis

GI losses of HCO₃	Diarrhea, intestinal or pancreatic fistulas or drainage
RTAs	*See section on renal tubular acidoses below*
Early renal failure	Impaired generation of ammonia
Ingestions	Acetazolamide, sevelamer, cholestyramine, toluene
Dilutional	Due to rapid infusion of bicarbonate-free IV fluids
Posthypocapnia	Respiratory alkalosis → renal wasting of HCO₃; rapid correction of resp. alk. → transient acidosis until HCO₃ regenerated
Ureteral diversion	Colonic Cl⁻/HCO₃⁻ exchange, ammonium reabsorption

Workup for non-AG metabolic acidosis (CJASN 2012;7:671)

- Evaluate history for causes (see above)
- ✓ **urine anion gap** (UAG) = $(U_{Na} + U_k) - U_{Cl}$
  UAG = unmeasured anions − unmeasured cations; as NH_4^+ is primary unmeasured cation, UAG is indirect assay for renal H^+ excretion as NH_4^+ (NEJM 1988;318:594)
- ⊖ UAG → ↑ renal NH_4^+ excretion → appropriate renal response to acidemia
  Ddx: GI causes, proximal RTA, ingestions or dilutional
- ⊕ UAG → failure of kidneys to generate NH_4^+
  Ddx: distal or hypoaldo RTA, early renal failure
  nb, plasma K usually ↓ in distal and ↑ in hypoaldo RTA
- UAG evaluation assumes Pt volume replete (U_{Na} >25), U_{pH} <6.5 & no AG met. acidosis (which causes ⊕ UAG due to excretion of organic anions)

Renal tubular acidoses (RTAs) (JASN 2002;13:2160; Int J Clin Pract 2011;65:350)

- **Proximal** (Type II): ↓ proximal reabsorption of HCO₃
  1° (Fanconi's syndrome = ↓ proximal reabsorption of HCO₃, PO₄, glc, amino acids), paraprotein (multiple myeloma, amyloidosis), meds (acetazolamide, heavy metals, ifosfamide), renal transplant, ↓ Vit D, NRTIs
- **Distal** (Type I): defective distal H^+ secretion
  1°, autoimmune (Sjögren's, RA), nephrocalcinosis, meds (ampho, Li, ifosfamide); normally a/w ↓ K; if with ↑ K → sickle cell, obstruction, SLE, renal transplant
- **Hypoaldo** (Type IV): ↑ K → ↓ NH₃ synthesis/delivery → ↓ urine acid carrying capacity
  ↓ renin: diabetic nephropathy, NSAIDs, chronic interstitial nephritis, HIV
  normal renin, ↓ aldo synthesis: 1° adrenal disorders, ACEI, ARBs, heparin
  ↓ response to aldosterone
    meds: K-sparing diuretics, TMP-SMX, pentamidine, calcineurin inhibitors
    tubulointerstitial disease: sickle cell, SLE, amyloid, diabetes
- Combined (Type III): rarely discussed or clinically relevant, also called juvenile RTA, has distal & proximal features, can be due to carbonic anhydrase II deficiency

Renal Tubular Acidosis						
Location	Type	Acidosis	UAG	UpH	Fe_{HCO_3}[b]	Serum K
Proximal	II	Moderate	±	<5.3[a]	>15%	↓
Distal	I	Severe	⊕	>5.3	<3%	↓[c]
Hypoaldo	IV	Mild	⊕	<5.3	<3%	↑

[a]Urine pH will rise above 5.3 in the setting of HCO_3 load
[b]Fe_{HCO_3} should be checked after an HCO_3 load
[c]See above for causes of distal RTA (Type I) associated with hyperkalemia

Figure 4-2 Approach to metabolic acidosis

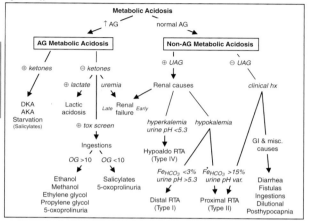

Treatment of severe metabolic acidoses (pH <7.2) (Nat Rev Nephol 2012;8:589)
- DKA: insulin & IVF; AKA: dextrose, IVF, replete K, Mg, PO_4 as needed
- Lactic acidosis: treat underlying condition, avoid vasoconstrictors, avoid "Type B" meds
- Renal failure: hemodialysis
- Methanol & ethylene glycol: early fomepizole, vit. B_6 (for ethylene glycol), folate
  (for methanol), hemodialysis (esp. if late presentation) (NEJM 2009;360:2216)
- Alkali therapy: $NaHCO_3$ (eg, three 50-mmol amps in 1 L D_5W) to get serum HCO_3 >8
  and pH >7.2 (estimate mmol of HCO_3 needed as 8 − [HCO_3]$_{serum}$ × wt × 0.5)
  side effects: ↑ volume, ↑ Na, ↓ iCa, ↑ P_aCO_2 (& ∴ intracellular acidosis), overshoot
  No proven benefit in lactic acidosis or DKA (Annals 1986;105:836 & 1990;112:492)
- THAM in Pts w/ ↑ P_aCO_2 (proton acceptor that generates HCO_3^- and consumes CO_2)

METABOLIC ALKALOSIS

Pathophysiology
- Saline-responsive etiologies require *initiating event* and *maintenance phase*
- *Initiating event*: gain of HCO_3 or loss of acid
  loss of H^+ from GI tract or kidneys
  exogenous alkali: iatrogenic HCO_3 administration, milk alkali syndrome
  contraction alkalosis: diuresis → excretion of HCO_3-poor fluid → extracellular fluid
    "contracts" around fixed amount of HCO_3 → ↑ HCO_3 concentration
  posthypercapnia: respiratory acidosis → renal compensation with HCO_3 retention;
    rapid correction of respiratory disorder (eg, with intubation) → transient excess HCO_3
- *Maintenance phase*
  volume depletion → ↑ proximal reabsorption of $NaHCO_3$ and ↑ aldosterone (see next)
  hyperaldosteronism (either 1° or 2°) → distal Na reabsorption in exchange for K^+ and
    H^+ excretion (and consequent HCO_3 retention)
  hypokalemia → transcellular K^+/H^+ exchange; intracellular acidosis in renal proximal
    tubular cells promotes bicarbonate reabsorption and ammoniagenesis

Etiologies of Metabolic Alkalosis	
Saline-responsive	**GI loss of H^+:** vomiting, NGT drainage, villous adenoma **Diuretic use** Posthypercapnia, laxatives, cystic fibrosis

Saline-resistant	*Hypertensive* **(mineralocorticoid excess)**
	    1° hyperaldosteronism (eg, Conn's)
	    2° hyperaldosteronism (eg, renovascular dis., renin-secreting tumor)
	    non-aldo (Cushing's, Liddle's, exogenous mineralocorticoids, licorice)
	Normotensive
	    severe hypokalemia; exogenous alkali load
	    Bartter's syndrome (loop-like); Gitelman's syndrome (thiazide-like)

Workup

• Check **volume status** and U_{Cl}

    U_{Cl} <20 mEq/L → saline-responsive
    U_{Cl} >20 mEq/L → saline-resistant (unless currently receiving diuretics)
    (U_{Na} unreliable determinant of volume status as alkalemia → ↑ HCO_3 excretion →
        ↑ Na excretion; negatively charged HCO_3^- "drags" Na^+ along)
    If U_{Cl} >20 and volume replete, ✓ **blood pressure**

Figure 4-3 Approach to metabolic alkalosis

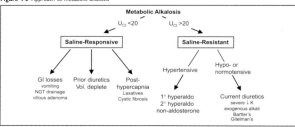

Metabolic Alkalosis

U_{Cl} <20 U_{Cl} >20

Saline-Responsive   Saline-Resistant

GI losses / Prior diuretics / Post-hypercapnia   Hypertensive / Hypo- or normotensive

GI losses: vomiting, NGT drainage, villous adenoma
Prior diuretics: Vol. deplete
Post-hypercapnia: Laxatives, Cystic fibrosis
Hypertensive: 1° hyperaldo, 2° hyperaldo, non-aldosterone
Hypo- or normotensive: Current diuretics, severe ↓ K, exogenous alkali, Bartter's, Gitelman's

Treatment of severe metabolic alkalosis (pH >7.6)

• If volume depletion: d/c diuretics and correct volume deficit with isotonic saline
    If cardiopulmonary disease precludes hydration, can use KCl, acetazolamide, HCl
• If NGT drainage that cannot be stopped: PPI
• Hyperaldosteronism: treat underlying condition

RESPIRATORY ACIDOSIS

Etiologies (also see "Hypercapnia")

• **CNS depression:** sedatives, CNS trauma, O_2 in chronic hypercapnia (↓ hypoxemic drive), central sleep apnea
• **Neuromuscular disorders:** myasthenia gravis, Guillain-Barré, poliomyelitis, ALS, muscular dystrophy, severe hypophosphatemia, high spinal cord injury, drugs (paralytics)
• **Upper airway abnormalities:** acute airway obstruction, laryngospasm, obstructive sleep apnea, esophageal intubation
• **Lower airway abnormalities:** asthma, COPD
• Lung parenchyma abnormalities (often cause hypoxia → ↑ RR → resp. alk., but eventual muscle fatigue → resp. acid.): pneumonia, pulmonary edema, restrictive lung disease
• Thoracic cage abnormalities: pneumothorax, flail chest, kyphoscoliosis
• Post infusion of bicarbonate in acidemic Pt w/ limited ability to ↑ minute ventilation

RESPIRATORY ALKALOSIS

Etiologies (*NEJM* 2002;347:43)

• **Hypoxia → hyperventilation:** pneumonia, pulm. edema, PE, restrictive lung disease
• **Primary hyperventilation**
    CNS stimulation, pain, anxiety, fever, trauma, stroke, voluntary
    drugs: salicylates, progesterone, methylxanthines, nicotine
    pregnancy, sepsis, hepatic failure, fever
• **Pseudorespiratory alkalosis:** ↓ perfusion w/ preserved ventilation (eg, CPR, severe HoTN) → ↓ delivery of CO_2 to lungs for excretion; low P_aCO_2 but ↑ tissue CO_2

OVERVIEW

General *(NEJM 2015;372:55 & 373:1350)*
- Disorders of serum sodium are generally due to Δs in *total body water,* not sodium
- Hyper- or hypo-osmolality → rapid water shifts → Δs in brain cell volume → Δ MS, seizures

Key hormones
- **Antidiuretic hormone (ADH):** primary hormone that regulates *sodium concentration*
  Stimuli for secretion: hyperosmolality, ↓↓ effective arterial volume (EAV), angiotensin II
  Action: insertion of aquaporin-2 channels in collecting ducts → passive water reabsorption
  urine osmolality is an indirect functional assay of the ADH-renal axis
  U_{osm} range: 60 mOsm/L (no ADH) to 1200 mOsm/L (maximal ADH)
- **Aldosterone:** primary hormone that regulates *total body sodium* (and ∴ volume)
  Stimuli for secretion: hypovolemia (via renin and angiotensin II), hyperkalemia
  Action: iso-osmotic reabsorption of sodium in exchange for potassium or H^+

HYPONATREMIA

Pathophysiology *(NEJM 2015;372:1349)*
- **Excess of water relative to sodium;** almost always due to ↑ **ADH**
- ↑ ADH may be *appropriate* (eg, hypovolemia or hypervolemia with ↓ EAV)
- ↑ ADH may be *inappropriate* (SIADH)
- Rarely, ↓ ADH (appropriately suppressed), but kidneys unable to maintain nl $[Na]_{serum}$
  ↑ H_2O intake *(1° polydipsia):* ingestion of massive quantities (usually >12 L/d) of free H_2O
  overwhelms diluting ability of kidney (normal dietary solute load ~750 mOsm/d,
  minimum U_{osm} = 60 mOsm/L → excrete in ~12 L; if H_2O ingestion exceeds this amount
  → H_2O retention)
  ↓ solute intake ("tea & toast" & "beer potomania"): ↓↓ daily solute load → insufficient solute
  to excrete H_2O intake (eg, if only 250 mOsm/d, minimum U_{osm} = 60 mOsm/L → excrete
  in ~4 L; if H_2O ingestion exceeds this amount → H_2O retention)

Workup *(JASN 2012;23:1140; Crit Care 2013;17:206; NEJM 2015;372:55)*
- **History:** (1) acute vs. chronic (>48 h); (2) sx severity; (3) risk for neuro complications
  (alcoholism, malnourished, cirrhosis, older females on thiazides, hypoxia, hypoK)
- Measure **plasma osmolality**
  Hypotonic hyponatremia most common scenario; true excess of free H_2O relative to Na
  Isotonic hyponatremia: rare lab artifact from hyperlipidemia or hyperproteinemia
  Hypertonic hyponatremia: excess of another effective osmole (eg, glucose, mannitol) that
  draws H_2O intravascularly; each 100 mg/dL ↑ glc >100 mg/dL → ↓ [Na] by 2.4 mEq/L
- For hypotonic hyponatremia, ✓ **volume status** (vital signs, orthostatics, JVP, skin
  turgor, mucous membranes, peripheral edema, BUN, Cr, uric acid)
- U_{osm} diagnostically useful in limited circumstances, because almost always >300
  exceptions: U_{osm} <100 in ↑ H_2O intake or ↓ solute intake
  moreover, U_{osm} >300 ≠ SIADH; must determine if ↑ ADH appropriate or inappropriate
  however, U_{osm} important when deciding on *treatment* (see below)
- If euvolemic and ↑ U_{osm}, evaluate for glucocorticoid insufficiency and hypothyroidism

Figure 4-4 Approach to hyponatremia

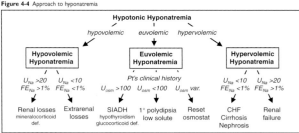

Hypovolemic hypotonic hyponatremia (ie, ↓↓ total body Na, ↓ TBW)

- **Renal losses** (U_{Na} >20 mEq/L, FE_{Na} >1%): diuretics (esp. thiazides, as loop diuretics ↓ tonicity of medullary interstitium and impair urine concentrating ability), salt-wasting nephropathy, cerebral salt wasting, mineralocorticoid deficiency
- **Extrarenal losses** (U_{Na} <10 mEq/L, FE_{Na} <1%): hemorrhage, GI loss (diarrhea), third-spacing (pancreatitis), ↓ PO intake, insensible losses

Euvolemic hypotonic hyponatremia (ie, ↑ TBW relative to total body Na)

- **SIADH** (euvolemia or mild hypervolemia, **inapprop ↑ U_{osm}**, approp. U_{Na}, ↓ BUN & UA)
  malignancy: lung, brain, GI, GU, lymphoma, leukemia, thymoma, mesothelioma
  pulmonary: pneumonia, TB, aspergillosis, asthma, COPD, PTX, ⊕ pressure ventilation
  intracranial: trauma, stroke, SAH, seizure, infxn, hydrocephalus, Guillain-Barré synd.
  drugs: antipsychotics, antidepress. (esp. *SSRIs*), chemotherapy, AVP, MDMA, NSAIDs
  miscellaneous: pain, nausea, postoperative state
- **Endocrinopathies:** ↑ADH activity seen in *glucocorticoid deficiency* (co-secretion of ADH & CRH) and *severe hypothyroidism/myxedema coma* (↓ CO & ↓ GFR)
- **Psychogenic polydipsia** (U_{osm} <100, ↓ uric acid): usually requires intake >12 L/d
- **Low solute** (↓ U_{Na}, ↓ U_{osm}) "tea & toast" "beer potomania"
- **Reset osmostat:** chronic malnutrition (↓ intracellular osmoles) or pregnancy (hormonal effects) → ADH physiology reset to regulate a lower $[Na]_{serum}$

Hypervolemic hypotonic hyponatremia (ie, ↑ total body Na, ↑ TBW)

- ↓ EAV → activation of RAAS → ↑↑ aldosterone *and* ↑↑ ADH
- **CHF** (↓ CO & renal venous congestion → ↓ EAV; U_{Na} <10 mEq/L, FE_{Na} <1%)
- **Cirrhosis** (splanchnic arterial vasodilation + ascites → ↓ EAV; U_{Na} <10 mEq/L, FE_{Na} <1%)
- **Nephrotic syndrome** (hypoalbuminemia → edema → ↓ EAV; U_{Na} <10 mEq/L, FE_{Na} <1%)
- **Advanced renal failure** (diminished ability to excrete free H_2O; U_{Na} >20 mEq/L)

Treatment (*Crit Care 2013;17:206; NEJM 2015;372:55*)

- **Approach:** depends on *volume status, acuity* of hyponatremia, and if *symptomatic*
  Acute sx: *initial rapid correction* of $[Na]_{serum}$ (2 mEq/L/h for the first 2–3 h) until sx resolve
  Asx or chronic symptomatic: correct $[Na]_{serum}$ at rate of ≤0.5 mEq/L/h
  Rate of ↑ Na *should not exceed 6* (chronic) to 8 (acute) mEq/L/d to avoid central pontine myelinolysis/osmotic demyelination syn. (CPM/ODS: paraplegia, dysarthria, dysphagia)
  If severe (<120) or neuro sx: consider use 3% NaCl + dDAVP (to prevent rapid overcorrection) in consultation w/ nephrology (*AJKD 2013;61:571*)
- **Frequent lab draws** and **IVF rate adjustments** are cornerstones of treatment
- **Overly rapid correction:** can lead to CPM/ODS. Should be emergently reversed w/ dDAVP ± D_5W; partial neurologic recovery possible (*CJASN 2014;9:229*)
- **Effect of IV fluids** (http://www.medcalc.com/sodium.html)

$$\text{initial } \Delta[Na]_{serum} \text{ per L infusate} = \frac{[Na]_{infusate} - [Na]_{serum}}{TBW + 1} \quad \begin{array}{l} TBW = wt \text{ (kg)} \times 0.6(\male) \text{ or } 0.5 \text{ ($\female$)}; \\ \text{if elderly use } 0.5 \text{ ($\male$) or } 0.45 \text{ ($\female$)} \end{array}$$

If $[Na]_s$ = 110 mEq/L in 70 kg male:			
IVF type	[Na]$_{content}$	1 L IVF ↑ [Na]$_s$	Rate to ↑ [Na]$_s$ by 0.5 mEq/L/h
5% NaCl	856 mEq/L	17.3 mEq/L	~25 mL/h
3% NaCl	513 mEq/L	9.4 mEq/L	~50 mL/h
0.9% NaCl	154 mEq/L	1 mEq/L	~500 mL/h
LR	130 mEq/L	0.5 mEq/L	~1000 mL/h

however, above assumes entire infusate retained *without any output of Na or H_2O*
if Pt euvolemic, as in SIADH, infused Na will be excreted
eg, 1 L NS (154 mEq of Na or 308 mOsm of solute) given to Pt with
SIADH with U_{osm} = 616 → 308 mOsm solute excreted in 0.5 L H_2O →
net gain 0.5 L H_2O → ↓ $[Na]_{serum}$
∴ normal saline can *worsen* hyponatremia from SIADH if U_{osm} > infusate$_{osm}$

- **Hypovolemic hyponatremia:** volume repletion with normal saline at a **slow rate**.
  Once volume replete → stimulus for ADH removed (w/ very short ADH $t_{1/2}$) → kidneys excrete free H_2O → serum Na will correct rapidly (D_5W ± dDAVP if overcorrection)
- **SIADH** (*NEJM 2007;356:2064; AJKD 2015;65:435*): **free water restrict** + treat underlying cause
  hypertonic saline (± loop diuretic) if sx or Na fails to ↑ w/ free H_2O restriction
  1 L hypertonic saline (3% NaCl) will raise $[Na]_{serum}$ by ~10 mEq (see above)
  ~50 mL/h will ↑ [Na] by ~0.5 mEq/L/h; 100–200 mL/h will ↑ [Na] by ~1–2 mEq/L/h
  formula only provides estimate; ∴ recheck serum Na frequently (at least q2h)
  NaCl tabs: particularly if chronic and no CHF
  aquaresis: ? vaptans (vasopressin receptor antag) for refractory SIADH (*NEJM 2015;372:23*)
  demeclocycline: causes nephrogenic DI, ↓ U_{osm} (rarely used)

- **Hypervolemic hyponatremia: free water restrict**
    mobilize excess Na & H_2O (use loop diuretics; avoid thiazides) & ↑ EAV (vasodilators to ↑ CO in CHF; colloid infusion in cirrhosis)
    aquaresis: vaptans sometimes used; however, no proven mortality benefit, hypoNa recurs after stopping drug, risk of overcorrection, contraindicated in cirrhosis, and expensive (*NEJM 2015;372:2207*)

HYPERNATREMIA

Pathophysiology (*Crit Care 2013;17:206; NEJM 2015;372:55*)
- Deficit of water relative to sodium; by definition, all hypernatremic Pts are hypertonic
- Usually **loss of hypotonic fluid** (ie, "dehydration"); occasionally infusion of hypertonic fluid
- *And* **impaired access to free water** (eg, intubation, Δ MS, elderly): hypernatremia is a powerful thirst stimulus, ∴ usually only develops in Pts w/o access to H_2O

Workup
- ✓ U_{osm}, U_{Na}, volume status (vital signs, orthostatics, JVP, skin turgor, BUN, Cr)

Figure 4-5 Approach to hypernatremia

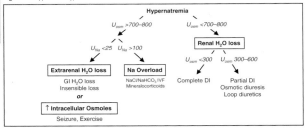

Extrarenal H_2O loss (U_{osm} >700–800)
- **GI H_2O loss:** vomiting, NGT drainage, osmotic diarrhea, fistula
- **Insensible loss:** fever, exercise, ventilation

Renal H_2O loss (U_{osm} <700–800)
- **Diuresis:** osmotic (glucose, mannitol, urea), loop diuretics
- **Diabetes insipidus** (*J Clin Endocrinol Metab 2012;97:3426*)
    ADH deficiency (central) or resistance (nephrogenic)
    Central: hypothalamic or posterior pituitary disease (congenital, trauma/surgery, tumors, infiltrative/IgG4); also idiopathic, hypoxic encephalopathy, anorexia, EtOH
    Nephrogenic (*Annals 2006;144:186*)
        congenital (ADH receptor V2 mutation, aquaporin-2 mutation; *Ped Nephrol 2012;27:2183*)
        drugs: **lithium,** amphotericin, demeclocycline, foscarnet, cidofovir
        metabolic: **hypercalcemia, severe hypokalemia,** protein malnutrition, congenital
        tubulointerstitial: **postobstruction, recovery phase of ATN,** PKD, sickle cell, Sjögren's, amyloid, pregnancy (placental vasopressinase)
    DI usually presents as *severe polyuria* and *mild hypernatremia*

Other (U_{osm} >700–800)
- **Na overload:** hypertonic saline (eg, resuscitation w/ $NaHCO_3$), mineralocorticoid excess
- **Seizures,** ↑ **exercise:** ↑ intracellular osmoles → H_2O shifts → transient ↑ $[Na]_{serum}$

Treatment
- **Restore access to H_2O** or supply daily requirement of H_2O (≥1 L/d)
- **Replace free H_2O deficit** (also replace concurrent volume deficit if appropriate):

$$\text{Free } H_2O \text{ deficit (L)} = \frac{[Na]_{serum} - 140}{140} \times TBW$$

TBW = wt (kg) × 0.6 (♂) or 0.5 (♀); if elderly use 0.5 (♂) or 0.45 (♀)

shortcut: for typical 70-kg man, free H_2O deficit (L) ~ ([Na]$_{serum}$ − 140)/3

$$\Delta [Na]_{serum} \text{ pe L infusate} = \frac{[Na]_{serum} - [Na]_{infusate}}{TBW + 1}$$

eg, 1 L D_5W given to 70-kg man w/ [Na] = 160 mEq/L will ↓ [Na]$_{serum}$ by 3.7 mEq
nb, do not forget to correct Na if hyperglycemia also present

- **Rate of ↓ of Na should not exceed 0.5 mEq/L/h** to avoid cerebral edema
  shortcut: in 70-kg man, 125 mL/h of free H_2O will ↓ [Na] by ~0.5 mEq/L/h
- ½ NS (77 mEq/L) or ¼ NS (38 mEq/L) provides both volume & free H_2O (500 or 750 mL of free H_2O per L, respectively); can give free H_2O via NGT/OGT
- Formulas provide only estimates; ∴ recheck serum Na frequently
- **DI and osmotic diuresis:** see "Polyuria" section below
- **Na overload:** D_5W + diuretic

POLYURIA

Definition and pathophysiology
- **Polyuria** defined as >3 L UOP per day
- Due to an *osmotic* or a *water diuresis*; almost always due to osmotic diuresis in inpatients

Workup
- Perform a timed urine collection (6 h sufficient) and measure U_{osm}
- 24-h osmole excretion rate = 24-h UOP (actual or estimate) × U_{osm}
  >1000 mOsm/d → osmotic diuresis
  <800 mOsm/d → water diuresis

Osmotic diuresis
- Etiologies:
  Glucose (uncontrolled diabetes mellitus)
  Mannitol
  Urea: recovering AKI, ↑ protein feeds, hypercatabolism (burns, steroids), GI bleed
  NaCl administration
  Propylene glycol

Water diuresis
- Etiologies: **diabetes insipidus (DI)** (Na_{serum} >143) or **1° polydipsia** (Na_{serum} <136)
  see "Hypernatremia" above for list of causes of central and nephrogenic DI
- Workup of DI: U_{osm} <300 (complete) or 300–600 (partial)
  water deprivation test (start in a.m., ✓ Na_{serum}, P_{osm}, U_{osm}, UOP q1–2h)
  Deprive until P_{osm} >295, then ✓ U_{osm}. If U_{osm} <300, then administer vasopressin (5 U SC) or dDAVP (10 µg intranasal), then check U_{osm} in 1–2 h:
  U_{osm} ↑ by >50% = central DI
  U_{osm} unchanged = nephrogenic DI
  ✓ADH level before and after water deprivation to evaluate proper response

Figure 4-6 Approach to polyuria

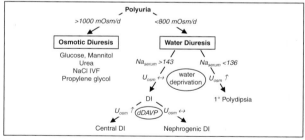

Treatment
- **1° polydipsia:** treat psychiatric illness, check meds, restrict access to free H_2O
- **Osmotic diuresis:** address underlying cause, replace free H_2O deficit (see "Hypernatremia" for formula to calculate) and ongoing losses
- **DI:**
  central DI: desmopressin (dDAVP)
  nephrogenic DI: treat underlying cause if possible; Na restriction + thiazide (mild volume depletion → ↓ delivery of filtrate to dysfunctional diluting segment of kidney), consider amiloride for lithium-induced DI (*Kid Int* 2009;76:44)
  pregnancy-induced DI: due to vasopressinase from placenta, ∴ Rx w/ dDAVP

Overview (NEJM 2015;373:60)
- Renal: potassium excretion regulated at **distal nephron** (collecting tubule)
    distal Na delivery & urine flow: Na absorption → lumen electronegative → K secretion
    metabolic alkalemia and aldosterone: increase Na absorption and K secretion
    nb, diurnal urinary K excretion (day > night), ∴ 24-h sample preferred over spot
- Transcellular shifts: most common cause of acute Δ in serum K (98% intracellular)
    Acid-base disturbance: K^+/H^+ exchange across cell membranes
    Insulin → stimulates Na-K ATPase → hypokalemia; reversed by β-blockers (mitigates postprandial ↑ K)
    Catecholamines → stimulate Na-K ATPase → hypokalemia; reversed by β-blockers
    Massive necrosis (eg, tumor lysis, rhabdo, ischemic bowel) → release of intracellular K
    Hypo- or hyperkalemic periodic paralysis: rare disorders due to channel mutations
- Diet: alone rarely causes ↑ or ↓ K (total body store ~3500 mEq, daily intake ~100 mEq)

HYPOKALEMIA

Transcellular shifts ($U_{K:Cr}$ <20 mEq/g)
- Alkalemia, insulin, catecholamines, hypokalemic/thyrotoxic periodic paralysis, acute ↑ in
    hematopoiesis (megaloblastic anemia Rx w/ B_{12}, AML crisis), hypothermia, chloroquine,
    barium/cesium intoxication, antipsychotic overdose (risperidone, quetiapine)

GI potassium losses (U_K <25 mEq/d, $U_{K:Cr}$ <20 mEq/g, TTKG <3)
- GI losses *plus* metabolic acidosis: diarrhea, laxative abuse, villous adenoma
- Vomiting & NGT drainage usually manifest as *renal losses* due to 2° hyperaldo & met. alk.

Renal potassium losses (U_K >30 mEq/d, ? $U_{K:Cr}$ >20 mEq/g, TTKG >7)
- Hypotensive or normotensive
    acidosis: DKA, RTA [proximal RTA (type II) and some distal RTAs (type I)]
    alkalosis: diuretics, vomiting/NGT drainage (via 2° hyperaldosteronism)
        Bartter's syndrome (loop of Henle dysfxn → furosemide-like effect; NEJM 1999;340:1177)
        Gitelman's syndrome (distal convoluted tubule dysfxn → thiazide-like effect)
    ↓ Mg: ? release Mg-mediated inhib. of ROMK channel ∴ ↑ K secretion (JASN 2007;18:2649)
- Hypertensive: mineralocorticoid excess
    1° hyperaldosteronism (eg, Conn's syndrome, glucocorticoid-remediable aldosteronism)
    2° hyperaldosteronism (eg, renovascular disease, renin-secreting tumor)
    nonaldosterone mineralocorticoid (eg, Cushing's, Liddle's, exogenous mineralocort.,
    licorice, congenital adrenal hyperplasia)

Clinical manifestations
- Nausea, vomiting, ileus, weakness, muscle cramps, rhabdomyolysis, polyuria
- ECG: can have no Δs, U waves, ↑ QT interval, ventricular ectopy (PVCs, VT, VF)

Workup (Nat Rev Neph 2011;7:75)
- Rule out transcellular shifts
- ✓ 24-h U_K and transtubular potassium gradient (TTKG) = $(U_K/P_K)/(U_{osm}/P_{osm})$
    U_K >30 mEq/d, ? $U_{K:Cr}$ >20 mEq/g, or TTKG >7 → suggests renal loss
    U_K <25 mEq/d, $U_{K:Cr}$ <20 mEq/g, or TTKG <3 → suggests extrarenal loss
- If renal losses, ✓ **BP, acid-base, U_{Cl}** (U_{Na} unreliable for volume status w/ alkalemia)

Figure 4-7 Approach to hypokalemia

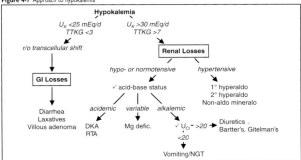

Treatment

- If true potassium deficit: **potassium repletion** (↓ 1 mEq/L ≈ 200 mEq total body loss)
  KCl 40 mEq PO q4–6h if nongurent, KCl 10 mEq/h IV if urgent, recheck K freq
- Beware of excessive potassium repletion if transcellular shift cause of hypokalemia
- Treat underlying cause (if hydration needed, avoid dextrose-containing solutions as dextrose → ↑ insulin → intracellular potassium shifts)
- Replete low Mg: IV Mg-SO₄ 1–2 g q2h (oral Mg-oxide poorly tolerated b/c diarrhea)
  Causes of low Mg: GI loss (diarrhea, bypass, pancreatitis, malnutrition, PPI); renal loss (diuretics, nephrotoxic drugs, EtOH, ↑ Ca, 1° wasting syndromes, volume expansion)

HYPERKALEMIA

Transcellular shifts (BMJ 2009;339:1019)

- Acidemia, insulin defic. (DM), β-blockers, dig intox. (blocks Na-K ATPase), massive cellular release (tumor lysis, rhabdo, ischemic bowel, hemolysis, transfusions, resorbing hematomas, hyperthermia, rewarming), hyperkalemic periodic paralysis, succinylcholine

Decreased GFR

- Any cause of oliguric or anuric AKI or any cause of end-stage renal disease

Normal GFR but with ↓ renal K excretion

- Normal aldosterone function
  ↓ EAV (K excretion limited by ↓ **distal Na delivery & urine flow**): CHF, cirrhosis
  excessive K intake: in conjunction with impairment in K excretion or transcellular shift
  ureterojejunostomy (absorption of urinary K in jejunum)
- **Hypoaldosteronism**: same as etiologies of hypoaldo RTA (type IV)
  ↓ renin: diabetic nephropathy, NSAIDs, chronic interstitial nephritis, HIV
  normal renin, ↓ aldo synthesis: 1° adrenal disorders, ACEI, ARBs, heparin
  ↓ response to aldosterone
    meds: K-sparing diuretics, TMP-SMX, pentamidine, calcineurin inhibitors
    tubulointerstitial disease: sickle cell, SLE, amyloid, diabetes

Clinical manifestations

- Weakness, nausea, paresthesias, palpitations
- ECG: peaked T waves, ↑ PR interval, ↑ QRS width, loss of P wave, sine wave pattern, PEA/VF (ECG: low sensitivity, cardiac arrest can be first clinical manifestation!)

Workup (Crit Care Med 2008;36:3246)

- Rule out pseudohyperkalemia (IVF with K, hemolysis during venipuncture, ↑ plt or WBC)
- Rule out transcellular shift
- **Assess GFR**, if normal, then consider ↓ distal Na delivery and urine flow. ✓ transtubular K gradient (TTKG) = $(U_K/P_K)/(U_{osm}/P_{osm})$ <6 c/w hypoaldo (JASN 2008;19:424).

Treatment of Hyperkalemia			
Intervention	**Dose**	**Onset**	**Comment**
Ca gluconate **Ca chloride**[a]	1–2 amps IV	<3 min	transient effect (30–60 min) stabilizes cell membrane
Insulin	reg. insulin 10 U IV + 1–2 amps D₅₀W	15–30 min	transient effect (30–60 min) drives K into cells
Bicarbonate (esp. if acidemic)	1–2 amps IV	15–30 min	transient effect (60 min) exchange K for H⁺ in cells
β2 agonists	albuterol 10–20 mg inh. or 0.5 mg IV	30–90 min	transient effect (~2 h) drives K into cells
K-binding resins	Kayexalate[b] 30–90g PO/PR ? Na zirconium 1.25–10 g/tid PO Patiromer 8.4–25.2 g/d PO	hrs hrs hrs-d	exchange K for cations in gut (Na, Ca, H); ↓ total body K; (NEJM 2015;372:211 & 222)
Diuretics	furosemide ≥40 mg IV	30 min	↓ total body K
Hemodialysis			↓ total body K

[a] Calcium chloride contains more calcium and is typically reserved for use in codes (↑ risk of tissue necrosis)
[b] rare a/w intestinal necrosis esp. with postoperative ileus or obstructive bowel disease (AJKD 2012;60:409)

- Rate of onset important to note when establishing a treatment plan
- Calcium helps prevent/treat cardiac complications; ∴ should be initial Rx, esp. if ECG Δs
- Insulin, bicarbonate (esp. if acidemic), and β2 agonists should follow to ↓ plasma K
- Treatments that **eliminate total body K essential**, as other Rxs will wear off with time; Kayexalate or Na diuretics may be effective in many cases, but emergent hemodialysis should be considered in life-threatening situations
- Patient information for diet education: http://www.kidney.org/atoz/content/potassium.cfm

ACUTE KIDNEY INJURY (AKI)

Definition (*CJASN* 2008;3:844; *KI Suppl* 2012;2:19)
- AKI: abrupt (<48 h) ↑ Cr ≥0.3 mg/dL, ↑ Cr ≥50%, or UOP <0.5 mL/kg/h for ≥6 h additional gradations based on further ↑ Cr & ↓ UOP but not used clinically
- *Cannot* estimate GFR using Cr in setting of AKI or Δ'ing Cr (requires steady state)

Workup (*NEJM* 2007;357:797; *Lancet* 2012;380:756)
- **H&P:** recent procedures & meds; thirst; VS & vol status; s/s of obstruction, vasc or systemic dis.; ischemia (prerenal & ATN) accounts for >50% of in-hospital AKI
- **Urine evaluation:** output, urinalysis, **sediment,** electrolytes, and osmolality
- **Fractional excretion of sodium (FE$_{Na}$)** = $(U_{Na}/P_{Na})/(U_{Cr}/P_{Cr})$
  <1% → prerenal, contrast, HRS or glomerulonephritis; >2% → ATN
  In setting of diuretics, ✓ FE$_{UN}$ = $(U_{UN}/P_{UN})/(U_{Cr}/P_{Cr})$; <35% → prerenal
- Renal U/S or CT: r/o obstruction & eval kidney size to estimate chronicity of kidney disease
- Serologies (if indicated): see "Glomerular Disease"
- Renal biopsy (light microscopy, IF, and EM): may be necessary if etiology remains unclear (esp. if hematuria and/or proteinuria). Relative contraindications: SBP>150, ASA/NSAID or anticoag use. Consider dDAVP (0.3 μg/kg 30–60 min prior) for severe uremia.

<table>
<tr><th colspan="3">Etiologies and Diagnosis of Acute Kidney Injury (Lancet 2012;380:756)</th></tr>
<tr><th colspan="2">Etiologies</th><th>U/A, Sediment, Indices</th></tr>
<tr>
<td rowspan="3">Prerenal</td>
<td>↓ Effective arterial volume (NEJM 2007;357:797)
Hypovolemia, ↓ cardiac contractility (eg, CHF),
systemic vasodilatation (eg, sepsis)</td>
<td rowspan="3">Bland
Transparent hyaline casts
FE$_{Na}$ <1%
BUN/Cr >20
U$_{Na}$ <20
U$_{osm}$ >500</td>
</tr>
<tr>
<td>Renal vasoconstriction: NSAIDs, ACEI/ARB,
contrast, calcineurin inhib., HRS, hyperCa</td>
</tr>
<tr>
<td>Large vessel: RAS (bilateral + ACEI), vasculitis,
dissection, abd compartment synd., renal
venous congestion, VTE</td>
</tr>
<tr>
<td rowspan="4">Intrinsic</td>
<td>Acute tubular necrosis (ATN)
Ischemia: progression of prerenal disease
Toxins
Drugs: AG, amphotericin, cisplatin, HES (starch)
Pigments: Hb, myoglobin (NEJM 2009;361:62)
Monoclonal: Ig light chains (Blood 2010;116:1397)
Crystals: UA, ACV, MTX, indinavir, oral NaPO$_4$
Contrast-induced AKI (CIAKI): ↓ RBF + toxin</td>
<td>Pigmented granular muddy
brown casts in ~75%
(± in CIAKI)
± RBCs & protein from tubular
damage
FE$_{Na}$ >2%, BUN/Cr <20, U$_{Na}$
>20 (except pigment, CIAKI)
U$_{osm}$ <350</td>
</tr>
<tr>
<td>Acute interstitial nephritis (AIN)
Allergic: β-lactams, sulfa drugs, NSAIDs, PPIs
Infection: pyelonephritis, legionella, TB, leptospirosis
Infiltrative: sarcoid, lymphoma, leukemia
Autoimmune: Sjögren's, TINU syndrome, IgG4, SLE</td>
<td>WBCs, WBC casts, ± RBCs
w/ neg UCx
⊕ urine eos in abx
⊕ lymphs in NSAIDs</td>
</tr>
<tr>
<td>Small-med vessel: chol emboli, PAN, TMAs (TTP,
HUS, atypical HUS, DIC, preeclampsia, APS,
malignant HTN, scleroderma renal crisis)</td>
<td>± RBCs
⊕ urine eos in chol emboli</td>
</tr>
<tr>
<td>Glomerulonephritis (see "Glomerular Disease")</td>
<td>Dysmorphic RBCs, RBC casts</td>
</tr>
<tr>
<td rowspan="2">Post</td>
<td>Bladder neck: BPH, prostate cancer, neurogenic
bladder, anticholinergic meds</td>
<td>Bland
± nondysmorphic RBCs</td>
</tr>
<tr>
<td>Ureteral (bilateral or unilateral in single kidney):
malig, LAN, retroperitoneal fibrosis, nephrolithiasis</td>
<td>FE$_{Na}$ variable</td>
</tr>
</table>

General treatment (*CJASN* 2008;3:962)
- Prerenal: isotonic IVF ≈ alb (*NEJM* 2004;350:22), HES (starch) nephrotoxic (*NEJM* 2012;367:124)
- Avoid nephrotoxic insults; review dosing of renally cleared drugs
- Optimize hemodynamics (both MAP & CO)
- No benefit to dopamine (*Annals* 2005;142:510), diuretics (*JAMA* 2002;288:2547), or mannitol

Managing complications
- May take 1–3 wk to recover from ATN; anticipate volume overload, ↑ K, ↑ PO$_4$, acidosis
- Episodes of AKI ↑ risk of CKD progression, even after recovery (*NEJM* 2014;371:58)
- Indications for urgent dialysis (when condition refractory to conventional therapy)
  Acid-base disturbance: refractory acidemia
  Electrolyte disorder: generally hyperkalemia; occasionally hypercalcemia, tumor lysis

Intoxications (http://www.extrip-workgroup.org/): contact Poison Control (1-800-222-1222)
  Indicated for: methanol, ethylene glycol, metformin, Li, valproic acid, salicylates, barbiturates, theophylline, thallium
  Also consider for: carbamazepine, acetaminophen, dig (also give Digibind), dabigatran (also give idarucizumab)
Overload of volume (CHF)
Uremia: pericarditis, encephalopathy, bleeding
- Data on benefit of early RRT remains mixed (*NEJM* 2016;375:122 & *JAMA* 2016;315:2190)

DISEASE-SPECIFIC MANAGEMENT

Cardiorenal syndrome (CRS) (*Nat Rev Neph* 2009;5:641 & 2013;9:99; *CJASN* 2013;8:1800)
- Multifactorial pathophys including: 1) ↓ CO, 2) ↑ renal venous congestion, 3) ↑ RAAS
- Bidirectionality: acute CHF → AKI, and oliguric AKI can worsen CHF (*JACC* 2008;52:1527)
- Treatment: **IV loop diuretics** (bypass potential gut edema; see below for dosing; no diff. between high vs. low dose and bolus vs. gtt (*NEJM* 2011;364:797). No clinical benefit w/ vaptans (ADH receptor antag; *JAMA* 2007;297:1319), dopamine or nesiritide (*NEJM* 2011;365:32; *JAMA* 2013;310:2533), or ultrafiltration (*NEJM* 2012;367:2296)
- Prognosis: 7% ↑ mortality a/w each 10 mL/min ↓ eGFR in ADHF (*JACC* 2006;47:1987)

Contrast-induced acute kidney injury (CIAKI; *Circ* 2015;132:1931)
- Risk factors: CKD, DM, CHF, age, hypotension, ↑ contrast volume (*JACC* 2004;44:1393)
- Clinical: AKI w/in 48 h of contrast exposure, peaks in 3–5 d, resolves in 7–10 d (if does not resolve, consider cholesterol emboli or other etiology)
- Prevention: consider when eGFR <60 or diabetes (*CJASN* 2013;8:1618)
  Isotonic IV fluids (unless contraindic, eg, CHF)
    Outpatients: 3 mL/kg/h × 1 h before, 1–1.5 mL/kg/h × 6 h after (*JAMA* 2004;291:2328)
    Inpatients: 1 mL/kg/h × 6–12 h before, during, and 6–12 h after;
      if undergoing cardiac cath, consider rate of IVF based on LVEDP:
      5, 3, or 1.5 mL/kg/h if LVEDP <13, 13–18, or >18 mmHg (*Lancet* 2014;383:1814)
    $NaHCO_3$ similar to NaCl (*CJASN* 2015;10:1519).
  Hold ACEI/ARB (*AJKD* 2012;60:576), NSAIDs, diuretics. ? high-dose statin (*Circ* 2012;126:3008)
  Minimize contrast volume and use iso-osmolar contrast (*JACC* 2006;48:692)
  N-acetylcysteine 600–1200 mg PO bid on day prior to & day of contrast; benefit in some but not all studies (*Annals* 2016;164:406); as safe, reasonable to consider in high-risk Pts
  No proven benefit to Ppx RRT in addition to above, may be harmful (*Am J Med* 2012;125:66)
- Gadolinium: can cause AKI in stage IV CKD (*Neph Dial Trans* 2006;21:697), no effective Ppx
  Nephrogenic systemic fibrosis: fibrosis of skin, joints, eyes, and internal organs ~2–4 wk post exposure in Pts w/ mod-severe CKD (*JACC* 2009;53:1621). Postgado HD encouraged albeit no data. Physical therapy. Can be irreversible.

Hepatorenal syndrome (HRS; see "Cirrhosis"; *AJKD* 2013;62(6):1198)
- Albumin + either octreotide & midodrine or IV vasopressors

Rhabdomyolysis (*NEJM* 2009;361:62)
- Multifactorial pathophys: myoglobin-induced oxidant injury, vasoconstriction, myoglobin precipitation & pre-renal (extravasation). Can lead to ↓ Ca, ↑ K, and ↑ PO_4.
- Diagnosis: UA ⊕ for heme but 0 RBCs (ie, myoglobinuria)
- Generally low risk of AKI when CK <5000, but correlation imperfect. Rhabdo & risk of AKI/death calculator: http://www.brighamandwomens.org/research/rhabdo/default.aspx
- Aggressive IVF resuscitation and augmenting UOP (tailor IVF to target UOP ~3 mL/kg and ensure ↓ CK). If urine pH <6.5, can consider $NaHCO_3$ solutions and watching pH.
  ✓ K & Ca frequently. Monitor for compartment syndrome.

Acute interstitial nephritis (AIN; *KI* 2008;73:940 & 2010;77:956)
- Commonly drug-induced: β-lactams, sulfa drugs, NSAIDs, PPIs
- If suspected, prompt removal of offending drug, consider early steroids w/in 7 d of dx

Thrombotic microangiopathies (TMAs): *please see "Hematology"*

Obstructive diseases
- Dx: imaging w/ renal U/S if undifferentiated or abd/pelvic CT (I⁻) if suspect nephrolithiasis
- Treatment: Foley catheter vs. percutaneous nephrostomy for decompression
- Following decompression, at risk of:
  Hypotonic diuresis (2° buildup of BUN, tubular damage); Rx w/ IVF (eg, ½ NS)
  Hemorrhagic cystitis (rapid Δ in size of bladder vessels); avoid by decompressing slowly

CHRONIC KIDNEY DISEASE (CKD)

Definition and etiologies (*Lancet* 2012;379:165; *JAMA* 2015;313:837)
- ≥3 mo of **reduced GFR** (<60) *and/or* **kidney damage** (path, markers, imaging)
- Prevalence 13% in U.S.

- Cr poor estimate of GFR, use equation (www.kidney.org/professionals/KDOQI/gfr_calculator.cfm) CKD-EPI preferred over MDRD as less likely to underestimate at normal GFRs cystatin-C–based formulae perform better than Cr-based *(NEJM 2012;367:20)*
- Etiologies: DM (45%), HTN/RAS (27%), glomerular (10%), interstitial (5%), PKD (2%) *(NEJM 2008;359:1477)*, congenital, drugs, myeloma, progression of AKI *(JAMA 2009;302:1179)*
- Presence and degree of albuminuria a/w worse outcomes independent of Cr
- Rates of all-cause mortality and CV events increase with each stage of CKD & albuminuria and are greater than rate of progression to kidney failure *(NEJM 2004;351:1296)*

Stages of CKD *(Kid Int 2013;[Suppl]:5)*		
GFR Stage	**GFR mL/min/1.73 m^2**	**Goals**
1 (nl or ↑ GFR)	>90	Dx/Rx of underlying condition & comorbidities, slow progression; cardiovascular risk reduction
2 (mild)	60–89	Estimate progression
3a (mild-mod)	45–59	Evaluate and treat complications
3b (mod-severe)	30–44	Evaluate and treat complications
4 (severe)	15–29	Prepare for renal replacement therapy (RRT)
5 (kidney failure)	<15 or dialysis	Dialysis if uremic

Albuminuria stage based on albuminuria (mg/d) or spot urine alb (μg) to Cr (mg) ratio: nl or mildly ↑ (<30); mod ↑ or microalbuminuria (30–299); or severely ↑ or macroalb (≥300)

Signs and Symptoms of Uremia *(NEJM 2007;357:1316)*	
General	Nausea, anorexia, malaise, fetor uremicus, metallic taste, susceptibility to drug O/D, decreased temperature
Skin	Uremic frost (white crystals in & on skin), pruritus, calciphylaxis, NSF
Neurologic	Encephalopathy (Δ MS, ↓ memory & attention), seizures, neuropathy, impaired sleep, restless leg syndrome
Cardiovascular	Pericarditis, accelerated atherosclerosis, hypertension, hyperlipidemia, volume overload, CHF, cardiomyopathy (esp. LVH)
Hematologic	Anemia, bleeding (due to platelet dysfunction and Epo deficiency)
Metabolic	↑ K, ↑ PO$_4$, acidosis, ↓ Ca, 2° hyperparathyroidism, osteodystrophy

Complications & treatment *(Annals 2009;150:ITC2-1; NEJM 2010;362:57)*
- **General:** nephrology referral when GFR <30 & access planning (avoid subclavian lines; preserve an arm for access by avoiding blood draws, BP measurements, IVs); Rx CV risk factors (eg, smoking, LDL-C; *Lancet 2011;377:2181*), vaccines (flu, PNA, HBV)
- **Dietary restrictions:** Na (if HTN), K (if oliguric or hyperkalemic), PO$_4$, ? moderate protein restriction, strict glc control in DM, avoid herbal and unknown OTCs
- **BP Control:** goal <130/80, ? <120/80 if tolerated *(NEJM 2015;373:2103)*; start w/ ACEI (or ARB), effective in DM & nondiabetic CKD *(NEJM 2004;351:1952)*; no benefit of ACEI + ARB combined and a/w adverse outcomes *(NEJM 2013;369:1892)*. For outPts, ✓ Cr & K in 1–2 wk, d/c if Cr ↑ 30% or K >5.4 (after dietary Δ & loop diuretic)
- **Metabolic acidosis:** sodium bicarbonate or sodium citrate if low HCO$_3$ *(JASN 2015;26:515)*
- **Hyperkalemia:** (qv)
- **Anemia:** goal Hb ~10 g/dL, worse outcomes if target higher *(NEJM 2009;361:2019)* epoetin (start 80–120 U/kg SC, divided 3×/wk) or darbepoetin (0.45 μg/kg q wk) iron supplementation to keep transferrin sat >20% (often given IV in HD Pts)
- **Uremic bleeding:** desmopressin (dDAVP) 0.3 μg/kg IV or 3 μg/kg intranasally
- **2° HyperPTH:** ↑ PO$_4$, ↓ Ca, ↓ calcitriol, ↑ FGF-23 → ↑ PTH → renal osteodystrophy

CKD stage	3	4	5
Target PTH (pg/mL)	35–70	70–110	150–300

  phosphorus binders (*take with meals!*) *(NEJM 2010;362:1312)*
  if ↑ PO$_4$ and ↓ Ca → calcium acetate (PhosLo) or calcium carbonate
  if refractory ↑ PO$_4$ or in setting of ↑ Ca → sevelamer (Renagel), lanthanum (Fosrenol)
  non-Ca–based binders a/w ↓ mort. compared to Ca-based *(Lancet 2013;382:1268)*
  if PTH above goal then start vit. D (if 25-(OH)D <30) before adding 1,25-(OH)D analogue (paricalcitol); stop if ↑ Ca *(AJKD 2013;63:408)*
  cinacalcet (parathyroid calcium-sensing receptor agonist) if ↑ PTH despite phosphorus binders ± vit. D analogue *(CJASN 2016;11:161)*; consider parathyroidectomy
- **Calciphylaxis** (calcific uremic arteriopathy):
  Pathophys: calcification of media of small- to med-sized blood vessels of dermis & SC fat → ischemia and skin necrosis w/ *painful* lesions *(NEJM 2007;356:1049)*
  Risk Factors: uremia in ESRD (↑ PO$_4$, ↑ Ca, ↑ PTH), ♀>♂, DM, obesity, warfarin
  Diagnosis: skin bx gold standard; bone imaging in support of dx

Treatment: multidisciplinary wound care, manage hyperPTH, avoid vit D & Ca suppl.,
IV & intralesional Na thiosulfate, cinacalcet; NOAC rather than warfarin
Prognosis: a/w 60% 1-y mort. in ESRD Pts *(AJKD 2015;66(1):133)*
• **Transplant evaluation**

DIURESIS

General considerations
• Increases Na excretion for treatment of HTN or edema in CHF, renal failure, and cirrhosis
• Daily wt most effective method of documenting successful diuresis

Loop diuretics *(NEJM 1998;339:387)*
• **Drugs:** furosemide (Lasix), torsemide, bumetanide (Bumex), ethacrynic acid
• **Mech:** inhib Na-K-2Cl transporter in thick ascending limb (ThAL); 20–25% Na reabsorp.
Transient, immediate venodilation may aid in pulmonary congestion *(NEJM 1973;288:1087)*
Response is fxn of amt of drug excreted; ∴ ↑ dose needed in renal insufficiency, CHF
Sigmoidal dose response curve; ∴ ↑ dose until induce diuresis, ↑↑ dose beyond that
point yields diminishing returns compared with ↑ frequency of dosing
• **Dosing:** PO bioavailability of furosemide ~50%, ∴ IV dose ~2× as potent as PO dose
torsemide & bumetanide ~90% bioavailability; use ethacrynic acid if sulfa allergy
40 mg furosemide PO ≈ 20 mg furosemide IV ≈ 20 mg torsemide PO ≈ 1 mg bumetanide
dose furosemide bid-qid; qd dosing can lead to initial diuresis → antinatriuresis
Continuous vs. bolus IV: similar results in acute CHF *(NEJM 2011;364:797)*
? ↑ diuresis w/ co-administration of albumin if ↓ serum albumin *(Crit Care Med 2005;33:1681)*

Thiazide diuretics *(NEJM 2009;361:2153)*
• **Drugs:** hydrochlorothiazide (HCTZ), chlorothiazide (Diuril), metolazone (Zaroxolyn)
• **Mech:** inhib Na-Cl cotransporter in the distal convoluted tubule (DCT); 5% Na reabsorp.
synergistic with loop diuretic, esp. if chronic loop use
↓ effect when GFR <30, *except metolazone* which is still effective in renal insufficiency
• **Dosing:** give prior to loop diuretic, typically ~30 min before

K-sparing diuretics
• **Drugs:** spironolactone (Aldactone), amiloride, triamterene, eplerenone
• **Mech:** ↓ Na reabsorption (~1%) in collecting duct (amiloride/triamterene inhibit principal
cell Na channel [ENaC]; spironolactone/eplerenone inhibit mineralocorticoid receptor).
Relatively weak natriuretic activity, useful in combination with thiazide or in cirrhosis.

Approach to Diuresis (if inadequate diuresis, go to next step)	
Step	Action
1	**Loop diuretic PO:** ✓ response at 3 h, redose at 2× prior dose if needed
2	**Add thiazide diuretic PO** (potentiates response to loop diuretic)
3	**Loop diuretic IV:** bolus bid–qid ± thiazide *(may start here if inPt)* ↑ dose needed w/ ↑ Cr; initial effective IV Lasix dose ≈ 30 × Cr (ie, if Cr = 4 → 120 mg IV lasix)
4	**Loop diuretic infusion:** bolus + continuous IV infusion ± thiazide (PO or IV)
5	**RRT:** consider ultrafiltration, CVVH, or HD

Disease state specific regimens
• Renal insufficiency: loop diuretic (↑ dose to achieve effective delivery to ThAL) ± thiazide
• CHF: loop diuretic (↑ frequency over ↑ dose) + thiazide (watch K & Mg)
• Nephrotic syndrome: urinary albumin binds secreted loop diuretic, use 2–3× normal dose
• Cirrhosis: spironolactone (blocks 2° hyperaldosteronism) + Lasix in 2.5:1 ratio
• Severe metabolic alkalosis: acetazolamide & treat underlying cause

Adverse effects
• Loop: ± ↑ Na, ↓ K, ↓ Mg, ↓ Ca, hyperuricemia, ototoxicity, hypersensitivity (sulfa)
• Thiazide: ↓ Na, ↓ K, ↓ Mg, ↑ Ca, hyperlipidemia, pancreatitis, ↑ glucose, hypersensitivity
• K-sparing: ↑ K (esp. w/ ACEI), metabolic acidosis, gynecomastia (spironolactone)

RENAL REPLACEMENT AND DIALYSIS

General
• Substitutes for renal solute and fluid removal
• Acute indications: see "AKI"; choices CVVH vs HD
• Chronic indications: time of RRT initiation should factor in Pt QoL, uremic sx, risk of
development of urgent/acute indications; choices PD vs. HD

Hemodialysis (HD) *(NEJM 2010;363:1833)*
• Physiology: blood flows along one side of *semipermeable* membrane, dialysate along other
Fluid removal (ie, Na + H_2O) via transmembrane pressure (TMP) gradient

Solute removal via transmembrane concentration gradient and inversely proportional to size (∴ effective removal of K, urea, and Cr, but not PO_4)
• Typical orders: duration, volume removal goals, K and Ca in dialysate bath, anticoagulation
• 6× vs. 3×/wk improved HTN, LV mass, QoL, but ↑ vasc issues (NEJM 2010;363:2287); w/ 3×/wk HD, ↑ adverse outcomes after 2-d interval (NEJM 2011;365:1099)
• Complications: HoTN, arrhythmia, access issues (clot, stenosis, infxn, recirculation), disequilibrium syndrome (sx of cerebral edema due to H_2O shifts after removal of plasma urea during dialysis, esp. in new HD Pts w/ ↑↑ BUN), high-output HF
• Fever w/ catheter: empiric abx (vanc + GNR coverage qHD). GPC > GNR > mixed/fungal. Catheter removal, replacement, or "lock" abx. Consider metastatic infxn w/u (AJKD 2004;44:779; JASN 2014;25:2927).

Vascular Access		
	Advantages	Disadvantages
AV fistula	Highest patency Lowest risk of bacteremia Lowest mortality (JASN 2013;24:465)	Long maturation time (2–6 mo) Primary nonfunction (20%)
AV graft	Easier to create than AVF Maturation time (2–3 wk)	Poor 1° patency, often requiring thrombectomy or angioplasty
Catheter	Immediate use Use as bridge to AVF/AVG	Highest risk of bacteremia ↓ blood flow → ↓ HD efficiency

Continuous veno-venous hemofiltration (CVVH) (NEJM 2012;367:26)
• Physiology: hemofiltration rather than dialysis. Blood under pressure passes down one side of highly permeable membrane allowing H_2O and solutes to pass across membrane via TMP gradient (convective clearance). Filtrate discarded. Replacement fluid infused (solute concentrations similar to plasma, except no urea, Cr, PO_4). Fluid balance precisely controlled by adjusting filtrate/replacement fluid.
• Access: double-lumen central venous catheter
• Typical orders: volume goals, replacement fluid buffer: HCO_3 (requires heparin to prevent machine from clotting, although can be run heparin-free) vs. citrate [hepatically metabolized (∴ cannot be given in cirrhosis/liver failure) to HCO_3; provides anticoagulation w/in machine via Ca chelation])
• Complications: hypotension, ↓ PO_4, access complications; ↓ ICa (citrate toxicity in Pts with hepatic dysfunction → look for ↓ ICa but normal ↑ serum Ca and AG met acidosis)
• Potential advantages over HD: less hypotension, better volume control, removal of inflammatory mediators; however, no survival advantage (Lancet 2006;368:379)
• No advantage for high-intensity CVVH over standard intensity (NEJM 2008;359:7)

Peritoneal dialysis (PD) (Perit Dial Int 2001;21:25; Perit Dial Int 2009;29:559)
• Physiology: peritoneum acts as membrane. Fluid balance controlled by choosing dialysate [glucose] (higher concentrations pull more fluid into peritoneum); longer dwell times pulls first more and then less fluid as glc equilibrates across peritoneum
• Access: permanent catheter inserted in OR
• Typical orders for CAPD (continuous ambulatory peritoneal dialysis):
PD fluid = dextrose (1.5%, 2.5%, or 4.25%), buffer (lactate), Na^+, Ca^{2+}, Mg^{2+} infuse 10 min, dwell 90 min–5.5 h, drain 20 min
• Can use overnight cycler device that infuses & drains more rapidly, with shorter dwells, while Pt sleeps. Called automated or continuous cycling peritoneal dialysis (APD, CCPD)
• Complications: hypoalbuminemia; right-sided pleural effusion
Peritonitis: abd pain, tenderness, cloudy drainage (WBC >100 and >50% PMNs)
spectrum: 60–70% GPC, 15–20% GNR, remainder no bacteria or fungal
Rx: abx IV or in PD, catheter removal for certain pathogens (eg, yeast, Pseudomonas)
Hyperglycemia: exacerbated by inflammation, long dwell times, and higher [glucose]

Kidney transplantation (Med Clin N Am 2016;100:435)
• Rx of choice for ESRD; contraindic: active malig, infxn, ischemia, noncompl, subst use
• Immunosupp.: calcineurin inhib (tacrolimus, CsA) or CTLA4 inhib (NEJM 2016;374:333), antimetabolite (AZA, MMF), prednisone, ± mTOR inhibitor (sirolimus) (NEJM 2004;351:2715)
• Late renal dysfxn: usual AKI causes + calcineurin tox, rejection (NEJM 2010;363:1451), BK virus, recurrence of 1° disease; usual w/u + immunosupp levels, BK virus load, U/S, then bx if no other cause (CJASN 2008;3:556; CJASN 2011;6:1971)
• ↑ risk of infxn (incl opportunistic such CMV, JC, BK viruses; CJASN 2012;7:2058) & malignancy (incl PTLD)
• ↑ CVD risk due to HTN (calcineurin inhib, RAS), DM & dyslipidemia (immunosupp meds)

GLOMERULONEPHRITIS (GN)

Definition (Lancet 2016;387:2036)
- *Pathologically*: intraglomerular inflammation (ranging from focal proliferative [<50% of glomeruli] to diffuse proliferative to crescentic) (Lancet 2006;368:404)
- *Clinically*: hematuria w/ dysmorphic RBCs or RBC casts, ± subnephrotic proteinuria often w/ AKI, HTN, edema
- *Progression*: acute GN ≈ days; rapidly progressive GN (RPGN) ~6 wks; chronic GN ≈ mos; can simply have asx hematuria
- Crescentic GN (pathologic description) ≈ RPGN (clinical description)

ANCA ⊕ Vasculitis (pauci-immune, minimal staining) ~40–45% of total

Pathogen:? bacterial infxn, drugs (hydral, allopurinol, contam cocaine) (CJASN 2011;6:2799)

Disease	Gran	Renal	Pulm	Asthma	ANCA Type[a]	ANCA ⊕
Granulomatosis with polyangiitis[b]	⊕	80%	90% (+ ENT)	—	anti-PR3 (c-ANCA)	90%
Microscopic polyangiitis	—	90%	50%	—	anti-MPO (p-ANCA)	70%
Eosinophilic gran with polyangiitis[b]	⊕	45%	70%	⊕	anti-MPO (p-ANCA)	50%

[a]Predominant ANCA type; either p- or c-ANCA can be seen in all three diseases (NEJM 2012;367:214)
[b]GPA is formerly Wegener's granulomatosis and EGPA is formerly Churg-Strauss

Anti-GBM Disease (linear staining) <15% of total

Disease	Glomerulonephritis	Pulm hemorrhage	Anti-GBM
Goodpasture's	⊕	⊕	⊕
Anti-GBM disease	⊕	—	⊕

Immune Complex (IC) Disease (granular staining) ~40–45% of total

Renal-limited diseases	Systemic diseases
Infection-related GN (Staph & Strep; ↓ C3, ± ASLO)	**SLE** (⊕ ANA, ⊕ anti-dsDNA, ↓ C3, ↓ C4)
Membranoproliferative GN (MPGN) (↓ C3)	**Cryoglobulinemia** (⊕ cryocrit, ⊕ RF, ⊕ HCV, SPEP, ↓ C3, ↓ C4)
Fibrillary and Immunotactoid GN (normal C3)	**Endocarditis** (fever, ⊕ BCx, valvular disease, ↓ C3)
IgA nephropathy (normal C3) (NEJM 2013;368:2402)	**Henoch-Schönlein purpura** (IgA nephropathy + systemic vasculitis w/ IgA deposits, nl C3)

Oncology-related glomerulopathy (Kid Int 2013;84:34; CJASN 2012;7:1701)
- Associations between malig (solid tumors & heme) and/or their Rx (HSCT & chemo-therapeutics) and GN, nephrotic syndrome, and thrombotic microangiopathies (TMA)
- Most common associations: membranous (solid tumors, HSCT), MCD (Hodgkin's, solid tumors), MPGN (CLL, MM), TMA (HSCT, VEGF, anti-EGFR, CNIs, TKIs, mTOR)

Workup (Archives 2001;161:25; AJKD 2014;63(4):656)
- *Acute GN/RPGN ± lung hemorrhage is an emergency* → requires early Dx and Rx
- ✓ ANCA (Lancet 2006;368:404), anti-GBM, complement levels
- Depending on clinical hx: ANA, ASLO, BCx, cryocrit, hepatitis serologies, skin bx
- Consider GN mimics: thrombotic microangiopathies (qv), myeloma, AIN, cholesterol emboli
- Renal biopsy with immunofluorescence (IF) ± electron microscopy (EM)

Figure 4-8 Approach to glomerulonephritis based on immunofluorescence pattern

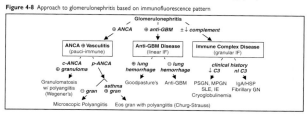

- If acute GN/RPGN suspected, give 500–1000 mg methylpred. IV qd × 3d ASAP while awaiting bx results. Consider plasmapheresis & further Rx based on underlying disease.
- SLE nephritis: induction w/ steroids + cyclophosphamide (CYC) or MMF (JASN 2010;21:2028)
- ANCA ⊕ or anti-GBM: pulse steroids + CYC (or rituximab) ± plasma exchange (JASN 2007;18:2180; NEJM 2010;363:221; AJKD 2011;57:566)
- See "Vasculitis" for further disease specific treatment details

ASYMPTOMATIC GLOMERULAR HEMATURIA

Definition and etiologies
- Hematuria ± proteinuria of glomerular origin w/o renal insufficiency or systemic disease (nonglomerular hematuria more common; see "Hematuria")
- Ddx: any cause of GN (esp. IgA); also consider Alport's (X-linked, deafness, renal failure), thin basement membrane nephropathy (autosomal dominant, benign; JASN 2006;17:813)

IgA nephropathy (NEJM 2013;368:25; KI Suppl 2012;2:143; CJASN 2014;9:617)
- Most common cause of GN; ♂ pred; peak incidence 20–30s; can also be post-infectious
- Wide range of clinical presentations: asx hematuria (30–40%), gross hematuria ~1–3 d after URI (30–40%), chronic GN (10%), nephrotic syndrome (5%), RPGN (<5%)
- Though clinical presentation can be highly suggestive, definitive dx only w/ bx
- Prognosis: 20–40% will reach ESRD w/in 20 y of presentation
- Rx:ACEI/ARB (JASN 1999;10:1772); steroids if proteinuria (JASN 2012;23:1108; NEJM 2015;373: 2225); ± cytotoxic Rx for crescentic GN & nephrotic sx, consider for prog. chronic GN

NEPHROTIC SYNDROME

Definition (NEJM 1998;338:1202)
- Pathologically: abnormal glomerular podocyte permeability to protein
- Clinically: proteinuria >3.5 g/d, albumin <3.5 g/dL, edema, ↑ cholesterol, hypertension

Primary glomerular diseases (grouped by pathology)
- **Focal segmental glomerulosclerosis** (40%; NEJM 2011;365:2398): 1° (? ↑ soluble urokinase receptor; Nat Med 2011;17:952), HIV (collapsing variant), NSAIDs, lymphomas, pamidronate, heroin, congenital, ↑ filtration from prior nephron loss, obesity, vesicoureteral reflux, anabolic steroids, ApoL 1 mutation in AA (JASN 2015;26:1443)
- **Membranous nephropathy** (30%; CJASN 2014;9:609; Lancet 2015;385:1983): idiopathic (auto Ab to phospholipase A_2 or thrombospondin; NEJM 2009;361:11 & 2014;371:2277), infxn (esp. HBV, also HCV, syphilis), autoimmune (eg, SLE), carcinomas, drugs (NSAIDs, penicillamine)
- **Minimal change disease** (20%, more common in children; NDT 2003;18:vi52) idiopathic, NSAIDs, Hodgkin's disease, & other lymphoproliferative disorders
- **Membranoproliferative GN** (5%, mixed nephrotic/nephritic features; CJASN 2014;9:600) Immune complex-mediated: infection (esp. HCV ± cryos, IE, HBV, "shunt" nephritis, other chronic infxns), SLE, cryos, Sjögren's, lymphomas, dysproteinemia, idiopathic Complement-med (rare); abnl C3 convertase activity, dense deposit dis, C3GN
- **Fibrillary-immunotactoid glomerulopathy** (1%; Kid Int 2003;63:1450)
- **Mesangial proliferative GN** (? atypical forms of MCD/FSGS, 5%) IgM, C1q nephropathy

Systemic diseases with secondary glomerular involvement
- **Diabetes mellitus**: nodular glomerulosclerosis (Kimmelstiel–Wilson lesion); large kidneys hyperfiltration → microalbuminuria → dipstick ⊕ → nephrotic range (10–15 y) concomitant proliferative retinopathy seen in 90% of type 1 and 60% of type 2
- **Amyloidosis**: AL or light chain amyloid or AA amyloid secondary to inflammation
- **SLE**: typically with membranous nephropathy (WHO class V)
- **Cryoglobulinemia**: typically with membranoproliferative GN

Workup (Archives 2001;161:25; BMJ 2008;336:1185)
- Urine sediment: usually benign; ± oval fat bodies ("Maltese crosses"; NEJM 2007;357:806)
- Measure proteinuria: 24-h urine collection or spot urine prot/Cr ratio (not accurate in AKI)
- r/o 2° causes: ↑ Hb_{A1c} + retinop. → presumpt. dx of diab. nephrop.; √ ANA, anti-dsDNA, C3/C4, SPEP/light chains, fat pad bx, cryocrit, HBV/HCV, HIV, RPR, APLA₂ recept. Ab
- Renal biopsy

Treatment (Kid Int Sup 2012;2:143; NEJM 2013;368:10)
- General: protein suppl.; diuretics for edema; treat hyperlipidemia, Na restriction (<2 g/d)
- **ACEI or ARB**: decrease proteinuria → slow nonimmunologic progression of renal disease
- 1° glomerular dis: steroids ± cytotoxic therapy; cancer screening if membranous neph.
- Secondary causes: treat underlying disease
- Watch for malnutrition (protein loss), thrombosis (in ~25%, esp. renal vein, b/c loss of ATIII & other endogenous anticoags), infxn (esp. encaps. organisms b/c loss of Ig)

Urine Dipstick

Measurement	Significance and uses
Specific gravity	Estimate U_{osm}: each 0.001 above 1 ≈ 30 osm (SG 1.010 → U_{osm} ≈ 300) SG and U_{osm} useful in evaluating AKI, dysnatremias, polyuria heavy substances (glucose, contrast) ↑ SG more than U_{osm}
pH	Range: 4.5–8.5; useful in evaluation of stones, RTAs, infection
Protein	Detects albumin (marker for glomerular dysfxn); see "Proteinuria"
Blood	See "Hematuria"; can also be ⊕ w/ few RBCs on sediment review in myoglobinuria (rhabdomyolysis) False ⊕: semen, dilute urine (→ osmotic cell lysis), ↑ pH, vaginal blood
WBC	Suggests inflammation (UTI, interstitial nephritis, GN)
Ketones	Detects acetoacetate (ie, ketoacidosis) but *not* β-hydroxybutyrate
Nitrite	Suggests presence of nitrate reductase ⊕ bacteria (most enteric GNRs)
Bilirubin	↑ in biliary or hepatic disease
Glucose	⊕ in hyperglycemia (>180 mg/dL), pregnancy, Fanconi's syndrome

Urine Sediment (microscopic examination) (Am J Kidney Dis 2008;51:1052)

Method: Centrifuge fresh sample (prox. port if Foley) × 3–5 min at 1500–3000 rpm; pour off supernatant in one motion; resuspend pellet by agitating base of tube; pour suspension onto slide w/ coverslip; view under "high dry" power; phase contrast for RBC morphology

Cells	RBCs: assess amount & morphology (many dysmorphic → glomerular) WBCs: PMNs (UTI) vs. eosinophils (AIN; may require special stain) Epithelial cells: tubular (ATN), transitional (bladder or ureters), squamous
Casts (see urinalysis photo inserts in appendix)	*Proteins molded in lumen of renal tubule ± entrapped cellular elements* RBC → GN WBC → AIN, pyelonephritis, GN Granular ("muddy brown"): degenerating cellular casts → ATN Tubular cell → ATN Hyaline: Tamm-Horsfall protein (nonspecific) Waxy and broad → advanced chronic kidney disease
Crystals (see urinalysis photo inserts in appendix)	Calcium oxalate monohydrate: spindle, oval, or dumbbell shaped Calcium oxalate dihydrate: envelope shaped or octahedral Uric acid: variable shape; polychromatic under polarized light Cystine: hexagon shaped Struvite: coffin-lid shaped; seen in chronic UTI with urea-splitting organisms Drugs: sulfa, protease inhibitors: "shocks of wheat"; acyclovir: fine needles

PROTEINURIA

Etiologies of Proteinuria

Category	Description	Etiologies
Glomerular (can be >3.5 g/d)	Disruption of filtration barrier → lose albumin	Glomerulonephritis Nephrotic syndrome
Tubulointerstitial (usually <1–2 g/d)	↓ reabsorption of freely filtered proteins → lose globulins	ATN; AIN Fanconi's syndrome
Overflow	↑ production of freely filtered proteins	Multiple myeloma Myoglobinuria
Isolated	By def'n: asx, normal renal fxn, sed, & imaging, no h/o renal disease	Functional (fever, exercise, CHF) Orthostatic (only when upright) Idiopathic (transient or persistent)

- **Urine dipstick**
  1+ ≈30 mg/dL, 2+ ≈100 mg/dL, 3+ ≈300 mg/dL, 4+ >2 g/dL; interpretation depends on SG; eg, 3+ in very concentrated urine might not indicate heavy proteinuria
  Insensitive for microalbuminuria and myeloma light chains (Bence-Jones protein)
- **Spot urine:** protein (mg/dL)/creatinine (mg/dL) = g/d of proteinuria (NEJM 1983;309:1543) unlike urine dipstick, will accurately measure myeloma light chains
  reliable surrogate for 24-hr urine, esp. 1st morning void (JASN 2009;20:436); inaccurate if AKI
  depends on Cr production, ∴ underestimates if muscular, overestimates if cachectic
- **Microalbuminuria** (30–300 mg/24h or mg/L or μg/mg of Cr): early sign of glomerular vascular disease; marker for ↑ risk of CV adverse outcomes (JAMA 2001;286:421)
- Orthostatic proteinuria: typically in adolescents; ~90% of young ♂ with isolated proteinuria have orthostatic proteinuria; typically resolves spontaneously

Etiologies of Hematuria	
Extrarenal (far more common)	**Intrarenal**
Nephrolithiasis	Nephrolithiasis or crystalluria
Neoplasm: transitional cell, prostate	Neoplasm
Infxn: cystitis, urethritis, prostatitis	Trauma/exercise (? extrarenal component)
Foley trauma	Vascular: renal infarcts, renal vein thromb., sickle
BPH	cell, ruptured hemangioma
Schistosoma haematobium	Glomerular: IgA, thin BM > others; ? loin pain synd.
	PKD (NEJM 2008;359:1477)

- Wide, overlapping ages for various etiologies, but general guide for common causes:
  <20 y: GN, UTI, congenital; 20–60 y: UTI, nephrolithiasis, cancer
  >60 y ♂: prostatitis, cancer, UTI; >60 y ♀: UTI, cancer

Workup (JAMA 2015;314:1865 & 2016;315:2726; Annals 2016;164:488)
- **Urine dipstick:** ⊕ if ≥3 RBCs; ⊕ dipstick and ⊖ sediment → myo- or hemoglobinuria
- **Urine sediment:** dysmorphic RBCs or RBC casts → GN → consider renal bx
- If no evidence of glomerulonephritis:
  r/o UTI and non-GU causes (GI or vaginal bleed)
  Urine cytology (Se ~70%, Sp ~95%), not adequate substitute for cystoscopy
  Renal imaging: helical CT ± contrast (r/o nephrolithiasis and neoplasia of upper tract),
  cystoscopy (r/o bladder neoplasia, esp. ≥35 y), ± MRI, retrograde pyelogram, U/S

NEPHROLITHIASIS

Types of stones and risk factors (J Clin Endocrinol Metabol 2012;97:1847)
- **Calcium** (Ca oxalate > Ca phosphate): **70–90% of kidney stones**
  Urine findings: ↑ Ca, ↑ oxalate (Ca-ox only), ↑ pH (Ca-phos only), ↓ citrate, ↓ volume
  2° hypercalciuria: 1° hyperparathyroidism, distal RTA, sarcoid
  2° hyperoxaluria: Crohn's, ileal disease w/ intact colon, gastric bypass, pancreatic insuffic.
  Diet: ↑ animal protein, ↑ sucrose, ↑ Na, ↓ K, ↓ fluid, ↓ fruits/vegetables, ↑ vit. C, ↓ Ca
- **Uric acid:** 5–10% of kidney stones, radiolucent on plain film
  Urine findings: ↑ uric acid, ↓ pH (eg, from chronic diarrhea)
- **Magnesium ammonium phosphate** ("struvite" or "triple phosphate")
  Chronic upper UTI w/ urea-splitting organisms (eg, Proteus, Klebs) → ↑ urine NH_3, pH >7
- **Cystine:** inherited defects of tubular amino acid reabsorption

Clinical manifestations
- Hematuria (absence does not exclude diagnosis), flank pain, N/V, dysuria, frequency
- Ureteral obstruction (stones >5 mm unlikely to pass spont.) → AKI if solitary kidney
- UTI: ↑ risk of infection proximal to stone; urinalysis of distal urine may be normal

Workup
- **Noncontrast helical CT scan** (ureteral dilation w/o stone suggests recent passage) 97%
  sens. 96% spec. (AJR 2008;191:396); U/S appears comparable (NEJM 2014;371:1100)
- Strain urine for stone to analyze; U/A & UCx; electrolytes, BUN/Cr, Ca, PO_4, PTH
- 24-h urine × 2 (>6 wk after acute setting) for Ca, PO_4, oxalate, citrate, Na, Cr, pH, K, vol.

Acute treatment (NEJM 2004;350:684)
- Analgesia (narcotics ± NSAIDs; combination superior, Ann Emerg Med 2006;48:173), ensure
  adequate fluid repletion, antibiotics if UTI
- Consider alpha blocker > CCB to promote ureteral relaxation (Lancet 2006;368:1171)
- Indications for **immediate urologic eval and/or hosp:** obstruction (esp. solitary or
  transplant kidney), urosepsis, intractable pain or vomiting, significant AKI
- Urologic Rx: lithotripsy (NEJM 2012;367:50), stent, perc nephrostomy, ureteroscopic removal

Chronic treatment (J Clin Endocrinol Metabol 2012;97:1847)
- Increase fluid intake (>2 L/d) for goal UOP 2 L/d
- Calcium stones: 24-h urine identifies **specific urinary risk factors to treat**
  ↓ Na and meat intake (NEJM 2002;346:77), thiazides: decrease urine Ca
  Depending on 24-h urine: K-citrate, dietary oxalate restriction, allopurinol
  High dietary Ca is likely beneficial by ↓ oxalate absorp., unclear role of Ca supplements
- Uric acid: urine alkalinization (K-citrate), allopurinol
- Magnesium ammonium phosphate: antibiotics to treat UTI, urologic intervention,
  acetohydroxamic acid: urease inhibitor, reserve for experienced clinician, poorly tolerated
- Cystine: urine alkalinization (K-citrate), D-penicillamine, tiopronin

ANEMIA

↓ in RBC mass: Hct <41% or Hb < 13.5 g/dL (men); Hct <36% or Hb < 12 g/dL (women)

Clinical manifestations

- Symptoms: ↓ O_2 delivery → fatigue, exertional dyspnea, angina (if CAD)
- Signs: pallor (mucous membranes, palmar creases), tachycardia, orthostatic hypotension
- Other findings: **jaundice** (hemolysis), **splenomegaly** (thalassemia, neoplasm, chronic hemolysis), **petechiae/purpura** (bleeding disorder), **glossitis** (iron, folate, vitamin B_{12} defic.), **koilonychia** (iron defic.), **neurologic abnormalities** (B_{12} defic.)

Diagnostic evaluation

- History: bleeding, systemic illness, drugs, exposures, alcohol, diet (including **pica**), FHx
- CBC w/ diff.; RBC params incl. retics, MCV (nb, mixed disorder can → nl MCV), RDW
- **Reticulocyte index (RI)** = [reticulocyte count × (Pt's Hct/nl Hct)]/maturation factor
  maturation factors for a given Hct: 45% = 1, 35% = 1.5, 25% = 2, 20% = 2.5
  RI >2% → adequate marrow response; RI <2% → hypoproliferation
- **Peripheral smear:** select area where RBCs evenly spaced and very few touch each other; ✓ RBC size, shape, inclusions (see "Appendix" & "Peripheral Smear" inserts), WBC morphology, plt count
- Additional labs as indicated: hemolysis labs (if RI >2%, see below), iron/TIBC, ferritin, folate, B_{12}, LFTs, BUN & Cr, TFTs, Hb electrophoresis, enzyme/gene mutation screens
- **Bone marrow (BM) aspirate and biopsy (bx)** with cytogenetics as indicated

Figure 5-1 Approach to anemia

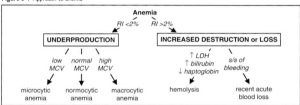

MICROCYTIC ANEMIAS

Figure 5-2 Approach to microcytic anemias (NEJM 2014;371:1324)

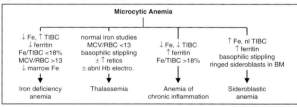

Iron deficiency (NEJM 2015;372:1832; Lancet 2016;387:907)

- ↓ marrow iron & depleted body iron stores → ↓ heme synthesis → microcytosis → anemia
- Special clinical manifestations: angular cheilosis, atrophic glossitis, pica (consumption of nonnutritive substances such as ice, clay), koilonychia (nail spooning)
  Plummer-Vinson syndrome (iron deficiency anemia, esophageal web & atrophic glossitis)
- Etiologies: **chronic bleeding** (GI—incl. cancer, menstrual, parasites, NSAIDs, etc.), ↓ **supply** (malnutrition; ↓ absorp. due to celiac sprue, Crohn's, ↑ gastric pH, subtotal gastrectomy), ↑ **demand** (preg., Epo). Iron-refractory iron-defic. anemia (IRIDA; rare Fe refractory genetic disorder due to hepcidin dysregulation; Nat Genet 2008;40:569).
- Diagnosis (eval ideally before Rx): ↓ **Fe**, ↑ **TIBC**, ↓ **ferritin** (esp. <15), ↓ **transferrin sat** (Fe/TIBC; esp. <15%), ↑ soluble transferrin receptor; ↑ plt
  Unless hx c/w other etiology, *initiate workup for GIB*, incl. H. pylori serology
  ? Celiac sprue labs (**anti-TTG**, antigliadin, antiendomysial Ab)
  Cytogenetics & molecular testing as indicated

- Treatment oral Fe tid (~6 wk to correct anemia; ~6 mo to replete Fe stores; nb, oral Fe does not give ⊕ Hemoccult). In excessive/persistent GI losses or dialysis, cancer, CHF, or prior to Epo Rx, *IV iron* (Fe-sucrose, -gluconate, -dextran) should be considered.

Thalassemias (Lancet 2013;379:373)
- ↓ synthesis of α- or β-globin chains of Hb → ≠ subunits → destruction of RBCs and erythroid precursors; ∴ anemia from hemolysis and *ineffective erythropoiesis*
- **α-thalassemia** (NEJM 2014;371:1908): deletions in α-globin gene complex (nl 4 α genes), seen w/ Southeast Asian, Mediterranean, African, Middle East ancestry
  - 3 α → α-thal-2 trait = silent carrier; 2 α → α-thal-1 trait or α-thal minor = mild anemia
  - 1 α → HbH (β₄) disease = severe anemia, hemolysis and splenomegaly
  - 0 α genes → Hb Barts (γ₄) = intrauterine hypoxia and hydrops fetalis
- **β-thalassemia**: mutations in β-globin gene → absent or ↓ gene product
  seen w/ Mediterranean (espec. Greek or Italian), African, or Asian ancestry
  - 1 mutated β gene → thal minor (or trait) = mild anemia (no transfusions)
  - 2 mutated β genes → thal intermedia (occasional transfusions) or thal major (= Cooley's anemia; transfusion dependent) depending on severity of mutations
- Severe clinical manifestations: chipmunk facies, pathologic fractures, hepatosplenomegaly (due to extramedullary hematopoiesis), high-output CHF, bilirubin gallstones, Fe overload
- Diagnosis: MCV <70, **normal Fe, MCV/RBC count <13** [Mentzer Index, 60% Se, 98% Sp; (Ann Hematol 2007;86:486)], ± ↑ retics, basophilic stippling; **Hb electrophoresis**: ↑ HbA₂ (α₂δ₂) in β-thal; *normal pattern in α-thal trait*, ∴ PCR or supravital stain for dx
- Treatment: folate; transfusions + Fe chelator [either deferoxamine (IV) or deferasirox (PO)]; ? splenectomy if ≥50% ↑ in transfusions; consider allo-HSCT in children w/ severe β-thal

Anemia of chronic inflammation (see below)

Sideroblastic anemia
- Defective heme biosynthesis within RBC precursors
- Etiologies: **hereditary/X-linked** (*ALAS2* mutations), **idiopathic, MDS-RARS, reversible** (alcohol, lead, isoniazid, chloramphenicol, copper deficiency, hypothermia)
- Special clinical manifestations: hepatosplenomegaly, iron overload syndromes
- Dx: social, work & TB hx; can be micro-, normo- or macrocytic; variable populations of hypochromic RBCs; ↑ Fe, nl TIBC, ↑ ferritin, basophilic stippling, RBC **Pappenheimer bodies** (Fe-containing inclusions); **ring sideroblasts** (w/ iron-laden mitochondria) in BM
- Treatment: treat reversible causes; trial of pyridoxine, supportive transfusions for severe anemia with chelation therapy; high-dose pyridoxine for some hereditary cases

NORMOCYTIC ANEMIAS

Pancytopenia (see below)

Anemia of chronic inflammation (ACI; NEJM 2012;366:4)
- ↓ RBC production due to impaired iron utilization and functional iron deficiency from ↑ **hepcidin**; cytokines (IL-6, TNF-α) cause ↓ Epo responsiveness/production
- Etiologies: autoimmune disorders, chronic infection, inflammation, HIV, malignancy
- Dx: ↓ **Fe, ↓ TIBC** (usually normal or low transferrin sat), ± ↑ **ferritin**; usually normochromic, normocytic (~70% of cases) but can be microcytic if prolonged
- Coexisting iron deficiency common. Dx clues include ↓ serum ferritin levels, absence of iron staining on BM bx, ⊕ response to a trial of oral iron and/or ↑ soluble transferrin receptor/ferritin index (Blood 1997;89:1052).
- Treatment: treat underlying disease ± iron and/or erythropoiesis-stimulating agent (ESA; eg, Epo). Iron if ferritin <100 or Fe/TIBC <20%. Consider ESA if Epo <500. Avoid ESA in cancer if treatment goal is cure (Lancet 2009;373:1532). Unclear if one should treat highly sx Pts w/ goal Hb 10–12 g/dL; weigh risk of thrombosis.

Anemias of other chronic disorders
- Anemia of chronic kidney disease: ↓ Epo; treat w/ Epo (see "Chronic Kidney Disease")
- Endocrine deficiencies: hypometabolism and ↓ O_2 demand with thyroid, pituitary, adrenal, or parathyroid disease → ↓ Epo; can be normocytic or macrocytic

Sideroblastic anemia (see above)

Pure red cell aplasia
- Destructive antibodies or lymphocytes → ineffective erythropoiesis
- Associated with thymoma, CLL and parvovirus infection, autoimmunity, drugs
- Diagnostic studies: **lack of erythroid precursors on BM bx**, other lines normal
- Treatment: thymectomy if thymus enlarged; IVIg if parvovirus infection; immuno-suppression/chemoRx if CLL or idiopathic; supportive care w/ PRBC transfusions; ? erythropoietin receptor agonist if due to antierythropoietin Ab (NEJM 2009;361:1848) consider hematopoietic cell transplantation.

MACROCYTIC ANEMIAS
includes megaloblastic and nonmegaloblastic causes

Megaloblastic anemia
- **Impaired DNA synthesis** → cytoplasm matures faster than nucleus → ineffective erythropoiesis and macrocytosis; due to **folate** or **B_{12} deficiency**; also in **MDS**
- ✓ folate and vitamin B_{12}; ↑ LDH & indirect bilirubin (due to ineffective erythropoiesis)
- Smear: **neutrophil hypersegmentation, macro-ovalocytes**, anisocytosis, poikilocytosis

Folate deficiency
- Folate present in leafy green vegetables and fruit; total body stores sufficient for **2–3 mo**
- Etiologies: **malnutrition** (alcoholics, anorectics, elderly), ↓ absorption (sprue), impaired metabolism (methotrexate, pyrimethamine, trimethoprim; *NEJM* 2015;373:1649), ↑ requirement (chronic hemolytic anemia, pregnancy, malignancy, dialysis)
- Diagnosis: ↓ folate; ↓ RBC folate, ↑ homocyst. but nl methylmalonic acid (unlike B_{12} defic.)
- Treatment: folate 1–5 mg PO qd for 1–4 mo or until complete hematologic recovery; *critical to r/o B_{12} deficiency first (see below)*

Vitamin B_{12} deficiency *(NEJM 2013;368:149)*
- B_{12} present only in foods of animal origin; total body stores sufficient for **2–3 y**
- Binds to **intrinsic factor** (IF) secreted by gastric parietal cells; absorbed in terminal ileum
- Etiologies: malnutrition (alcoholics, vegans), **pernicious anemia** (PA, autoimmune disease against gastric parietal cells, a/w polyglandular endocrine insufficiency and ↑ risk of gastric carcinoma), other causes of ↓ absorption (gastrectomy, sprue, Crohn's disease), ↑ competition (intestinal bacterial overgrowth, fish tapeworm)
- Clinical manifestations: **neurologic** changes (**subacute combined degeneration**) affecting peripheral nerves, posterior and lateral columns of the spinal cord and cortex → numbness, paresthesias, ↓ vibratory and positional sense, ataxia, dementia
- Dx: ↓ B_{12}; ↑ homocysteine and methylmalonic acid; anti-IF Ab; Schilling test; ↑ gastrin in PA
- Treatment: 1 mg B_{12} IM qd × 7 d → q wk × 4–8 wk → q month for life
  neurologic abnormalities are reversible if treated w/in 6 mo
  folate can reverse *hematologic* abnormalities of B_{12} deficiency but not *neurologic* changes (and can lead to "steal" of B_{12} stores → worsening of neuro complications)
  oral supplementation (2 mg qd) appears feasible as well *(Cochrane Rev CD004655)* even w/o IF

Nonmegaloblastic macrocytic anemias
- **Liver disease:** often macrocytic, may see target cells, or spur cell anemia w/ hemolysis
- **Alcoholism:** BM suppression & macrocytosis independent of folate/B_{12} defic. or cirrhosis
- **Reticulocytosis**
- **Other causes:** hypothyroidism; MDS; meds that impair DNA synthesis (zidovudine, 5-FU, hydroxyurea, Ara-C); hereditary orotic aciduria; Lesch-Nyhan syndrome

---

PANCYTOPENIA

Etiologies
- Hypocellular bone marrow (nl cellularity ~100 – age): **aplastic anemia,** hypoplastic MDS
- Cellular bone marrow: **MDS,** aleukemic leukemia, PNH, severe megaloblastic anemia
- Marrow replacement (myelophthisis): **myelofibrosis,** metastatic solid tumors, granulomas
- Systemic diseases: hypersplenism, sepsis, alcohol, toxins

Clinical manifestations
- Anemia → fatigue
- Neutropenia → recurrent infections
- Thrombocytopenia → mucosal bleeding & easy bruisability

Aplastic anemia = stem cell failure *(NEJM 2015;373:35)*
- Epidemiology: 2–5 cases/10^6/y; biphasic (major peak in adolescents, 2nd peak in elderly)
- Diagnosis: pancytopenia w/ ↓ retics, BM bx w/ cytogenetics showing hypocellularity
- Etiologies: **idiopathic** ($\frac{1}{2} - \frac{2}{3}$ of cases)
  stem cell destruction: radiation, chemotherapy, chemicals (eg, benzene)
  idiosyncratic **med rxn** (eg, chloramphenicol, NSAIDs, sulfa drugs, gold, carbamazepine, antithyroid)
  viruses (HHV-6, HIV, EBV, parvovirus B19); **post-viral hepatic failure** (not Hep A/B/C)
  immune disorders (SLE, GVHD post-HSCT, thymoma)
  PNH (see below); Fanconi's anemia (congenital disorder w/ pancytopenia, macrocytic anemia, ↑ risk of MDS, AML, & SCC of head & neck, and multiple physical anomalies);
  shortened telomeres: seen w/ telomerase (*TERT, TERC*) mut. (10% of aplastic anemia), dyskeratosis congenita/DKC1 mut; a/w IPF, cirrhosis *(NEJM 2009;361:2353)*
  somatic mutations: PNH clones in ~50% of aplastic anemia *(Haematologica 2010;95:1075)*

- Treatment and prognosis

  allogeneic HSCT: for *young* Pts → ~80% long-term survival and significantly ↓ risk of malignant evolution, but has risk of transplant-related morbidity & mortality; if possible avoid transfusions (and alloimmunization) pretransplant

  immunosuppression (CsA/tacrolimus, ATG): 70–80% respond, with 80–90% 5-y survival in responders (96% vs. 76% w/ horse vs. rabbit ATG; *NEJM 2011;365:430*);
  15–20% 10-y incidence of clonal disorders (mostly MDS, AML, PNH)

  TPO mimetics (eg, eltrombopag) an option in refractory disease (*Blood 2014;123:1818*)

  supportive care: transfusions, antibiotics, possible utility of G-CSF and Epo (if Epo <500)

Myelodysplastic syndromes (MDS) (qv)

Paroxysmal nocturnal hemoglobinuria (PNH) (*Blood 2009;113:6522*)

- Acquired clonal stem cell disorder = inactivating somatic mutation of *PIG-A* gene → deficiency of GPI-anchor for CD55 & CD59 (inhib of complement) → complement-mediated RBC lysis, plt aggreg., & hypercoagulability
- Clinical: intravascular **hemolytic anemia, hypercoagulability** (venous > arterial; esp. intraabdominal, cerebral), smooth muscle dystonias; **deficient hematopoiesis** (cytopenias); a/w aplastic anemia, MDS and evolution to AML
- Dx: **flow cytometry** (↓ CD55 & CD59) on RBCs and granulocytes; urine hemosiderosis
- Treatment: supportive care (iron, folate, transfusions); consider anticoagulation

  allogeneic HSCT for hypoplasia or severe thrombosis

  eculizumab (Ab inactivates terminal complement C5s): ↓ hemolysis, improves QoL & stabilizes Hb levels (*NEJM 2004;350:552 & 2006;355:1233; Lancet 2009;373:759*); effective in pregnancy (*NEJM 2015;373:1032*); must have meningococcal vaccination

Myelophthisic anemia (see also "Primary Myelofibrosis")

- Infiltration of bone marrow by cancer, leukemia, infection, fibrosis (primary myelofibrosis), granulomas, lysosomal storage disorders

HEMOLYTIC ANEMIAS

Causes of Hemolytic Anemia by Mechanism (Lancet 2000;355:1169 & 1260)			
Location	**Mechanism**	**Examples**	**Mode**
Intrinsic	Enzyme deficiency	G6PD deficiency	**Hereditary**
	Hemoglobinopathies	Sickle cell anemia, thalassemia	
	Membrane abnormalities	Hereditary spherocytosis	
		PNH, spur cell anemia in liver disease	
Extrinsic	Immune-mediated	Autoimmune; drug-induced, tx rxn	**Acquired**
	Traumatic	MAHA; prostheses (valves, TIPS)	
	Direct infections, toxins	Malaria, babesiosis; snake & spider venoms; Wilson's; hypotonic infusions	
	Entrapment	Hypersplenism	

Diagnostic evaluation

- ↑ reticulocyte count (RI >2%), ↑ LDH, ↓ haptoglobin (83% Se, 96% Sp), ↑ indirect bili
- Autoimmune hemolysis: Coombs' test = direct antiglobulin test (DAT) → ⊕ if agglutination occurs when antisera against Ig or C3 are applied to patient RBCs
- Intravascular: ↑↑ LDH, ↓↓ haptoglobin; hemoglobinemia, hemoglobinuria, hemosiderinuria
- Extravascular: splenomegaly
- Family h/o anemia; personal or family h/o cholelithiasis

Glucose-6-phosphate dehydrogenase (G6PD) deficiency (*Lancet 2008;371:64*)

- X-linked defect of metabolism (*G6PD* mutations) w/ ↑ susceptibility to oxidative damage
- Most common in ♂ of African or Mediterranean descent (malaria-endemic areas)
- Hemolysis precipitated by **drugs** (sulfonamides, dapsone, nitrofurantoin, rasburicase, primaquine, doxorubicin, methylene blue), **infection, DKA** or **foods** (fava beans)
- Diagnosis: smear may show RBC **Heinz bodies** (oxidized Hb) that result in **bite cells** once removed by spleen; ↓ G6PD levels (*may be normal after acute hemolysis* as older RBCs have already lysed and young RBCs may still have near normal levels)

Sickle cell anemia (*Lancet 2016;387:2545, 2554 & 2565*)

- Recessive β-globin mutation → usually abnl hemoglobin (HbS). ~8% African Americans heterozygotes ("sickle trait"; usually w/o sx); ~1/400 homozygotes (sickle cell disease).
- ↓ O_2 → HbS polymerizes → RBC sickles, ↓ RBC deformability → **hemolysis & microvascular occlusion** due to endothelial activ. & PMN adhesion (*Blood 2013;122:3892*)
- **Anemia:** chronic hemolysis ± acute aplastic (parvo. B19) or splenic sequestration crises

- **Vaso-occlusion and infarction:** painful crises, acute chest syndrome, CVA, splenic sequestration, hand-foot syndrome, renal papillary necrosis, aseptic necrosis, priapism
- **Infection:** splenic infarction → overwhelming infection by **encapsulated organisms;** infarcted bone → **osteomyelitis** (*Salmonella, Staph. aureus*)
- Diagnosis: sickle-shaped RBCs with Howell-Jolly bodies on smear; Hb electrophoresis
- Treatment: **hydroxyurea** causes ↑ HbF → ↓ painful crises, acute chest episodes and may ↓ mortality (*NEJM 2008;358:1362*); allogeneic HSCT may have a role in young Pts w/ severe disease (*Blood 2000;95:1918*) and adults (*NEJM 2009;361:2309; Blood 2012;120:4285*)
- Supportive care: folic acid qd; pneumococcal, meningococcal, *H. flu* & HBV vaccination; pain crises Rx'd w/ **hydration, O₂** & **analgesia;** simple or exchange transfusion for TIA or stroke, severe acute chest syndrome, or preop (goal Hb 10 g/dL; *Lancet 2013;381:930*)

Hereditary spherocytosis (HS) (*Br J Hematol 2004;126:455*)
- Defect in a cytoskeletal protein of RBC membrane → membrane loss
  mutations in ankyrin, α- and β-spectrin, band 3, and pallidin have been identified
- Most common in N. European populations (1/5000 births); ⊕ FHx (75% of Pts)
- Anemia, jaundice (mostly neonates), splenomegaly, pigmented gallstones
- Diagnosis: spherocytes on smear, ↑ osmotic fragility test (~80% Se), ↓ eosin-5-maleimide (EMA) binding (93% Se; 99% Sp; *Haemat 2012;97:516*), acidified glycerol lysis test (Se 95%)
- Treatment: folate, transfusions, splenectomy for moderate and severe HS (balance w/ ↑ risk of future thrombosis and infection; *J Thromb Haemost 2008;6:1289*)

Paroxysmal nocturnal hemoglobinuria (see above)

Autoimmune hemolytic anemia (AIHA)
- Acquired, antibody-mediated RBC destruction
- **Warm AIHA: IgG** Abs opsonize RBCs *at body temp* → removal by spleen
  Etiologies: idiopathic, lymphoproliferative (CLL, NHL), autoimmune (SLE), drugs, HIV
- **Cold AIHA: IgM** Ab binds to RBCs *at temp <37°C* → **complement fixation**
  → intravascular hemolysis and acrocyanosis on exposure to cold
  Etiologies: idiopathic, lymphoprolif. disorders (eg, Waldenström's; monoclonal),
  Mycoplasma pneumoniae infxn and infectious mononucleosis (polyclonal)
- Diagnosis: spherocytes on smear, ⊕ **Coombs';** ✓ cold agglutinin titer, splenomegaly
- Treatment: treat underlying disease
  warm AIHA: corticosteroids ± splenectomy, IVIg, cytotoxic agents, rituximab
  cold AIHA: avoid cold; steroids ineffective; rituximab (*Blood 2004;103:2925*)

Drug-induced hemolytic anemia
- Acquired, antibody-mediated, RBC destruction precipitated by a medication:
  abx: cephalosporins, sulfa drugs, rifampin, ribavirin
  CV: methyldopa, procainamide, quinidine, thiazides
  TCAs, phenothiazines, NSAIDs, sulfonylureas, MTX, 5-FU, rasburicase (G6PD defic.)
- Diagnosis: Coombs' usually negative, ↑ LDH
- Treatment: discontinue offending agent

Microangiopathic hemolytic anemia (MAHA; *NEJM 2014;371:654*)
- Intra-arteriolar fibrin damages RBCs → acquired intravascular hemolysis
- Etiologies: **hemolytic-uremic syndrome (HUS), thrombotic thrombocytopenic purpura (TTP), disseminated intravascular coagulation (DIC),** malignancy, malignant HTN, eclampsia/HELLP, mech. cardiac valves, infected vascular prostheses
- Diagnosis: **schistocytes** ± thrombocytopenia ± abnormalities a/w specific disorders (eg, ↑ PT in DIC, ↑ Cr in HUS, ↑ LFTs in HELLP)
- Rx underlying dx; **urgent plasma exchange w/ TTP** (replace low ADAMTS13)

Hypersplenism
- Stasis/trapping in spleen → Mφ attack & remodeling of RBC → spherocytosis → hemolysis

Causes of Splenomegaly	
Etiology	**Comments***
RES hyperplasia	Hemolytic anemia, sickle cell disease, **thalassemia major**
Immune hyperplasia	Infxn [HIV, EBV, CMV, TB, **malaria, kala azar** ("black water fever" from visceral leishmaniasis), ***Mycobacterium avium*** complex], autoimmune disorders (SLE, RA w/ Felty's syndrome), sarcoidosis, serum sickness
Congestion	Cirrhosis, CHF, portal/splenic vein thrombosis, **schistosomiasis**
Infiltration (nonmalignant)	Lysosomal storage disorders (**Gaucher's,** Niemann-Pick), glycogen storage diseases, histiocytosis X, splenic cysts
Neoplasm	**MPN (CML, PMF, PV, ET), CMML, leukemia, lymphoma (NHL, HL, hairy cell leukemia, CLL, PLL, WM),** T-LGL, myeloma, amyloid

RES = reticuloendothelial system; ***boldface** = causes of massive splenomegaly.

Clinical Characteristics of Bleeding Disorders		
Feature	**Platelet/vascular defect**	**Coagulation defect**
Site	Skin, mucous membranes	Deep in soft tissues (muscles, joints)
Lesions	Petechiae, ecchymoses	Hemarthroses, hematomas
Bleeding	After minor cuts: yes	After minor cuts: unusual
	After surgery: immediate, mild	After surgery: delayed, severe

Figure 5-3 Approach to abnormal hemostasis (NEJM 2014;370;847)

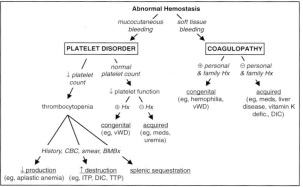

Figure 5-4 Coagulation Cascade (NEJM 2008;359:938)

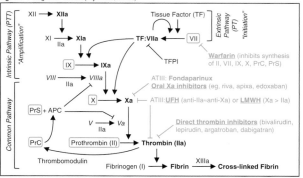

APC, activated protein C; AT, antithrombin; PrC, protein C; PrS, protein S; TF, tissue factor; TFPI, tissue factor pathway inhib.

Purpura (*nonblanching* purple/red lesions due to extravasation of RBCs into dermis)
- **Nonpalpable** (macular; ≤3 mm in diameter = petechiae; >3 mm = ecchymoses)
  platelet disorder: thrombocytopenia, defect in platelet fxn
  thromboemboli: DIC, TTP, cholesterol or fat emboli
  trauma or vascular fragility: amyloidosis, Ehlers-Danlos, scurvy
- **Palpable** (papular); **vasculitis:** leukocytoclastic, HSP, PAN, RMSF;
  infectious emboli: meningococcemia, bacterial endocarditis
- ***Purpura fulminans*** (aka retiform purpura): **purpura + hypotension + DIC;**
  typically due to infxn/sepsis, protein C or S deficiency or APS (see section on DIC)

PLATELET DISORDERS

THROMBOCYTOPENIA (PLT COUNT <150,000/μL)

Thrombocytopenia and Risk of Bleeding	
Platelet count (cells/μL)	**Risk**
50,000–100,000	Risk with major trauma; can proceed with general surgery
20,000–50,000	Risk with minor trauma or surgery
<20,000	Risk of *spontaneous* bleeding (less so with ITP)
<10,000	Risk of severe, life-threatening bleeding

Etiologies
- ↓ **production**
  hypocellular bone marrow: aplastic anemia (qv), rarely MDS, drugs (eg, thiazides, antibiotics), alcohol, cirrhosis
  hypercellular bone marrow: MDS, leukemia, severe megaloblastic anemia
  marrow replacement: myelofibrosis, hematologic and solid malignancies, granulomas
- ↑ **destruction**
  immune-mediated (distinguish primary from secondary; *Blood* 2009;113:2386)
  Primary (idiopathic): immune thrombocytopenic purpura (**ITP**, see below)
  Secondary: infxn (**HIV, HCV,** HSV), collagen vascular diseases (**SLE**), APS, lymphoproliferative (**CLL,** lymphoma), drugs (*many,* including **heparin,** abciximab, quinidine, sulfonamides, vancomycin), alloimmune (posttransfusion)
  non–immune-mediated: MAHA (DIC, HUS, TTP), ticlopidine/clopidogrel, vasculitis, preeclampsia/HELLP, cardiopulm bypass, CVVH, IABP, cavernous hemangioma
- **Abnormal distribution or pooling:** splenic sequestration, dilutional, hypothermia
- **Unknown:** ehrlichiosis/anaplasmosis, babesiosis, RMSF

Diagnostic evaluation
- H&P: meds, infxns, underlying conditions, splenomegaly, lymph nodes, **bleeding hx**
- **CBC with differential:** isolated thrombocytopenia *vs.* multilineage involvement
- **Peripheral smear**
  ↑ destruction → look for large plts, **schistocytes** (see "Peripheral Smear" inserts)
  ↓ production → rarely limited to platelets → look for **blasts,** hypersegmented PMNs, leukoerythroblastic Δs; can see inclusion bodies (anaplasma), parasites (*Babesia*)
  r/o **pseudothrombocytopenia** due to platelet clumping (✓ platelet count in non–EDTA-containing tube, eg, citrate or heparin-containing tube)

Figure 5-5 Approach to thrombocytopenia

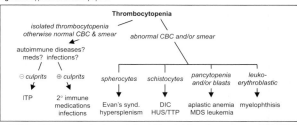

- Additional laboratory evaluations as indicated (eg, viral titers, flow cytometry, ANA, APLA)
  if anemia: ✓ reticulocyte count, LDH, haptoglobin, bilirubin to detect hemolysis
  if hemolytic anemia: ✓ PT, PTT, fibrinogen, D-dimer, Coombs, ANA
  BM bx for unexplained thrombocytopenia, esp. if associated with splenomegaly

Primary immune thrombocytopenic purpura (ITP) (*Blood* 2010;115:168)
- Primary ITP: isolated thrombocytopenia due to immune plt *destruction* & ↓ *production* (auto-Ab to megakaryocytes); (2° ITP a/w disease/drug exposure; Rx underlying disorder)
- Primary ITP is *diagnosis of exclusion*; no robust clinical or lab parameters, but typically:
  CBC: isolated ↓ plt (<100,000/μL); 10% have ITP + AIHA = Evans syndrome
  Peripheral smear: large platelets
  BM bx: ↑ megakaryocytes; perform in adults >60 y to r/o myelodysplasia
  R/o other etiologies: viral serologies (**HIV, HCV,** HBV, EBV), *H. pylori* Ab, ANA, pregnancy test, APLA, TSH, parvovirus, & CMV PCR. *Anti-plt Ab tests not useful.*

- Clinical manifestations: insidious onset of mucocutaneous bleeding; ♀:♂ = 3:1
- Treatment: goals based on individual Pt
  rarely indicated w/ plt >50,000/μL unless bleeding, trauma/surgery, anticoag, comorbidities
  steroids, IVIg, & splenectomy mainstay of initial Rx; romiplostim/eltrombopag if refractory

Treatment of Primary ITP in Adults		
Approach	**Treatment**	**Notes**
First-line	**Steroids:** prednisone 0.5–2 mg/kg/d PO tapered ~4 wk, or dexamethasone 40 mg PO × 4 d	↓ Mϕ FcR & ↓ anti-plt Ab 70–90% initial response ~20% sustained remission
	Anti-Rh(D) Ig 75 μg/kg/d IV	For Rh(D) ⊕ Pts w/ spleen Ab-coated RBCs overwhelm Mϕ FcR
	IVIg (1 g/kg/d IV × 2–3 d) *consider if need rapid ↑ in plt*	Blocks Mϕ FcR, ↓ anti-plt Ab Up to 80% initial response
Second-line	**Splenectomy** (? for ITP >6 mo)	~65% long-term remission
	Rituximab (anti-CD20) ± dex	anti-B-cell Ab
	Romiplostim or **eltrombopag**	TPO-R agonists → ↑ plt prod
	Azathioprine, cyclophosphamide	Immunosuppressants
	Danazol, vincristine	↓ plt clearance
Bleeding	Aminocaproic acid	Inhibits plasmin activation
	Methylprednisolone 1g/d IV × 3 d	See above
	IVIg	See above
	Platelet transfusion	Given w/ IVIg or anti-Rh(D)
Refractory	Romiplostim or eltrombopag	See above
	Autologous HSCT	Limited data, investigational

(NEJM 2003;349:831; 2010;464:1889 & 2011;365:734; Blood 2013;121:537)

Overview of Heparin-Induced Thrombocytopenias		
Feature	**Type I (historic)**	**HIT (formerly type II)**
Mechanism	Direct effect of heparin (nonimmune)	Immune (Ab)-mediated IgG against plt factor 4—heparin complex
Incidence	10–20%	1–3% with UFH, 0–0.8% LMWH
Onset	After 1–4 d of heparin therapy	After 4–10 d; but can occur in <24 h if prior exposure w/in 100 d (persistent Ab). Postop highest risk. Can occur after heparin d/c.
Platelet nadir	>100,000/μL	~60,000/μL, ↓ >50%
Sequelae	None	Thrombotic events (**HITT**) in 30–50% Rare hemorrhagic complications
Management	Can continue heparin and observe	**Discontinue heparin** Alternative anticoagulation

(Chest 2012;141:e495S; NEJM 2015;373:252)

- Pathophysiology (type II): Ab binds heparin-PF4 → immune complex binds to plt → **plt activation**, further PF4 release → plt aggregates removed from circulation → **thrombocytopenia**; procoagulants released by plts and tissue factor released by endothelial cells damaged by HIT Abs → **prothrombotic state**
- Diagnosis (need clinical + pathologic)
  Clinical: plt <100k or ↓ 50% from baseline; or **venous** (DVT/PE) or **arterial** (limb ischemia, CVA, MI) thrombosis (4:1 ratio); skin necrosis; ? ↑ heparin resistance
  Pathologic: ⊕ HIT Ab using PF4-heparin ELISA (≥90% Se, IgG-specific ELISA Sp 94%), may confirm w/ functional plt aggregation (serotonin-release) assay (>95% Se/Sp)
  Clinical context important: HIT Ab (esp. IgM ELISA) may be ⊕ in 10–20% of Pts on UFH/LMWH (Am J Hem 1996;52:90), up to 50% of cardiac bypass Pts (Circ 1997;95:1242)
  Pretest prob w/ "4 T's" criteria (Blood 2012;120:4160): ≤3 points → 99% NPV, investigate other causes; 4–5 points 22% PPV & 6–8 points 64% PPV, ✓ lab test & replace UFH

Evaluation of Suspected HIT ("4T's")			
Factor	**2 points**	**1 point**	**0 points**
Thrombo-cytopenia	↓ >50% and nadir ≥20k	↓ 30–50% or nadir 10–19k	↓ <30% or nadir <10k
Timing	5–10 d or ≤1 d if heparin w/in 30 d	? 5–10 d (but not clear), >10 d or ≤1 d if hep w/in 30–100 d	≤4 d w/o recent hep
Thrombosis	New thromb, skin necrosis, acute rxn after IV UFH	Prog/recurrent thromb, suspect thromb or non-nec skin lesion	None
Other cause	None apparent	Possible	Definite

- Treatment of HIT (type II) *(Chest 2012;141:e495S; Blood 2012;119:2209; NEJM 2013;368:737)*
  - **Discontinue heparin** *(incl. flushes, LMWH Ppx, heparin lines)*. Avoid plts (anecdotal link w/ thrombosis); if given warfarin, give vit K to reverse, prevent warfarin skin necrosis.
  - **Nonheparin anticoag** (argatroban, bivalirudin; *NEJM 2013;368:737)* *regardless of thrombosis*; start warfarin when plt >150k, overlap ≥5 d (✓ chromogenic Xa to titrate)
    - ⊕ thrombosis (HITT): anticoagulate for ≥3–6 mo
    - ⊖ thrombosis (HIT): screen for DVT; unclear duration of subsequent anticoag (until plt count recovers, often ~2–3 mo if no clot); 25–50% thrombosis rate w/in 30 d
- H/o HIT: if PF4 Ab ⊖ or SRA ⊖ (typically >100 d after dx) → may consider re-exposure to UFH (eg, for surgery); HIT recurrence low but can be seen *(Blood 2014;123:2485)*

Thrombotic microangiopathies *(NEJM 2014;371:654)*

- Includes hemolytic-uremic syndrome (HUS) & thrombotic thrombocytopenic purpura (TTP)
- Definition: vascular occlusive disorders w/ systemic (TTP) or intrarenal (HUS) plt aggreg. → thrombocytopenia & mechanical injury to RBCs (MAHA) *(NEJM 2002;347:589)*
  - **HUS triad** = thrombocytopenia + MAHA + renal failure
  - **TTP pentad** (all 5 in only ~5%) = ↓ plts + MAHA (100%) ± Δ MS (65%) ± renal failure (50%, late feature) ± fever (25%)
- Pathophysiology: mechanism in most HUS cases is distinct from TTP *(NEJM 1998;339:1578)*
  - **HUS:** Shiga toxin binds & activates renal endothelial cells & plts → intrarenal thrombi
  - **TTP:** ↓ ADAMTS13 protease activity *or* inhibitor → persistence of large vWF multimers on endothelial surface → adhesion and aggregation of passing platelets → thrombosis
- Clinical manifestations and associations
  - **HUS:** usually in children; prodrome of bloody diarrhea due to enterohemorrhagic *E. coli*
  - **TTP (low ADAMTS13):** usually in adults; **idiopathic**, autoimmune dis., familial, preg
  - **TTP-like (nl ADAMTS13): drugs** (CsA, tacrolimus, gemcitabine, mitomycin-C, ticlopidine, clopidogrel, quinine), HIV, HSCT, malig
- Dx: unexplained **thrombocytopenia** (typically <20k) + **MAHA** → sufficient for dx
  - ⊕ **schistocytes** (>2–3/hpf), ⊖ Coombs, normal PT/PTT & fibrinogen, ↓↓ ADAMTS13
  - ↑↑ LDH (tissue ischemia + hemolysis), ↑ indirect bili., ↓↓ haptoglobin, ↑ Cr (esp. in HUS)
  - Biopsy: arterioles filled with platelet hyaline thrombi
  - Ddx: DIC, vasculitis, malignant hypertension, preeclampsia/HELLP syndrome
- Rx: **urgent plasma exchange** ± glucocorticoids if ? TTP; FFP if delay to plasma exchange *(Blood 2010;116:4060);* ? eculizumab in HUS & ? caplacizumab in TTP *(NEJM 2013;368:2169 & 2016;374:511);* plt transfusions contraindic. → ↑ microvascular thromb *(NEJM 2006;354:1927)*

Disseminated intravascular coagulation (DIC): see "Coagulopathies"

DISORDERS OF PLATELET FUNCTION

Mechanisms and Etiologies of Platelet Function Abnormalities

Function	Inherited	Acquired
Adhesion	Bernard-Soulier; vWD	Uremia; acquired vWD
Aggregation	Afibrinogenemia Glanzmann's thrombasthenia	Ticlopidine, clopidogrel, GP IIb/IIIa Dysproteinemias (myeloma)
Granule release	Chediak-Higashi syndrome Hermansky-Pudlak syndrome	Drugs (ASA, NSAIDs); liver disease; MPN; cardiopulmonary bypass

Tests of platelet function

- Platelet aggregation tests: measure aggregation in response to agonists (eg, ADP)

von Willebrand's disease (vWD) *(NEJM 2004;351:683 & 2012;367:1954)*

- von Willebrand factor (vWF) function = platelet glue & plasma carrier of factor VIII
- vWD most common inherited (usually auto dom) bleeding disorder; ~85% (type 1) have partial quantitative defic of vWF, ~15% (type 2) have qualitative defic in vWF
- Acquired vWD: a/w many disorders (malig, MPN w/ ↑ plt count; autoimmune; hypo-thyroidism; drugs) and caused by different mechanisms (anti-vWF Abs, ↑ clearance, ↓ synthesis); Heyde's syndrome = vWF destruction by severe AS, a/w GI AVMs/bleed
- Diagnosis: ↓ vWF:Ag, ↓ **vWF activity** (measured by ristocetin cofactor assay), ↓ **factor VIII**, ± ↑ PTT, ↓,↑,↔ platelets; confirm with **vWF multimer analysis**
- Clinical condition, factor VIII levels and ristocetin cofactor assay useful to guide Rx decision
- Rx: **desmopressin** (dDAVP, IV/IN) → ↑ endothelial cell release of vWF; efficacy depends on type (avoid in type 2), ∴ ✓ response before use w/ subseq. bleeding or procedures; **vWF replacement:** cryoprecipitate, factor VIII concentrates rich in vWF, recomb. vWF

Uremic bleeding

- Uremia → platelet dysfunction including ↓ aggregation, impaired adhesiveness
- Treatment: dDAVP, cryoprecipitate, correct anemia (improves plt aggregation and adhesion by increasing plt interactions with endothelium), consider holding anti-plt agents

COAGULOPATHIES

Screening Test Abnormalities in Inherited and Acquired Coagulopathies

PT	PTT	Factors	Inherited	Acquired
↑	↔	VII	FVII defic.	**Vit. K defic.; liver dis.;** factor inhib.
↔	↑	VIII or IX	Hemophilias, vWD	**Antiphospholipid Ab;** factor inhib.
↑	↑	I, II, V or X	Fbgn, FII or FV defic.	**DIC; liver dis.;** factor inhib.

Further coagulation tests
- Mixing study: useful if ↑ PT or PTT; mix Pt's plasma 1:1 w/ normal plasma and retest
  PT/PTT normalizes → factor **deficiency;** PT/PTT remains elevated → factor **inhibitor**
- Coagulation factor levels: useful if mixing study suggests factor deficiency
  DIC → all factors consumed; ∴ ↓ factors V and VIII
  liver disease → ↓ all factors *except* VIII; ∴ ↓ factor V, normal factor VIII
  vitamin K deficiency → ↓ factors II, VII, IX, X (and protein C, S); ∴ normal V and VIII
- **DIC screen:** fibrinogen (consumed), fibrin degradation products (FDPs, ⊕ due to intense fibrinolysis), D-dimer (more specific FDP test that detects degradation of X-linked fibrin)

Hemophilias (Lancet 2016;388:187)
- X-linked recessive **factor VIII** (hemophilia A) or **factor IX** (hemophilia B) **deficiency**
- Classification: mild (5–25% normal factor activity), moderate (1–5%) or severe (<1%)
- Clinical manifestations: hematomas, hemarthroses, bruising, bleeding (mucosal, GI, GU)
- Diagnosis: ↑ PTT (normalizes w/mixing study), normal PT & vWF, ↓ factor VIII or IX
- Rx: purified/recomb. factor VIII (NEJM 2016;374:2054) or IX; desmopressin (mild dis.); amino-caproic acid; cryo (FVIII); recomb. factor VII or IX-Fc fusion proteins have ↑ $t_{1/2}$, so 1–2×/wk dosing for Ppx (NEJM 2013;369:2313); ? emicizumab (binds FIX & X; NEJM 2016;374:2044)

Coagulation factor inhibitors (most commonly anti–factor VIII)
- Etiologies: hemophilia; postpartum; lymphoproliferative & autoimmune disorders; cancers
- Diagnosis: ↑ PTT (does *not* normalize w/mixing study); Bethesda assay quantitates titer
- Treatment: if high titer → **recomb. factor VIIa,** porcine factor concentrates, activated prothrombin complex; for others → high-purity human factor, plasmapheresis, immunosupp. w/ steroids, CYC and/or RTX (Curr Opin Hematol 2008;15:451)

Disseminated intravascular coagulation (DIC) (NEJM 2014;370:847)
- Etiologies: trauma, shock, infection, malignancy (esp. APL), obstetric complications
- Pathogenesis: *massive activation of coagulation that overwhelms control mechanisms*
  thrombosis in microvasculature → ischemia + microangiopathic hemolytic anemia
  acute consumption of coagulation factors and platelets → **bleeding**
  chronic DIC → able to compensate by ↑ factors and platelets → **thrombosis**
- Diagnosis: ↑ PT, ↑ PTT, ↓ **fibrinogen** (may be *nl* b/c acute phase), ⊕ FDP/D-dimer, ↓ plts, ⊕ schistos, ↓ LDH, ↓ hapto; *chronic* DIC: ⊕ FDP/D-dimer, variable plts, other labs nl
- Treatment: Rx underlying process; support w/ **FFP, cryo** (goal fbgn >100 mg/dL) & **plts**

Vitamin K deficiency
- Etiologies: malnutrition, ↓ absorption (antibiotic suppression of vitamin K-producing intestinal flora or malabsorption), liver disease (↓ stores), warfarin

Properties and Antidotes for Anticoagulants & Fibrinolytics (Circ 2016;134:248)

Anticoag.	$t_{1/2}$	Labs	Rx for O/D w/ serious bleeding (+ d/c anticoag)
UFH	60–90', RES	↑ PTT	**Protamine** IV 1 mg/100 U UFH (max 50 mg). For infusions, dose to reverse 2× UFH given per h.
LMWH	2–7°, K	anti-Xa*	Protamine reverses ~60%
Bivalirudin	25', K	↑ PTT	Dialysis
Argatroban	45', L	↑ PTT	? Dialysis
Fondaparinux	24°, K	anti-Xa*	? Dialysis
Warfarin	36', L	↑ PT	*No bleeding:* INR 4.5–10, Ø Rx or **vit. K** 2.5 mg PO; INR >10 give 5 mg PO (sup to SC, ≈ IV at 24 h) *Bleeding:* **vit. K** 10 mg IV + **FFP** 2–4 U IV q6–8h; PCC (eg, KCentra) faster, ↓ tfn (Circ 2013;128:360)
Fibrinolytic	20', LK	↓ fbgn	**Cryoprecipitate, FFP,** ± aminocaproic acid
Dabigatran	~12°, K	↑ PTT*	Idarucizumab (NEJM 2015;373:511)
Rivaroxaban Apixaban Edoxaban	8–12°, K > L	↑ PT* anti-Xa*	Anti-fibrinolytic agent; consider PCC; specific reversal agents (eg, andexanet) under development (NEJM 2015;373:2413; J Thromb Haemost 2015;13:S187)

*Routine monitoring not performed. Mode of excretion: K, kidney; L, liver; RES, reticuloendothelial system. PCC: prothrombin complex concentrate (FII, VII, IX, X; Protein C & S). Anti-fibrinolytics: tranexamic, aminocaproic acid.

HYPERCOAGULABLE STATES

Suspect in Pts with venous or arterial thrombosis at young age or unusual locations, recurrent thromboses or pregnancy loss, or ⊕ FHx

Inherited Hypercoagulable States

Risk factor	Prevalence	VTE	Comments
Factor V Leiden	3–7%	4.3×	Activated protein C (APC) resist.
Prothrombin mutation	2%	2.8×	G20210A → ↑ prothrombin level
Hyperhomocysteinemia	5–10%	2.5×	Inherited or acquired
Protein C deficiency	0.02–0.05%	11×	Warfarin-induced skin necrosis risk
Protein S deficiency	0.01–1%	32×	Warfarin-induced skin necrosis risk
Antithrombin III def.	0.04%	17.5×	May be heparin-resistant

Prevalence is in Caucasians. (*NEJM* 2001;344:1222; *JAMA* 2005;293:2352)

Vascular Beds Affected by Inherited and Acquired Hypercoagulable States

	Venous	Venous and Arterial
Inher.	**Factor V Leiden** Prothrombin mutation ↓ protein C, S or AT III	? factor V Leiden + smoking Hyperhomocysteinemia (inherited or acquired) Dysfibrinogenemia
Acquired	Stasis: immobilization, surgery, CHF Malignancy Hormonal: OCPs, HRT, tamoxifen, pregnancy Nephrotic syndrome	Platelet defects: myeloproliferative disorders, HIT, PNH (viscosity: venous > arterial) Hyperviscosity: polycythemia vera, Waldenström's macroglobulinemia, sickle cell, acute leukemia Vessel wall defects: vasculitis, trauma, foreign bodies Others: **antiphospholipid syndrome**, IBD

Diagnostic evaluation (not routinely required for initial VTE)
- APC resistance screen; prothrombin PCR test; functional assays for proteins C and S, ATIII; homocysteine level; factor VIII levels; anticardiolipin and lupus anticoagulant Ab. Also consider nephrotic syndrome, PNH (esp. if mesenteric thrombus).
- Consider *JAK2* mutation testing if suspect MPN or splanchnic thrombosis
- Proteins C & S and ATIII levels are affected by acute thrombosis and anticoagulation ∴ levels best assessed ≥2 wk after completing anticoagulation course
- Age-appropriate malignancy screening (occult cancer in ~4% of initial unprovoked VTE; no benefit of routine abd/pelvis CT; *NEJM* 2015; 373:697)

Treatment
- Asx w/ inherited risk factor: consider prophylactic anticoag. if develops acquired risk factor
- Thrombosis w/ inherited risk factor: see "Venous Thromboembolism"

Antiphospholipid syndrome (APS) (*J Thromb Haemost* 2006;4:295; *NEJM* 2013;368:1033)
- Definition: dx requires ≥1 clinical & ≥1 laboratory criteria
  Clinical: thrombosis (any) or complication of pregnancy (≥3 spont. abortions before 10 wk or ≥1 fetal loss after 10 wk or premature birth before 34 wk)
  Laboratory: ⊕ moderate–high titer anticardiolipin (ACL), ⊕ lupus anticoagulant (LA), or ⊕ β_2-glycoprotein-I (β_2-GP-I) Ab, on ≥2 occasions, at least 12 wk apart
- Clinical: **DVT/PE/CVA**, recurrent fetal loss, ↓ plts, hemolytic anemia, livedo reticularis; "**catastrophic APS**": ≥3 organ systems in <1 wk w/ APLA & tissue microthrombi; 44% mortality (*Arth Rheum* 2006;54:2568); Rx w/ plasmapheresis, rituximab
- **Antiphospholipid antibodies (APLA)**
  ✓ if: SLE, age <40 y & arterial thromb, recurrent venous thromb, spontaneous abortion
  ACL: Ab against cardiolipin, a mitochondrial phospholipid; IgG more specific than IgM
  LA: Ab that prolongs phospholipid-dependent coagulation reactions; ∴ ↑ **PTT** that does not correct with mixing study but does correct with excess phospholipids or platelets; PT not affected b/c the reaction contains much more phospholipid
  β_2-GP-I: Ab against β_2-glycoprotein-I, IgG or IgM (uncertain role of Abs in pathogenesis)
  False ⊕ VDRL: nontreponemal test for syphilis in which cardiolipin is part of Ag complex
  Risk of thromboembolic phenomena may increase with titer of APLs
- Etiologies: primary (idiopathic) or secondary due to **autoimmune syndromes** (eg, SLE), **malignancy, infections**, drug reactions
- Treatment: UFH/LMWH → warfarin after thromboembolic event (lifelong for most Pts)
  Intensity of anticoagulation controversial (*Nat Rev Rheum* 2015;11:586)
  Initial *venous* thrombosis: INR 2–3 (*NEJM* 2003;349:1133; *J Thromb Haemost* 2005;3:848)
  Initial *arterial* thrombosis: typically INR 2–3 + ASA 81, although some treat to INR 3–4
  Recurrent thrombosis on warfarin: consider INR 3–4 vs. LMWH or fondaparinux (*Arth Rheum* 2007;57:1487)
  Consider ASA prophylaxis for high-risk asx Pt (eg, SLE); no current evidence for NOACs

DISORDERS OF LEUKOCYTES

Neutrophilia (>7500–10,000/μL)

Infection	Usually bacterial; ± toxic granulations, Döhle bodies
Inflammation	Burn, tissue necrosis, MI, PE, collagen vascular disease
Drugs and toxins	Corticosteroids, β-agonists, lithium, G-CSF; cigarette smoking
Stress	Release of endogenous glucocorticoids and catecholamines
Marrow stimulation	Hemolytic anemia, immune thrombocytopenia
Asplenia	Surgical, acquired (sickle cell), congenital (dextrocardia)
Neoplasm	Can be 1° (MPN) or paraneoplastic (eg, carcinomas of lung, GI)
Leukemoid reaction	>50,000/μL + left shift, not due to leukemia; unlike CML, ↑ LAP

Neutropenia (ANC <1000/μL)

Congenital	Myelokathexis, Shwachman-Diamond-Oski, Chédiak-Higashi, retic dysgen., WHIM syndrome, cyclic neutropenia, monoMAC syndrome (↓ monos, NKs)
Infection	Viral (CMV, EBV, HIV); bacterial (brucella, *Rickettsia*, TB); malaria
Nutritional	Vit B$_{12}$ defic., copper defic.
Drugs and toxins	Chemotherapeutics, clozapine, methimazole, TMP-SMX, NSAIDs, sulfasalazine, phenytoin (*Am J Hem* 2009;84:428), alcohol
Neoplasm	MDS, leukemia (AML, ALL, hairy cell, LGL, others)

Lymphocytosis (>4000–5000/μL)

Infection	Usually viral; "atypical lymphocytes" with mononucleosis syndromes Other: pertussis, toxoplasmosis
Hypersensitivity	Drug-induced, serum sickness
Stress	Cardiac emergencies, trauma, status epilepticus, postsplenectomy
Autoimmune	Rheumatoid arthritis (large granular lymphocytes), malignant thymoma
Neoplasm	Leukemia (eg, CLL, hairy cell, LGL), lymphoma (eg, mantle cell, folic.)

Monocytosis (>500/μL)

Infection	Usually TB, SBE, *Listeria, Brucella, Rickettsia,* fungi, parasites
Inflammation	IBD, sarcoidosis, collagen vascular diseases
Neoplasm	Hodgkin lymphoma, leukemias, MPD, carcinomas

Eosinophilia (>500/μL)

Infection	Usually parasitic (helminths)
Allergic	Drugs; asthma, hay fever, eczema; ABPA
Collagen vasc dis.	RA, Churg-Strauss syndrome, eosinophilic fasciitis, PAN
Endocrine	Adrenal insufficiency
Neoplasm	HL, CML, mycosis fungoides, carcinomas, systemic mastocytosis
Atheroembolic dis.	Cholesterol emboli syndrome
Hypereosinophilic syndrome	Multiorgan involvement incl. heart & CNS, a/w FIP1L1-PDGFRA fusion (*NEJM* 2003;348:1201)

Basophilia (>150/μL)

Neoplasm	MPN, Hodgkin lymphoma
Alteration in BM or reticuloendothelial compartment	Hemolytic anemia, splenectomy
Inflammation or allergy	IBD, chronic airway inflammation

Lymphadenopathy

Viral	HIV, EBV, CMV, HSV, VZV, hepatitis, measles, rubella
Bacterial	Generalized (brucellosis, leptospirosis, TB, atypical mycobacteria, syphilis) Localized (streptococci, staphylococci, cat-scratch disease, tularemia)
Fungal and parasitic	Histoplasmosis, coccidioidomycosis, paracoccidioidomycosis Toxoplasmosis
Immunologic	Collagen vascular disease, drug hypersensitivity (eg, phenytoin), serum sickness, histiocytosis X, Castleman's and Kawasaki disease
Neoplasm	Lymphoma, leukemia, amyloidosis, metastatic carcinoma
Other	Sarcoidosis; lipid storage diseases
Factors that favor biopsy	Age (>40 y), size (>2 cm), location (supraclavicular is always abnormal), duration (>1 mo) Consistency (hard *vs.* rubbery *vs.* soft) & tenderness are not reliable

TRANSFUSION THERAPY

Blood Products and Indications (Lancet 2013;381:1845)	
Packed red blood cells (PRBCs) (Annals 2012;157:49)	For acute blood loss or to ↑ O₂-carrying capacity if end organ ischemia. 1 U PRBC → ↑ Hb by ~1 g/dL. Conservative Hb goal >7 g/dL adequate for UGIB & critically ill Pts (NEJM 2013;368:11 & 2014;371:1381; BMJ 2015;350:h1354). Controversy remains re: coronary ischemia, although Hb >8 may be adequate (JAMA Int Med 2013;173:132), but perhaps not peri-cardiac surgery (NEJM 2015;372:997; Anesth 2016;125:46).
Platelets (plts) (Annals 2014;162:205)	For plts <10k (NEJM 2010;362:600) or <20k w/ infxn or ↑ bleeding risk or <50k w/ active bleeding or preprocedure. 6 U pooled donor plts ≈ 1 single donor plt apheresis unit (↓ alloimmunization) → ↑ plts ~30–60k. Contraindic: TTP/HUS, HELLP, HIT. Refractory if ↑ <5k 30–60′ post-plts. Suggests alloimmunization → trial ABO-matched plts. If still refractory ✓ panel reactive Abs to assess utility of HLA-matched plts.
Fresh frozen plasma (FFP)	Contains all coagulation factors. For bleeding due to deficiency of multiple coagulation factors (eg, DIC, TTP/HUS, liver disease, warfarin excess, dilution) or INR >2 preprocedure (Transfusion 2006;46:1279).
Cryoprecipitate	Enriched for fibrinogen, vWF, VIII and XIII. For bleeding in vWD, factor XIII deficiency or fibrinogen <100 mg/dL.
Irradiated	Prevents donor T-cell proliferation. Use if risk of transfusion-assoc. GVHD (HSCT, heme malignancy, congenital immunodeficiency).
CMV-negative	From CMV-negative donors. For CMV-seronegative pregnant women, transplant candidates/recipients, SCID, AIDS Pts.
Leuko-reduced	WBCs cause HLA alloimmunization and fever (cytokine release) and carry CMV. For chronically transfused Pts, potential transplant recipients, h/o febrile nonhemolytic transfusion reaction, cases in which CMV-negative products are desired but unavailable.
Intravenous immune globulin (IVIg)	Polyvalent IgG from >1000 donors. For postexposure prophylaxis (eg, HAV), certain autoimmune disorders (eg, ITP, Guillain-Barré, MG, ? CIDP), congenital or acquired hypogammaglobulinemia (CVID, CLL).
Therapeutic apheresis	Removes large molec wt subst. (eg, cryoglobulinemia, Goodpasture's, Guillain-Barré, hyperviscosity syndrome, TTP) or cells (eg, leukemia w/ hyperleukocytosis, sx thrombocytosis, sickle cell) from plasma.
Massive transfusion	Large-vol. PRBC → ↓ Ca, ↑ K, ↓ plt, ↑ coags; ratio of PRBC:plt:FFP repletion controversial, follow labs (J Trauma 2006;60:S91 & 2008;65:272).

Transfusion Complications (NEJM 1999;340:438; JAMA 2003;289:959)

Noninfectious	Risk (per unit)	Infectious	Risk (per unit)
Febrile	1:100	CMV	Common
Allergic	1:100	Hepatitis B	1:220,000
Delayed hemolytic	1:1000	Hepatitis C	1:1,600,000
Acute hemolytic	<1:250,000	HIV	1:1,800,000
Fatal hemolytic	<1:100,000	Bacteria (PRBCs)	1:500,000
TRALI	1:5000	Bacteria (platelets)	1:12,000

Transfusion reactions
- For all reactions (except minor allergic): **stop transfusion;** send remaining blood product and fresh blood sample to blood bank
- **Acute hemolytic:** fever, HoTN, flank pain, AKI w/in 24 h. Due to ABO incompatibility → preformed Abs vs. donor RBCs. Rx: IVF, ↑ UOP w/ diuretics, mannitol or dopamine
- **Delayed hemolytic:** generally less severe than acute hemolytic; 5–7 d after transfusion Due to undetected allo-Abs against minor antigens → anamnestic response. Rx: usually no specific therapy required; dx is important for future transfusion
- **Febrile nonhemolytic:** fever, rigors 0–6 h post transfusion. Due to Abs vs donor WBCs and cytokines in blood product. Rx: acetaminophen ± meperidine; r/o infection, hemolysis
- **Allergic:** urticaria; rarely, **anaphylaxis:** bronchospasm, laryngeal edema, hypotension Reaction to transfused proteins; anaphylaxis seen in IgA-deficient Pts w/ anti-IgA Abs. Rx: urticaria → diphenhydramine; anaphylaxis → epinephrine ± glucocorticoids
- **Transfusion-associated circulatory overload (TACO):** ↑ volume → pulm edema, ↑ BP. Rx: slow transfusion rate, diuretics, O₂, ± nitrates, ± positive pressure ventilation
- **Transfusion-related acute lung injury (TRALI):** noncardiogenic pulmonary edema Due to donor Abs that bind recipient WBCs, which then aggregate in pulmonary vasculature and release mediators causing ↑ capillary permeability. Rx: see "ARDS."

Myeloid neoplasm overview (Blood 2016;127:2391)
• Categories based on clinical features, morphology, immunophenotyping, and genetics

WHO 2016 classification of myeloid neoplasms & acute leukemia	
Acute myeloid leukemia	Clonal myeloid stem cell (SC) disorder w/ ≥20% blasts
Myelodysplastic syndromes	Dysplastic clonal myeloid SC disorder → cytopenias; <20% blasts, risk of leukemic transformation
Myeloproliferative neoplasms	Nondysplastic multipotent myeloid SC clonal expansion
MDS/MPN neoplasms	Features of MDS & MPN (eg, CMML, atypical CML)
Myeloid/lymphoid malig. w/ eos & rearrangements of PDGFR or FGFR1 or w/ PCM1-JAK2	May be responsive to TKI therapy (eg, imatinib) for PDGFR rearrangement
Mastocytosis	Systemic disease, assoc w/ KIT mutations
Myeloid neoplasms w/ germ line predisposition	MDS, MDS/MPN, acute leukemias in background of predisposing germline mutations

Myelodysplastic syndromes (MDS) overview (Lancet 2014;383:2239)
• Acquired clonal stem cell disorder → ineffective hematopoiesis → **cytopenias, dysmorphic blood cells and precursors,** variable risk of **leukemic transformation**
• Epidemiology: >10,000 cases/y; median age ~70 y; male predominance (1.8×)
• **Idiopathic** or 2° to chemo w/ **alkylating agents;** ↑ risk w/ radiation, benzene
• Clinical manifestations: **anemia** (85%), neutropenia (50%), thrombocytopenia (40–65%)
• Diagnosis: dysplasia (usually multilineage) in peripheral smear (oval macrocytes, **pseudo-Pelger-Huët anomaly**) and bone marrow (≥10% dysplasia with blasts ± RS)
• Both **cytogenetic** [eg, del(5q), mono 7, del(7q), trisomy 8, del(20q)] and **molecular** abnl (**TP53**, EZH2, ETV6, RUNX1, ASXL1, SF3B1, DNMT3A) may carry prognostic signif
• Prior to dx MDS: exclude AML (≥20% blasts) and CMML (monos >1 × 10⁹/L); r/o 2° BM Δs (defic. of B₁₂, folate, copper); viral infx (eg, HIV); chemo; EtOH; lead, arsenic exposures

WHO 2016 Classification Systems for MDS (Blood 2016;127:2391)		
Classification	**WHO 2008**	**Features**
MDS w/ single lineage dysplasia (MDS-SLD)	RCUD (RA/RN/RT)	1 dysplastic lineage, 1–2 cytopenias, <15% RS*, <5% BM/<1% PB blasts, no Auer rods
MDS w/ multilineage dysplasia (MDS-MLD)	RCMD	2–3 dysplastic lineages, 1–3 cytopenias, <15% RS*, <5% BM/<1% PB blasts, no Auer rods
MDS w/ ring sideroblast (MDS-RS)	RARS	≥15% RS or ≥5% RS if SF3B1 mut. is present, <5% BM/<1% PB blasts
MDS w/ isolated del(5q)	Del(5q)	Del(5q) alone or w/ 1 abnl except −7 or del(7q)
MDS w/ excess blasts (MDS-EB)	RAEB-1 RAEB-2	EB-1: 5–9% BM/2–4% PB blasts, no Auer rods EB-2: 10–19% BM/5–19% PB blasts or Auer rods
MDS, unclassifiable (MDS-U)	MDS-U	w/ 1% PB blasts, single lineage dysplasia & pancytopenia, or defining cytogenetic alteration

Certain cytogenetics [eg, t(15;17), t(8;21), inv16, t(16;16), or MLL rearrangement] classified as AML, regardless of BM blast count. RS, ring sideroblast; BM, bone marrow; PB, peripheral blood. * <5% RS if SF3B1 mutation.

• Rx (Am J Hematol 2012;87:692): intensity based on IPSS-R (qv), age, performance status (PS)
   Poor PS, any risk → supportive care (transfusions, G-CSF, Epo, TPO-mimetic, abx prn)
   Low/intermediate risk → Epo (if Epo level <500); lenalidomide (esp. for 5q syndrome; NEJM 2006;355:1456); DNA hypomethylating agents (azacitidine or decitabine)
   Intermediate/high risk → DNA hypomethylating agents (survival advantage w/ azacitidine; Lancet Oncol 2009;10:223), combination **chemo** (akin to AML Rx) or **allogeneic HSCT**
   Hypoplastic MDS (rare) → consider **immunosuppression** (CsA,ATG, pred), HSCT
• Prognosis: IPSS-R correlates with **survival** and **progression to AML**

Revised International Prognostic Scoring System (IPSS-R) (Blood 2012;120:2454)								
Variable	**0**	**0.5**	**1**	**1.5**	**2**	**3**	**4**
Cytogenetics	Very good	-	Good	-	Intermed	Poor	Very poor
BM blasts (%)	≤2	-	>2 to <5	-	5–10	>10	-
Hb (g/dL)	≥10	-	8 to <10	<8	-	-	-
Plt (k)	≥100	50 to <100	<50	-	-	-	-
ANC	≥0.8	<0.8	-	-	-	-	-
Total score	≤1.5		>1.5 to 3		>3 to 4.5	>4.5 to 6	>6
Category	Very low		Low		Intermed	High	Very high
Median survival (y)	8.8		5.3		3.0	1.6	0.8

General (Am J Hematol 2012;87:285; JAMA Oncol 2015;1:97; Blood 2016;127:2391)
- Results from clonal expansion of multipotent hematopoietic stem cell
- Different from MDS in that the cells are not dysplastic (ie, normally developed)
- Categories of MPN: polycythemia vera (PV); essential thrombocythemia (ET); primary myelofibrosis (PM); chronic myelogenous leukemia (CML), BCR-ABL1 ⊕; chronic neutrophilic leukemia (CNL); chronic eosinophilic leukemia, not otherwise specified; myeloproliferative neoplasms, unclassifiable
- Mutations useful as clonal markers & dx tools:
  Gain of fxn mutations in **JAK2** V617F (Janus kinase) frequently present (PV ~95%, ET ~50%, PMF ~50%; NEJM 2005;352:1779)
  BCR-ABL fusion in **all** cases of CML
  CALR exon 9 mutation (most MPNs w/o JAK2 or MPL mutation, including ~25% of ET, ~35% of myelofibrosis Pts; NEJM 2013;369:2379 & 2391)
  MPL, TET2, & ASXL1 mutation w/ lower frequency
  CSF3R mutation present in ~60% of CNL

Definition
- ↑ in RBC mass ± ↑ granulocytes and platelets in the absence of physiologic stimulus

Etiologies of erythrocytosis
- Relative ↑ RBC (↓ plasma): dehydration; "stress" erythrocytosis (Gaisböck's syndrome)
- *Absolute* ↑ RBC: 1° (PV, other MPD) or 2° due to **hypoxia; carboxyhemoglobinemia; inappropriate erythropoietin** (renal, hepatic, cerebellar tumors); Cushing's syndrome

Clinical manifestations (common between PV and ET)
- Symptoms → often termed "vasomotor symptoms"
  hyperviscosity (erythrocytosis): headache, dizziness, tinnitus, blurred vision
  thrombosis (hyperviscosity, thrombocytosis): transient visual disturbances (amaurosis, ocular migraine); Budd-Chiari syndrome; erythromelalgia = intense burning, pain and erythema of extremities due to microvascular ischemia; ↑ risk of **DVT, MI, stroke.** Risk of thrombosis highly correlated with ↑ WBC in PV and ET (see below).
  bleeding (abnormal platelet function): easy bruising, epistaxis, GI bleeding
  ↑ histamine from basophils → **pruritus**, peptic ulcers; ↑ uric acid (cell turnover) → gout
- Signs: **plethora, splenomegaly,** hypertension, engorged retinal veins
- Expression profiling beyond JAK2 may define different phenotypes (NEJM 2014;371:808)

Diagnostic evaluation
- Men: Hb >16.5 g/dL or HCT >49%, women: Hb >16 g/dL or HCT >48%, or ↑ red cell mass
- BM bx → hypercellularity for age, trilineage growth, pleomorphic mature megakaryocytes
- **JAK2 V617F** mutation in ~95% of PV; other Pts typically harbor JAK2 exon 12 mutations
- ✓ Epo to rule out secondary causes of erythrocytosis; **if Epo ↓, PV more likely** If Epo ↑, then ✓ SaO₂ or PaO₂, carboxyhemoglobin, BM exam
- ± ↑ WBC, platelets, basophils; ↑ uric acid, leukocyte alkaline phosphatase, vit B₁₂
- Peripheral smear → no morphologic abnormalities

Treatment
- **Phlebotomy** to goal Hct <45% (NEJM 2013;368:22), consider <42% in women
- **Low-dose ASA** in all Pts (NEJM 2004;350:114)
- **Hydroxyurea** if high risk of thrombosis (age ≥60, prior thrombosis) or symptomatic thrombocytosis (plt >1.5 × 10⁶/μL), or if inadequate Hct by phlebotomy alone
- Ruxolitinib (JAK1/2 inhibitor) if poor response, intolerant of hydroxyurea (NEJM 2015;372:426)
- PEG IFNα-2a yields high response rate w/ limited toxicity (Blood 2008;112:3065)
- Supportive: allopurinol (gout), H₂-blockers/antihistamines (pruritus)

Prognosis
- Median survival w/ Rx ~13.5 y (Blood 2014;124:2507); ↑ age, WBC, additional acquired somatic mutations → worse prognosis (Haematol 2013;160:251)
- Post-PV myelofibrosis (spent phase) occurs in 10–20% of cases, usually after 10 y
- Risk of transformation into acute leukemia (<2–5%; higher if previous cytoreductive chemo)

Definition
- Sustained ↑ in platelets (>450,000/μL) ± ↑ RBC and granulocytes

Etiologies of thrombocytosis
- 1° = ET or other MPN; myelodysplastic syndromes (5q-syndrome); RARS-T
- 2° = **reactive thrombocytosis:** inflammation (RA, IBD, vasculitis), infection, acute bleeding, iron deficiency, postsplenectomy, neoplasms (eg, Hodgkin lymphoma)
- Of patients with plt >10⁶/μL, <1 in 6 will have ET

Clinical manifestations (also see "Polycythemia Vera")
- Thrombosis with erythromelalgia (risk of thrombosis highest in Pts with leukocytosis), bleeding, pruritus; mild splenomegaly; migraine, TIA; early fetal loss

Diagnostic evaluation
- Peripheral smear: large hypogranular platelets
- BM bx: megakaryocytic hyperplasia; absence of Philadelphia chromosome and very rarely, minor increase in reticulin fibers; normal iron stores
- **JAK2 V617F** present in ~50% of ET; **MPL** or **CALR** mutations in majority of JAK2 wt
- Patients should not meet WHO criteria for diagnosis of CML, PV, PMF or MDS

Treatment of ET			
Risk	**Features**	**ASA 81 mg qd**	**Cytoreduction**
Low	Age <60 and no h/o thrombosis and plt <1.5 × 10⁶/μL and no CV risk factors	Consider for vasomotor symptoms	No
Int.	Neither low nor high	±	Consider if plt >1.5 × 10⁶/μL
High	Age ≥60 or h/o thrombosis or plt >1.5 × 10⁶/μL	⊕ (consider holding if plt >1 × 10⁶/μL and lab evid. of acquired vWD)	**Hydroxyurea.** Goal plt <0.4 × 10⁶/μL or sx free. IFNα if young or pregnant.

Imetelstat (telomerase inhib) under investigation (NEJM 2015;373:92)

Prognosis
- Low-risk Pts have overall survival = control population
- Risk of transformation into acute leukemia <2%; risk of progression to MF similar

PRIMARY MYELOFIBROSIS (PMF)

Definition
- Clonal myeloproliferation with reactive marrow fibrosis & extramedullary hematopoiesis
- Prefibrotic stage (pre-PMF): megakaryocyte prolif, grade 1 reticulin fibrosis, ↑ BM cellularity. Important to distinguish from ET: ↑ thrombosis, ↑ progression, ↓ survival (Blood 2012;120:569)

Etiologies of myelofibrosis
- Myeloproliferative neoplasm = primary myelofibrosis; post-PV/ET myelofibrosis
- Other hematologic (CML, AML, ALL, MDS) and solid cancers (breast, prostate)
- Autoimmune (SLE and other collagen vascular disorders)
- Toxins (benzene); radiation; granulomas (TB, fungal, sarcoid); deposition dis. (Gaucher's)

Clinical manifestations (BJH 2012;158:453)
- Ineffective erythropoiesis → anemia; extramedullary hematopoiesis → **massive splenomegaly** (abdominal pain, early satiety) ± hepatomegaly
- Tumor bulk and ↑ cell turnover → fatigue, weight loss, fever, sweats

Diagnostic evaluation (JAMA 2010;303:2513; Blood 2016;127:2391)
- Anemia with variable WBC and platelet counts
- Peripheral smear → **"leukoerythroblastic"** (**teardrop cells,** nucleated RBCs, immature WBCs); large abnormal platelets
- BM aspirate → **"dry" tap;** BM bx → **severe fibrosis,** replacement by reticulin & collagen
- **JAK2 V617F** in 45–50%; **CALR** mut in 45–50%, **MPL** mut in 7–10%, triple neg in 1–2%
- No BCR-ABL translocation; also does not meet criteria for PV or MDS

Treatment (Blood 2011;117:3494)
- In absence of adverse prognostic factors (eg, anemia or sx) → no treatment
- Allogeneic HSCT only potential cure → consider in young Pts with poor prognosis
- Supportive care: **transfusions;** inconsistent benefit from androgens or Epo;
  ? splenectomy if refractory to transfusions, failed chemoRx, painful splenomegaly
- Hydroxyurea for significant leukocytosis or thrombocytosis
- Ruxolitinib (JAK1/JAK2 inhibitor) ↓ sx, ↓ splenomegaly, ↑ survival (NEJM 2012;366:787 & 799)
- Thalidomide and lenalidomide ± steroids may improve red cell count
- Imetelstat (telomerase inhibitor) under investigation (NEJM 2015;373:908)

Complications and prognosis
- Median survival ~6 y; transformation into AML occurs at a rate of ~8%/y
- Dynamic International Prognostic Scoring System (DIPPS plus): age >65, WBC >25k, Hgb <10, blasts >1%, ⊕ symptoms, RBC Tx, Plt <100K, karyotype (JCO 2011;29:392). IWG-MRT allows prognostication at any point during clinical course (Blood 2010;115:1703).

ACUTE LEUKEMIA

Definition
- Clonal proliferation of hematopoietic progenitor with failed differentiation into mature elements → ↑ blasts in bone marrow and periphery → ↓ RBCs, platelets and neutrophils

Epidemiology and risk factors
- Acute myelogenous (AML): ~21k cases/y in U.S.; median age 67 y; >80% of adult acute leukemias
- Acute lymphocytic (ALL): ~6k cases/y in U.S.; median age 14 y but 2nd peak in older adults
- Risk factors: **radiation, chemo** (alkylating agents, topo II inhib), benzene, smoking, ? rising from acquired somatic mutations and clonal hematopoiesis (NEJM 2014;371:2477)
- Secondary to acquired hematopoietic dis.: MDS, MPN (esp. CML), aplastic anemia, PNH
- Inherited: Down's, Klinefelter's, Fanconi's anemia, Bloom syndrome, ataxia telangiectasia

Clinical manifestations
- Cytopenias → **fatigue** (anemia), **infection** (neutropenia), **bleeding** (thrombocytopenia)
- More common in **AML**
  - **leukostasis** (more often when blast count >50,000/μL): occluded microcirculation → local hypoxemia and hemorrhage → dyspnea, hypoxia, headache, blurred vision, TIA/CVA; look for *hyperviscosity retinopathy* (vascular engorgement, exudates, hemorrhage)
  - **DIC** (esp. with APL); leukemic infiltration of skin, gingiva (esp. with monocytic subtypes); chloroma: extramedullary tumor of leukemic cells, virtually any location
- More common in **ALL**:
  - bony/lumbar pain, lymphadenopathy, hepatosplenomegaly (also in monocytic AML)
  - CNS involvement (up to 10%): cranial neuropathies, N/V, headache
  - anterior mediastinal mass (esp. in T-cell); tumor lysis syndrome (qv)

Diagnostic evaluation (Blood 2009;114:937)
- **Peripheral smear:** anemia, thrombocytopenia, variable WBC + circulating **blasts** (seen in >95%; ⊕ Auer Rods in AML), peripheral flow cytometry for blast origin (ALL vs. AML)
- **Bone marrow:** hypercellular with >20% blasts; test for cytogenetics and flow cytometry
- Presence of certain **cytogenetic anomalies**, eg, t(15;17), t(8;21), inv(16) or t(16;16), are sufficient for dx of AML *regardless of the blast count*
- ✓ for tumor lysis syndrome (rapid cell turnover): ↑ UA, ↑ LDH, ↑ K, ↑ PO₄, ↓ Ca
- Coagulation studies to r/o DIC: PT, PTT, fibrinogen, D-dimer, haptoglobin, bilirubin
- LP (w/ **co-admin of intrathecal chemotherapy** to avoid seeding CSF w/ circulating blasts) for Pts w/ ALL (CNS is sanctuary site) and for Pts w/ AML w/ CNS sx
- TTE if prior cardiac history or before use of anthracyclines
- **HLA typing** of Pt, siblings > parents/children for potential allogeneic HSCT candidates

ACUTE MYELOGENOUS LEUKEMIA (AML; NEJM 2015;373:1136)

Classification (WHO; Blood; 2016;127:2391)
- Features used to confirm myeloid lineage and subclassify AML to guide treatment: morphology: **blasts**, ⊕ **granules**, ± **Auer rods** (eosinophilic needle-like inclusions) cytochemistry: ⊕ **myeloperoxidase** and/or **nonspecific esterase**
- Immunophenotype: myeloid: CD13, CD33, CD117; monocyte: CD11b, CD64, CD14, CD15
- Cytogenetics: important for prognosis. Intermed. risk = no favorable/unfavorable features.

WHO 2016 Classification of AML (Blood 2016;127:2391)	
4 Major Subtypes	**Examples**
Recurrent genetic abnl	t(8;21); inv(16); *PML-RARA*; t(9;11), t(6;9), inv(3), t(1;22), mutation in *NPM1*, biallelic mutation in *CEBPA*
Myelodysplasia-related Δ	w/ or w/o antecedent MDS or MPN
Therapy-related	eg, alkylating agents or topoisomerase inhibitors
Not otherwise specified	w/ min differentiation; w/ or w/o maturation; myelomonocytic; monoblastic/cytic; pure erythroid; megakaryoblastic
Also: myeloid sarcoma, myeloid proliferations of Down's syndrome	

AML Genetics (Blood 2010;115:453 & 116:354; NEJM 2016;374:2209)		
	Favorable prognosis	**Unfavorable prognosis**
Karyotype	t(15;17) in APL; t(8;21); inv(16)/t(16;16)	−5; −7; 3q26 aberrations; t(6;9); 11q23 aberrations; complex karyotype
Gene mutations	*NPM1*+; biallelic *CEBPA*	*FLT3* ITD; *MLL-PTD*; *TP53*, *RUNX1*
Recurrent somatic mutations: *DNMT3A*; *TET2*; *ASXL1*; *RAS*; *WT1*; *IDH1/2*; spliceosome		

- Induction chemo followed by consolidation; if unfit, hypomethylating agents or clinical trial
- **Induction chemo:** "7 + 3" = cytarabine × 7 d + ida/daunorubicin × 3 d. Daunorubicin dose: age <60 → high (90 mg/m²); age >60 → standard (60 or 45 mg/m²) (NEJM 2009;361:1249). Gemtuzumab ozogamicin (α-CD33) ? benefit in fav/int risk AML (Lancet 2012;379:1508).
- ✓ for complete remission (CR) = ANC >1000, plts >100, off RBC Rx, <5% BM blasts **CR ≠ cure;** ∴ must always f/u induction with **consolidation Rx**
- If ⊕ CR: consolidation Rx per Pt risk (age, genetics, PS); chemo (eg, high-dose cytarabine, HiDAC) if favorable risk; poor risk → allo-HSCT; int risk depends on mutat., donors, PS
- If ⊖ CR: reinduce w/ altern. Rx [eg, MEC (mitoxantrone, etoposide, cytarabine)], HiDAC
- If relapse after CR: salvage chemo or clinical trial → allogeneic HSCT
- Supportive care: hydration + allopurinol or rasburicase for tumor lysis prophylaxis; transfusions; antibiotics for fever and neutropenia; antifungals for prolonged fever & neutropenia; hydroxyurea ± leukapheresis for leukostasis (avoid pheresis in APL)

Prognosis
- CR achieved in 70–80% of Pts <60 y and in 40–50% for Pts >60 y
- Overall survival variable, depends on prognostic factors: ranges from <10% of older Pts w/ poor risk tumor genetics to >75% for younger Pts w/ favorable prognostic factors
- Poor prog. factors: age >60, unfavorable cytogenetics, poor performance status, antecedent MDS/MPN, tAML; genetics (NEJM 2016;374:2209; JAMA 2015;314:811); residual dis. eg, persistent NPM 1-mut. transcripts a/w ↑ relapse, ↓ survival (NEJM 2016;374:422)

Acute promyelocytic leukemia (APL) (Blood 2009;113:1875)
- Rare disease, approx. 8% of total AML cases in U.S. but biologically and clinically distinct
- Atypical promyelocytes (large, granular cells; bilobed nuclei) in blood and bone marrow
- Defined by translocation of retinoic acid receptor: **t(15;17); PML-RARα** (>95% of cases)
- **Medical emergency** with **DIC** and **bleeding** common; supportive care measures crucial
- Remarkable responses to **all-trans-retinoic acid (ATRA)**, which induces differentiation, and **arsenic trioxide (ATO)**; early initiation of ATRA critical as soon as APL suspected; ATO highly effective as first-line therapy or in treatment of refractory disease
- Induction: ATRA + ATO → CR ~100%, ↑ 2-y event-free survival (NEJM 2013;362:111); anthracycline + ATRA ± cytarabine → CR in ~90%, favored in high-risk APL (WBC >10k)
- Differentiation (ATRA) syndrome: ~25% of Pts; fever, pulm infiltrates, SOB, edema, HoTN, AKI; tx w/ dexamethasone 10 mg bid, supportive care (± diuresis) (Blood 2008;113:775)
- Consolidation: daunorubicin + ATRA (Blood 2010;116:3751) or ATRA+ATO (NEJM 2013;369:111)
- Role of maintenance Rx (eg, ATRA + 6MP + MTX) controversial; not w/ ATRA/ATO Rx
- Best prognosis of all AMLs: >90% cure; WBC >10,000/μL = ↓ prognosis (Blood 2000;96:1247)

ACUTE LYMPHOBLASTIC LEUKEMIA (ALL)

Classification
- Lymphoblastic neoplasms may present as acute leukemia (ALL) with **>20% BM blasts** or as lymphoblastic lymphoma (LBL) w/ mass lesion & <20% BM blasts. ALL and LBL are considered the same disease with different clinical presentations.
- Morphology: **no granules** (granules seen in myeloid lineage)
- Cytochemistry: ⊕ terminal deoxynucleotidyl transferase (TdT) in 95% of ALL
- Cytogenetics (Blood 2010;115:206): t(9;22) = Philadelphia chrom (Ph) ~25% of adults w/ ALL; "Ph-like" ALL gene expression: worse prognosis, ? role of TKI (NEJM 2014;371:1005)
- Immunohistochem.: 2 major phenotypes (Burkitt's treated differently; see "Lymphoma")

WHO Immunophenotype Classification of ALL (Blood 2016;127:2375)		
WHO type	**Adult freq.**	**Immunohistochemistry**
B cell	75%	⊕ TdT, ⊕ CD19; variable CD10, CD20
T cell	25%	⊕ TdT, ⊕ T-cell Ag (CD2, cytoplasmic CD3, CD5, CD7)

Treatment (JCO 2011;29:532; Leukemia 2015;29:526)
- **Induction chemo:** regimens typically include combination of anthracycline, vincristine, steroids, cyclophosphamide, ± asparaginase; based on pediatric regimens
- **CNS prophylaxis:** intrathecal MTX/cytarabine ± cranial irradiation or systemic MTX
- **Postremission therapy** options:
  consolidation/intensification chemo (~7 mo) followed by maintenance chemo (~2–3 y) high-dose chemo w/ allo HSCT considered for Pts in CR1 w/ available donor pediatric regimens in adults (Leukemia 2015;29:526); consider allo SCT if <50 (controversial)
- If relapse → salvage (chemo or CAR-T or inotuzumab), then allogeneic HSCT if able
- Ph ⊖ t(9;22) primary refractory/relapsed B-cell ALL: blinatumomab (Lancet Oncol 2015;16:57)
- Ph ⊕ t(9;22) → add imatinib or dasatinib, followed by allogeneic HSCT

- MLL-AF4 t(4;11), hypodiploidy (<44 chromosomes), min residual disease → consider allo-HSCT
- Infusion of chimeric antigen receptor–modified T cells promising *(NEJM 2014;371:1507)*

Prognosis
- Morphologic CR in >80% of adults; but minimal residual disease (MRD) at CR = poor prog.
- Cure achieved in 50–60% if good prog. factors vs. 10–30% w/ poor prog. factors
- Good prognostic factors: younger age, WBC <30,000/μL, T-cell immunophenotype, absence of Ph chromosome or t(4;11), early attainment of CR w/ MRD negative

Chronic Myelogenous Leukemia (CML)

Definition *(Blood 2009;114:937)*
- **Myeloproliferative neoplasm** with clonal overproduction of hematopoietic myeloid stem cells that can differentiate
- **Philadelphia chromosome** (Ph) = t(9;22) → **BCR-ABL** fusion → ↑ Abl kinase activity *BCR-ABL* **required for Dx** (make via karyotyping or FISH; PCR useful but not adequate)
- "Atypical CML" (BCR-ABL ⊖) now considered a separate disease and reclassified as MDS/MPN (qv) w/ many Pts ⊕ for *CSF3R* or *SETBP1* mutations

Epidemiology and risk factors
- ~6600 new cases/y in U.S.; median age ~64 at presentation; ~15% of adult leukemias
- ↑ risk with irradiation; no clear relation to cytotoxic drugs

Clinical manifestations
- Triphasic clinical course; 85% present in the chronic phase
- **Chronic phase:** often asymptomatic but common features are fatigue, malaise, weight loss, night sweats, abdominal fullness (**splenomegaly** 50%)
- **Accelerated phase:** refractory leukocytosis, ↓ plt and worsening sx → fever, wt loss, ↑ splenomegaly, bone pain, bleeding, infections, pruritus (basophilia)
- **Blastic phase** ≈ acute leukemia → severe constitutional symptoms, infection, bleeding, and possible **leukostasis** (see "Acute Leukemia")

Diagnostic evaluation
- **Peripheral smear: leukocytosis,** left-shifted with *all stages of myeloid maturation;* anemia, thrombocytosis, **basophilia**
- **Bone marrow:** hypercellular, ↑ myeloid to erythroid ratio, ↓ leuk alkaline phosphatase
- **Chronic:** <10% blasts (peripheral or BM)
- **Accelerated:** 10–19% blasts, ≥20% basos, plts <100k, ↑ spleen size, karyotypic prog.
- **Blastic:** ≥20% blasts (²⁄₃ myeloid, ¹⁄₃ lymphoid), may see extramedullary leukemia

Treatment *(Lancet 2015;385:1447)*
- **Tyrosine kinase inhibitor (TKI):** imatinib, dasatinib, nilotinib, bosutinib, & ponatinib are selective inhibitors of BCR-ABL *(JCO 2010;28:428; Blood 2012;120:1390).*
  Imatinib, nilotinib, & dasatinib approved as initial Rx.
  Resistance = recurrent dis. on TKI, often result of *BCR-ABL* mutation or amplification.
  Nilotinib, dasatinib, bosutinib, & ponatinib approved for resistant disease, w/ only ponatinib effective on T315I resistance mutation *(NEJM 2012;367:2075 & 2013;369:1783).*
  Side effects: nausea, diarrhea, muscle cramps, cytopenias, ↓ PO₄, ↑ QT, rarely CHF; dasatinib: pericardial & pleural effusions and pulm HTN; nilotinib: ↑ bili & lipase, CV toxicity; ponatinib: thrombosis, pancreatitis and CV toxicity
- **Chronic phase:** TKI; continued indefinitely in responders *(Blood 2012;120:1390)*
- **Accelerated phase:** TKI upfront, consider allogeneic HSCT
- **Blastic phase:** TKI vs. TKI + either ALL or AML induction (based on cell type); then HSCT
- **Allogeneic HSCT:** possibility of cure, consider for Pts w/ available donor; Pts who present in accelerated or blastic phase; or Pts with relapsed/refractory disease to TKIs

Goals of TKI Therapy *(Blood 2013;122:872)*		
Response	**Definition**	**Optimal time**
Hematologic	WBC <10k, plt <450k, no immature cells in blood, basophils <5%, spleen nonpalpable	3 mo
Cytogenetic	Absence of the Ph chromosome in metaphase cells	12 mo
Molecular	<0.1% BCR-ABL = 3-log reduction by quantitative PCR	12 mo

Prognosis *(Cancer 2013;119:2620)*
- Chronic phase CML Rx'd w/ imatinib: 89% 5-y overall survival, 95% survival free of CML-related deaths, 7% progression to blast phase at 5 y *(NEJM 2006;355:2408)*
- Accelerated phase CML Rx'd w/ imatinib: ~50% overall survival at 4 y *(Cancer 2005;103:2099)*
- Poor prognostic factors: ↑ age, ↑ platelet count, ↑ spleen size, ↑% of blasts/basophils

CHRONIC LYMPHOCYTIC LEUKEMIA (CLL)

Definition (NEJM 2005;352:804; Blood 2008;111:5446)
- Monoclonal accumulation of functionally incompetent mature B lymphocytes
- CLL (>5000/μL malignant cells) & small lymphocytic lymphoma (SLL; <5000/μL malignant cells, with + LAN ± splenomegaly) classified as same disease
- Monoclonal B lymphocytosis (<5000/μL, nodes <1.5 cm, nl RBC and Plt counts): observe

Epidemiology and risk factors
- ~15,000 new cases/y; median age at dx is 71 y; most common adult leukemia
- ↑ incidence in 1st-degree relatives; no known association with radiation, chemicals, drugs

Clinical manifestations
- Symptoms: **often asx** & identified when CBC reveals lymphocytosis; 10–20% p/w fatigue, malaise, night sweats, weight loss (ie, lymphoma "B" sx)
- Signs: **lymphadenopathy** (80%) and **hepatosplenomegaly** (50%)
- **Autoimmune hemolytic anemia** (AIHA) (~10%) or **thrombocytopenia** (ITP) (~1–2%)
- Hypogammaglobulinemia ± neutropenia → ↑ susceptibility to **infections**
- Bone marrow failure in ~13%; monoclonal gammopathy in ~5%
- Aggressive transformation: ~5% develop **Richter's syndrome** = transformation into high-grade lymphoma (usually DLBCL) and sudden clinical deterioration

Diagnostic evaluation (see "Lymphoma" for general approach)
- **Peripheral smear: lymphocytosis** (>5000/μL, mature-appearing small cells) "smudge" cells from damage to abnl lymphs from shear stress of making blood smear
- **Flow cytometry:** clonality with dim surface Ig (sIg); CD5+, CD19+, CD20(dim), CD23+. CD38+ or ZAP70+ a/w unmutated Ig variable heavy chain region & worse prog.
- **Bone marrow:** normo- or hypercellular; infiltrated w/ small B-cell lymphocytes (≥30%)
- **Lymph nodes:** infiltrated w/ small lymphocytic or diffuse small cleaved cells = SLL
- **Genetics:** del 11q22-23 & 17p13 unfavorable; trisomy 12 neutral; del 13q14 and mut *IgVH* favorable. Nine significantly mutated genes, including *TP53*, *NOTCH 1*, *MYD88* and *SF3B 1*. Key role for spliceosome mutations (NEJM 2011;365:2497; JCI 2012;122:3432).

	CLL Staging			
Rai system		**Median survival**	**Binet system**	
Stage	**Description**		**Description**	**Stage**
0	Lymphocytosis *only*	>10 y	<3 node areas	A
I	⊕ lymphadenopathy	7–10 y	>3 node areas	B
II	⊕ hepatosplenomegaly			
III	⊕ anemia (not AIHA)	1–2 y	Anemia or thrombocytopenia	C
IV	⊕ thrombocytopenia (not ITP)			

Treatment (JAMA 2014;312:2265)
- Treatment is primarily *palliative* → early stage disease can be followed w/o Rx
- Indications for treatment: Rai stages III/IV, Binet stage C, disease-related sx, progressive disease, AIHA or ITP refractory to steroids, recurrent infections
- Options: combo superior to monoRx (Lancet 2007;370:230), but comorbidities/age important
  purine analogues: fludarabine ("F"), pentostatin ("P")
  alkylating agents: cyclophosphamide ("C"), bendamustine ("B"), CVP, CHOP
  ± **monoclonal Ab** against CD20 (**rituximab**, "R"; ofatumumab) or CD52 (alemtuzumab)
- Healthy/younger (<70y): FCR ↑ survival vs. FC (Lancet 2010;376:1164); FR also acceptable
- Infirm/elderly: many options incl. ibrutinib (NEJM 2015;373:2425); chlorambucil + anti-CD20 [eg, obinutuzumab (NEJM 2014;370:1101) or ofatumumab (Lancet 2015;385:1873)], BR
- Refractory disease: ibrutinib > ofatumumab (NEJM 2014;371:213); acalabrutinib (BTK; NEJM 2016;374:323), idelalisib (PI3K; NEJM 2014;370:997); venetoclax (α-BCL2; NEJM 2016;374:311)
- 17p- or *TP53* mutat.: venetoclax, idelalisib, or ibrutinib ± rituximab (J Clin Oncol 2014;10:1090)
- Consider allo-HSCT in 17p-, *TP53* mutation or refractory CLL (BJH 2012;158:174)
- Supportive care: PCP, HSV, VZV prophylaxis; CMV monitoring for Pts receiving anti-CD52; AIHA/ITP → steroids; recurrent infections → IVIg

Prognosis (NEJM 2004;351:893; JCO 2006;24:4634)
- Survival varies substantially. Median overall survival ~10 y (Am J Hematol 2011;12:985)
- Favorable prognosis: 13q14 deletion (~50% of CLL cases)
- Factors a/w worse prognosis include:
  unfavorable cytogenetics: eg, 17p- or *TP53* mutation (JCO 2010;28:4473)
  unmutated (<2% c/w germline) *IgVH* gene (<8–10 y vs. >20–25 y if mutated)
  high (>20–30%) Zap-70 expression (part of T cell receptor; correlated w/ unmutated *IgVH*)
  CD38 >30% or CD49d <30%: correlated with unmutated *IgVH* (Blood 2008;111:865)
  higher β2-microglobulin levels (correlate with disease stage and tumor burden)

LYMPHOMA

Definition
- Malignant disorder of lymphoid cells that reside predominantly in lymphoid tissues
- Generally characterized as **Hodgkin lymphoma** (HL) or **non-Hodgkin lymphoma** (NHL)

Clinical manifestations
- Lymphadenopathy (nontender)
  - **HL**: Reed-Sternberg (**RS**) **cells**; superficial (usually **cervical/supraclavicular**) ± mediastinal LAN; **nodal disease with orderly, anatomic spread** to adjacent nodes
  - **NHL**: diffuse; **nodal and/or extranodal** disease with **noncontiguous spread**; symptoms reflect involved sites (abdominal fullness, bone pain)
- Constitutional ("B") symptoms: **fever** (>38°), drenching **sweats**, ↓ **weight** (>10% in 6 mo)
  - **HL**: periodic, recurrent "Pel-Ebstein" fever; 10–15% have pruritus; ~35% "B" symptoms
  - **NHL**: "B" symptoms vary between subtypes; ~15–50%

Diagnostic and staging evaluation
- Physical exam: lymph nodes, liver/spleen size, Waldeyer's ring, testes (~1% of NHL), skin
- Pathology: excisional lymph node bx (not FNA b/c need surrounding architecture) with immunophenotyping and cytogenetics; BM bx or PET (except in HL clinical stage IA/IIA w/ favorable features or CLL by flow); LP if CNS involvement clinically suspected
- Lab tests: CBC, BUN/Cr, LFTs, ESR, LDH, UA, Ca, alb; ✓ HBV & HCV (and must ✓ HBsAg & anti-HBc if planning rituximab Rx, as can lead to HBV reactivation); consider HIV, HTLV, & EBV serologies and connective tissue diseases autoAbs
- Imaging: PET-CT scans as CT alone does not reliably detect spleen/liver involvement (espec. in HL, DLBCL). PET response to Rx can be prognostic & possibly guide Rx (NEJM 2015;372:1598 & 2016;374:2419). Head CT/MRI only if neurologic symptoms.

Ann Arbor Staging System with Cotswolds Modifications	
Stage	**Features**
I	Single lymph node (LN) region
II	≥2 LN regions on the same side of the diaphragm
III	LN regions on both sides of the diaphragm
IV	Disseminated involvement of one or more extralymphatic organs

Modifiers: A = no symptoms; B = fever, night sweats or weight loss; X = bulky disease = greatest transverse diam. of mediastinal mass/max diam. of chest wall >⅓ on CXR or >10 cm if in abd; E = involves single contiguous extranodal site; H = hepatic; S = splenic

HODGKIN LYMPHOMA (HL) (NEJM 2010;363:653)

Epidemiology and risk factors
- ~9,000 cases/y; bimodal distribution (15–35 & >50 y); ↑ ♂; role of EBV in subsets of HL, esp. immunocompromised patients (eg, HIV)

Pathology
- Affected nodes show RS cells (<1%) in background of non-neoplastic inflammatory cells
- Classic RS cells: bilobed nucleus & prominent nucleoli with surrounding clear space ("owl's eyes"). RS cells are **clonal B-cells**: CD15+, CD30+, CD20− (rarely +).

WHO Histologic Classification of Classical HL		
Nodular sclerosis	60–80%	Collagen bands; frequent mediastinal LAN; young adults; female predominance; usually stage I or II at dx
Mixed cellularity	15–30%	Pleomorphic; older age; male predominance; ≥50% stage III or IV at presentation; intermediate prognosis
Lymphocyte rich	5%	Abundant normal-appearing lymphocytes; mediastinal LAN uncommon; male predominance; good prognosis
Lymphocyte depleted	<1%	Diffuse fibrosis and large numbers of RS cells; older, male patients; disseminated at dx; seen in HIV; worst prognosis

- **Nonclassical** (5%): nodular lymphocyte predominant (NLP); involves peripheral LN 80% present in stages I–II and Rx can be RT alone or combination chemo + RT w/ 80% 10-y progression-free survival, 93% overall survival (JCO 1997;15:3060)
  - Consider rituximab as most NLP RS cells are CD20+
  - Stages III–IV treated with combination chemo (see below)

Treatment (*Lancet* 2012;380:836)

- **Stages I–II: ABVD** (doxorubicin, bleomycin, vinblastine, dacarbazine) ± RT
  Lower intensity regimens comparable efficacy if favorable prognosis (*NEJM* 2010;363:640)
- **Stages III–IV: ABVD** × 6 cycles or **escalated BEACOPP** (bleomycin, etoposide, doxorubicin, cyclophosphamide, vincristine, procarbazine and prednisone)
- Refractory/relapsed disease: salvage chemo + auto HSCT, ± RT
  brentuximab vedotin (CD30 antibody-drug conjugate): salvage (*NEJM* 2010;363:1812), or post-ASCT consolidation (*Lancet* 2015;385:1853)
  PD1/PDL1 blockade (eg, pembrolizumab or nivolumab) (*NEJM* 2015;372:311)
- Late effects include ↑ risk for:
  second cancers: ~4.6× risk for up to 40 y (*NEJM* 2015;373:2499)
    breast (if RT) ∴ annual screening at age 40 or 8–10 y post RT
    lung, ? role of screening CXR or CT (controversial)
    acute leukemia/MDS; NHL
  cardiac disease (if RT or anthracycline), ? role of echo/stress at 10 y (controversial)
  pulmonary toxicity (if bleomycin)
  hypothyroidism (if RT) ∴ annual TSH (if neck RT)

International Prognostic Score (IPS) (*JCO* 2012;30:3383)		
Negative prognostic indicators	**Total # of indicators**	**5-y PFS**
Albumin <4 g/dL; Hb <10.5 g/dL	0	88%
Male; Age >45 y	1	84%
Stage IV	2	80%
WBC ≥15k/μL	3	74%
Lymphocytes <600/μL or <8% of differential	4	67%
	≥5	62%

Non-Hodgkin Lymphoma (NHL)

Epidemiology and risk factors

- ~70,000 new cases/y; median age at dx ~65 y; ♂ predominance; 85% B-cell origin
- Associated conditions: immunodeficiency (eg, HIV, posttransplant); autoimmune disorders (eg, Sjögren's, RA, SLE); infection (eg, EBV, HTLV-I, *H. pylori*)
- Burkitt lymphoma: (1) endemic or African (jaw mass, 80–90% EBV-related); (2) sporadic or American (20% EBV-related); (3) HIV-related

WHO Classification of Lymphoid Malignancies (*Blood* 2016;127:2375)		
Type	**Examples**	**Associated abnormalities**
Mature B cell	Diffuse large B-cell lymphoma (DLBCL)	*BCL2, MYC, MLL2, CREBBP, etc.*
	Follicular lymphoma	*IGH-BCL2, MLL2*
	CLL/small lymphocytic lymphoma	*IGVH, ZAP70, TP53, SF3B1, etc.*
	Mantle cell	*t(11;14) BCL1-IgH → cyclin D1 dysreg*
	Marginal zone lymphoma (nodal, extranodal [MALT ✓ *H. pylori*], splenic)	*AP12-MALT1 & BCL-10-Ig enhancer*
	Burkitt's lymphoma	*8q24, c-MYC*
	Hairy cell leukemia (p/w fatigue, ↓ monos, massive splenomegaly; ⊕ TRAP)	*BRAF V600E*
Mature T cell & NK cell	Peripheral T-cell lymphoma	*TET2 and DNMT3A*
	Mycosis fungoides (cutaneous lymphoma)/Sézary syndrome (+ LAN)	
	Anaplastic large-cell lymphoma	Some *ALK1* ⊕
	Angioimmunoblastic T-cell lymphoma	

Treatment (*Lancet* 2012;380:848)

- Treatment and prognosis determined by histopathologic classification rather than stage
- Rituximab (antibody to CD20; *NEJM* 2012;366:2008) if CD20+; no role if tumor is CD20–
- **Indolent:** goal is sx mgmt (bulky dis., cytopenias, "B" sx); not curable (except allo HSCT)
  Options include RT for localized disease, rituximab ± chemo (bendamustine, CVP, fludarabine), ibrutinib
  For MALT → treat *H. pylori* if ⊕
  Rituximab maintenance ↑ survival in relapsed disease (*JNCI* 2009;101:248); growing role for rituximab maintenance in indolent and aggressive disease (*Lancet* 2011;377:42)
  Hairy cell: cladribine; oral BRAF inhibitor if relapsed/refractory (*NEJM* 2015;373:1733)
- **Aggressive** (DLBCL, 30–40% of NHL): goal is cure (*JCO* 2005;23:6387)
  R-CHOP (<u>R</u>ituximab, <u>c</u>yclophosphamide, doxorubicin = <u>h</u>ydroxydaunorubicin, vincristine = <u>O</u>ncovin, <u>p</u>rednisone) (*NEJM* 2002;346:235 & 2008;359:613)
  10-y progression-free survival = 45%; overall survival = 55% (*Blood* 2010;116:2040)

? R-ACVBP (rituxim, doxorubicin = <u>A</u>driamycin, <u>c</u>yclophosph, <u>v</u>indesine, <u>b</u>leo, <u>p</u>rednisone) ↑ 3-y OS vs. R-CHOP, but ↑ adverse events *(Lancet 2011;378:1858)*

+ **Radiation** for localized or bulky disease

Consider **CNS prophylaxis** w/ intrathecal or systemic high-dose methotrexate if paranasal sinus, testicular, breast, periorbital, paravertebral, or bone marrow involved; ≥2 extranodal sites + ↑ LDH may also warrant

Refractory/relapsed disease: salvage chemo; high-dose chemo + auto-HSCT *(NEJM 1995;333:1540)*; allo-HSCT if beyond 2nd relapse *(JCO 2011;29:1342)*

Mantle cell: ibrutinib for relapsed/refractory disease *(Lancet 2016;387:770)*

- **Highly aggressive** (Burkitt, lymphoblastic lymphoma, high-grade B-cell lymphoma w/ rearrangements of MYC and BCL2 and/or BCL6)

  Burkitt: intensive short-course chemo *(Blood 2004;104:3009)* + rituximab *(BJH 2014;165:102)*
    Low risk defined as nl LDH & single focus of disease <10 cm; all others high risk
    Low-risk Rx: CODOX-M (cyclophosphamide, vincristine, doxorubicin, high-dose methotrexate ± rituximab) *(Leuk Lymph 2004;45:761)*
    High-risk Rx: CODOX-M/IVAC (above w/ ifosfamide, etoposide, high-dose cytarabine), hyper-CVAD (cyclophosphamide, vincristine, doxorubicin, dexamethasone)
    Dose-adjusted EPOCH-R w/ promise (see below; titrate to ANC) *(NEJM 2013;369:1915)*
    All Pts receive CNS prophylaxis & tumor lysis syndrome prophylaxis
    Addition of rituximab improves EFS *(Lancet 2016;387:2402)*

  Lymphoblastic lymphoma (B or T cell): treated like ALL (see "Acute Leukemia")

  High-grade B-cell lymphoma w/ rearrangements of MYC and BCL2 and/or BCL6: previously "double-/triple-hit" lymphoma, assoc. w/ poor prognosis.

Prognosis

- Indolent: typically incurable, but long median survival

Follicular Lymphoma International Prognostic Index (FLIPI) *(Blood 2004;104:1258)*		
Factors: age >60, stages III/IV, Hb <12 g/dL, >4 nodal areas, LDH >nl		
# factors	5-y overall survival	10-y overall survival
0–1	90%	71%
2	78%	51%
≥3	52%	35%

- Aggressive: ↑ chance of cure, but overall worse prognosis

International Prognostic Index (IPI) for Aggressive NHL *(Blood 2007;109:1857)*		
Factors: age >60, stage III/IV, ≥2 extranodal sites, performance status ≥2, LDH > nl		
# factors	Complete response	5-y overall survival
0–1	87%	73%
2	67%	51%
3	55%	43%
4–5	44%	26%
Revised IPI Prognosis in Patients Rx'd with CHOP-R		
Factors	% at dx	4-y overall survival
0	10%	94%
1–2	45%	79%
3–5	45%	55%

HIV-associated NHL *(Blood 2006;107:13)*

- HIV ⊕ imparts 60–100× relative risk
- NHL is an AIDS-defining malignancy along with Kaposi's, cervical CA, anal CA
- Concurrent HAART & chemotherapy likely provide survival benefit
- DLBCL & immunoblastic lymphoma (67%): CD4 <100, EBV-associated
    Treat as immunocompetent (CHOP-R), but avoid rituximab if CD4 <100
    Alternative regimens include R-EPOCH (etop, pred, vincristine, cyclophos, doxorubicin)
- Burkitt lymphoma (20%): can occur with CD4 >200
    Treat as immunocompetent; prognosis is not significantly worse
- Primary CNS lymphoma (16%): CD4 <50, EBV-associated (also seen in Pts w/o HIV). Rx w/ high-dose MTX-based regimen + steroids ± temozolomide ± RT, consider auto HSCT.
- Primary effusion lymphoma (<5%): HHV8 driven; also can be seen in other immuno-supp. Pts such as s/p solid organ transplant or w/ chronic HBV. Treat with standard CHOP (often CD20–) or consider EPOCH, overall poor prognosis.

MULTIPLE MYELOMA (MM)

Definition and epidemiology (NEJM 2011;364:1046)
- Malignant neoplasm of **plasma cells** producing a monoclonal Ig = "**M protein**"
- ~27,000 new cases/y; median age at diagnosis 69 y; more common in African-Americans

Clinical manifestations (CRAB criteria and other less common features)
- Hyper**C**alcemia due to ↑ osteoclast activity
- **R**enal disease: multiple mechanisms include toxic effect of filtered light chains → *renal failure* (cast nephropathy) *or* type II RTA; amyloidosis or light chain deposition disease → *nephrotic syndrome*; hypercalcemia, urate nephropathy, type I cryoglobulinemia
- **A**nemia (normocytic) due to bone marrow involvement; rarely, may see AIHA
- **B**one pain due to ↑ osteoclast activity → lytic lesions, pathologic fx
- Recurrent infxns due to relative hypogammaglob. (clonal plasma cells suppress nl Ig)
- Neurologic: cord compression; POEMS (**p**olyneuropathy, **o**rganomegaly, **e**ndocrinopathy, **M** protein, **s**kin changes) syndrome
- Hyperviscosity: usually when IgM >4 g/dL, IgG >5 g/dL, or IgA >7 g/dL
- Coagulopathy: inhibition of or Ab against clotting factor; Ab-coated platelets
- AL Amyloidosis (see "Amyloidosis")

Diagnostic and staging evaluation (Lancet Onc 2014;15:e538)
- **MM criteria:** clonal BM plasma cells ≥10% or bx-proven plasmacytoma and ≥1 myeloma-defining event:
  (a) myeloma-related organ or tissue impairment (**ROTI**) = lytic bone lesions, Ca >11 mg/dL, Cr >2 mg/dL, or Hb <10 g/dL
  (b) any of the following biomarkers: BM plasma cells ≥60%, serum free light chain (FLC) ratio ≥100:1, >1 focal lesion on MRI studies
- **Variants**
  smoldering MM: M protein >3 g/dL or plasmacytosis >10%, no myeloma-defining event or amyloidosis; risk of prog. 10%/y, depends on M protein concen., subtype, FLC ratio
  solitary bone plasmacytoma: 1 lesion w/o plasmacytosis or other ROTI
  extramedullary (nonosseous) plasmacytoma: usually upper respiratory tract
  plasma cell leukemia: plasma cell count >2000/μL in peripheral blood
  nonsecretory MM (~2% of MM Pts): no M protein, but marrow plasmacytosis & ROTI
- Ddx of M component: MM, MGUS (see below), CLL, lymphoma, sarcoidosis, AL. Polyclonal hypergam can be seen in inflammatory states: HIV, rheumatic dis., cirrhosis.
- Peripheral smear → rouleaux (see insert); ✓ Ca, alb, Cr; ↓ anion gap, ↑ globulin, ↑ ESR
- **Protein electrophoresis and immunofixation**
  serum protein electrophoresis (**SPEP**): quantitates M component; ⊕ in >80% of Pts
  urine protein electrophoresis (UPEP): detects Pts who secrete only light chains (= Bence Jones proteins), which are filtered rapidly from the blood
  immunofixation: shows component is monoclonal and identifies Ig type → IgG (50%), IgA (20%), IgD (2%), IgM (0.5%), light chain only (20%), nonsecretors (<5%)
  serum FLC assay: important for Pts (esp. ligh chain only Pts) and f/up response to Rx
- β_2-microglobulin and LDH levels reflect tumor burden
- **BM bx cytogenetics:** normal karyotype better than abnl. **Standard risk** = hyperdiploidy or t(11;14); **high risk** = hypodiploidy, del. 17p13 (~10% of Pts), t(4;14) & t(4;16)
- Gene mutations include TP53, NRAS, KRAS, BRAF, & NK-κB pathway (Nature 2011;471:467)
- **Skeletal survey** (plain radiographs) to identify lytic bone lesions and areas at risk for pathologic fracture; *bone scan is not useful for detecting lytic lesions*

Multiple Myeloma Staging Systems (OS does not account for cytogenetics)			
Stage	ISS criteria*	Durie-Salmon (DS) criteria	ISS Median OS
I	β_2-microglobulin <3.5 mg/L *and* **albumin** >3.5 g/dL	*all of the following:* Hb >10 g/dL; Ca ≤12 mg/dL; 0–1 lytic bone lesions; IgG <5 g/dL or IgA <3 g/dL or urine light chain <4 g/24 h	62 mo
II	fulfilling criteria for neither I nor III		44 mo
III	β_2-microglobulin >5.5 mg/L	*any of the following:* Hb <8.5 g/dL; Ca >12 mg/dL; >5 lytic bone lesions; IgG >7 g/dL or IgA >5 g/dL or urine light chain >12 g/24 h	29 mo (30 mo if Cr < 2 mg/dL; 15 mo if Cr ≥2 mg/dL)

*Consider R-ISS incl chrom abnl & LDH (JCO 2005;23:3412 & 2015;61:2267).

Treatment *(NEJM 2011;364:1046; Am J Hematol 2012;87:79)*

- Decisions generally dictated by *risk stratification* and *transplant eligibility*
- Active drugs incl. **proteasome inhibitors:** bortezomib (V), carfilzomib (Cz), ixazomib (I); **immunomodulators:** lenalidomide (R), thalidomide (T), pomalidomide; **immunotherapy:** daratumumab (anti-CD38), elotuzumab (SLAMF7)
  Other active drugs incl. prednisone (P), dexamethasone (D), melphalan (M), panobinostat, cyclophosphamide (Cy);
  CAR-T cells promising *(NEJM 2015;373:621&1207; Lancet 2016;387:1551)*
- Induction Rx regimens w/ best response rate combine proteasome inhib (V, Cz) & immunomod (R). Common induction regimens include doublets (RD, VD) or triplets (RVD, CyBorD), based on comorbidities and risk *(NEJM 2014;371:906 & 2016;374:1621)*.
- If *not* transplant eligible: **induction chemo** ↑ survival, not curative; consider maint chemo
- If transplant *eligible:* induction chemo (eg, RVD, VCD, RD; *Lancet 2010;376:2075*) then **high-dose melphalan + auto-HSCT.** Not curative, but ↑ survival c/w chemo *(NEJM 2014;371:895, Lancet Onc 2015;16:1617).* Offer if good perf. status & no prohibitive comorbid. Maint Rx w/ R improves PFS/OS *(NEJM 2014;371:10).* Timing of HSCT (upfront vs. relapse) debatable. Tandem auto-HSCT & allo-HSCT ↑ survival for some *(NEJM 2003;349:2495).*
- Relapsed/refractory: based on prior response & HSCT eligibility: HSCT (if good prior response, no prior HSCT), RD, CVD, VRD, CzRD, IRD, pomalidoimide+D, daratumumab
- Local radiation for solitary or extramedullary plasmacytoma
- Adjunctive Rx: bone: **bisphosphonates** *(JCO 2007;25:2464),* XRT for sx bony lesions
  renal: avoid NSAIDs & IV contrast; consider plasmapheresis for acute renal failure
  hyperviscosity syndrome: plasmapheresis; *infxns:* suppression; consider IVIg for recurrent infections
- Common **toxicities** of Rx: melphalan → myelosuppression; lenalidomide → low plts & thromboembolism; bortezomib → periph. neuropathy; steroids → hyperglycemia, infxn

MONOCLONAL GAMMOPATHY OF UNCERTAIN SIGNIFICANCE (MGUS)

Definition and epidemiology *(NEJM 2006;355:2765)*

- M prot. <3 g/dL, marrow plasmacytosis <10%, neither myeloma ROTI nor amyloidosis
- Prevalence ~3% in population >50 y of age, ~5% in population >70 y of age, and 7.5% in population >85 y of age *(NEJM 2006;354:1362)*

Management

- ✓ CBC, Ca, Cr, SPEP, serum free light chains, UPEP w/ immunofixation (to exclude MM)
- Close observation: repeat SPEP in 6 mo, then yearly thereafter if stable

Prognosis *(NEJM 2002;346:564)*

- ~1%/y or ~25% lifetime risk → MM, WM, amyloidosis, or malign. lymphoproliferative dis.
- Abnormal serum free light chain ratio: ↑ risk of progression to MM *(Blood 2005;105:812)*

WALDENSTRÖM'S MACROGLOBULINEMIA (WM)

Definition *(Blood 2009;114:2375)*

- B-cell neoplasm (lymphoplasmacytic lymphoma) that secretes monoclonal IgM
- 91% w/ *MYD88* (NF-κB pathway) L265P mut., may distinguish from MM *(NEJM 2012;367:826)*
- *No evidence of bone lesions* (IgM M component + lytic bone lesions = "IgM myeloma")

Clinical manifestations

- **Fatigue** from anemia is most common sx
- **Tumor infiltration:** BM (cytopenias), hepatomegaly, splenomegaly, lymphadenopathy
- **Circulating monoclonal IgM**
  hyperviscosity syndrome (~15%): *Neurologic:* blurred vision ("sausage" retinal veins), HA, dizziness, Δ MS. *Cardiopulmonary:* congestive heart failure, pulm. infiltrates.
  type I **cryoglobulinemia** → **Raynaud's phenomenon**
  platelet dysfxn → mucosal bleeding
- **IgM deposition** (skin, intestine, kidney); amyloidosis and glomerulopathy
- **Autoantibody activity of IgM:** Chronic AIHA (prominent **rouleaux;** 10% Coombs' ⊕ = AIHA). *Peripheral neuropathy:* may be due to IgM against myelin-associated glycoprotein.

Diagnostic evaluation

- SPEP + immunofixation with IgM >3 g/dL; 24-h urine for UPEP (only 20% have ⊕ UPEP)
- Bone marrow biopsy: ↑ plasmacytoid lymphocytes; β₂-microglobulin for prognostic eval
- **Relative serum viscosity:** defined as ratio of viscosity of serum to H₂O (nl ratio 1.8) hyperviscosity syndrome when relative serum viscosity >5–6

Treatment

- Hyperviscosity: **plasmapheresis**
- Sx (eg, prog. anemia): rituximab ± chemo (eg, bendamustine, Cy, etc.); ibrutinib esp. in *MYD88* mut/*CXCR4* wt *(NEJM 2015;372:1430).* Everolimus or HSCT in salvage.

Transplantation of donor pluripotent cells that can reconstitute all recipient blood lineages

Categories of Stem Cell Transplantation		
Feature	**Allogeneic (Allo)**	**Autologous (Auto)**
Donor-recipient relationship	Immunologically distinct	Donor is also recipient
Graft-vs.-host disease	Yes	No
Graft-vs.-tumor effect	Yes	No
Risk of graft contam. w/ tumor	No	Yes
Relapse risk (leukemia)	Lower	Higher
Transplant-related mortality	Higher	Lower

- **Types of Allo HSCT:** *based on donor/recipient matching of major HLA antigens on Chr. 6* (4 principal genes for serotyping: *HLA-A, -B, -C, & -DR*; each w/ 2 alleles ∴ 8 major Ag)
  Matched related (sibling matched at 8/8 major Ag): lowest risk of GVHD; preferred donor
  Mismatched related (eg, 1/8 Ag mismatch) or *haploidentical* (mismatch at 4/8 Ag):
    easiest to find, but ↑ risk of GVHD, rejection; ∴ need additional immunosuppression
  Matched unrelated: ↑ risk of GVHD; ∴ matching of 10 HLA alleles (*DQ* also) to ↓ risk;
    chance of match correlates w/ ethnicity (*NEJM 2014;371:339*)
  Umbilical cord blood: HSC processed at birth & stored; ↓ risk of GVHD; tolerate mismatch
    but much slower immune reconstitution (*Blood 2010;116:4693*)
- **Graft-vs.-host disease (GVHD):** *undesirable* side effect of allo HSCT
  allogeneic T cells view host cells as foreign; ↑ incid. w/ mismatch or unrelated donors
- **Graft-vs.-tumor (GVT):** *desired* effect in allo-SCT; graft T cells attack host tumor cells

Indications (*BBMT 2015;21:1863; BMT 2015;50:1037*)
- **Malignant disease:**
  Auto HSCT allows **higher ablative chemo doses** and then rescues the hematopoietic
    system (used for lymphoma, multiple myeloma, testicular cancer, neuroblastoma)
  Allo HSCT produces **graft-vs.-tumor** (GVT) effect, in addition to
    hematopoietic rescue (used for AML, ALL > CML, CLL, MDS, lymphoma)
- **Nonmalignant disease:** allo HSCT replaces abnl lymphohematopoietic system w/ one
    from nl donor (eg, immunodef., aplastic anemia, hemoglobinopathies, ? autoimmune dis.)

Transplantation procedure
- **Preparative regimen:** *chemotherapy and/or immunosuppression prior to transplantation*
  myeloablative conditioning ("MAC"): chemotherapy and/or total body irradiation. Goal is
    eradication of underlying disease for which transplant is being performed.
  reduced intensity conditioning ("RIC" or "mini"): lower dose conditioning → ↓ toxicity to
    allow Pts w/ comorbidities or ↑ age to tolerate HSCT. Goal = transplant when in
    remission. Depends mostly on GVT; ↓ transplant-related mortality, but ↑ relapse (*Blood
    2015;126:23*). Otherwise eligible candidates should have MAC.
- **Sources of stem cells:**
  bone marrow (BM): original source of HSCT, now less commonly used than PBSC
  peripheral blood stem cells (PBSC): easier to collect, more commonly used. BM vs.
    PBSC ≈ survival; BM ↓ chronic GVHD, PBSC ↓ graft failure, faster engraftment (*NEJM
    2012;367:1487*)
  umbilical cord blood (UCB): less stringent HLA-matching requirements, but fewer cells
    per donor (∴ 2 donors combined); slower engraftment, delayed immune recovery
  haploidentical: most available; new conditioning makes safer/more common
- **Engraftment:** absolute neutrophil count (ANC) recovers to 500/μL w/in ~2 wk w/ PBSC,
  ~2.5 wk w/ BM, ~4 wk w/ UCB. G-CSF accelerates recovery by 3–5 d in all scenarios.
  Engraftment syndrome: fever, rash, noncardiogenic pulm edema, abnl LFTs, AKI, wt gain.
    Dx of exclusion: r/o infection, GVHD; Rx w/ 1 mg/kg steroids, rapid taper over 3–4 d.

Complications
- Either **direct chemoradiotoxicities** associated with preparative regimen or consequences
  of **interaction between donor and recipient immune systems**
- **Sinusoidal obstruction syndrome (SOS):** incidence ~10%, mortality ~30%
  Previously known as **veno-occlusive disease (VOD)** (*BBMT 2016;22:400*). Mechanism:
    direct cytotoxic injury to hepatic venules → *in situ* thrombosis.
  Symptoms: tender hepatomegaly, ascites, jaundice, fluid retention
    with severe disease → liver failure, encephalopathy, hepatorenal syndrome
  Diagnosis: ↑ ALT/AST, ↑ bilirubin; ↑ PT with severe disease; Doppler U/S *may* show
    reversal of portal vein flow; ↑ hepatic wedge pressure; abnl liver bx
  Treatment: supportive; prophylaxis with **ursodiol**; treat w/ defibrotide (*Blood 2016;127:1656*)

- **Idiopathic pneumonia syndrome (IPS):** 5–25% of Pts, >50% mortality *(Blood 2003;102:2777)*
  Alveolar injury 2/2 direct toxicity → fever, hypoxia, diffuse infiltrates; occult infxn frequent
- **Diffuse alveolar hemorrhage (DAH):** Diagnosis: bronchoscopy to exclude infection;
  ↑ bloody lavage fluid seen with DAH. Treatment: pulse 500–1000 mg Solu-Medrol × 3 d
  ± etanercept *(BBMT 2015;1:67)*.
- **Acute GVHD** (usually within 6 mo of transplant; *Lancet 2009;373:1550*)
  Clinical grades I–IV based on scores for **skin** (severity of maculopapular rash), **liver**
  (bilirubin level) & **GI** (volume of diarrhea); bx supports diagnosis
  Prevention: **immunosuppression** (MTX + CsA or tacrolimus) or T-cell depletion of graft
  Treatment: grade I → topical Rx grades II–IV → associated with ↓ survival and ∴ treated
  with immunosuppressants (corticosteroids, CsA, tacrolimus, rapamycin, MMF)
- **Chronic GVHD** (developing or persisting beyond 3 mo posttransplant; *BMT 2009;43:149*)
  Clinical: malar rash, sicca syndrome, arthritis, obliterative bronchiolitis, bile duct
  degeneration, cholestasis and many others. More common w/ PBSC than BM.
  Treatment: immunosuppression; rituximab; photopheresis
- **Graft failure**
  Primary = persistent neutropenia without evidence of engraftment
  Secondary = delayed pancytopenia after initial engraftment; either immune mediated
  via immunocompetent host cells (**graft rejection**) or non–immune mediated (eg, CMV)
- **Infectious complications**
  due to regimen-induced pancytopenia and immunosuppression
  auto HSCT recipients: no immunosuppression ∴ at ↑ risk only pre-/postengraftment
  both primary infections and reactivation events occur (eg, CMV, HSV, VZV)

Timing of Complications following Allogeneic HSCT			
Time after transplant and associated risk factors			
	Days 0–30 Mucositis Organ dysfunction Neutropenia	**Days 30–90** Acute GVHD ↓ cellular immunity	**>90 days** Chronic GVHD ↓ cellular & humoral immunity
Viral infection	Respiratory and enteral viruses, BK virus		
	HSV*	CMV*, HHV 6 & 7	
		EBV-related lymphoma	
			VZV*, JC
Bacterial infection	Gram ⊕ cocci (coagulase-negative *Staph.*, *S. aureus, S. viridans*) GNRs (Enterobacteriaceae, *Pseudomonas*, *Legionella, S. maltophilia*)		Encapsulated bacteria
Fungal infection	*Candida* spp.		
		Aspergillus spp.	
Parasitic infection		*T. gondii* *P. carinii* *S. stercoralis*	*T. gondii* *P. carinii*
Regimen-related	Pancytopenia		Growth failure
	Mucositis, rash, alopecia		Hypogonadism/infertility
	Nausea, vomiting, diarrhea		Hypothyroidism
	Peripheral neuropathies		Cataracts
	Hemorrhagic cystitis		Avascular necrosis of bone
	Veno-occlusive disease		2nd malignancy
	IPS/Interstitial pneumonitis		
Immune-mediated	Acute GVHD		Chronic GVHD
	Primary graft failure	Secondary graft failure	

*Primarily among persons who are seropositive before transplant.

Prophylaxis/Supportive Medications during HSCT		
Medication	**Prophylaxis against**	**Duration**
Fluconazole or posaconazole	*Candida*	75 d
Acyclovir	HSV/VZV	365 d
Valganciclovir or ganciclovir if CMV ⊕	CMV	100 d or when no longer immunosuppressed
Antibiotics (eg, fluoroquinolone)	Bacterial infxn	While neutropenic
TMP-SMX	PCP	365 d or when off immunosupp.
Allopurinol	Hyperuricemia	Until d −1
Ursodiol	SOS/VOD	60 d

Pathology and Genetics				
	Pathology	**%**	**Typ locat.**	**Genetic mutations in**
Non-small cell	Adeno-carcinoma (incl. bronchioalveolar)	40	Peripheral	*KRAS* (20–30%), *EGFR* (15–20%, esp. ♀, Asian, never smokers), *HER2* (6%) or rearrang. in *ALK* (~4%), *ROS 1* (~2%) and *RET* (~1%)
	Squamous	20	Central	*FGFR1, SOX, PIK3CA, PTEN, TP53, SOX2, DDR2, BRAF*
	Large cell	5	Peripheral	
	Other/not classifiable	20		
Small cell		15	Central	Complex; most have inactiv. of *TP53* and *RB1*

(*NEJM* 2008;359:1367; *JCO* 2012;30:863; *J Thorac Oncol* 2012;7:924; *Nature* 2011;489:519; *Cell* 2012;150:1107)

Epidemiology and risk factors
- Most common cause of cancer-related death for both men and women in the U.S.
- **Cigarette smoking:** 85% of lung cancers occur in smokers; risk ∝ total pack-yrs,
  ↓ risk after quitting/reducing but not to baseline (*Int J Cancer* 2012;131:1210)
  squamous & small cell almost exclusively in smokers
  adenocarcinoma most common type in nonsmokers
  bronchioalveolar carcinoma associated with women, nonsmokers, *EGFR* mutations
- **Asbestos:** when combined with smoking, synergistic ↑ in risk of lung cancer
- Radon: risk to general population unclear

Clinical manifestations
- ~10% are asx at presentation and are detected incidentally by imaging
- **Endobronchial growth** of 1° tumor: **cough, hemoptysis, dyspnea,** wheezing, post-obstructive pneumonia; more common with squamous or small cell (central location)
- **Regional spread**
  pleural effusion, pericardial effusion, hoarseness (recurrent laryngeal nerve palsy), dysphagia (esophageal compression), stridor (tracheal obstruction)
  Pancoast's syndrome: apical tumor → brachial plexus involvement (C8,T1,T2) →
  Horner's syndrome, shoulder pain, rib destruction, atrophy of hand muscles
  SVC syndrome (*NEJM* 2007;356:1862): central tumor → SVC compression → face or
  arm swelling (>80%), venous distention of neck & chest wall (~60%),
  dyspnea/cough (~50%), HA (~10%); Rx = steroids & diuretics, RT ± chemo
  after tissue dx, SVC stent for severe sx, fibrinolytic + anticoag if thrombus
- **Extrathoracic metastases:** brain, bone, liver, adrenal
- **Paraneoplastic syndromes**
  Endocrine:
  ACTH (SCLC) → **Cushing's syndrome;** ADH (SCLC) → **SIADH**
  PTH-rP (squamous cell) → **hypercalcemia**
  Skeletal: digital clubbing (non–small cell), **hypertrophic pulmonary osteoarthropathy** (adenocarcinoma) = symmetric polyarthritis and proliferative periostitis of long bones
  Neurologic (SCLC): **Eaton-Lambert,** peripheral neuropathy, cerebellar degeneration, limbic encephalitis
  Cutaneous: acanthosis nigricans, dermatomyositis
  Hematologic: hypercoagulable state (adenocarcinoma), DIC, marantic endocarditis

Screening (*Lancet* 2014;382:732)
- No benefit to CXR or sputum cytology, even in high-risk Pts
- Annual low-dose chest CT in ≥30 pack-yr in current or former (quit w/in 15 y) smokers, age
  55–74 y → 20% ↓ in lung cancer–related mortality (*NEJM* 2011;365:395 & USPSTF)
  number needed to screen = 320; high false ⊕ rate
  consider risk scores to target screening (*NEJM* 2013;369:245 & 910; *JAMA* 2016;315:2300)

Diagnostic and staging evaluation (*NCCN Guidelines* v.2.2016)
- **Initial imaging:** chest CT (include liver and adrenal glands) w/ contrast if possible
- **Tissue: bronchoscopy** (central lesions) or **CT-guided needle bx** (peripheral
  lesions or accessible sites of suspected metastasis); mediastinoscopy (LN bx), VATS
  (eval. of pleura peripheral lesions), thoracentesis (cell block for cytology) or
  sputum cytology (central lesions)
- **Staging**
  Intrathoracic: **mediastinoscopy** (± preceded by U/S-guided transesoph. or transbronch.
  needle aspiration; *JAMA* 2010;304:2245) or **VATS;** thoracentesis if pleural effusion

Extrathoracic: **PET-CT** more Se than CT alone for detecting mediastinal and distant mets as well as bone mets in all Pts (except A) (*NEJM* 2009;361:32); **brain MRI** for all Pts

- **Genetics:** ✓ *EGFR* mut. & *ALK, ROS 1* or *RET* rearrang. for stage IV nonsquam NSCLC
- PFTs w/ quantitative V/Q if planned treatment includes surgical resection; need to have 30% of normal, predicted lung fxn *after* resection

TNM Staging System for NSCLC (7th Edition)

T/M stage	Definition	N stage N0 no ⊕ nodes	N1 ipsilat. hilar	N2 ipsilat. mediast.	N3 contralat. or supraclav.
T1	T ≤2 cm (T1a) or T >2–3 cm (T1b)	IA	IIA		
T2	T ≤5 cm (T2a) or T 5–7 cm (T2b)	IB/IIA	IIA/B		
T3	T >7 cm or invasion of chest wall, diaph., mediast. pleura, pericard.	IIB	IIIA		
T4	Invasion of mediast., heart, great vessels, trachea, esoph, vertebrae; separate tumor nodule ipsilat. lobe				IIIB
M1a	Nodules contralat lobe; pleural nodules or malignant effusion	IV			
M1b	Distant metastasis				

NSCLC treatment (*NCCN Guidelines* v.2.2016)

- **Stages I & II: surgical resection** + **adjuvant chemo** (surgery alone for stage IA) (*NEJM* 2004;350:351 & 2005;352:2589)
- **Stage III: chemoradiation** is main treatment modality
  IIIA viewed as potentially resectable (*Lancet* 2009;374:379) and IIIB as unresectable
  neoadjuvant chemoradiation may convert unresectable → resectable
- **Stage IV: chemotherapy** ↑ survival; early palliative care also ↑ survival (*NEJM* 2010;363:733)
  backbone of therapy is platinum-based doublet; cisplatin/pemetrexed better for adenocarcinoma; cisplatin/gemcitabine better for squamous (*JCO* 2008;26:3543)
    PD-1 inhib (eg, nivolumab, pembrolizumab, atezolizumab) if progression on chemo (*NEJM* 2015;373:123; *Lancet* 2016;387:1540 & 1837); immune-related adverse events include pneumonitis, consider Rx w/ high-dose corticosteroids
    bevacizumab (anti-VEGF mAb) + chemo ↑ survival by 2 mo; ↑ bleeding risk, ∴ avoid if untreated, brain mets (*JCO* 2009;27:5255), hemoptysis or squamous (*NEJM* 2006;355:2542)
    if EGFR mut.: EGFR tyrosine kinase inhibitor (TKI, eg, erlotinib) 1st-line Rx; next-gen EGFR TKI for those who develop resistance mutations (*NEJM* 2015;372:1689 & 1700)
    if ALK rearrang.: ALK TKI (crizotinib 1st-line Rx; *NEJM* 2014;371:2167); ceritinib 2nd-line TKI toxicities: rash & diarrhea (common); lung & liver injury (rare but potentially serious)
    palliative radiation used to control lung sx caused by tumor or metastasis
    solitary brain metastasis: surgical resection + brain radiation may ↑ survival

NSCLC Simplified Staging Schema, Treatment and 5-y Survival

Stage	% at dx	Definition	Treatment	5-y (%)
I	10–20	Isolated lesion	Surgery + chemo	>60
II	10–20	Hilar node spread	Surgery + radiation ± chemo	40–50
IIIA	15	Mediast. spread but resectable	Chemoradiation ± surgical resection	25–30
IIIB	15	Unresectable	Chemoradiation ± biologic ± surgery (selected cases)	10–20
IV	40	Metastatic	Chemo ± bevacizumab or tyrosine kinase inhibitor and/or supportive care	4

SCLC treatment (*NCCN Guidelines* v.1.2016)

- SCLC usually disseminated at presentation but can be very responsive to chemoradiation
- **Chemotherapy** (platinum + etoposide) is primary treatment modality
- **Thoracic radiation** added to chemotherapy improves survival in limited-stage disease
- **Prophylactic cranial irradiation** (PCI) ↑ survival for limited disease in complete remission (*NEJM* 1999;341:476) & ↓ symptomatic brain mets in extensive disease (*NEJM* 2007;357:664)

SCLC Staging Schema and Treatment

Stage	% at dx	Definition	Treatment	Median survival
Limited	30–40	Confined to ipsilat. hemithorax w/in 1 radiation port	Radiation + chemotherapy ± PCI	1–2 y
Extensive	60–70	Beyond 1 radiation port	Chemotherapy ± PCI	~1 y

BREAST CANCER

Epidemiology and genetics (risk assessment tool: www.cancer.gov/bcrisktool/)
- In U.S., most common cancer in women; 2nd leading cause of cancer death in women
- Age: incidence rates ↑ with age, with possible ↓ in slope after menopause
- **Genetics** (Nature 2012;490:61): mutations in TP53, PIK3CA, and GATA3; HER2 amplified. 15–20% have ⊕ FHx → 2× ↑ risk; ~45% of familial cases a/w known germline mutation **BRCA1/2**: 35–85% lifetime risk of breast cancer & ↑ risk of **ovarian cancer;** ↑ ? colon & prostate cancer; prog not worse than in noncarriers w/ breast cancer (NEJM 2007;357:115); BRCA2: a/w ↑ **male** breast cancer & pancreatic cancer. Germline loss-of-function mutations in PALB2 a/w 35% ↑ risk of breast cancer by age 70 (NEJM 2014;371:497).
- **Estrogen:** ↑ risk with early menarche, late menopause, late parity or nulliparity (NEJM 2006;354:270); ↑ risk with prolonged HRT (RR = 1.24 after 5.6 y; JAMA 2003;289:3243); no ↑ risk shown with OCP use (NEJM 2002;346:2025)
- Benign breast conditions: ↑ risk w/ atypia (atypical ductal or lobular hyperplasia; NEJM 2015;372:78) & proliferative (ductal hyperplasia, papilloma, radial scar, or sclerosing adenosis) features; no ↑ risk w/ cysts, fibroadenoma, or columnar changes
- ↑ risk with h/o ionizing radiation to chest for treatment of Hodgkin lymphoma

Prevention (with selective estrogen receptor modulator or AI; Annals 2013;159:698)
- **Tamoxifen:** ↓ risk contralat. breast CA as adjuvant Rx. Approved for $1°$ prevent. if ↑ risk: ↓ invasive breast cancer, but ↑ DVT & uterine CA; ? ↑ in mortality (JAMA 2006;295:2727)
- **Raloxifene:** ↓ risk of invasive breast cancer & vertebral fx, ↑ risk of stroke & DVT/PE (NEJM 2006;355:125); ≈ tamoxifen in prevention of breast cancer & ↓ risk of DVT/PE & cataracts, trend toward ↓ uterine cancer (JAMA 2006;295:2727)
- AIs in high-risk postmeno ↓ breast cancer by >50% (NEJM 2011;364:2381; Lancet 2014;383:1041)
- BRCA 1/2 ⊕: intensified surveillance. Prophylactic bilat. mastectomy → ~90% ↓ risk; bilat. salpingo-oophorectomy ↓ risk of ovarian and breast cancer (NEJM 2016;374:454).

Clinical manifestations
- Breast mass (hard, irregular, fixed, nontender), nipple discharge (higher risk if unilateral, limited to 1 duct, bloody, associated with mass)
- Special types: **Paget's** disease → unilateral nipple eczema + nipple discharge; **inflammatory** breast cancer → skin erythema and edema (peau d'orange)
- Metastases: lymph nodes, bone, liver, lung, brain

Screening (JAMA 2015;314:1599; Annals 2016;164:279)
- **Mammography:** ~20–30% ↓ in breast cancer mortality (smaller abs. benefit in women <50 y) (Lancet 2006;368:2053; Annals 2009;151:727); 75% of all abnl findings benign; suspicious: clustered **microcalcifications, spiculated, enlarging**
- ACS recommends annual mammogram beginning at age 45 (consider biennial after age 54)
- USPSTF recommends beginning at 50 and biennially (some may want to begin at age 40)
- ↑ risk: screen earlier w/ CBE and mammo (age 25 in BRCA 1/2 carrier, 5–10 y before earliest FHx case, 8–10 y after thoracic RT, upon dx of ↑ risk benign disease)
- **MRI:** superior to mammo in high-risk Pts; consider annually if >20% lifetime risk (eg, ⊕⊕ FHx, BRCA 1/2, prior chest RT) (Lancet 2011;378:1804)
- **Genetic testing** should be considered in women with strong FHx

Diagnostic evaluation
- **Palpable breast mass:** age <30 y → observe for resolution over 1–2 menstrual cycles; age <30 y, unchanging mass → **U/S** → aspiration if mass not simple cyst; age >30 y or solid mass on U/S or bloody aspirate or recurrence after aspiration → **mammo** (detect other lesions) and either **fine-needle asp.** or **core-needle bx** clearly cancerous on exam or indeterminate read or atypia on bx → **excisional bx**
- **Suspicious mammogram** with normal exam: stereotactically guided bx
- MRI: detects contralateral cancer in 3% of Pts w/ recently dx breast cancer & ⊖ contra-lateral mammo (but PPV only 21%) (NEJM 2007;356:1295); utility remains unclear

Staging
- **Anatomic:** tumor size, chest wall invasion, axillary LN mets (strongest prognostic factor)
- **Histopathologic:** type (little prognostic relevance) & grade; lymphatic/vascular invasion
  In situ carcinoma: no invasion of surrounding stroma
    Ductal (DCIS): ↑ risk of invasive cancer in ipsilateral breast (~30%/10 y)
    Lobular (LCIS): marker of ↑ risk of invasive cancer in either breast (~1%/y)
  Invasive carcinoma: infiltrating ductal (70–80%); invasive lobular (5–10%); tubular, medullary and mucinous (10%, better prognosis); papillary (1–2%); other (1–2%)
  Inflammatory breast cancer (see above): not a histologic type but a clinical reflection of tumor invasion of dermal lymphatics; very poor prognosis
  Paget disease: ductal cancer invading nipple epidermis ± associated mass

- **Biomarkers**: ✓ estrogen, progesterone receptor (ER/PR) and *HER2/neu* status
- Oncotype DX 21-gene risk recurrence score has predictive and prognostic value in ER ⊕, HER2 ⊖, and node ⊖ Pts (NEJM 2015;373:2005)
- Circulating tumor DNA may serve as biomarker of met tumor burden (NEJM 2013;368:1199)

Simplified Staging System for Breast Cancer			
Stage	Characteristics	Description	5-y surv.
I	Tumor ≤2 cm	Operable locoregional	90%
IIA	Tumor >2 cm or *mobile* axillary nodes	Operable locoregional	80%
IIB	Tumor >5 cm		65%
IIIA	Internal mammary or *fixed* axillary nodes	Locally advanced	50%
IIIB	Direct extension to chest wall or skin	Inoperable locoregional	45%
IIIC	Infraclavicular or supraclavicular nodes		40%
IV	Distant metastases	Metastatic	25%

Treatment

- **Local control: surgery and radiation therapy (RT)**
  - *Breast-conserving* usual approach w/ lumpectomy + breast RT + axillary node dissection (ALND), unless multicentric dis., diffuse microCa²⁺, BRCA1/2 ⊕, prior RT, pregnant, ? tumor >5 cm; cavity shaving ↓ risk of need for re-excision (NEJM 2015;373:503)
  - *Sentinel lymph node dissection (SLND)* prior to ALND preferred if w/o palp axillary LNs; T1-2 w/ ⊕ SLND & Rx w/ lumpect./RT/chemo may not need ALND (JAMA 2011;305:569)
  - *Radiation therapy* (RT) after mastectomy for ≥4 ⊕ LN, tumor >5 cm, or ⊕ surgical margins → ↓ locoregional recurrence and ↑ survival (Lancet 2011;378:1707); regional nodal RT ↓ recurrence and breast cancer mortality (NEJM 2015;373:307 & 317)
- **Systemic therapy**: for stage I-III except tumors <1 cm (complex risk assessment needed). http://www.adjuvantonline.com/index.jsp can guide use of chemo and/or hormonal Rx.
  - *Chemotherapy:* neoadjuvant (to ↑ breast conservation; path complete response a/w ↑ disease-free survival; Lancet 2014;384:164) or *adjuvant* (anthracycline-based). Addition of taxane (eg, paclitaxel) → small ↑ survival (NEJM 2010;362:2053 & 2010;363:2200). Consider platinum in triple ⊖ cancers (JCO 2015;33:13).
  - *Anti-HER2 therapy* (growing list of agents) in *HER2* ⊕ tumors (NEJM 2012;366:176)
    - **trastuzumab** (anti-*HER2* mAb) ↑ survival (NEJM 2011;365:1273); 1 y = 2 yr (Lancet 2013;382:1021); after anthracycline or w/ taxane to ↓ cardiotox (JCO 2002;20:1215)
    - **lapatinib** (tyrosine kinase inhib. of *HER2* & *EGFR*) + trastuzumab ↑ survival after failing trastuzumab (JCO 2012;30:2585); dual inhib. initial Rx ↑ response (Lancet 2012;379:633)
    - **pertuzumab** (anti-*HER2* mAb, prevents dimerization) ↑ progression-free survival when added to trastuzumab as 1ˢᵗ-line Rx for metastatic dis. (NEJM 2015;372:724)
    - **trastuzumab emtansine** (T-DM1, *HER2* mAb conjugated to microtubule inhibitor) ↑ survival compared to 2ⁿᵈ-line lapatinib + capecitabine (NEJM 2012;367:1783)
  - *Bevacizumab* (anti-VEGF): ? in neoadjuvant Rx if *HER2* ⊖ (NEJM 2012;366:299 & 310)
  - *Hormonal* (in ER/PR ⊕ or unknown status)
    - **tamoxifen:** 39% ↓ recurrence and 30% ↓ breast cancer mortality in pre- and post-menopausal patients; 10 y of Rx superior to 5 y (Lancet 2011; 378:771 & 2013;381:805)
    - **aromatase inhibitors (AI)** (anastrozole, letrozole, exemestane): ~18% ↓ recurrence vs. tamoxifen in *postmenopausal* Pts (NEJM 2005;353:2747 & 2016;375:209)
    - 2ⁿᵈ-line: ovarian ablation with LHRH agonists (goserelin) or oophorectomy if *premenopausal;* pure antiestrogens (fulvestrant) if *postmenopausal*
  - *Cell proliferation inhibitors* (if postmenopausal & failed hormonal Rx)
    - **palbociclib** (CDK 4/6 inhib): ↑ progression-free survival (NEJM 2015;373:209)
    - **everolimus** (mTOR inhib): ↑ progression-free survival (NEJM 2012;366:520)

Treatment of Carcinoma *in situ* and Invasive Carcinoma of the Breast	
LCIS	Close surveillance + chemoprevention; ? prophylactic bilat. mastectomy
DCIS	Mastect. or lump. + RT; ALND *not* indic.; + chemoprev (Lancet 2016;387:849 & 866)
I II	Surgery + RT + Adjuvant chemo if ↑ risk: tumor >1 cm or ⊕ LN or ER/PR ⊖ (Lancet 1998;352:930) + Hormonal therapy if ER/PR ⊕ (or unknown status) (Lancet 2009;374:2055) + anti-*HER2* Rx if *HER2* ⊕ and tumor ≥1 cm or ⊕ LN
III	Neoadjuvant chemo → surgery + RT ± adjuvant chemotherapy + Hormonal therapy for ER/PR ⊕ (or unknown status) tumors + anti-*HER2* Rx if *HER2* ⊕
IV	ER/PR⊕: hormonal Rx (NEJM 2012;367:435) or chemo ± everolimus/palbociclib ER/PR⊖: *HER2* ⊕ → chemo + anti-*HER2* therapy; *HER2* ⊖ → chemotherapy Bony mets: bisphosphonates & denosumab ↓ fractures (Cochrane 2012;CD003474)

PROSTATE CANCER

Epidemiology and risk factors (NEJM 2003;349:366)
- Most common cancer in U.S. men; 2nd most common cause of cancer death in men
- Lifetime risk of prostate cancer dx ~16%; lifetime risk of dying of prostate cancer ~3%
- ↑ risk with ↑ age (rare if <45 y), in African Americans, ⊕ FHx, BRCA mutations

Clinical manifestations (usually asymptomatic at presentation)
- **Obstructive sx** (more common with BPH): hesitancy, ↓ stream, retention, nocturia
- **Irritative sx** (also seen with prostatitis): frequency, dysuria, urgency
- Periprostatic spread: hematuria, hematospermia, new-onset erectile dysfunction
- Metastatic disease: bone pain, spinal cord compression, cytopenias

Screening (NEJM 2012;367:e11; JAMA 2014;311:1143; Lancet 2014;384:2027)
- **Digital rectal exam** (DRE): size, consistency, lesions
- **PSA:** 4 ng/mL cut point neither Se nor Sp; can ↑ with BPH, prostatitis, acute retention, after bx or TURP, and ejaculation (no significant ↑ after DRE, cystoscopy);
  15% of men >62 y w/ PSA <4 & nl DRE have bx-proven T1 cancer (NEJM 2004;350:2239)
- ACS rec: ≥50 y (or ≥ 45 y if African-Am or ⊕ FHx) should discuss PSA screening w/ MD; USPSTF rec. against screening in asx males (no ↓ in prostate cancer-related mort.)

Diagnostic and staging evaluation
- **Transrectal ultrasound** (TRUS) **guided biopsy**, with 6–12 core specimens
- **Histology: Gleason grade** (2–10; low grade ≤6) = sum of the differentiation score (1 = best, 5 = worst) of the 2 most prevalent patterns in the bx; correlates with prognosis
- **Imaging:** to evaluate extraprostatic spread
  bone scan: for PSA >10 ng/mL, high Gleason grade or clinically advanced tumor
  abdomen-pelvis CT: inaccurate for detecting extracapsular spread and lymph node mets
  endorectal coil MRI: improves assessment of extracapsular spread

Stage	Tumor	Nodes, Mets	Treatment

TNM Staging & Treatment of Prostate Cancer (Lancet 2015;387:70)

Stage	Tumor	Nodes, Mets	Treatment
I	T1a = non-palp., not visible on imaging	N0, M0, Gleason 2–4	**Surveillance:** consider if life expect. <10 y. Dutasteride ↓ risk of progression (Lancet 2012;379:1103). **Radiation** (external or brachy; NEJM 2006;355:1583). Short-term androgen deprivation ↓ mort. (NEJM 2011;365:107)
II	T1/T2 = w/ in prostate	N0, M0	**Radical prostatectomy** (± RT and/or hormonal Rx if high-risk features): ↓ prostate cancer mortality, espec. if <65 y and not low risk (NEJM 2014;370:932)
III	T3 = extends thru capsule	N0, M0	**Radiation** + androgen deprivation (see below) (Lancet 2011;378:2104)
IV	T4 = invades adjacent structures	N0, M0	**Radiation** (for M0 disease) **Androgen deprivation Rx (ADT)** (NEJM 2009;360:2516) **GnRH analogues** (leuprolide, goserelin) **antiandrogens** (flutamide, bicalutamide).
		N1, M0	
	Any T	Any N, M1	**Docetaxel** added to ADT improves overall survival in metastatic disease (NEJM 2015;373:737) **If castrate resistant:** chemo (eg, docetaxel); androgen synthesis inhib. (abiraterone; NEJM 2011;364:1995) or receptor signaling inhib. (enzalutamide; NEJM 2012;367:1187) ↓ mort.; immuno Rx (NEJM 2010;363:411); olaparib (PARP inhib) if BRCA ⊕ (NEJM 2015;373:1697) **Bone mets:** bisphosph or denosumab, latter ↓ bone mets & fx (NEJM 2009;361:745; Lancet 2011;377:813 & 2012;379:39); radium-223 ↓ mortality by 30% (NEJM 2013;369:213)

Prognosis
- PSA level, Gleason grade and age are predictors of metastatic disease
- In surgically treated Pts, 5-y relapse-free survival >90% if disease confined to organ, ~75% if extension through capsule, and ~40% if seminal vesicle invasion
- PSA doubling time, Gleason, & time to biochemical recurrence predict mortality following recurrence. For local recurrence following RP, salvage RT may be beneficial if low PSA.
- Metastatic disease: median survival ~44-57 mo (NEJM 2015;373:737); all become castrate resistant (in 15–20% discontinuation of antiandrogens results in paradoxical ↓ in PSA)

Prevention
- Finasteride and dutasteride ↓ prostate cancers detected by bx, but ↑ # of high Gleason grade tumors; no Δ in overall mortality (NEJM 2003;349:215; 2010;362:1192; 2013;369:603)

COLORECTAL CANCER (CRC)

Epidemiology and risk factors (Lancet 2010;375:1030; CA Cancer J Clin 2011;61:212)

- 4th most common cancer in U.S. men & women; 2nd leading cause of all cancer death
- Rare before age 40, w/ 90% of cases occurring after age 50. ~75% are sporadic.
- **Family history:** up to 25% of Pts have ⊕ FHx. Risk depends on # of 1st-degree relatives (w/ CRC or polyp) and their age at dx; ~5% have an identifiable germline mutation

  Familial adenomatous polyposis (FAP): mutation in *APC* gene → 1000s of polyps at young age → ~100% lifetime risk; ↑ risk of thyroid, stomach, small bowel cancers

  Hereditary nonpolyposis colorectal cancer (HNPCC): most common hereditary CRC (~3% of all CRC); mutations in DNA mismatch repair genes (eg, *MSH2, MLH1*) → microsatellite instability (MSI) → ↑ tumor progression → ~80% lifetime risk.

  Predom. **right-sided** tumors; ↑ risk of **endometrial**, ovarian, stomach, urothelial, small bowel and pancreatic cancers.

  Amsterdam criteria: ≥3 family members w/ HNPCC-related cancer, one of which is dx before age 50, affecting 2 successive generations.

  MAP (MYH-assoc polyposis): autosomal *recessive*; consider if mult. polyps but ⊖ for FAP
- **Inflammatory bowel disease:** ↑ risk with ↑ extent and duration of disease
- **COX-2:** ↓ risk of adenomas w/ ASA & NSAIDs. ASA a/w ↓ CRC incidence, mets and mort. (Lancet 2010;376:1741; 2012;379:1591 & 1602). ASA effect limited to *PIK3CA*-mut CRC (NEJM 2012;367:1596). ASA rec for 1° prevention if age 50–59 (69?) y & ≥10% 10-y risk of CRC.

Pathology and genetics (NEJM 2009;361:2449; Nature 2012;487:330)

- **Adenoma → carcinoma sequence** reflects accumulation of multiple genetic mutations. ↑ risk of malig. w/ large (>2.5 cm), villous, sessile adenomatous polyps. Adenomas typically observed ~10 y prior to onset of cancer (both sporadic & familial).
- Genetic profile in sporadic CRC: *APC* (~80%), *KRAS* (~40%), *TP53* (50–70%), *DCC* or *SMAD4*, or *BRAF* (~15%); chrom instability (majority) or mismatch repair defic (10–15%)
- Upfront genotyping may guide Rx; eg, benefit of anti-EGFR Ab cetuximab greater in *KRAS* wild-type than KRAS mutant (NEJM 2008;359:1757). *BRAF* mutation may guide clinical trials. Lack of CDX2 a/w ↑ benefit from chemo (NEJM 2016;374:211).

Clinical manifestations

- Distal colon: Δ **bowel habits, obstruction,** colicky abdominal pain, **hematochezia**
- Proximal colon: **iron defic. anemia,** dull vague abd pain; obstruction atypical due to larger lumen, liquid stool and polypoid tumors (*vs.* annular distal tumors)
- Metastases: nodes, **liver,** lung, peritoneum → RUQ tenderness, ascites, supraclavicular LN
- Associated with *Streptococcus bovis* bacteremia and *Clostridium septicum* sepsis

Screening (JAMA 2016;315:2564)

- **Average risk:** colonoscopy starting at age 50 & repeat q10y strongly preferred method
- **↑ risk:** earlier and/or more frequent screening. → FHx: age 40 or 10 y before index dx, then q5y. IBD: 8–10 y after dx, then q1–2y. Known or suspected familial syndrome: genetic counseling & very early screening (eg, age 20–25 y), then q1–2y.
- **Imaging**

  Colonoscopy: test of choice as examines entire colon; 90% Se for lesions >1 cm. Flex sig less Se vs. colo and CTC (Gut 2009;58:241). If polyp found, re ✓ in 3–5 y. Removal of adenomatous polyps associated with lower CRC mortality (NEJM 2012;366:687).

  Sigmoidoscopy: 21% ↓ incidence in CRC & 26% ↓ mortality in distal CRC (NEJM 2012;366:2345). Benefit may also be seen w/ 1-time flex-sig (Lancet 2010;375:9726).

  CT colonography (CTC): c/w colonoscopy, ~90% Se for lesions ≥1 cm but considerably less for smaller lesions (NEJM 2008;359:1207). In high-risk Pts, Se only 85% for advanced neoplasia ≥6 mm (JAMA 2009;301:2453). At population level, ↑ participation w/ CTC, but ↓ yield vs colonoscopy; ∴ similar screening overall (Lancet 2012;13:55).
- **Biochemical fecal testing**

  Occult blood (FOBT): ↓ mortality (NEJM 1993;328:1365 & 2000;343:1603); 3 card home testing more Se (24% vs. 5%) than DRE/FOBT (Annals 2005;142:81). Repeat q1y.

  DNA: ↑ Se, ≈ Sp c/w FOBT but less Se than colonoscopy (NEJM 2004;351:2704) Combo DNA + Hb immunoassay w/ ~90% Se & Sp (NEJM 2014;370:1287)

Staging (AJCC Cancer Staging Manual, 7th ed, 2010)

- TNM staging: Size/depth of primary (T), locoregional nodes (N), distant metastases (M). Staging is complex and based on pathologic correlation with observed survival data.
- **Colonoscopy + biopsy/polypectomy + intraoperative** and **pathologic** staging essential for evaluating extracolonic spread
- CT scans of chest and abdomen/pelvis (inaccurate for depth of invasion & malignant LN)
- Baseline **CEA** in Pt *with known CRC* has prognostic significance and is useful to follow-low response to therapy and detect recurrence; *not* a screening tool

Treatment Based on TNM and Modified Dukes Staging of Colorectal Cancer

TNM	Dukes	Path. criteria	5-y surv.	Treatment
I	A	Into submucosa or muscularis	94–97%	Surgery alone (resection and analysis of ≥12 LN)
IIA	B	Into serosa	83%	Surgery; no established role for adjuvant chemo for colon cancer[a]
IIB	B	Into peritoneum	74%	
IIC	B	Direct invasion	56%	Preop RT or 5-FU/RT added for rectal cancer → postop chemo
IIIA	C	≤6 ⊕ LNs	86%	Surgery + chemotherapy[b]
IIIB	C	Varying # ⊕ LNs	51–77%	Preop RT or chemorad added for rectal cancer (NEJM 2006;355:1114)
IIIC	C	& local invasion	15–47%	
IV	D	Distant metastases	5%	Chemotherapy ± surgical resection for isolated mets (~30% 5-y surv) Consider resection of 1° tumor if perf, obstruction or bleeding

NCCN Clinical Practice Guidelines, www.nccn.org. 5-y survival data are approx. equivalent for colon and rectal cancers, shown as average, w/ ranges for TNM substaging, adapted from SEER data (JCO 2010;28:256 & 264). [a]Consider adjuvant chemo for high-risk stage II (obstruction, perf, adherence to adjacent structures, inadequate nodal sampling, lymphovasc invasion, poorly differentiated). MSI-high CRC benefit less from adjuvant chemo (NEJM 2003;349:247). [b]Adjuvant FOLFOX (see below) is standard of care chemo (NEJM 2004;350:2343).

- Chemotherapy (Lancet 2014;383:1490)
  FOLFOX (**5-FU + leucovorin + oxaliplatin**), FOLFIRI or CapeOx (NEJM 2004;350:2343)
  ± Bevacizumab (anti-VEGF, NEJM 2004;350:2335) or cetuximab/panitumumab (anti-EGFR mAb, NEJM 2004;351:337; benefit limited to Pts w/o RAS mutations; NEJM 2013;369:1023)
  Consider FOLFOXIRI-bevacizumab particularly if BRAF⊕ mutations or needing response for potentially curative resection (NEJM 2014;371:1609)
  Regorafenib (multikinase inhib.) and TAS102 (trifluridine + tipiracil) ↑ survival in progressive metastatic CRC (Lancet 2013;381:303; NEJM 2015;372:1909)

CHEMOTHERAPY SIDE EFFECTS

Nausea & vomiting common (NEJM 2016;374:1356; 375:134 & 177)

Select Adverse Effects from Chemotherapy

Toxicity	Common Agents	Comments
Cardiotoxicity (JCO 2005;23:7685; NEJM 2013;368:1154) Stop agent if adverse event; ? role for ACEI in prevention (Circ 2006;114:2474).	**Anthracyclines**	Dose-dependent CMP; ✓ EF pre-Rx; via topoisomerase IIb (Nat Med 2012;18:1639)
	5-FU	Spasm → ischemia; CCB may prevent
	Trastuz. & PD-1 inhib	CMP, esp. w/ concom anthracycline
	Tyrosine kinase inhib. (TKI)	QTc prolongation, CMP, angina
	Cyclophosphamide	Myopericarditis (esp. in BMT)
	Cisplatin	HypoMg → arrhythmia, ischemia
Pulmonary (Sem Oncol 2006;33:98)	Busulfan	~8% fibrosis or DAH; if severe → steroids
	Bleomycin	~10% IPF; d/c drug, Rx w/ steroids
	TKI (esp. dasatinib)	Pulmonary effusion
	Cyclophosphamide (<1%)	Pneumonitis, progressive fibrosis; d/c drug
	Bevacizumab	Pulm hemorrhage (esp. NSCLC)
	Anti-PD1 (eg, nivolumab)	Pneumonitis
	Anti-CTLA-4 (ipilimumab)	Organizing pneumonia, sarcoidosis
Nephrotoxicity/ urologic toxicity	Platinum Rx (**cisplatin**)	Esp. proximal tubule; pretreat w/ IV saline
	Methotrexate	Rx deposition; alkalinize urine, hydration
	Cyclophosphamide	Hemorrhagic cystitis; give Mesna
Neurotoxicity (Sem Oncol 2006;33:324)	Platinum Rx (**cisplatin**)	"Stocking-glove;" vit. E Ppx (JCO 2003;21:927)
	Cytarabine	Cerebellar toxicity (irreversible 5–10%)
	Methotrexate (esp. intrathecal)	Late leukoenceph, meningitis; reverse w/ intrathecal glucarpidase, leucovorin
	Ifosfamide	Enceph (10–30%); ? Rx w/ methylene blue, thiamine, dexmedetomidine
	Taxanes, vincristine	Sensorimotor long fiber neuropathy
Hepatotoxicity (Sem Oncol 2006;33:50)	TKI (eg, imatinib, nilotinib)	↑ LFTs, rarely necrosis; hold Rx, ? steroids
	Gemcitabine	Common ↑ ALT/AST; ↓ dose if ↑ bili
	Methotrexate	↑ ALT/AST, rarely fibrosis
Dermatologic	TKI (eg, imatinib)	Dermatitis, can be severe (eg, SJS)

PANCREATIC TUMORS

Pathology and genetics (Ann Rev Pathol 2008;3:157; Nature 2012;491:399)
- Histologic types: adenocarcinoma, acinar cell carcinoma, endocrine tumors, cystic neoplasms (eg, IPMN, see below); rarely, mets to pancreas (eg, lung, breast, renal cell)
- Pancreatic adenocarcinoma accounts for majority of pancreatic cancer (~85%)
- Location: ~60% in head, 15% in body, 5% in tail; in 20% diffuse infiltration of pancreas
- Mutations in adenoca.: KRAS (>90%), p16 (80–95%), p53 (50–75%), SMAD4 (~55%)

Epidemiology and risk factors (NEJM 2014;371:1039; Lancet 2016;388:73)
- Pancreatic adenocarcinoma 4th leading cause of cancer death in U.S. men and women
- 80% of pancreatic adenocarcinomas occur in Pts 60–80 y
- Acquired risk factors: **smoking** (RR ~1.5; 20% Pts), obesity, chronic pancreatitis, ? diabetes
- Hereditary risk factors: genetic susceptibility may play a role in 5–10% of cases
  Hereditary chronic pancreatitis: mutation in cationic trypsinogen gene (PRSS 1), SPINK 1
  Familial cancer syndromes and gene mutations with ↑ risk: familial atypical multiple mole melanoma (CDKN2A/p16), familial breast and ovarian cancer (BRCA2), Peutz-Jeghers (LKB 1), ataxia-telangiectasia (ATM), ? hereditary colorectal cancer (HNPCC and FAP)

Clinical manifestations
- **Painless jaundice** (w/ pancreatic head mass), **pain** radiating to back, ↓ **appetite & wt**
- New-onset atypical diabetes mellitus (25%); unexplained malabsorption or steatorrhea
- Migratory thrombophlebitis (Trousseau's sign), not specific to panc cancer (JCO 1986;4:509)
- Exam: abd mass; nontender, palpable gallbladder (Courvoisier's sign, but more often seen w/ biliary tract cancers); hepatomegaly; ascites; left supraclavicular (Virchow's) node & palpable rectal shelf (both nonspecific signs of carcinomatosis)
- Laboratory tests may show ↑ bilirubin, ↑ alk phos, anemia

Diagnostic and staging evaluation (NCCN Guidelines v.2.2012)
- **Pancreatic protocol CT scan** (I⁺ w/ arterial & venous phase imaging) **or MRI**
- If no lesion seen, → EUS, ERCP, MRI/MRCP may reveal mass or malignant ductal strictures
- Biopsy pancreatic lesion via EUS-guided FNA (preferred in potential surgical candidates) or CT-guided (potential risk of seeding) or biopsy of possible metastasis
- ↑ CA19-9 (nb, also ↑ in benign liver/biliary disease); may be useful to follow dis. postop

Clinical (Radiologic) Staging & Prognosis of Pancreatic Adenocarcinoma		
Stage (% at dx)	**Criteria**	**Median Survival**
Resectable, 15–20%	No extrapanc. dis. or bulky LAN Patent SMV & portal vein; celiac axis & SMA not involved	10–20 mo (favorable: tumor <3 cm, ⊖ marg., well-differen.) 5-y ~30% node ⊖ vs. ~10% if ⊕
Locally advanced (unresect.), 40%	Extensive PV/SMV, celiac axis or SMA involvement	8–12 mo
Metastatic, 40%	Usually liver & periton.; occ lung	Up to 11 mo w/ FOLFIRINOX

Treatment of pancreatic adenocarcinoma (NEJM 2014;371:1039; Lancet 2016;388:73)
- Resectable: surgery ± adjuvant (neoadjuvant or postoperative) therapy
  pancreaticoduodenectomy = **Whipple procedure** = resection of pancreatic head, duodenum, CBD and gallbladder ± partial gastrectomy
  adjuvant therapy: ↑ survival, but choice of regimen controversial (chemo vs. chemo/RT and gemcitabine vs. 5-FU (J Surg Oncol 2013;107:78; JAMA 2013;310:1473)
- Locally advanced: optimal strategy controversial. Gemcitabine alone vs. gemcitabine + RT (JCO 2008;26:214s; Ann Oncol 2008;19:1592; JCO 2011;29:4105).
- Metastatic: **FOLFIRINOX** (5-FU + leucovorin, irinotecan, oxaliplatin) if good perform. status (NEJM 2011;364:1817); **gemcitabine** + nab-paclitaxel (NEJM 2013;369:1691) or gemcitabine monotherapy if poor performance status (JCO 1997;15:2403). Offer clinical trials.
- Palliative and supportive care:
  obstructive jaundice or gastric outlet obstruction: endoscopic stenting or surgical bypass
  pain: opiates, celiac plexus neurolysis, radiation therapy
  weight loss: pancreatic enzyme replacement, nutrition consult, end-of-life discussions

Cystic lesions of the pancreas (NEJM 2004;351:1218; Oncologist 2009;14:125)
- <10% of pancreatic neoplasms. Dx w/ CT, ERCP, MRCP, or EUS.
- **Serous cystadenoma**: usually benign; central scar or honeycomb appearance on imaging
- **Mucinous cystic neoplasm** (MCN): predominantly young females; multiloculated tumors in body or tail w/ ovarian-type stroma and mucin-rich fluid w/ ↑ CEA levels; precancerous
- **Intraductal papillary mucinous neoplasm** (IPMN): neoplasm arising in main pancreatic duct or a branch; a/w ductal dilation w/ extrusion of mucinous material. Uncertain progression to cancer (? 5–20 y). Surgery based on age, size, location, & dysplasia.

FEVER AND NEUTROPENIA (FN)

Definition
- Fever: single oral temp ≥38.3°C (101°F) or ≥38°C (100.4°F) for ≥1 h
- **Neutropenia:** ANC <500 cells/μL or <1000 cells/μL with predicted nadir <500 cells/μL

Pathophysiology and microbiology
- Predisposing factors: catheters, skin breakdown, GI mucositis, obstruction (lymphatics, biliary tract, GI, urinary tract), immune defect a/w malignancy
- Most episodes thought to result from seeding of bloodstream by GI flora
- Neutropenic enterocolitis (typhlitis): RLQ pain, watery/bloody diarrhea, cecal wall thickening
- GNRs (esp. *P. aeruginosa*) were historically most common
- Gram ⊕ infections have recently become more common (60–70% of identified organisms)
- Fungal superinfection often results from prolonged neutropenia & antibiotic use
- Infection with atypical organisms and bacterial meningitis is rare

Prevention
- Levofloxacin (500 mg qd) ↓ febrile episodes & bacterial infections in chemo-related high-risk neutropenic patients; no difference in mortality (*NEJM 2005;353:977 & 988*)

Diagnostic evaluation
- Exam: skin, oropharynx, lung, perirectal area, surgical & catheter sites; avoid DRE
- Labs: CBC with differential, electrolytes, BUN/Cr, LFTs, U/A
- Micro: blood (peripheral & through each indwelling catheter port), urine, & sputum cx; for localizing s/s ✓ stool (*C. difficile*, cx), peritoneal fluid, CSF (rare source)
- Imaging: CXR; for localizing s/s → CNS, sinus, chest or abdomen/pelvis imaging
- Caveats: neutropenia → impaired inflammatory response → *exam and radiographic findings may be subtle*; absence of neutrophils by Gram stain does *not* r/o infection

Risk stratification (factors that predict lower risk)
- History: age <60 y, no symptoms, no major comorbidities, cancer in remission, solid tumor, no h/o fungal infection or recent antifungal Rx
- Exam: temp <39°C, no tachypnea, no hypotension, no Δ MS, no dehydration
- Studies: ANC >100 cells/μL, anticipated duration of neutropenia <10 d, normal CXR

Initial antibiotic therapy (Clin Infect Dis 2011;52:e56, NCCN Guidelines v.2.2015)
- Empiric regimens including drug w/ **antipseudomonal activity;** consider VRE coverage if colonized; OR 3.8 for VRE if VRE ⊕ (*B&MT 2010;16:1576*)
- PO abx may be used in low-risk Pts (<10 d neutropenia, nl hep/renal fxn, no N/V/D, no active infxn, stable exam): cipro + amoxicillin-clavulanate (*NEJM 1999;341:305*)
- IV antibiotics: no clearly superior regimen; monotherapy or 2-drug regimens can be used
  Monotherapy: ceftazidime, cefepime, imipenem, or meropenem
  2-drug therapy: aminoglycoside + antipseudomonal β-lactam
  PCN-allergic: levofloxacin + aztreonam or aminoglycoside
- **Vancomycin** in select cases (HoTN, PNA, clinically apparent catheter-related or soft-tissue infxn, MRSA colonization, gram ⊕ BCx, h/o quinolone ppx); d/c when cultures ⊖ × 48 h

Modification to initial antibiotic regimen
- Low-risk Pts who become afebrile w/in 3–5 d can be switched to PO antibiotics
- Empiric antibiotics changed for fever >3–5 d or progressive disease (eg, add vancomycin)
- Antifungal therapy is added for neutropenic fever >5 d
  liposomal amphotericin B, caspofungin, micafungin, anidulafungin, voriconazole, & posaconazole are all options (*NEJM 2002;346:225; 2007;356:348*)

Duration of therapy
- Known source: complete standard course (eg, 14 d for bacteremia)
- Unknown source: continue antibiotics until afebrile *and* ANC >500 cells/μL
- Less clear when to d/c abx when Pt is afebrile but prolonged neutropenia

Role of hematopoietic growth factors (NEJM 2013;368:1131)
- Granulocyte (G-CSF) and granulocyte-macrophage (GM-CSF) colony-stimulating factors can be used as 1° prophylaxis when expected FN incidence >20% or as 2° prophylaxis after FN has occurred in a previous cycle (to maintain dose-intensity for curable tumors). CSFs ↓ rate of FN but have not been shown to impact mortality.
- Colony-stimulating factors can be considered as adjuvant therapy in high-risk FN Pts

SPINAL CORD COMPRESSION

Clinical manifestations (Lancet Neuro 2008;7:459)
- Metastases located in vertebral body extend and cause epidural spinal cord compression

- **Prostate, breast** and **lung** cancers are the most common causes, followed by renal cell carcinoma, NHL and myeloma
- **Site of involvement: thoracic** (60%), lumbar (25%), cervical (15%)
- Signs and symptoms: **pain** (>95%, *precedes neuro ∆s*), **weakness, autonomic dysfunction** (urinary retention, ↓ anal sphincter tone), **sensory loss**

Diagnostic evaluation
- Always take back pain in Pts with solid tumors very seriously
- Do *not* wait for neurologic signs to develop before initiating evaluation b/c duration & severity of neurologic dysfunction before Rx are best predictors of neurologic outcome
- Urgent **whole-spine MRI** (Se 93%, Sp 97%); CT myelogram if unable to get MRI

Treatment
- **Dexamethasone** (10 mg IV × 1 stat, then 4 mg IV or PO q6h)
  initiate immediately while awaiting imaging if back pain + neurologic deficits
- Emergent RT or surgical decompression if confirmed compression/neuro deficit
- Surgery + RT superior to RT alone for neuro recovery in solid tumors (Lancet 2005;366:643)
- If pathologic fracture causing compression → surgery; if not surgical candidate → RT

TUMOR LYSIS SYNDROME

Clinical manifestations (NEJM 2011;364:1844; BJH 2010;149:578)
- Large tumor burden or a rapidly proliferating tumor → spontaneous or chemotherapy-induced release of intracellular electrolytes and nucleic acids
- Most common w/ Rx of high-grade lymphomas (**Burkitt's**) and leukemias (**ALL, AML, CML in blast crisis**); rare with solid tumors; rarely due to spontaneous necrosis
- Electrolyte abnormalities: ↑ K, ↑ uric acid, ↑ PO_4 → ↓ Ca
- **Renal failure** (urate nephropathy)

Prophylaxis
- Allopurinol 300 mg qd to bid PO or 200–400 mg/m² IV (adjusted for renal fxn) & aggressive hydration prior to beginning chemotherapy or RT
- Rasburicase (recombinant urate oxidase) 0.15 mg/kg or 6-mg fixed dose (except in obese Pts) & aggressive hydration prior to beginning chemotherapy or RT (see below)

Treatment
- *Avoid IV contrast and NSAIDs*
- Allopurinol + aggressive IV hydration ± diuretics to ↑ UOP for goal 80–100 cc/h
- Consider alkalinization of urine w/ isotonic $NaHCO_3$ to ↑ UA solubility, ↓ urate nephropathy risk (controversial: avoid w/ rasburicase; may cause met. alkalosis or $Ca_3(PO_4)_2$ precip.)
- Rasburicase (0.1–0.2 mg/kg × 1, repeat as indicated) for ↑↑ UA, esp. in aggressive malig; UA level must be drawn on ice to quench *ex vivo* enzyme activity (JCO 2003;21:4402; Acta Haematol 2006;115:35). Avoid in G6PD deficiency as results in hemolytic anemia.
- Treat hyperkalemia, hyperphosphatemia and symptomatic hypocalcemia
- Hemodialysis may be necessary; early renal consultation for Pts w/ renal insuffic. or ARF

CANCER OF UNKNOWN PRIMARY SITE

Evaluation of Cancer of Unknown Primary (Lancet 2012;379:1428)

Path	Possible sources	Markers	Imaging	Additional path
Adeno.	Colon, upper GI, panc.	CEA, CA19-9	Endoscopy/EUS	CDX1, CK7/20
	HCC	AFP	Abd/pelvic CT	
	Breast	CA15-3	Mammography	ER/PR, GCDFP
	Ovarian, prostate	CA125, PSA	Pelvic U/S	CA125, PSAP
	Lung		Chest CT	TTF1, CK7
Squam.	Lung	None	Chest CT	TTF1, CK7
	Head & neck		Laryngoscopy	
	Esophageal		Endoscopy	
	Cervix, anus			
Poorly Differen.	Germ cell	hCG, AFP	Testicular U/S	PLAP, isochrom 12p
	Lymphoma	LDH	PET	LCA, flow, cytogenetics
	Thyroid	Thyroglob.	Thyroid U/S	Thyroglobulin
	GIST, sarcoma		Abd/pelvic CT	c-KIT, desmin, vimentin
	Neuroendocrine			NSE, chromogranin
				Consider EM for all

Additional studies for each possible source listed in same row.

- Bony mets: common primary tumors include breast, lung, thyroid, kidney, prostate

Microbiology of Pneumonia	
Clinical setting	**Etiologies**
Community-acquired (CAP) (*NEJM* 2014;371:1619 & 373:415; *Lancet* 2015;386:1097)	No pathogen identified in 50–60%, virus alone in ~25%, bacteria alone in ~10%, virus-bacteria coinfection in <5% Viruses: influenza, RSV, hMPV, rhinovirus (unknown significance), parainfluenza virus, coronavirus S. pneumoniae (most common bacterial cause) S. aureus (esp. postinfluenza) Mycoplasma, Chlamydia (esp. in young & healthy) H. influenzae, M. catarrhalis (esp. in COPD) Legionella (esp. in elderly, smokers, ↓ immunity, TNF inhibitors) Klebsiella & other GNR (esp. in alcoholics & aspiration)
Hospital-acquired or health care-assoc (HAP/HCAP)	S. aureus, Pseudo., Klebsiella, E. coli, Enterobacter, Acinetobacter (HCAP risk factors: hosp or abx w/in 90 d, nursing home, home infusion Rx or dialysis w/in 30 d, home wound care, family member w/ MDR pathogen, immunosupp)
Immunosuppressed	Above + PCP, fungi, Nocardia, non-TB mycobacteria (NTM), CMV

Aspiration
(*NEJM* 2001;334:665; *Curr Opin Pulm Med* 2011;17:148)
	Chemical pneumonitis due to aspiration of gastric contents
	Bacterial pneumonia ≥24–72 h after aspiration event
	  outPt: oral flora (strep, S. aureus, anaerobes)
	  inPt or chronically ill: GNR (Pseudomonas) and S. aureus

Clinical manifestations
- Presenting features are variable and depend upon several host factors (esp. age)
- Classically (eg, w/ S. pneumo): fever, cough w/ purulent sputum, consolidation on CXR
- Atypical pathogens (Legionella, Mycoplasma, Chlamydia, virus): historically classified as "atypical" b/c they failed to grow on routine cx. Presentation varies from insidious to acute; imaging features vary from interstitial infiltrates to tree-in-bud opacities, to dense consolid.
- Clinical and imaging features do NOT distinguish "typical" from "atypical"
- Aspiration pneumonitis/PNA: can be infectious or non-infectious; may p/w acute inflammatory syndrome (fever, ↑WBC, etc.) or insidious course (typically w/ putrid breath)

Diagnostic studies
- **Sputum Gram stain/Cx:** reliable if high quality (ie, sputum not spit; <10 squamous cells/lpf) & if PNA should be purulent (>25 PMNs/lpf). Yield ↓ >10 h after abx (*CID* 2014:58:1782).
- **Blood cultures** (*before antibiotics!*): ⊕ in ~10% of inPts, depending on pathogen
- **CXR** (PA & lateral; see Radiology inserts) → tap effusions if >5 cm or severe PNA
- Other: **S,O₂** or P,O₂, arterial pH (if severe), CBC w/ diff, Chem-20; HIV test (if unknown)
- Other micro based on clinical suspicion (paired serologies available for most atypicals):
Mycoplasma: PCR of throat or sputum/BAL before first dose abx
Legionella urinary Ag (detects L. pneumophila L1 serotype, 60–70% of clinical disease)
S. pneumoniae urinary Ag (Se 70%, Sp >90%)
MTb: induced sputum for AFB stain and mycobacterial cx (empiric respiratory isolation while pending); avoid quinolones if suspect TB; request rapid DNA probe if stain ⊕
Induced sputum for PCP if HIV ⊕ or known ↓ cell-mediated immunity
- Viral testing (DFA or PCR) on nasopharyngeal swab or sputum
- Bronchoscopy: consider if immunosupp., critically ill, failing to respond, or chronic pneumonia. Also if suspected TB or PCP, or inadequate or ⊖ sputum cx. Some pathogens need specific cx media (eg, Legionella on BCYE).
- Reasons for failure to improve on initial Rx:
Insufficient time: may take ≥72 h to see improvement (fever persists >4 d in ~20%)
Insufficient drug levels for lung penetration (eg, vanco trough <15–20 μg/mL)
Resistant organisms (or superinfxn): eg, MRSA, Pseudo.; consider **bronchoscopy**
Wrong dx: fungal/viral, chemical pneumonitis, PE, CHF, ARDS, DAH, ILD; **consider CT**
Parapneumonic effusion/empyema/abscess: if CXR ⊖, **consider CT** (dx tap ± chest tube if effusion present, esp. if loculated)
Metastatic infection (eg, endocarditis, meningitis, septic arthritis)

Prevention
- Pneumococcal vaccine (PPSV23): all persons >65 y of age. If high-risk comorbidity, give at younger age and consider additional vaccination with PCV13.
- VAP precautions (or equivalent): HOB >30°, chlorhexidine rinse; aspiration precautions in high-risk Pts.
- Tdap booster: 1-time dose in adults with uncertain vaccination history (*MMWR* 2012; 61:468)

Prognosis
- For low-risk Pts, can discharge immediately after switching to PO abx (*CID* 2007;44:S27)
- CXR resolves in most by 6 wk; consider f/u to r/o underlying malig (esp. if >50 y or smoker)

Pneumonia Severity Index, Prognosis, & Recommended Triage (NEJM 1997;336:243)			
Class	**Score**	**Mortality**	**Suggested Triage**
I & II	≤70	<1%	Outpatient
III	71–90	3%	? Brief inpatient
IV	91–130	8%	Inpatient
V	>130	29%	ICU
Variables	**Points**		
Demograph.	Men (age in y), women (age – 10), nursing home resident (+10)		
Coexist. probs	Neoplasm (+30), liver dis. (+20), CHF (+10), CVA (+10), renal dis. (+10)		
Exam	Δ MS (+20), RR >30 (+20), SBP <90 (+20), T <35°/>40° (+15), HR >125 (+10)		
Laboratory	pH <7.35 (+30), BUN >30 (+20), Na <130 (+20), glc >250 (+10), Hct <30 (+10), P_aO_2 <60 or S_aO_2 <90 (+10), pleural effusion (+10)		

Treatment (CID 2007;44 Suppl:S27; JAMA 2016;315:593)		
Scenario	**Regimen**	**Special considerations**
CAP (outPt)	Azithro or doxy	Recent abx or multiple comorbidities: respiratory FQ or [azithro + amox/clav]
CAP (ward)	Resp FQ or [3rd-gen ceph + azithro]	Doxy can replace azithro
CAP (ICU)	Resp FQ + [3rd-gen ceph or amp-sulbactam]	Only cover MRSA or Pseudomonas if risk factors. If resp FQ contraindic., use azithro
HCAP (incl. VAP)	[Pip-tazo or cefepime or carbapen.] + [vanco or linezolid]	May add resp FQ (or azithro) when concerned re: atypicals
Aspiration	Clindamycin, amox-clav, or β-lactam + metronidazole	

- Consider TMP-SMX if PCP suspected in immunosupp. host. Consider oseltamivir for flu.
- Steroids (pred 50 mg × 7 d or methylpred 0.5 mg/kg q12h × 5 d) *may* speed clinical
  stabilization and ↓ late resp failure (Lancet 2015;385:1511; JAMA 2015;313:677; Annals
  2015;163:519), but not well studied in flu and not widely embraced yet
- Duration: CAP: 5–7 d if stable & afebrile for 48–72 h
  HCAP: 8 d (exception: 15 d for Pseudomonas or other nonfermenting GNR)
- When possible, de-escalate abx based on sensitivities

VIRAL RESPIRATORY INFECTIONS
URI, bronchitis, bronchiolitis, pneumonia (Lancet 2011;377:1264)

Microbiology & epidemiology (http://www.cdc.gov/flu/weekly)
- Typical pathogens: short, mild = rhinovirus; coronavirus; longer, more severe or
  complicated = **influenza**, parainfluenza, respiratory syncytial virus (RSV), adenovirus,
  metapneumovirus. Can be esp. severe in immunosupp.
- Seasonal flu: 365,000 hosp, 51,000 deaths per y in U.S.; most >65 y (NEJM 2008;359:2579)
- Pandemic 2009 H1N1 (swine): more severe in younger and obese Pts (JAMA 2009;302:1896)
- Sporadic 2011 H3N2: adults exposed to swine (also human-to-human) (MMWR 2011;60:1615)
- H5N1 influenza (avian): ongoing small outbreaks globally

Diagnosis
- Primarily clinical: **cough, fever, myalgias**, arthralgias, rhinorrhea, pharyngitis
  (in contrast, viral bronchitis p/w cough ± low-grade temp; usually benign & self-limited)
- Respiratory viral panel on nasal washing or sputum/BAL
- Rapid influenza test on nasal swab: Se ~50–70% (? lower for pandemic flu), Sp >95%
- DFA (Se ~85%), RT-PCR (gold standard) avail. for influenza (PCR distinguishes type)

Treatment (NEJM 2008;359:2579; Lancet 2015;385:1729)
- Seasonal influenza: treat with neuraminidase inhib. (oseltamivir, zanamivir), which are
  effective vs. A & B (shortens sx by ~1 d), but resistance emerging. M2 inhib. (amantadine,
  rimantadine) not recommended due to widespread resistance (MMWR 2011;60:1).
- Pandemic H1N1: nearly 100% sens. to **oseltamivir**. H5N1: Uncertain resistance pattern.
  H7N9: newly emerging in Asia (NEJM 2013;368:1888)
- Oseltamivir dosed 75 mg PO bid × 5 d. Must start w/in 48 h of sx for low-risk; for critically ill
  or immunosupp., start ASAP even if >48 h.
- Consider inhaled ribavirin for RSV in immunosupp. (eg, BMT, lung tx); limited adult data

Prevention
- Inactivated **influenza vaccine:** incl. H1N1. Rec for *all* >6 mo of age and esp. if pregnant,
  >50 y, immunosupp., or HCW (MMWR 2012;61:613)
- Isolation, droplet precautions for inPts strongly recommended
- Prophylaxis for high-risk contacts of confirmed influenza: oseltamivir 75 mg PO daily × 10 d

FUNGAL INFECTIONS

Candida species
- **Microbiology:** normal GI flora; *C. albicans* & nonalbicans spp. (consider azole resistance if h/o Rx or nonalbicans; *C. parapsilosis* ↑ echinocandin resistant). Sensi testing available.
- **Risk factors:** neutropenia, immunosupp., broad-spectrum abx, intravascular catheters (esp. if TPN), IVDU, abd surgery, DM, renal failure, age >65
- **Clinical manifestations**
  Mucocutaneous: cutaneous (eg, red, macerated lesions in intertriginous zones); oral thrush (exudative, erythematous or atrophic; if unexplained, r/o HIV); esophageal (odynophagia; ± oral thrush); vulvovaginal, balanitis
  Candiduria: typically colonization due to broad-spectrum abx and/or indwelling catheter
  Candidemia: r/o retinal involvement (ophtho consult in all cases, req ↑ Rx duration); endocarditis rare but serious (esp. w/ nonalbicans & prosthetic valve). May present with erythematous papules or pustules in immunocompromised.
  Hepatosplenic: occurs w/ neutrophil recovery

Treatment (CID 2016;62:409)	
Mucocutaneous	Clotrimazole, nystatin, fluconazole, itraconazole
Candiduria (*must determine colonization vs. infection*)	Fluconazole or intravesical ampho* if sx, severely immunosupp. or will undergo GU procedure
Candidemia w/o neutropenia	**Echinocandin** or fluconazole or ampho, *remove any intravascular catheters if possible*
Febrile neutropenia	**Echinocandin** or ampho

*See IDSA guidelines for ampho dosing. Liposomal preparation preferred, if available.

Cryptococcus (CID 2010;50:291)
- **Epidemiology:** immunosupp. (esp. AIDS) most susceptible; can occur in healthy host, esp. elderly, EtOH, DM. Consider *C. gattii* (typically in healthy host).
- **Clinical manifestations**
  CNS (meningitis): HA, fever, meningismus, ↑ ICP, CN abnl, ± stupor, often subacute. Dx: CSF CrAg, India ink stain, fungal cx. Cell counts vary; serum CrAg >1:8 Se/Sp in AIDS.
  Other sites: pulm, GU, cutaneous, CNS cryptococcoma. *With any crypto dx, LP all Pts.*
- **Treatment**
  CNS: If ↑ ICP, repeat large-volume LPs or temp. lumbar drain; few require VP shunt
  In HIV ⊕ or immunosupp. Pts, CNS Rx has induction (ampho ± flucytosine), consolidation and maintenance (fluconazole) phases (*NEJM* 2013;368:1291). If r/o CNS disease, then fluconazole. Dosing and duration vary by host.
  Non-CNS disease in healthy Pts: fluconazole vs. observation, based on clinical setting

Histoplasmosis (CID 2007;45:807)
- **Hyperendemic** to central & SE US, but sporadic cases throughout U.S.
- **Clinical manifestations**
  Acute: often subclinical, but may see mild to severe PNA ± cavitary & hilar LAN
  Chronic pulm: ↑ productive cough, wt loss, night sweats, apical infiltrates, cavitation
  Disseminated (typically in immunosupp.): fever, wt loss, HSM, LAN, oral ulcers, skin lesion, fibrosing mediastinitis, reactive arthritis, pericarditis
- **Treatment:** itraconazole (monitor levels); ampho ± steroids if severe or immunosupp.

Coccidioidomycosis (CID 2005;41:1217)
- **Endemic:** SW U.S. (San Joaquin or "Valley" fever)
- **Clinical manifestations**
  Acute: 50–67% subclinical; PNA w/ cough, chest pain, fever, arthralgias, *fatigue*
  Chronic pulm: nodule(s), cavity or progressive fibrocavitary PNA (can be asx or sx)
  Disseminated (typically in immunosupp.): fever, malaise, diffuse pulmonary process, bone, skin, & meningeal involvement
- **Treatment:** monitor mild disease closely q3–6mo; for severe disease: fluconazole, itraconazole or amphotericin

Blastomycosis (CID 2008;46:1801)
- **Endemic:** south central, SE and Midwest U.S.
- **Clinical manifestations**
  Acute: 50% subclinical; cough, multilobar PNA; can progress to ARDS
  Chronic pulm: cough, wt loss, malaise, CT w/ masses & fibronodular infiltrates
  Disseminated: (25–40% of all but ↑ immunosupp.): verrucous & ulcerated skin lesions, bone, & GU involvement; CNS rare unless immunosupp.
- **Treatment:** itraconazole (monitor levels); ampho B if severe, disseminated or immunosupp.

Aspergillosis (CID 2008:46:327; NEJM 2009:360:1870)
- **ABPA; hypersensitivity pneumonitis:** see "Interstitial Lung Disease"
- **Aspergilloma:** usually in pre-existing cavity (from TB, etc.); most asx, but can lead to hemoptysis; sputum cx ⊕ in <50%; CT → mobile intracavitary mass with air crescent Rx: antifungals w/o benefit; embolization or surgery for persistent hemoptysis
- **Necrotizing tracheitis:** white necrotic pseudomembranes in Pts w/ AIDS or lung Tx
- **Chronic necrotizing:** mild immunosupp.; sputum production, fever, wt loss; CT: infiltrate ± nodule ± thick pleura; lung bx → invasion
- **Invasive:** seen if immunosupp. (neutropenia for >10 d, transplant, high-dose corticosteroids, AIDS); s/s PNA w/ chest pain & hemoptysis; CT: nodules, halo sign (cavitates w/ Rx → air crescent sign); dx w/ galactomannan >0.5 (serum or BAL)
- Rx (necrotizing/invasive): voriconazole (or isavuconazole) superior to ampho; ✓ drug levels

Zygomycetes (eg, Mucor, Rhizopus)
- **Epidemiology:** diabetes (70%, esp. DKA), heme malignancy, s/p transplant, chronic steroids, deferoxamine or iron overload, trauma, h/o voriconazole Rx or Ppx
- **Clinical manifestations: rhinocerebral** = periorbital/forehead pain when w/ orbital cellulitis), ± fever (may appear nontoxic at first), exophthalmos, ↓ EOM, CNs (V > VII); nasal turbinates ± black eschar but exam can be quite nl. Also, **pulmonary** (PNA w/ infarct & necrosis); **cutaneous** (indurated painful cellulitis ± eschar); **GI** (necrotic ulcers).
- **Treatment:** debridement + Rx (ampho, posaconazole, or isavuconazole); high mortality

Fungal diagnostics
- **Culture:** Candida grows in blood/urine Cx, but ↓ Se of BCx in deep tissue infection; others (eg, Crypto, Histo) ↓↓ Se of BCx; if suspect Coccidio alert lab (biohazard)
- **Antibody detection:** only clinically useful for Coccidio
- **Antigen detection**
  Histo urine/serum Ag: Se of urine Ag 90% (serum 80%) if dissem; Sp limited by X-react
  Crypto Ag (serum, CSF): serum Ag >90% Se & Sp in invasive infxn, less for pulm only
  1,3-β-D-glucan: Se for many fungal infxns (Candida, Aspergillus, Histo, Coccidio, Fusarium, Pneumocystis, Sporothrix), but not Crypto, Blasto, Mucor, Rhizopus; not Sp
  Galactomannan: serum levels Se ~65%, Sp ~90% for invasive aspergillosis. BAL levels in Pts w/ hematologic malignancy ↑ Se, but ↓ Sp (false ⊕ seen w/ colonization)
  Blastomyces: urine > serum Ag, high Se but modest Sp given X-react w/other fungi
- **Biopsy** (ie, histopathology): nb, no grinding of tissue if Zygomycetes suspected

INFXNS IN IMMUNOSUPPRESSED HOSTS

Overview
- Many Pts have ≥1 risk (eg, DM, ESRD, transplant, extremes of age)
- The following is not an exhaustive list, but a delineation of common or classic etiologies

Predisposition	Classic Infectious Etiologies
Humoral immune dysfunction (eg, CVID, myeloma) and asplenia	**Encapsulated bacteria:** S. pneumo, H. flu, N. meningitidis (vaccinate against these 3, ideally prior to splenectomy) **Other bacteria:** E. coli and other GNRs, Capnocytophaga **Parasites:** Babesia, Giardia; **Viruses:** VZV, echovirus, enterovirus
Granulocytopenia or neutropenia (includes DM, ESRD → functional impairment)	**Bacteria:** Gram positive: coag ⊖ staph, S. aureus, viridans strep, S. pneumo, other strep; Corynebacterium spp., Bacillus spp. Gram negative: E. coli, Klebsiella, Pseudomonas **Fungi:** Yeast: Candida albicans and other Candida spp. Molds: Aspergillus, Mucor spp., endemic fungi and others **Viruses:** VZV, HSV1 and 2, CMV
Impaired cell-mediated immunity (CMI) (eg, HIV, chronic steroids, posttransplant, DM, ESRD)	**Bacteria:** Salmonella spp., Campylobacter, Listeria, Yersinia, Legionella (Lancet 2016:387:376), Rhodococcus, Nocardia, TB, non-TB mycobacteria **Fungi:** Candida, Crypto, Histo, Coccidio, Aspergillus, Pneumocystis, Zygomycetes spp. and other molds **Viruses:** HSV,VZV, CMV, EBV, JC virus, BK virus **Parasites:** Toxoplasma, Cryptosporidium, Isospora, Microsporidia Babesia; Strongyloides
Organ dysfunction	**Liver (esp. cirrhosis):** Vibrio spp., encapsulated bacteria **ESRD:** impaired granulocyte fxn and CMI as above **Iron overload (or deferoxamine Rx):** Yersinia, Zygomycetes
Biologics (eg, TNF inhibitors, anti-B-cell Rx; ✓ for TB before starting)	**Bacteria:** sepsis, septic arthritis, TB, NTM, Listeria, Legionella **Fungi:** Pneumocystis, Histo, Coccidio, Aspergillus, endemic fungi **Viruses:** JC virus (PML), EBV, HSV, VZV, HBV **Parasites:** Strongyloides reactivation

(NEJM 2007; 357:2601; Am J Med 2007;120;764; CID 2011;53:798)

Definitions
- **Anatomic**
  - **lower:** urethritis, cystitis (superficial infection of bladder)
  - **upper:** pyelonephritis (inflam of renal parenchyma), renal/perinephric abscess, prostatitis
- **Clinical**
  - **uncomplicated:** cystitis in immunocompetent ♀ w/o underlying structural/neuro disease
  - **complicated:** upper tract infection in women or any UTI in men or pregnant women or UTI with underlying structural/neuro disease, bladder dysfxn or immunosuppression

Microbiology
- Uncomplicated UTI: **E. coli** (80%), *Proteus, Klebsiella, S. saprophyticus* (CID 2004;39:75). In healthy, nonpregnant women, lactobacilli, enterococci, Group B strep and coag-neg staph (except *S. saprophyticus*) usually contaminants (Annals 2012;156:ITC3).
- Complicated UTI: *E. coli* (30%), enterococci (20%), PsA (20%), *S. epi* (15%), other GNR
- Catheter-associated UTI: **yeast** (30%), E. coli (25%), other GNR, enterococci, *S. epi*
- Urethritis: *Chlamydia trachomatis, Neisseria gonorrhoeae, Ureaplasma urealyticum, Trichomonas vaginalis, Mycoplasma genitalium,* HSV
- *S. aureus:* uncommon primary urinary pathogen in absence of catheter or recent instrumentation; ∴ consider bacteremia w/ hematogenous seeding

Clinical manifestations
- **Cystitis: dysuria, urgency, frequency,** hematuria, suprapubic pain; fever usually *absent.* R/o vaginitis if symptoms of cystitis and urethritis.
- **Urethritis:** similar to cystitis except *urethral discharge* can be present
- **Prostatitis**
  - **chronic:** similar to cystitis except *symptoms of obstruction* (hesitancy, weak stream)
  - **acute:** perineal pain, fever, tenderness on prostate exam
- **Pyelonephritis:** fever, chills, flank or back pain, nausea, vomiting, diarrhea
- **Renal abscess** (intrarenal, perinephric): identical to pyelonephritis w/ *persistent fever despite appropriate antibiotics*

Diagnostic studies (NEJM 2016;374:562)
- **Urinalysis:** pyuria + bacteriuria ± hematuria ± nitrites
- **Urine Cx** (clean-catch midstream or straight-cath): obtain cx only if sx
  Significant bacterial counts: typically ≥10^5 CFU/mL in women, ≥10^3 CFU/mL in men or catheterized Pts. Counts may vary depending on dilution & stage of infxn; interpret in context of sx and host.
  Pyuria & ⊖ UCx = sterile pyuria → urethritis, nephritis, renal tuberculosis, foreign body
- Blood cultures: obtain in febrile Pts; consider in complicated UTIs
- DNA detection/cx for *C. trachomatis/N. gonorrhoeae* in high-risk Pts or sterile pyuria
- If ? prostatitis: 1st void, midstream, prostatic expressage & postprostatic massage UCx
- Abdominal CT: r/o abscess in Pts with pyelo who fail to defervesce after 72 h
- Urologic w/u (renal U/S w/ PVR, abd CT, voiding cystography) if recurrent UTIs in men

Treatment of UTIs

Scenario	Empiric treatment guidelines[a]
Cystitis (JAMA 2014;16:1677)	Uncomp: nitrofurantoin[b] 100 mg × 5 d or TMP-SMX DS PO × 3 d or fosfomycin (3 g × 1). Refer to dosing guidelines for ↑ Cr. Complicated: FQ or TMP-SMX PO × 7–14 d Asx bacteriuria in pregnancy or prior to urologic surgery → abx × 3 d
Catheterized	Abx as above & **remove catheter.** Exchange if removal impossible.
Urethritis	Treat for both *Neisseria* and *Chlamydia* *Neisseria:* CTX 250 mg IM × 1 and 1 g azithro PO × 1 *Chlamydia:* doxy 100 mg PO bid × 7 d or azithro 1 g PO × 1 *M. genitalium:* 1 g azithro PO × 1
Prostatitis	FQ or TMP-SMX PO × 14–28 d (acute) or 6–12 wk (chronic)
Pyelonephritis	OutPt: FQ × 7 d or TMP-SMX PO × 14 d (Lancet 2012;380:452) InPt: CTX or amp/sulbactam or aminoglycoside × 14 d (Δ IV → PO when clinically improved & afebrile 24–48 h)
Renal abscess	Drainage + antibiotics as for pyelonephritis

[a]Choice of agent individualized based on h/o allergies and adherance, local practice patterns, community prevalence and uropathogen resistance patterns, availability, cost, and Pt and provider threshold for failure. For empiric outPt Rx, community resistance to abx should be <20% for cystitis or <10% for pyelonephritis. Beta-lactams have less efficacy than other abx for UTI (CID 2011;52:e103; NEJM 2012;366:1028)
[b]Note risk of pulmonary fibrosis with prolonged or recurrent use.

SKIN AND SOFT TISSUE INFECTIONS (SSTI; CID 2014;59:e10)

Clinical
- Cellulitis: infxn of dermis/sc fat, w/ erythema, edema, warmth, pain (rubor, tumor, calor, dolor)
- Erysipelas: infxn of upper dermis (more superficial than cellulitis), often caused by strep, w/ raised erythematous lesion w/ clear demarcation from normal skin
- Impetigo: infxn of superficial layers, often caused by staph, typically in children, w/ purulent lesions, often on face/extrem, ± bullae, ± gold crust
- Lymphangitis: proximal red streaking ± regional lymphadenopathy
- **Toxic shock syndrome** can occur w/ staph or strep infxn. Fever, HA, N/V, diarrhea, myalgias, pharyngitis, diffuse rash w/ desquamation, HoTN, shock. BCx may be ⊖.

Microbiology (CID 2014;59:e10)
- Primarily strep and staph, including MRSA; may include GNRs in diabetics/immunosupp.
- **MRSA** (NEJM 2005;352:1485 & 2006;355:666) causes up to 75% of purulent skin/soft tissue infxns, depending on local epi (rapidly increasing), often assoc. w/ purulent drainage or exudate. Often TMP-SMX sensitive; variably clindamycin sensitive (may falsely appear susceptible on lab testing, requires confirmation w/ D-test; NEJM 2007;357:380).
- Bites: skin and oral flora (incl anaerobes) + special exposures:

Feature	Microbiology	Clinical
Cat bite	P. multocida	Rapid onset
Dog bite	P. multocida	
	C. canimorsus	Sepsis w/ symmetric, peripheral gangrene in asplenic/cirrhosis and other immunosupp.
Penetrating injury	Pseudomonas	Can be a/w deep tissue abscess
Gardening	Sporothrix	Ulcerating nodules, lymphatic spread
Salt H$_2$O or raw oysters/fish	V. vulnificus	Hemorrhagic bullae & sepsis (esp. in cirrhotics). If suspected, Rx w/ doxy + ceftaz
	Erysipelothrix	Rapid onset, endocarditis can develop
Fresh H$_2$O	Aeromonas	Myonecrosis/rhabdo can occur. If suspected, Rx w/ doxy + cipro.

Diagnosis
- Largely clinical diagnosis; BCx low yield (~5–10%) but useful if ⊕
- Aspirate of bulla or pus from furuncle or pustule may provide microbiologic dx

Cellulitis Treatment (NEJM 2014;370:2238; CID 2014;59:e10; JAMA 2016;316:325)			
Purulent	Micro	Severity	Treatment
No	β-hemolytic Strep > S. aureus	Mild	PCN, diclox, cephalosporin or clinda
		Mod	PCN, CTX, cefazolin or clinda
		Severe	Vanc + pip/tazo
Yes	S. aureus (incl. MRSA) >> β-hemolytic Strep.	Mild	I&D only
		Mod	TMP-SMX or doxy; some data for clinda (NEJM 2015;372:1093), but MRSA sensitivity variable
		Severe	Vanc, dapto, linezolid, ceftaroline, or telavancin

Mild: no systemic signs of infection; moderate: systemic signs; severe: SIRS or immunocompromised
Narrow abx per Cx data. Dalbavancin & oritavancin being studied (NEJM 2014;370:2169 & 2180).

- **Limb elevation;** erythema may *worsen* after starting abx b/c bacterial killing → inflam.
- In obese Pts, adequate drug dosing important to avoid treatment failure (J Infect 2012;2:128)

NECROTIZING FASCIITIS

Definition
- Infection and necrosis of superficial fascia, subcutaneous fat and deep fascia (necrosis of arteries and nerves in subcutaneous fat → gangrene)
- Fournier's gangrene: necrotizing fasciitis of the male genitalia or female perineum

Epidemiology
- Affects healthy individuals but ↑ risk: DM, PVD, EtOH abuse, IVDU, immunosupp., cirrhosis

Microbiology
- Type I (after abd/perineal surgery or trauma; in DM, PVD): polymicrobial (w/ anaerobes)
- Type II (usually extremities): Strep pyogenes ± MRSA, often healthy w/o obvious portal of entry; up to ½ have toxic shock syndrome (TSS)

- Need *high degree of clinical suspicion* because of nonspecific physical exam
- Most common sites: extremities, abdominal wall, and perineum, but can occur anywhere
- **Cellulitic skin Δs with poorly defined margins + rapid spread + systemic toxicity**
- **Pain out of proportion** to apparent cellulitis; skin hyperesthetic and later anesthetic
- **Bullae, darkening of skin to bluish-gray ± crepitus** or radiographically visible gas

Diagnostic signs
- Clinical dx sufficient to initiate **urgent surgical exploration**
- Aspiration of necrotic center; BCx; Gram stain; ✓ CK for tissue necrosis
- Imaging: **noncontrast CT,** but do not delay therapy *(Arch Surg 2010;145:452)*
- Microbiologic dx from Gram stain and culture of surgical specimens

Treatment
- Definitive treatment is **surgical débridement** of necrotic tissue and fasciotomy
- Type I: empiric Tx w/vanc + pip-tazo
- Type II: PCN + clinda. If ↑ risk of CA-MRSA, + vanco. If concern for strep, IVIG.

Prognosis
- Generally fatal if untreated; reported mortality 20–50%

CLOSTRIDIAL MYONECROSIS (GAS GANGRENE)

Definition
- Life-threatening, fulminant clostridial infection of skeletal muscle
- **Wound contamination** w/ clostridial spores after **trauma** (penetrating or crush injury)
- Most commonly *C. perfringens; C. septicum* assoc w/ cancer (GI, heme), even w/o trauma

Clinical manifestations
- Incubation period 6 h to 2–3 d
- Sense of heaviness/pain, often at site of trauma; rapid worsening; marked systemic toxicity
- Bronze skin discoloration, tense bullae, serosanguineous or dark fluid and necrotic areas
- **Crepitus** present but not prominent (gas in muscle), may be obscured by edema

Diagnostic studies
- Gram stain: **large, Gram ⊕ rod w/ blunt ends** *(can be Gram-variable)*, few polys
- Bacteremia in ~15%
- Plain radiographs: gas dissecting into muscle

Treatment
- **Surgical exploration with débridement,** fasciotomies and amputation if necessary
- **Antibiotics:** high-dose **penicillin G** 24 MU IV divided q2–3h + **clinda** 900 mg IV q8h

NEUROPATHIC FOOT ULCER
Leading cause of DM-related hosp. days & nontrauma amputations

Microbiology
- **Mild** (superficial, no bone or joint involvement): usually *S. aureus* or aerobic streptococci
- **Limb- or life-threatening** = deep, bone/joint involvement, systemic tox., limb ischemia
- Mono- or polymicrobial with aerobes + anaerobes
  aerobes = *S. aureus*, strep, enterococci and GNR (including *Pseudomonas*)
  anaerobes = anaerobic streptococci, *Bacteroides, Clostridium* (rare)

Clinical manifestations
- Clinical dx: ≥2 classic s/s of inflammation (erythema, warmth, tenderness [may be absent in neuropathy], pain or induration) or purulent secretions ± crepitus (indicating gas and ∴ mixed infection w/ GNR & anaerobes or *Clostridium*)
- Complications: osteomyelitis, systemic toxicity (fever, chills, leukocytosis, hyperglycemia)

Diagnostic studies
- Avoid superficial swabs (*only helpful if* ⊕ for *S. aureus* and suspect infxn); **wound cx** (eg, deep tissue sample or curettage at ulcer base after débridement) has ↑ Se
- Blood cx should be obtained in all Pts, ⊕ in 10–15%
- **Osteomyelitis should always be ruled out:** probe to bone test for all open wounds in a diabetic foot (high Sp but low Se); imaging (see below); **bone biopsy** best

Treatment *(CID 2012;54:e132)*

Severity of Infxn	Empiric Antibiotics
Mild	PCNase-resistant PCN or 1ˢᵗ-gen. ceph. (TMP-SMX if ? MRSA)
Chronic, previously treated or serious	(FQ or ceftriaxone + clinda) or amp-sulbactam or ticar-clav or ertapenem. If MRSA, add vanco or TMP-SMX or linezolid or televancin or dapto or ceftaroline.
Limb or life-threatening	Vanco + anti-*Pseudomonal* agent: imipenem or pip-tazo or (aztreonam + metronidazole)

- Elevation, non–weight-bearing status, **wound care,** glycemic control
- Evaluation and treatment for venous insufficiency and arterial ischemia
- **Many require surgery:** early, aggressive and repeated débridement; revascularization or amputation may be necessary
- Management by multidisciplinary team improves outcomes

OSTEOMYELITIS

Infection of bone due to hematogenous seeding or direct spread from contiguous focus

Microbiology (NEJM 1997;336:999; Lancet 2004;364:369)

- **Hematogenous:** *S. aureus;* mycobacterial infection of vertebral body = Pott's disease
- **Contiguous focus** (may be acute or chronic)
  open fracture, orthopedic surgery, etc.: *S. aureus* and *S. epi*
  skin breakdown + vasc. insuffic. (eg, diabetic foot): **polymicrobial**
  GU source (GNR, *Enterococcus*)

Clinical manifestations

- Surrounding soft tissue compromise ± fistula to superficial skin
- ± Fever, malaise and night sweats (more common in hematogenous than contiguous)
- Vertebral osteomyelitis (esp. IVDU): unremitting, focal back pain, usually febrile (NEJM 2010;362:1022)

Diagnostic studies (JAMA 2008;299:806)

- Identification of the causative organism is key
- **Tissue cx** (aspiration bx Se 30–74%) unless ⊕ blood Cx. Do not rely on swabs of ulcers or fistulae drainage.
- High suspicion in diabetic foot (see above) if can probe ulcer to bone or ulcer >2 cm^2
- **Blood cultures** (more often ⊕ with acute hematogenous osteomyelitis)
- **ESR** >70 greatly increases likelihood of osteo (JAMA 2008;299:806)
- Imaging
  Plain radiographs: normal early in disease; lytic lesions seen after 2–6 wk
  MRI: most sensitive imaging study (overall Se 90%, Sp 82%; Archives 2007;167:125)
  CT: can demonstrate periosteal reaction and cortical and medullary destruction
  CT & MRI very Se but ↓ Sp; false ⊕ if contig focus w/ periosteal reaction, Charcot Δs
  Radionuclide imaging: very Se but non-Sp (false ⊕ if soft tissue inflammation)

Treatment

- **Antibiotics:** based on cx data. Duration depends on Rx strategy/goals of Rx management (eg, 6 wks for vertebral osteo; Lancet 2015;385:875).
- **Surgery** should be considered for any of the following: acute osteo that fails to respond to medical Rx, chronic osteo, complications of pyogenic vertebral osteo (eg, neurologic compromise, spinal instability, epidural abscess) or infected prosthesis

---

EPIDURAL ABSCESS

Etiology

- Hematogenous spread (²/₃): skin infection, soft tissue (dental abscess) or endocarditis
- Direct extension (¹/₃): vertebral osteo, sacral ulcer, spinal anesthesia or surgery, LP
- Risk factors: diabetes, renal failure, alcoholism, IVDU, immunosupp.
- *S. aureus* most common pathogen, increasing incidence of MRSA

Clinical manifestations

- **Back pain** (unremitting including midline) + often **fever** ± nerve root or cord signs

Diagnostic studies

- **MRI**
- Aspiration of abscess fluid for Gram stain & cx or operative Gram stain & cx
- Blood cx (frequently ⊖)

Treatment

- **Antibiotics ± surgery** (decompressive laminectomy and débridement) for failure to improve on medical Rx. Emergent surgery for early s/s of cord compression (w/ vertebral osteo and epidural abscess, may see paraplegia 48–72 h after first signs)

ACUTE BACTERIAL MENINGITIS

Clinical manifestations (NEJM 2006:354:44; Lancet 2012;380:1684)
- **Fever** (77%), **headache** (87%), **stiff neck** (31%), **photosensitivity**, Δ **MS** (69%) (defined as GCS <14), **seizures** (5%); 2 of 4 (fever, HA, stiff neck, Δ MS) present in 95%
- Presentation may be *atypical* (eg, lethargy w/o fever) in elderly and immunosupp.

Physical exam
- **Nuchal rigidity** (Se 31%), **Kernig's sign** (Pt supine, hip flexed at 90°, knee flexed at 90°; ⊕ if passive extension of knee → resistance), **Brudzinski's sign** (Pt supine and limbs supine; ⊕ if passive neck flexion → involuntary hip and/or knee flexion) nb, Kernig's or Brudzinski's signs ⊕ in only ~10% of Pts (Lancet 2012;380:1684)
- ± Focal neuro findings (~30%; hemiparesis, aphasia, visual field cuts, CN palsies)
- ± Funduscopic findings: papilledema, absent venous pulsations
- ± HEENT findings: sinus tenderness, clear rhinorrhea (CSF leak)
- ± Skin findings: petechial rash (*N. meningitidis*), genital or oral ulcers (HSV)

Microbiology in Bacterial Meningitis (NEJM 2011;364:2016)	
Etiology	**Comments**
S. pneumoniae (30–60%)	Assess for distant infxn (eg, Osler's triad = meningitis, PNA, IE) Drug-resistant *S. pneumoniae*: ~40% PCN-resistant (even *intermediate* resistance problematic) ~<10% 3rd-gen. cephalosporin-resistant Vaccine may have reduced rate of invasive disease
N. meningitidis (10–35%)	Primarily in those <30 y; may be a/w petechiae or purpura. Deficiencies in terminal complement predispose to recurrent meningococcemia & rarely meningitis. Vaccine rec for all adolescents, college freshmen living in dorm, military recruits, s/p splenectomy or C5-9 deficiency
H. influenzae (<5%)	↓ Incidence in children b/c vaccine. Look for risk factors in adults (eg, CSF leak, neurosurgical procedure, trauma, mastoiditis).
L. monocytogenes (5–10%)	↑ Incid in elderly, alcoholics or Pts w/ cancer, immunosupp. or iron overload. Outbreaks a/w contaminated dairy & raw vegetables. Despite name, a/w *poly-predominant* pleocytosis.
GNRs (1–10%)	Usually health care associated, postprocedure or in elderly or immunosuppressed
Staphylococci (5%)	Seen with indwelling CSF shunt (*S. epidermidis*) or following neurosurgery or head trauma (*S. aureus*)
Mixed infection	Suspect parameningeal focus or CSF leak
Fungal	Seen if immunosuppressed or after neurosurgery

Sequential approach to bacterial meningitis
(1) Stat **BCx** → **antibiotics + corticosteroids** (see below)
(2) **CT head** (if indicated, see below)
(3) **LP** (if not contraindicated); yield of CSF cx unlikely to be changed if obtained w/in ~4 h of initiation of abx

Diagnostic studies (Lancet 2012;380:1684)
- **Blood cultures** ×2 *before abx*
- **WBC count**: >10,000 in >90% of bacterial meningitis in healthy hosts
- *Consider* head CT to r/o mass effect before LP *if* ≥ 1 high-risk feature (age >60 y, immunosupp., h/o CNS disease, new-onset seizure, Δ MS, focal neuro findings, papilledema); absence of all these has NPV 97%; however, in Pts w/ mass effect, herniation may occur w/o LP and may not occur even w/ LP (NEJM 2001;345:1727)
- **Lumbar puncture** (NEJM 2006;355:e12)
  CSF Gram stain has 30–90% Se; cx 80–90% Se if LP done prior to abx opening pressure typically ↑ in bact meningitis; must measure w/ Pt's legs extended *rule of 2s*: CSF WBC >2k, glc <20, & TP >200 has >98% Sp for bacterial meningitis repeat LP only if no clinical response after 48 h of appropriate abx or CSF shunt
- Additional CSF studies based on clinical suspicion: AFB smear & cx, India ink prep, cryptococcal Ag, fungal cx, VDRL, PCR (HSV, VZV, enteroviral), cytology

Typical CSF Findings in Meningitis

Type	Appearance	Pressure (cm H$_2$O)	WBC/mm^3 *Predom type*	Glc (mg/dL)	TP (mg/dL)
Normal	Clear	9–18	0–5 lymphs	50–75	15–40
Bacterial	Cloudy	18–30	100–10,000 polys	<45	100–1000
TB	Cloudy	18–30	<500 lymphs	<45	100–200
Fungal	Cloudy	18–30	<300 lymphs	<45	40–300
Aseptic	Clear	9–18	<300 polys → lymphs	50–100	50–100

Treatment of Bacterial Meningitis (Lancet 2012;380:1693)

Clinical scenario	Empiric treatment guidelines*
Normal adult	**Ceftriaxone 2 g IV q12h + Vancomycin 15–20 mg/kg IV q12h** If >50 y or alcoholic: add ampicillin 2 g IV q4h for *Listeria* β-lactam allergy: substitute cipro 400 mg q8h or aztreonam 2 g q6h for CTX. Substitute TMP/SMX for amp.
Immunosuppressed	Ampicillin + ceftazidime 2 g IV q8h + vancomycin
CSF shunts, recent neurosurgery or head trauma	Vancomycin + ceftazidime 2 g IV q8h (NEJM 2010;362:146)

Corticosteroids: dexamethasone 10 mg IV q6h × 4 d → ↓ neuro disability & mortality by ~50% w/ *S. pneumo* & GCS 8–11. Consider steroids in all bacterial meningitis prior to organism identification. **Must start before or w/ 1st dose of abx** (NEJM 2002;347:1549). Nb, do *not* give steroids in cryptococcal meningitis (NEJM 2016;374:542).

Prophylaxis: rifampin (600 mg PO bid × 2 d) or ciprofloxacin (500 mg PO × 1) or ceftriaxone (250 mg IM × 1) for close contacts of Pt w/ *N. meningitidis* meningitis

Precautions: droplet precautions until *N. meningitidis* is r/o

*When possible, organism-directed Rx, guided by sensitivities or local patterns of drug resistance should be used

Prognosis
- For community-acquired *S. pneumo* mort. 19–37%; 30% have long-term neuro sequelae

ASEPTIC MENINGITIS

Definition
- CSF pleocytosis w/ ⊖ blood & CSF cx; typically lymphocyte predominant
- Less likely to be bacterial, but can be infectious or noninfectious

Etiologies (Neurology 2006;66:75)
- **Viral:** enteroviruses (most common), HIV, HSV (type 2 > 1), VZV, mumps, lymphocytic choriomeningitis virus, encephalitis viruses, adenovirus, polio, CMV, EBV, WNV
- **Parameningeal focus of infection** (eg, brain abscess, epidural abscess, septic thrombophlebitis of dural venous sinuses or subdural empyema)
- **Partially treated bacterial meningitis**
- **TB, fungal, spirochetal** (Lyme, syphilis, leptospirosis), **rickettsial,** *Coxiella, Ehrlichia*
- **Medications:** TMP/SMX, NSAIDs, IVIG, PCN, INH, lamotrigine
- **Systemic illness:** SLE, sarcoidosis, Behçet's, Sjögren's syndrome, RA
- **Neoplasm:** intracranial tumors (or cysts), lymphomatous or carcinomatous meningitis (CSF cytology or flow may be reactive and dx may require meningeal bx)

Empiric treatment
- No abx if suspect viral (cell count <500 w/ >50% lymphs, TP <80–100 mg/dL, normal glc, ⊖ Gram stain, not elderly/immunosupp.); o/w start empiric abx, wait for cx data
- If suspect MTb: antimycobacterial Rx + dexamethasone (NEJM 2004;351:1741)
- If suspect fungal: ampho lipid formulation, ± 5-fluorouracil

Definition
- Infection of brain parenchyma with evidence of neurologic dysfunction

Etiologies (specific etiology found in <20% of cases; *Neurology* 2006;66:75; *CID* 2008;47:303)
- **HSV-1** (~9%): all ages/seasons; MRI: temporal lobe lesions/edema; EEG: temporal focus
- **VZV** (~9%): 1° or reactivation; ± vesicular rash; all ages (favors elderly), all seasons
- **Arboviruses** (~9%): Eastern/Western equine, St. Louis, Japanese, Powassan, W. Nile (*NEJM* 2005;353:287): fever, HA, **flaccid paralysis**, rash. Risk factors for severe dis: renal dis., cancer, EtOH, DM, HTN (*Am J Trop Med Hyg* 2012;87:179).
- **Enteroviruses** (coxsackie, echo): viral syndrome; peaks in late summer/early fall
- Others: CMV, EBV, HIV, JC virus (PML), measles, mumps, rubella, rabies, flu, adenovirus
- Nonviral mimics: autoimmune/paraneoplastic (anti-NMDAR, anti-Hu, anti-Ma2, anti-CRMP5), bacterial endocarditis, brain abscess, toxoplasmosis, TB, toxins, vasculitis, Whipple's disease, subdural hematoma, encephalomyelitis (eg, ADEM), seizure

Clinical manifestations
- **Fever, HA, Δ MS,** ± seizures and focal neuro findings (latter atypical for viral *meningitis*)

Diagnostic studies (*CID* 2013; 57:1114)
- **Lumbar puncture:** lymphocytic pleocytosis; PCR for HSV (95% Se & Sp at 2–3 d), VZV, CMV, EBV, HIV, JC, adeno/enterovirus, W. Nile (<60% Se); W. Nile CSF IgM 80% Se
- Consider testing for autoimmune etiologies (anti-NMDAR, etc.) in approp. setting
- **MRI** (CT if MRI unavailable); HSV w/temporal lobe involvement; W. Nile w/ thalamic hyperintensity
- EEG to r/o seizure; findings in encephalitis are nonspecific

Treatment
- HSV, VZV: acyclovir 10 mg/kg IV q8h (often empiric Rx given frequency of HSV/VZV)
- CMV: ganciclovir ± foscarnet; supportive care for most other etiologies

Definition & etiology
- Acute idiopathic unilat. **facial nerve palsy** (CN VII), often presumed HSV-1 reactivation

Clinical manifestations
- Unilateral **facial muscle weakness, hyperacusis,** ↓ taste/lacrimation/salivation

Diagnosis
- Dx of exclusion: r/o brainstem lesion, Lyme (often bilateral), zoster (incl *sine herpete*), HIV/AIDS, sarcoid (often bilateral)

Treatment (*NEJM* 2007;357:1598; *JAMA* 2009;302:985)
- ~80% recover spontaneously by 9 mo (much lower rate in DM)
- Corticosteroids (prednisolone 25 mg PO bid × 10 d) started w/in 72 h of sx onset improve odds of recovery (note: no conclusive data for use in DM, immunosupp.)
- No conclusive data to support the use of acyclovir or valacyclovir

Definition & etiology
- Zoster = herpes zoster = shingles: acute, unilat., **painful dermatomal skin eruption**
- VZV reactivation in peripheral nerve distribution from latency in dorsal root ganglion

Clinical manifestations
- **Neuritic pain in a dermatomal distribution,** then acute **dermatomal eruption of clustered rash** (vesicles > papules/pustules > macules) in varying stages of evolution
- Consecutive dermatomes may be seen in all Pts; more widespread in immunosupp.
- Lesions in V1 distribution of facial nerve require urgent ophthalmologic evaluation
- Post-herpetic neuralgia (PHN) = severe pain lasting >90 d after episode; may last mos to y, more frequent w/ ↑ age and delay of antiviral Rx

Diagnosis
- Appearance of rash; DFA is most Se from scrape of newly unroofed vesicle. Tzanck does not distinguish HSV or VZV; cx insensitive for VZV (unlike HSV).

Treatment
- Rx if can initiate w/in 72 h of skin lesions in healthy Pt or at *any time* in immunosupp.
- Valacyclovir or famciclovir × 7–14 d, or until lesions fully crusted; acyclovir 10 mg/kg IV q8h if dissem. or high-risk Pt (medically ill, immunosupp., V1 zoster w/ ophthalmic s/s., etc.)
- Prevention: vaccine approved for Pts >50 y (↓ lifetime risk from 20% to 10%, also ↓ PHN)

BACTERIAL ENDOCARDITIS

Definition
- Infection of endothelium of heart (including but not limited to the valves)
- **Acute (ABE):** infxn of normal valves w/ virulent organism (eg, *S. aureus*, β-hemolytic strep, *Strep pneumo*)
- **Subacute (SBE):** more indolent infxn w/ less virulent organism (eg, *S. viridans*, *Enterococcus*); often abnl valves

Predisposing conditions
- **Abnormal valve**
    High risk: prior endocarditis, rheumatic heart disease, AoV disease (incl. bicuspid), complex cyanotic lesions, prosthesis (annual risk 0.3–1%)
    Medium risk: MV disease (including MVP w/ MR or thickened leaflet), HCMP
- **Risk of bacteremia:** IVDU, indwelling venous catheters, poor dentition, hemodialysis, DM, prosthetic material in heart (eg, pacemaker, ICD, graft)

Modified Duke Criteria

Major	Minor
• **BCx** with common endocarditis pathogen (grown in 2 separate cultures) • *Coxiella* serology ≥1:800 • **Endocardial involvement,** w/ either: echocardiogram w/ vegetation, abscess, or prosthetic dehiscence <u>new</u> valvular regurgitation	• Predisposing condition (see above) • Fever • **Vascular phenomena:** septic arterial or pulmonary emboli, mycotic aneurysms, ICH, Janeway lesions • **Immune phenomena:** ⊕ RF, GN, Osler's nodes, Roth spots • ⊕ BCx not meeting major criteria

Definitive (ie, highly probable): 2 major *or* 1 major + 3 minor *or* 5 minor criteria
Possible: 1 major + 1 minor or 3 minor criteria

See ~90%, Sp >95%, NPV ≥92% (CID 2000;30:633). *Serologic or molecular tests for other known agents of Cx ⊖ endocarditis (see below) not yet included as major criterion, but may help dx.

Microbiology of Endocarditis

Etiology	Native valve endocarditis (NVE)		Prosthetic valve endocarditis (PVE)	
	Non-IVDA	**IVDU**	**Early** (≤60 d post)	**Late** (>60 d post)
S. viridans et al.	**36%**	**13%**	<5%	20%
Enterococcus	**11%**	**5%**	8%	13%
S. aureus	**28%**	**68%**	36%	20%
S. epidermidis	**9%**	<5%	17%	20%
GNR	<5%	**<5%**	6%	<5%
Other	<5%	<5%	10%	10%
Fungal[a]	1%	1%	9%	3%
Culture ⊖[b]	11%	<5%	17%	12%

[a] ↑ risk w/ DM, indwelling lines, immunosupp. [b] Cx w/ ⊖ = abiotrophic strep, HACEK (*Haemophilus para- influenzae & aphrophilus, Actinobacillus, Cardiobacterium, Eikenella* and *Kingella*), *T. whipplei, Bartonella, Coxiella, Chlamydia, Legionella, Brucella* (JAMA 2007;297:1354; Annals 2007;147:829; J Clin Microbiol 2012;50:216)

Clinical manifestations (Lancet 2016;387:882)
- **Persistent bacteremia:** fever (80–90%), rigors, night sweats, anorexia, wt loss, fatigue
- **Valvular or perivalvular infection:** CHF, conduction abnormalities
- **Septic emboli:** systemic emboli (eg, to periphery, CNS, kidneys, spleen, or joints; JACC 2013;62:1384), stroke, PE (if right-sided), mycotic aneurysm, MI (coronary artery embolism)
- **Immune complex phenomena:** arthritis, glomerulonephritis, ⊕ RF, ↑ ESR
- **SBE:** can p/w fatigue, nonspecific sx in Pts w/o risk factors; ∴ need high index of suspicion

Physical exam
- **HEENT: Roth spots** (retinal hemorrhage + pale center), **petechiae** (conjunctivae, palate)
- **Cardiac: murmur** (85%), **new valve regurgitation** (40–85%) ± thrill (fenestrated valve or ruptured chordae), muffled sounds (PV). *Frequent exams for Δ murmurs, s/s CHF.*
- **Abdomen:** tender splenomegaly; **musculoskeletal:** arthritis, vertebral tenderness
- **Extremities** (*typically seen in SBE, not ABE*)
    Janeway lesions (septic emboli → nontender, hemorrhagic macules on palms or soles)
    Osler's nodes (immune complexes → tender nodules on pads of digits)
    proximal nail bed splinter hemorrhages (8–15%); petechiae (33%); clubbing
- **Neuro:** Δ MS or focal deficits
- **Devices:** erythema, tenderness or drainage at catheter site, PM/ICD pocket tenderness

- **Blood cultures** *(before abx):* at least 3 sets (aerobic & anaerobic bottles) from different sites, ideally spaced ≥1 h apart. ✓ BCx (at least 2 sets) after appropriate abx have been initiated to document clearance; repeat q24–48h until ⊖.
- CBC w/ diff (↑WBC common in ABE; anemia in 90% SBE), ESR, RF, BUN/Cr, U/A, & UCx
- **ECG** (on admission and at regular intervals) to assess for new conduction abnormalities
- **Echocardiogram:** obtain TTE if low clinical suspicion, expect good image quality; TEE if (i) mod-to-high suspicn, expect ⊖ image quality (prosthetic valve, prior IE, congenital heart dis), (iii) TTE nondx, (iv) TTE ⊖ but high-risk endocarditis, or (v) suspect progressive or invasive infection (eg, persistent bacteremia or fever, new conduction abnl, etc.) *(Circ 2015;132:1435)*

Method	Sensitivity		
	NVE	**PVE**	**Abscess**
Transthoracic (TTE)	50–65%	36–69%	28–36%
Transesophageal (TEE)	>90%	~90%	80–87%

(EHJ 1999;20:232; J Am Soc Echo 2003;16:67; Heart 2004;90:614)

- ^{18}F-FDG PET/CT may have utility in assessing PVE *(JACC 2013;61:2374)*
- Brain MRI may be useful to detect silent cerebral emboli *(Circ 2009;120:585)*
- **Cx ⊖ endocarditis:** may be due to abx prior to BCx. PCR, bacterial 16S ribosomal RNA, serologies may be helpful. Detailed hx: animal exposure, travel, unpasteurized dairy, etc. Seek ID eval *(NEJM 2007;356:715; CID 2010;51:131).*

Treatment *(Circ 2015;132:1435; EHJ 2015;36:3075)*
- **Obtain culture data first**
  ABE → abx should start promptly after cx data obtained
  SBE → if hemodynamically stable, may defer abx until BCx properly obtained
- **Suggested empiric therapy**
  NVE: vanco ± nafcillin (or cefazolin)
  PVE: *early* (≤60 d): **vanco + cefepime + gent;** *intermediate* (60–365 d): **vanco + gent;** *late* (>1 y): **vanco + CTX + gent**
- **Adjust abx regimen & duration** based on valve (NVE vs. PVE)
  if possible, de-escalate abx to organism-directed Rx guided by *in vitro* sensi's or local patterns of Rx-resist
  add rifampin for PVE due to staph spp. (usually after BCx ⊖ to ↓ risk resistance develops)
  combination therapy for *Enterococcus* (amp + gent or amp + CTX)
- Repeat BCx q24-48h until Pt defervesces and BCx ⊖; usually 2–3 d
- Fever may persist even >1 wk after appropriate abx. *Consider metastatic infxn if >1 wk.*
- Systemic anticoagulation relatively *contraindicated* given risk of hemorrhage in cerebral embolic strokes; w/o stroke, can continue short-acting anticoag for a pre-existing indication
- Monitor for complications of endocarditis (CHF, conduction block, new emboli, etc., which can occur even on abx) and of abx Rx (interstitial nephritis, ARF, neutropenia, etc.)
- Duration of Rx: usually **4–6 wk.** With NVE & sx <3 mo → 4 wk of abx; sx >3 mo → ≥6 wk. Uncomplicated right-sided NVE or PCN-S strep spp → 2 wk may be comparable.
- Posthospitalization outPt IV abx monitoring; future endocarditis Ppx

Indications for surgery *(EHJ 2015;36:3075)*
- **Severe valvular dysfunction → refractory CHF:** *emergent* if refractory cardiogenic shock (ie, despite ICU-level Rx); *urgent* (w/in days) if persistent refractory heart failure; *elective* (w/in wks) if asx severe AI or MR
- **Uncontrolled infxn** (urgent surgery w/in days): periannular abscess (10–40% NVE, 60–100% PVE), fistula, worsening conduction, PVE w/ dehiscence, ↑ veg. size or persistent sepsis (eg, ⊕ BCx after ~1 wk of appropriate IV abx and no drainable metastatic focus or other identifiable cause)
- **Organism:** consider surgery for *S. aureus,* fungal or multiRx-resistant organisms
- **Systemic embolism** (20–50%): risk 4.8/1000 Pt days in 1st wk, 1.7/1000 thereafter urgent surgery if L-sided w/ >10 mm veg & severe AI/MR *(NEJM 2012;366:2466)* or if recurrent emboli, embolism & >10 mm veg, or >15 mm veg despite approp. abx *cerebral emboli* no longer considered contraindic to surgery unless hemorrhage (then ideally wait 1 mo) or severe stroke *(Stroke 2006;37:2094)*
- **PVE:** esp. w/ valve dysfxn or dehiscence or *S. aureus* or GNR infection. Seek ID eval.

Prognosis
- NVE: non-IVDU *S. aureus* → 30–45% mortality; IVDU *S. aureus* (often right-sided) → 10–15% mortality; SBE → 10–15% mortality
- PVE → 23% mortality
- Aortic valve worse prognosis than mitral valve

Endocarditis Prophylaxis (Circ 2007;116:1736)	
Cardiac conditions*	**Prosthetic valve; previous NVE; congenital heart disease** (CHD) including unrepaired or incompletely repaired cyanotic CHD (palliative shunts or conduits), 1st 6 mo after completely repaired CHD using prosthetic material; **cardiac transplant recipients w/ valvulopathy** (Prophylaxis no longer rec. in acquired valvular dysfxn, bicuspid AoV, MVP with leaflet thickening or regurgitation, HCMP)
Procedures*	**Dental:** manipulation of gingival tissue or periapical region of teeth or perf oral mucosa (eg, extraction, periodontal, implant, root canal, cleaning) **Respiratory:** incision or biopsy of respiratory mucosa (no prophylaxis for GI or GU procedures)
Regimens	Oral: **amoxicillin 2 g 30–60 min before** Unable to take PO: amp 2 g IM/IV or cefazolin or Cftx 1 g IM/IV PCN-allergic: clinda 600 mg PO/IM/IV

*Pts should meet both indications (high-risk condition & high-risk procedure) to qualify for Ppx

BACTEREMIA (JAMA 2014;312:1330)

Etiologies
- 1° infxn due to direct inoculation of the blood, frequently assoc w/ intravascular catheters. Catheter-related bloodstream infection = same org from peripheral cx *and* cath tip cx or cx drawn from catheter (CID 2009;49:1).
- 2° infxn due to infection in another site (eg, UTI, lung, biliary tree, skin) spreading to blood

Microbiology
- 1° infxn/indwelling catheters (ICHE 2008;29:996): coag-neg staph (incl S. epi and others) 34%, S. aureus 10%, enterococci 16%, Candida spp. 12%, Klebsiella spp. 5%
- 2° infxn: dependent on source

Risk factors for true bacteremia (JAMA 2012;308:502)
- **Pt:** fever, rigors, SIRS (96% sens.), IVDU, comorbidities, immunosupp, indwelling lines
- **Organism**
  more likely pathogenic: S. aureus, β-hemolytic strep, enterococci, GNR, S. pneumo, Neisseria
  less likely pathogenic: coag-neg staph (~10%), diphtheroids, Propionibacterium (~0%)
- **Time to growth:** <24 h → higher risk, >72 h → lower risk (except for slow-growing organisms such as HACEK group)
- **Factors increasing the likelihood of endocarditis:** high-grade bacteremia w/o source, persisting after line removal or drainage of focal source, in hosts at risk for endocarditis or w/ organisms known to cause IE; emboli

Diagnosis
- Obtain BCx prior to abx if possible, ≥2 sets (2 bottles in each set, each w/ 10 cc blood)
- If S. aureus, **obtain TEE** (TTE only if nosocomial, no intracardiac device, no e/o IE, no HD)

Treatment
- **1° infxn:** antibiotics based on Gram stain/culture results; tailor abx to sensitivities empiric therapy for GPC: vanco to cover coag-neg staph and MRSA while awaiting sensi
- **S. aureus bacteremia:** if uncomplicated (*all of followng:* ⊖ echo, no prosthetic material, no signs of metastatic infxn, after starting abx defervesce w/in 2–3 d and BCx ⊖ w/in 2–4 d) then 2 wks of abx, o/w 4 wks min. (depends on site of infxn, see individual sections)

Short-Term Central Venous Catheter-Related Bloodstream Infections (CID 2009;49:1)	
S. aureus	**Risk of endocarditis in bacteremia:** ~25% (JACC 1997;30:1072) D/c CVC, TEE to r/o endocarditis; if echo ⊖ and not immunosupp. and no intravasc prosthesis, Rx × 2 wk from first ⊖ BCx. If no echo obtained, Rx × 4–6 wk. **Preferred abx:** MSSA → nafcillin or cefazolin; MRSA → vancomycin
Coag-neg staphylococci	May consider keeping catheter. Catheter retention does not ↓ rate of bacteremia resolution, but a/w ↑ rate of recurrence (CID 2009;49:1187). If catheter left in place, Rx × 10–14 d and consider abx or ethanol lock If catheter d/c, Rx × 5–7 d
Enterococcus	**D/c catheter** & Rx × 7–14 d
GNR	Rx × 7–14 d. Abx based on sensitivities. **D/c catheter** if Pseudomonas.
Fungi	**D/c catheter** & Rx × 14 d from first ⊖ BCx

- **2° infxn:** assess for primary source of infection and treat. Source control essential for cure and to prevent recurrence.
- **Persistently ⊕ BCx:** d/c indwelling catheters, consider metastatic infxn, infected thrombosis or infected prosthetic material (joint, abscess, vascular graft, PPM, etc.)

Epidemiology

- U.S.: 10–15 million infected (10× ↑ risk if foreign-born or minority); worldwide: ~2 billion
- After resurgence in U.S. 1984–1992, rates have declined
- Multidrug resistant (**MDR**) **TB**: resistant to isoniazid (INH) and rifampin (RIF). Can occur as primary infxn if exposed in former Soviet Republics, China
- Extensively drug resistant (**XDR**) **TB** resistant to INH, RIF, FQ and injectables
- Pts more likely to develop **TB** disease (NEJM 2011;364:1441)
    High-prevalence populations (more likely to be exposed & infected): immigrant from high-prevalence area, homeless, IVDU or medically underserved, resident or worker in jail or long-term facility, HCW at facility w/ TB, close contact to Pt w/ active TB
    High-risk populations (infected & likely to progress to active disease): HIV ⊕, immunosupp. incl. biologics, uncontrolled DM & smoking, close contact w/ active TB Pt, underweight, CKD, organ Tx, IVU, EtOH, malnourished, cancer, gastrectomy

Microbiology & natural history

- Transmission of *Mycobacterium tuberculosis* via small-particle aerosols (droplet nuclei)
- 90% of infected normal hosts will never develop clinically evident disease
- Localized disease: healing & calcification *or* progressive 1° TB (at site of infection)
- Hematogenous spread: latent infection ± reactivation TB *or* progressive dissem. TB

Screening for latent infection

- **Whom to screen:** high-prevalence and high-risk populations (HIV ⊕ Pts should have PPD testing as part of initial evaluation and annually thereafter)
- **How to screen:** Mantoux tuberculin test (ie, purified protein derivative or PPD) inject 5-TU (0.1 mL) intermed. strength PPD *intradermally* → wheal; examine 48–72 h
- **How to interpret a PPD:** determine max. diameter of *induration* by palpation

Size of reaction	Persons considered to have ⊕ test
>5 mm	HIV ⊕ or immunosupp (eg, prednisone 15 mg/d × >1 mo) Close contacts of Pt w/ active TB; CXR w/ apical fibrosis c/w TB
>10 mm	All other high-risk or high-prevalence populations Recent conversion (↑ in induration by >10 mm in last 2 y)
>15 mm	Everyone else
False ⊖	Faulty application, anergy (including from active TB), acute TB (2–10 wk to convert), acute non-TB mycobacteria (NTM), malignancy
False ⊕	Improper reading, cross-reaction with NTM, BCG vaccination (although usually <10 mm by adulthood)
Booster effect	↑ induration b/c immunologic boost by prior skin test in prev sensitized individual (by TB, NTM or BCG). Test ⊖ → ⊕ but *not* true conversion due to *recent* infxn. 2nd test true baseline. Can be 1 y after initial test.

(NEJM 2002;347:1860)

- **IFN-γ release assays (IGRA):** (Ag-stimulated IFN-γ release from Pt's T-cells): can use to screen when PPD could be used (MMWR 2010;59:1); ↑ Sp, esp. in BCG Rx'd Pts (Annals 2008;149:177). Does not distinguish active vs. latent or past infxn. Relies on host immune fxn; is limited in immunosupp. (J Clin Epi 2010;63:257; CID 2011;52:1031).

Clinical manifestations (Lancet 2016;387:1211)

- **Primary TB pneumonia:** middle or lower lobe **consolidation**, ± effusion, ± cavitation
- **TB pleurisy:** can occur w/ primary or reactivation. Due to breakdown of granuloma w/ spilling of contents into pleural cavity and local inflammation. **Pulmonary effusion** ± pericardial and peritoneal effusions (tuberculous polyserositis).
- **Reactivation TB pulmonary disease:** apical infiltrate ± volume loss ± cavitation
- **Miliary TB:** acute or insidious; due to hematogenous dissemination; usually in immunosupp, DM, EtOH, elderly or malnourished. **Constitutional sx** (fever, night sweats, weight loss) usually prominent. Pulm disease w/ millet seed-like lesions (2–4 mm) on CXR or chest CT (latter more Se) present in 60–80% of those w/ miliary TB.
- **Extrapulmonary TB:** lymphadenitis, pericarditis, peritonitis, meningitis, nephritis ± sterile pyuria, osteomyelitis (vertebral = Pott's disease), hepatitis, splenitis, cutaneous, arthritis
- **TB and HIV:** HIV ⊕ at ↑ risk infxn, progressive 1° infxn & reactivation. Risk of progression from infxn to disease >8–10%/y, higher risk with ↓ CD4. Reinfection (also w/ MDR) significant, esp. in hyperendemic areas.

Diagnostic studies for active TB (high index of suspicion is key!)

- **AFB smear** (rapid dx) and **culture** (↑ Se & allows sensitivity testing) of sputum, BAL, pleura, etc.; *avoid FQ* if considering TB (can compromise dx yield)

- Gene Xpert PCR (rapid dx) can also detect INH resistance; validated on nonbloody sputum only. Sp 98% & Se 74% independent of HIV status (*AJRCCM* 2014;189;1426).
- PCR: 94–97% Se c/w smear; 40–77% Se c/w culture (*JAMA* 2009;301:1014).
- CXR: classically fibrocavitary apical disease in reactivation vs. middle & lower lobe consolidation in 1° TB but distinction imperfect. HIV ⊕ assoc. w/ nonapical disease regardless of timing (*JAMA* 2005;293:2740).
- Adenosine deaminase testing: useful in extrapulmonary sites; best validated for ascites

Preventive therapy (prevent progression to active disease)
- Prophylaxis reduces incidence of active disease by 65–75%
- Treat Pts who are ⊕ based on guidelines (*NEJM* 2015;372:2127; *Eur Respir J* 2015;46:1563) or any exposed HIV ⊕ or immunocompromised Pt
- **R/o active disease** in any Pt w/ suggestive s/s before starting INH. If HIV ⊕, routinely ask if cough, fever or night sweats; if yes → ✓ sputum smear, CXR, CD4

Scenario	Prophylaxis Regimen
Likely INH sensitive	INH 300 mg PO qd + pyridoxine 25 mg PO qd × 6–9 mo or 12-wk observed combo Rx (INH + rifapentine) (*NEJM* 2011;365:2155)
HIV ⊕	INH 300 mg PO qd + pyridoxine 25 mg PO qd × 9 mo
Contact case INH resistant	RIF × 4 mo
Contact case known or suspected to have MDR TB	No proven regimen: ? PZA + EMB, ? PZA + FQ

(INH, isoniazid; RIF, rifampin; PZA, pyrazinamide; EMB, ethambutol; FQ, fluoroquinolone)

- ✓ LFTs monthly (risk ↑ w/ age; *Chest* 2005;128:116): if 5× ULN or sx → stop TB meds & re-eval

Treatment of active tuberculosis (*NEJM* 2015;373:2149; *Lancet* 2016;387:1211)
- Isolate Pt per infection control if hospitalized, modified isolation per Dept of Health if outPt
- Use multiple drugs (see below) to which organism susceptible; consult ID before empiric Rx if possible MDR-TB (suspect if prior TB Rx, from or travel to area w/ ↑ rates of MDR, exposure to person w/ likely MDR-TB, poor Rx adherence) or if INH resistance in community ≥4% (includes most of U.S.), extrapulm. TB or HIV ⊕ (*NEJM* 2008;359:636)
- Screen for HIV in Pts starting TB Rx; if HIV ⊕, consult ID re: timing of concurrent HIV Rx
- Promote adherence to Rx; directly observed Rx cost-effective if high risk for nonadherence
- Obtain monthly smears/cx on treatment until 2 consecutive are ⊖ for TB
- Monthly clinical evaluation to monitor for Rx response and adverse drug rxns
- "Paradoxical *worsening*" of sx can occur after starting Rx. More common w/ extrapulm. TB (eg, tuberculoma, LAN) likely due to hypersensitivity response to killing of bacilli. More frequent/severe w/ concurrent immune reconstitution (eg, HIV ⊕ Pts started on ARVs, Pts taken off immunosuppression). Must r/o Rx failure (repeat Cx, imaging, etc.).

Antituberculous Medications		
Drug	Dose	Adverse effects*
Isoniazid (INH)	300 mg PO qd	Hepatitis, periph neuropathy (↓ risk by suppl. vit B₆), drug-induced lupus
Rifampin (RIF)	600 mg PO qd	Orange tint of body fluids, GI upset, hepatitis, hypersensitivity, fever, drug interactions, avoid EtOH
Pyrazinamide (PZA)	25 mg/kg PO qd	Hepatitis, hyperuricemia, arthritis
Ethambutol (EMB)	15–25 mg/kg PO qd	Optic neuritis
Streptomycin (SM)	15 mg/kg IM qd	Ototoxicity, nephrotoxicity
Amikacin (AMK)	15 mg/kg IM qd	Ototoxicity, nephrotoxicity
Quinolone (moxifloxacin)	400 mg PO qd	GI upset, tendinopathy, ↑ QTc

*Risk of hepatitis ↑ w/ pre-existing liver disease. Consult ID if mod to severe liver disease, and consider holding/replacing PZA or INH.

Scenario	Antituberculous Treatment Regimens*
Pulmonary TB ≥4% INH-resist. in community (includes most of U.S.)	INH + RIF + PZA + (EMB) until suscept. known If *sensitive* to INH & RIF → INH + RIF + PZA × 2 mo, then → INH + RIF × 4 mo If *resistant*, see next row
Drug-resistant TB (INH-R, RIF-R or MDR/XDR)	*Consult ID specialist* (*NEJM* 2008;359:636)
Extrapulmonary TB	*Consult ID specialist*
TB in HIV ⊕ patient	*Consult ID specialist*

*Individualize duration based on host, disease form, and rate of clinical/microbiologic improvement

Definition
- AIDS: HIV + CD4 <200/mm³ *or* AIDS-defining opportunistic infection (OI) *or* malignancy

Epidemiology
- ~1 million Americans living w/ HIV; ~36 million worldwide
- 13% in U.S. unaware of infxn, many dx w/ late disease. CDC rec testing all people for HIV.
- Routes: sexual (risk is 0.3% for male-to-male, 0.2% for male-to-female, 0.1% for female-to-male transmission), IVDU, transfusions, needlesticks (0.3%), vertical (15–40% w/o ARV)

Prophylaxis (*JAMA* 2014:312:390)
- Postexposure (PEP): risk infxn ~0.3%; Rx: 2 NRTIs + II × 4 wks
- Preexposure (PrEP): TDF/FTC qd or on-demand effective (44-86% ↓) & safe in high-risk, adherent populations w/o renal insufficiency (*NEJM* 2010:363:2587 & 2015:373:2237; *Lancet* 2016:387:53). Monitor renal fxn, STDs, preg, & HIV status.

Acute retroviral syndrome
- Occurs in ~40–90% of Pts ~2–6 wk after infxn; ± ELISA ⊕, ⊕ viral load (2 wk after infxn); early ART may be beneficial (*NEJM* 2013:368:207 & 218)
- Mono-like syndrome (↑ mucocut. & neuro manifestations compared to EBV or CMV)

Diagnostic studies
- **ELISA** for HIV-1 Ab/Ag: ⊕ 1–12 wk after acute infxn; >99% Se; 1° screening test
- If ⊕, Ab differentiation assay confirms and differentiates HIV-1 vs. -2 (*MMWR* 2013:62:489)
- **Rapid tests:** Ab tests; use saliva, plasma, blood or serum; 99% Se & 96–99% Sp (*Annals* 2008:149:153); PPV in low prev populations is low; needs confirmation
- **PCR (viral load):** detects HIV-1 RNA in plasma; assay range is 20–10 million copies/mL ~2% false ⊕, but usually low # copies; in contrast, should be very high (>750 k) in 1° infxn
- **At least 1-time HIV screening recommended for all adults** (*Annals* 2013:159:51)
- **CD4 count:** not a dx test, b/c can be HIV ⊕ w/ normal CD4 or be HIV ⊖ w/ low CD4

Approach to newly diagnosed HIV ⊕ Pt (*Lancet* 2014:384:258)
- **Document HIV infection;** counseling re: treatment options, adherence, & disclosure
- **H&P** (including focus on h/o OIs, STDs); **review all current meds**
- **Lab evaluation:** CD4 count, PCR, HIV genotype, CBC w/ diff., Cr, lytes, LFTs, A1c, & fasting lipids; PPD or IGRA, syphilis & toxo screen & CMV IgG; HAV, HBV, & HCV serologies; *Chlamydia* & gonorrhea screen; baseline CXR; Pap smear/anal pap in ♀/♂

	Common Antiretrovirals (ARVs)	Common Side Effects
NRTI	abacavir (ABC; Ziagen) emtricitabine (FTC; Emtriva) lamivudine (3TC; Epivir) tenofovir (TAF or TDF) zidovudine (AZT; Retrovir)	*Class:* GI intol, lipoatrophy, lactic acidosis ABC: hypersensitivity (3%), ✓ HLA-B*5701 AZT: BM suppression (esp. macrocytic anemia) TDF: renal toxicity TAF: minimal renal toxicity
NNRTI	efavirenz (EFV; Sustiva) etravirine (ETR; Intelence) nevirapine (NVP; Viramune) rilpivirine (RPV; Edurant)	*Class:* rash, hepatitis, mixed CYP450 inducer/inhib EFV: CNS effects (incl depression) NVP: rash and hypersensitivity [risk factors are female, CD4 >250, pregnancy (∴ avoid)]
PI	atazanavir (ATV; Reyataz) darunavir (DRV; Prezista) lopinavir/riton. (LPV/r; Kaletra) ritonavir (RTV; Norvir)	*Class:* GI intol; hepatotoxicity; inhibit CYP450 (caution w/ statins); T2DM; truncal obesity; hyperlipid (less w/ ATV); MI (*NEJM* 2007:356:1723) ATV: crystalluria → nephrolithiasis DRV: rash (10%); possible sulfa cross-reactivity
FI	enfuvirtide (T20; Fuzeon)	injection site reaction
EI	maraviroc (MVC; Selzentry)	dizziness, hepatotoxicity; ✓ CCR5 tropism assay
II	dolutegravir (DTG; Tivicay) elvitegravir (EVG; Vitekta) raltegravir (RAL; Isentress)	*Class:* diarrhea & other GI intol; ↑ CPK DTG + metformin requires glc monitoring
B	ritonavir (r); cobicistat (COBI)	drug interactions (inhibit CYP450)

NRTI, nucleoside/tide reverse transcriptase inhibitor; NNRTI, nonnucleoside RTI; PI, protease inhibitor; FI, fusion inhibitor; EI, entry inhibitor (CCR5 antagonist); II, integrase inhibitor; *booster to give w/ other ARVs; several multiclass combination pills exist

- **ARVs should be given in consultation w/ HIV specialist** (*JAMA* 2016:316:191)
- Counseling re: strict adherence to ARVs is essential; genotype prior to ART-initiation
- All HIV ⊕ Pts should be treated w/ ARVs (*NEJM* 2015:373:795; http://aidsinfo.nih.gov); especially those w/ AIDS-defining illness, preg, HIV-assoc. nephropathy, HCV/HBV co-infxn
- Rec regimens include: 2 NRTI (eg, TAF + FTC) + *either* II *or* boosted PI (eg, DRV/r)

- Initiation of ARVs may *transiently worsen* existing OIs for several wks due to immune reconstitution inflammatory syndrome (IRIS)

Approach to previously established HIV ⊕ Pt
- **H&P** (mucocutaneous, neurocognitive, OIs, malignancies, STDs); meds
- **Review ARVs** (past and current); if any must be interrupted, *stop all* to ↓ risk of resistance
- Failing regimen = unable to achieve undetectable viral load, ↑ viral load, ↓ CD4 count or clinical deterioration (with detectable viral load consider genotypic or phenotypic assay)

OI Prophylaxis (https://aidsinfo.nih.gov/guidelines)		
OI	**Indication**	**1° Prophylaxis**
Tuberculosis	⊕ PPD (≥5 mm)/IGRA or high-risk exposure	INH + vit B_6 × 9 mo
Pneumocystis jiroveci (PCP)	CD4 <200/mm³ or CD4 <14% or thrush	TMP-SMX DS or SS qd or DS tiw or dapsone 100 mg qd or atovaquone 1500 mg qd or pentamidine 300 mg inh q4wk
Toxoplasmosis	CD4 <100/mm³ and ⊕ Toxo IgG	TMP-SMX DS qd or dapsone 50 mg qd + pyrimethamine 50 mg qwk + leucovorin 25 qwk
MAC	CD4 <50/mm³	azithro 1200 mg qwk or clarithro 500 mg bid
Stop 1° prophylaxis if CD4 >initiation threshold >3–6 mo on ARVs		
Stop 2° prophylaxis (maintenance therapy for prior OI; drugs and doses differ by OI) if clinical resolution or stabilization and CD4 thresholds have been exceeded × 3–6 mo		

COMPLICATIONS OF HIV/AIDS

CD4 Count	Complications
<500	Constitutional sx; noninfectious disease (CVD, bone, oncologic) Mucocutaneous: Kaposi's sarcoma; seborrheic dermatitis; oral hairy leukoplakia; lymphoma; candidiasis; HSV; VZV Recurrent bacterial infections, TB (pulm and extrapulm); neurosyphilis
<200	PCP, Toxo, Bartonella, Crypto, Histo, Coccidio
<50–100	CMV, MAC, CNS lymphoma, PML, death (<50 is medical emergency) Invasive aspergillosis, bacillary angiomatosis (disseminated Bartonella)

Fever
- Etiologies (Infect Dis Clin North Am 2007;21:1013)
  infxn (82–90%): MAC, TB, CMV, early PCP, Histo, Crypto, Coccidio, Toxo, endocarditis
  noninfectious: lymphoma, drug reaction. Non 1° HIV itself rarely (<5%) cause of fever.
- Workup: guided by CD4 count, s/s, epi, & exposures
  CBC, chem, LFTs, BCx, CXR, UA, mycobact. & fungal cx, ✓ meds, ? ✓ chest & abd CT
  CD4 <100–200 → serum crypto Ag, LP, urinary Histo Ag, CMV PCR or antigenemia
  pulmonary s/s → CXR; ABG; sputum for bacterial cx, PCP, AFB; bronchoscopy
  diarrhea → stool cx, O&P, AFB; direct visualization with bx on colonoscopy
  cytopenias → BM bx for, path & cx of aspirate including for mycobacteria & fungi
  abnormal LFTs → abd CT, liver bx for path & cx including for mycobacteria & fungi

Cutaneous
- Seborrheic dermatitis; eosinophilic folliculitis; **warts** (HPV); HSV & VZV; MRSA skin & soft tissue infxns; scabies; candidiasis; eczema; prurigo nodularis; psoriasis; drug eruptions
- Dermatophyte infx: prox subungual onychomycosis (at nail bed); pathognomonic for HIV
- **Molluscum contagiosum** (poxvirus): 2–5 mm pearly papules w/ central umbilication
- **Kaposi's sarcoma** (KSHV or HHV8): red-purple nonblanching nodular lesions
- **Bacillary angiomatosis** (disseminated Bartonella): friable violaceous vascular papules

Ophthalmologic
- **CMV retinitis** (CD4 usu <50): Rx: gan- or valganciclovir, ganciclovir implant or cidofovir
- HZV, VZV, syphilis (at any CD4 count) or Toxo: CD4 usually <100

Oral
- **Aphthous ulcers; KS; thrush** (oral candidiasis): curd-like patches typically w/ burning or pain; **oral hairy leukoplakia:** painless proliferation of papillae w/ adherent white coating usually on lateral tongue, caused by EBV but not precancerous

Endocrine/metabolic
- **Hypogonadism;** adrenal insufficiency (CMV, MAC, TB, HIV or med-related); wasting osteopenia/porosis (at all CD4 counts); fragility fractures
- **Lipodystrophy:** central obesity, peripheral lipoatrophy, dyslipidemia, hyperglycemia

- Dilated CMP (10–20%); PHT; CAD); pericarditis/effusion
- Higher rates of VTE, stroke, worse outcomes after MI *(JAIDS 2012;60:351; Circ 2013;127:1767)*

Pulmonary

Radiographic Pattern	Common Causes
Normal	Early PCP
Diffuse interstitial infiltrates	PCP, TB, viral or disseminated fungal
Focal consolidation or masses	Bacterial or fungal, TB, KS
Cavitary lesions	TB, non-TB mycobacteria, aspergillus, other fungal, bacterial (incl MRSA, *Nocardia*, *Rhodococcus*)
Pleural effusion	TB, bacterial or fungal, KS, lymphoma

- *Pneumocystis jiroveci* **(PCP)** pneumonia **(CD4 <200)** *(NEJM 1990;323:1444)* constitutional sx, fever, night sweats, dyspnea on exertion, nonproductive cough CXR w/ interstitial pattern, ↓ P_aO_2, ↑ A-a ∇, ↑ LDH, ⊕ PCP sputum stain, ⊕ β-glucan Rx if P_aO_2 >70: **TMP-SMX** 15–20 mg of TMP/kg divided tid, avg dose = DS 2 tabs PO tid Rx if P_aO_2 <70 or A-a gradient >35: **prednisone** before abx (40 mg PO bid; ↓ after 5 d). Alternative Rx if sulfa-allergy or renal insufficiency.

Gastrointestinal & hepatobiliary

- **Esophagitis:** *Candida,* CMV, HSV, aphthous ulcers, pills; EGD if no thrush or no response to empiric antifungals
- **Enterocolitis:** *bacterial* (esp. if acute: shigella, salmonella, *C. diff*); *protozoal* (esp. if chronic: Giardia, Entamoeba, etc.); *viral* (CMV, adeno); *fungal* (histo); MAC; AIDS enteropathy
- **GI bleeding:** CMV, KS, lymphoma, histo; **proctitis:** HSV, CMV, *LGV, N. gonorrhoeae*
- **Hepatitis:** HBV, HCV, CMV, MAC, TB, histo, drug-induced
- **AIDS cholangiopathy:** often a/w CMV or *Cryptosporidium* or *Microsporidium* (at ↓ CD4)

Renal

- **HIV-associated** nephropathy (collapsing FSGS); nephrotoxic drugs (incl TDF)

Hematologic/oncologic *(Lancet 2007;370:59; CID 2007;45:103)*

- **Anemia:** ACD; BM infiltration by infxn or tumor, drug toxicity, hemolysis
- **Leukopenia; thrombocytopenia** (bone marrow involvement, ITP); infection, ↑ **globulin**
- **Non-Hodgkin lymphoma:** ↑ frequency w/ any CD4 count, but incidence ↑ with ↓ CD4
- **CNS lymphoma:** CD4 count <50, EBV-associated
- **Kaposi's sarcoma** (HHV-8): at any CD4 count, incidence ↑ as CD4 ↓, usu. MSM *Mucocut.* (violaceous lesions); *pulmonary* (nodules, infiltrates, LAN); *GI* (bleed, obstruct.)
- **Cervical/anal CA** (HPV); ↑ rates of liver (a/w HBV/HCV), gastric, & lung CA

Neurologic

- **Meningitis:** Crypto (p/w HA, ↓ MS, CN palsy ± meningeal s/s; dx w/ CSF; serum CrAg 90% Se), bact (inc. *Listeria*), viral (HSV, CMV, 1° HIV), TB, histo, *Coccidio,* lymphoma
- **Neurosyphilis:** meningitis, cranial nerve palsies, dementia, otic or ophtho s/s
- **Space-occupying lesions:** may present as HA, focal deficits or ∆ MS. Workup: MRI, brain bx if suspect non-*Toxo* etiology (*Toxo* sero ⊖) or no response to 2 wk of empiric anti-*Toxo* Rx (if *Toxo,* 50% respond by d3, 91% by d14; *NEJM 1993;329:995*)

Etiology	Imaging appearance	Diagnostic studies
Toxoplasmosis	Enhancing lesions, typically in basal ganglia (can be multiple)	⊕ *Toxo* serology (Se ~85%)
CNS lymphoma	Enhancing ring lesion (single 60% of the time)	⊕ CSF PCR for EBV ⊕ SPECT or PET scan
Progressive multifocal leukoencephalopathy (PML)	Multiple nonenhancing lesions in white matter	⊕ CSF PCR for JC virus
Other: abscess, nocardiosis, crypto, TB, CMV, HIV	Variable	Biopsy

- **AIDS dementia complex:** memory loss, gait disorder, spasticity (usually at CD4 ↓)
- **Myelopathy:** infxn (CMV, HSV), **cord compression** (epidural abscess, lymphoma)
- **Peripheral neuropathy:** meds, HIV, demyelinating

Disseminated *Mycobacterium avium* complex (DMAC)

- Fever, night sweats, wt loss, HSM, diarrhea, pancytopenia. Enteritis and mesenteric lymphadenopathy if CD4 <150, bacillemia if <50. Rx: clarithromycin + ethambutol ± rifabutin.

Cytomegalovirus (CMV)

- Usually reactivation with ↓ CD4. Retinitis, esophagitis, colitis, hepatitis, neuropathies, encephalitis. Rx: ganciclovir, valganciclovir, foscarnet or cidofovir.

Distinguishing Features of Tick-Borne Illnesses					
Disease	**Rash**	**↓WBC**	**Anemia**	**↓ Plts**	**↑ LFTs**
Lyme	80%: erythema migrans	–	–	–	+
RMSF	90%: petechiae, palms/soles	–	+	+	+++
Borrelia miyamotoi	<10%	++	+	+++	+++
Ehrlichiosis (HME)	25%: maculopapular, petechiae	+++	++	++++	++++
Anaplasmosis (HGA)	<5%	+++	+	+++	++++
Babesia	–	+	++++ (lysis)	++++	+++

-: <15%, +: 15–25%, ++: 25–50%, +++: 50–75%, ++++: > 75%

LYME DISEASE

Microbiology
- **Spirochete** *B. burgdorferi* (consider coinfection w/ *Ehrlichia, Babesia, B. miyamotoi*)
- Transmitted by **ticks** (*Ixodes*, deer tick); infxn usually requires **tick attached >36–48 h**

Epidemiology
- Most common vector-borne illness in U.S.; peak incidence in summer (May–Aug)
- Majority of cases in MN, WI, New England, northern mid-Atlantic, northern CA
- Humans contact ticks usually in fields with low brush near wooded areas

Clinical Manifestations	
Stage	**Manifestations**
Stage 1 (early localized) 3-30d after bite	Pathogenesis: local effects of spirochete. *General:* flu-like illness *Derm* (~80%): **erythema migrans** (EM) = erythematous patches w/ central clearing, often popliteal, axilla, or inguinal; 6–38 cm in size
Stage 2 (early dissem.) wks to mos after bite	Pathogenesis: spirochetemia and immune response *General:* fatigue, malaise, LAN, HA; fever uncommon *Derm:* **multiple (1–100) annular lesions ≈ EM** *Rheum* (~10%): **migratory arthralgias** (knee & hip) **& myalgias** *Neurologic* (~15%): cranial neuropathies (esp. **CN VII**), aseptic meningitis, mononeuritis multiplex (± pain), transverse myelitis *Cardiac* (~8%): **conduction block,** myopericarditis
Stage 3 (late persistent) mos to y after bite	Pathogenesis: immune response *Derm:* **acrodermatitis chronica atrophicans,** panniculitis *Rheum* (~60%): **recurrent mono- or oligoarthritis of large joints** (classically knee), synovitis *Neurologic:* subacute encephalomyelitis, polyneuropathy, dementia

(*CID* 2006;43:1089; *Lancet* 2012;379:461; *NEJM* 2014;370:1724)

Diagnostic studies (*NEJM* 2014;370:1724; *JAMA* 2016;315:1767 & 2461)
- EM present: confirmed in appropriate geographic setting; no need for testing (ie, clinical dx)
- EM absent (ie, stage 2 or 3 disease): 2-step testing
  - 1st step: ELISA screen (false ⊕ common, false ⊖ w/ early abx or <6 wk after tick bite)
  - 2nd step: if ⊕ ELISA, confirm with Western blot (↑ Sp)
- ✓ CSF if suspected neuro disease: ⊕ CSF Ab if (IgG$_{CSF}$/IgG$_{serum}$)/(alb$_{CSF}$/alb$_{serum}$) >1

Treatment (*NEJM* 2014;370:1724; *JAMA* 2016;315:1767 & 2461)
- Prophylaxis: tick avoidance, protective clothing, tick ✓ q24h, DEET
  Chemoprophylaxis w/ doxycycline 200 mg PO × 1 *only* if *all* of the following:
  1. *Ixodes scapularis* tick attached ≥36 h
  2. Local Lyme carriage in ticks ≥20% (peak season in New England, mid-Atl, MN, WI)
  3. Abx can be given w/in ≤72 h of tick bite
  4. No contraindication to doxy (eg, preg, allergy, age <8 y)
  If criteria 1–4 met, NNT to prevent 1 case ~50; w/o doxy, risk of Lyme after tick bite 1–3%
  Regardless of Ppx, monitor for fever, flu-like sx, rash (erythema migrans) × 30 d
- Antibiotics: *if clin. manifestations and* ⊕ serology in endemic area
  Stage 1 or stage 2 w/o meningitis, arthritis, or carditis: **doxy** 100 mg PO bid × 2–3 wk;
    alternative (eg, preg, doxy allergy): amox 500 mg PO tid or cefuroxime 500 mg PO bid
  Meningitis, arthritis, carditis: CTX 2 g IV qd × 2–4 wk;
    alternative (eg, severe β-lactam allergy): doxy 100–200 mg PO bid × 2–4 wk
- Consider coinfection if severe/refractory sx, persistent fever, cytopenias

Rocky Mountain Spotted Fever (RMSF)

Microbiology & epidemiology
- Infection with *Rickettsia rickettsii* (Gram ⊖ obligate intracellular bacterium)
- Transmitted by *Dermacentor variabilis, D. andersoni* (dog tick); peak in spring/early summer
- Occurs in **mid-Atl, SE, Midwest**, New Engl, NW, Canada, Mexico, Central & S.America
- Consider other rickettsial spp.: *R. akari* (Rickettsial pox), *R. conorii* (Mediterranean spotted fever), *R. africae* (African tick bite fever), *R. felis* (Flea rickettsiosis)

Clinical manifestations (typically w/in 1 wk of tick exposure)
- Nonspecific: **fever, HA,** ΔMS, myalgias, N/V, occasionally abdominal pain
- **Rash** (2–5 d *after* onset) = *centripetal*: starts on ankles and wrists → trunk, palms, & soles; progresses from macular to maculopapular to petechial
- Severe cases ⇒ vasculitis, hypoperfusion/shock, end-organ damage; more likely in elderly
- Up to 75% mortality if untreated, 5–10% even w/ Rx (esp. if delayed) (*NEJM 2005;353:551*)

Diagnosis
- Usually a clinical dx; *requires early clinical suspicion* given risks of delayed Rx
- Acute illness dx by **skin bx** for rickettsiae (Se ~70%); 7–10 d after sx onset, serology ⊕

Treatment
- Doxycycline 100 mg PO bid (*give empirically if clinical suspicion*)

Ehrlichiosis/Anaplasmosis

Microbiology
- Gram ⊖ obligate intracellular bacterium; **human monocytic ehrlichiosis** (*E. chaffeensis,* HME); **human granulocytic anaplasmosis** (*A. phagocytophilum,* HGA)
- Transmission: HME by *Amblyomma americanum, Dermacentor variabilis*; HGA by *Ixodes*

Epidemiology
- HGA cases typically in New Engl, mid-Atl, MN; HME in SE and south central US
- Peak incidence spring and early summer; can be transmitted by blood transfusion

Clinical manifestations (typically w/in 3 wk of tick exposure)
- Asx or nonspecific: fever, myalgias, malaise, HA, cough, dyspnea; onset often acute
- Laboratory: leukopenia, thrombocytopenia, ↑ aminotransferases, LDH, AΦ, renal insuff
- More severe disease can occur with bacterial superinfection in HGA

Diagnosis
- Acute: intraleukocytic morulae on peripheral blood smear (rare); **PCR**; later: serology

Treatment (*JAMA 2016;315:1767*)
- Start Rx based on clinical suspicion; definitive dx requires PCR (may not detect all spp.)
- Doxycycline 100 mg PO bid (often × 10 d); should defervesce in ≤48 h, else reconsider dx

Babesiosis

Microbiology & epidemiology
- Infxn w/ parasite *Babesia microti* (U.S.), transmitted by *Ixodes* ticks; also a/w transfusion
- Europe & U.S. (more commonly MN, WI, **coastal areas & islands of MA**, NY, NJ, RI, CT)
- Peak incidence June–August (*MMWR 2012;61:505*)

Clinical manifestations (typically 1–4 wk after tick exposure; <9 wk if transfusion)
- Range from asx to fevers, sweats, myalgias, & HA to severe hemolytic anemia, hemoglobinuria, & death (degree of parasitemia correlates roughly with severity)
- Risk factors for severe disease: asplenia, ↓ cellular immunity, TNF inhib, ↑ age, pregnancy

Diagnosis (*NEJM 2012;366:2397*)
- Clinical syndrome + **blood smear w/ intraerythrocytic parasites**
- Repeat smears (q12–24h) if sx persist despite negative initial smear
- PCR serum if smear ⊖ and high clinical suspicion; serum IgG can help but some false ⊕

Treatment (*JAMA 2016;315:1767*)
- Atovaquone & azithro for mild/mod illness; clinda & quinine if severe (more toxic)
- Duration depends on host; immunosupp Pts often need longer Rx
- Exchange transfusion if parasitemia >10%, severe hemolysis or SIRS

Tularemia

Microbiology
- Infxn w/ *Francisella tularensis* via contact w/ animal tissue, aerosol, tick/insect bite

Clinical manifestations (typically w/in 2–10 d of exposure)
- Acute onset of fever, HA, nausea; ulcer w/ black eschar at site of entry; LAN; PNA

Diagnosis & treatment
- Hazardous and difficult to Cx, alert lab. Serology ⊕ by wk 2. PCR by research lab.
- Streptomycin or gentamicin × 7–14 d; empiric Rx may be needed given challenges in dx

FEVER SYNDROMES

Temperature ≥ 100.4°F or ≥38°C

Diagnostic approach

- Thorough history including ROS, PMH/PSH, immunizations, including from childhood
- **Fever curve** (consider holding antipyretics); less likely to mount fever if: chronic renal or liver dis., extremes of age, protein calorie malnutrition, immunosupp., steroid use
- **Exposures:** travel, occupation or hobbies, animals and insects, sexual contacts, TB; consider age, geography, season and incubation time in relation to exposures
- **Physical exam:** complete exam w/ focus on mucous membranes & conjunctiva; cardiac murmurs; liver and spleen size; skin, genitals, lymph nodes, & joints; complete neuro exam incl cranial nerves and meningeal signs
- **If rash:** location, duration, progression/Δ in appearance, was prodrome present

FEVER OF UNKNOWN ORIGIN (FUO)

Definition & etiologies

- **Fever** (as per above def) on >1 occasion during ≥3 wk & **no dx** despite 1 wk of evaluation
- More likely to be *unusual manifestation of common disease* than an uncommon disease
- In Pts with HIV: >75% causes are infectious, but *rarely due to HIV itself*
- **Frequent reassessment needed** to identify focal signs and progression of disease

Category	Etiologies of Classic FUO (Archives 2003;163:545; Medicine 2007;86:26)
Infection ~30%	**Tuberculosis:** disseminated or extrapulm disease can have normal CXR, PPD, sputum AFB; bx (lung, liver, bone marrow) for granulomas has 80–90% yield in miliary disease **Abscess:** dental, paraspinal, hepatic, splenic, subphrenic, pancreatic, perinephric, pelvic, prostatic abscess or prostatitis, appendicitis **Endocarditis:** consider HACEK orgs, Bartonella, Legionella, Coxiella Osteomyelitis, sinusitis, Lyme, typhoid, 1° CMV or EBV, malaria, Babesia
Connective tissue disease ~30%	**Giant cell arteritis/PMR:** headache, scalp pain, jaw claudication, visual disturbances, myalgias, arthralgias, ↑ ESR **Adult-onset Still's:** evanescent truncal rash, LAN, pharyngitis, ↑↑ ferritin **PAN, ANCA ⊕, other vascul.;** SLE, RA, psoriatic or reactive arthritis
Neoplasm ~20%	**Lymphoma:** LAN, HSM, ↓ Hct or plt, ↑ LDH; leukemia, myelodysplasia **Renal cell carcinoma:** microscopic hematuria, ↑ Hct **HCC, pancreatic and colon cancers, sarcomas, mastocytosis** Atrial myxomas: obstruction, embolism, constitutional symptoms
Misc ~20%	Drugs, factitious, DVT/PE, hematoma Thyroiditis or thyroid storm, adrenal insufficiency, pheochromocytoma Granulomatous hepatitis (many causes), sarcoidosis, Kikuchi's, Behçet's Familial Mediterranean fever (peritonitis, episodic fever, pleuritis; ↑ WBC & ESR during attacks); other defects in innate immunity

Workup

- Focus by H&P, incl: CBC w/ diff, lytes, BUN, Cr, LFTs, ESR, CRP, ANA, RF, cryoglobulin, LDH, CK, SPEP, 3 sets BCx (off of abx), U/A, UCx, PPD or IGRA, HIV Ab ± PCR, heterophile Ab (EBV serologies if ⊖), CMV antigen, Hep serologies if LFTs abnl
- Stop unnecessary meds (only 20% with a med cause have eos or rash), reassess 1–3 wk
- Imaging: CXR, chest & abd CT, consider tagged WBC, gallium scan, PET, TTE, LENI
- Consider temporal artery bx if ↑ ESR and age >60, particularly if other s/s
- Consider BM aspirate & bx (esp. if signs of marrow infiltration) or liver bx (esp. if ↑ Aφ): even w/o localizing s/s, yield may be up to 24% (path and cx) (Archives 2009;169:2018)
- Pursue abnormalities raised by above w/u (eg, bx, MRI, etc., for dx, *not* screening)

Treatment

- Empiric abx *not* indicated (unless Pt neutropenic)
- Empiric glucocorticoids not indicated unless strong suspicion for specific rheumatologic dx
- Up to 30% of cases remain undiagnosed, most spontaneously defervesce (wks to mos)

FEVER AND RASH

Approach to diagnostic workup

- **Meningococcemia, endocarditis, RMSF, sepsis, toxic shock need urgent dx & Rx**
- Workup: CBC w/ diff, lytes, BUN/Cr, LFTs, LDH, CK, U/A, HIV Ab ± PCR, BCx (off abx)
- To narrow Ddx: characterize time course of rash, progression & morphology

- **Erythema multiforme:** symmetric "target" lesions often of palms, soles, & mucous memb
  Infxn etiol: HSV ½, *Mycoplasma*, syphilis, tick-borne diseases, etc.
  Non-infxn etiol: meds (eg, NSAIDs, sulfa), malignancy, autoimmune & rheum disease
- **Erythema nodosum:** tender erythematous or violaceous nodules usually symmetric on LE
  Infxn etiol: Strep, TB, EBV, *Bartonella*, HBV, psittacosis, fungal, *L. venereum*, etc.
  Non-infxn etiol: sarcoidosis, IBD, Behçet's, other rheum, pregnancy/OCP use
- Pursue specific dx based on exposure hx & exam, including serologies, viral swab PCR,
  antigen tests and possibly skin biopsy ± culture of vesicular or bullae fluid if present
- Etiologies more broad in immunosupp. Pts, dx testing should be earlier and more
  extensive; higher risk of critical illness due to disseminated or rapidly progressive infxns

Variable	Possible Etiology
Summer/fall > other seasons	Enterovirus
Winter	Parvovirus, Meningococcemia
Spring/summer	Measles/rubella, Lyme, RMSF
Year-round	Adenovirus, *Mycoplasma*
Cat and dog exposure	*Bartonella, Pasteurella, Toxoplasma, Capnocytophaga*
Tick exposure	Lyme, RMSF, Ehrlichiosis, Anaplasmosis
Adult <30 y	Mononucleosis (EBV or CMV)
Inadequate immunization	Measles, Rubella, VZV, influenza
Sexually active	HIV, syphilis, disseminated gonococcal infection, HSV2
Consider noninfectious causes: allergy/DRESS, DVT, phlebitis, vasculitides, neutrophilic dermatoses, gout, connective tissues dis., malignancy, foreign body rxn	

Treatment
- Empiric abx *not* indicated (unless Pt neutropenic or critically ill)

FEVER 6-23

FEVER IN A RETURNED TRAVELER

Region or Exposure	Common Etiologies
Sub-Saharan Africa	**Malaria** >> dengue, rickettsial disease, enteric disease
Southeast Asia	Dengue > malaria, enteric disease (*S. typhi*), Chikungunya
Central & S. America	Enteric disease, malaria, dengue, Zika
Caribbean & Mexico	Dengue >> Chikungunya > malaria. Also consider Zika.
Middle East & S. Korea	Middle East Respiratory Syndrome
Freshwater swimming	Schistosomiasis, leptospirosis
Unpurified drinking water	Enteric disease (*E. coli* >> *S. typhi, Campylobacter,* hepatitis E > *Vibrio cholerae*), amebic liver abscess
Lacking immunizations	HAV/HBV, *S. typhi,* influenza, measles, rubella, yellow fever
Animal bite	Rabies
African "safari"	Rickettsial disease, African trypanosomiasis
Adult <30 years	Mononucleosis (EBV or CMV)

(*NEJM* 2002;347:505; *CID* 2007;44:1560; *Curr Opin Infect Dis* 2007;20:449)

- Pts visiting friends and relatives abroad are most likely to contract illness during travel
- Geography influences Ddx in returned travelers: http://www.nccdc.gov/travel/notices
- Emerging pathogens: Influenza occurs year-round in the tropics. Chikungunya and dengue w/ ↑ areas of transmission, hemorrhagic fevers primarily in Central Africa.
- Consider domestic infxns, STIs, & non-infxn causes. Enteric parasites rarely cause fever.

Select clinical manifestations
- **Ebola:** fever in traveler from area with active transmission of Ebola w/in 21 d: isolate & contact state health department (http://www.cdc.gov/vhf/ebola)
- **Malaria:** nonspecific symptoms including diarrhea, myalgias, cough, altered mental status
- **Dengue:** nonspecific symptoms including headache, severe myalgias, rash/petechiae
- **Chikungunya:** nonspecific symptoms including joint pain, moderate myalgias, fever
- **Typhoid** (*Lancet* 2015;385:1136): constipation, abd pain, possible rash, relative bradycardia
- **Rickettsial disease:** headache, myalgias, lymphadenopathy, possible rash/eschar
- **Zika:** fever, rash, arthralgia, H/A, conjunctivitis (http://www.cdc.gov.zika)

Workup
- Routine testing: CBC w/ diff, lytes, LFTs, BCx, UA, rapid malaria test
- **Fever in a traveler from a malaria zone is malaria until proven otherwise; consider hospitalization and empiric Rx.** One ⊖ smear does *not* r/o malaria.
- Other tests based on s/s, labs, exposure, incubation period, geography and seasonality. O&P exam, CXR, blood smears for filaria/Babesiosis/*Borrelia,* serologies, STI & HIV, PPD or IGRA, bone marrow aspirate, bx of lymph nodes or skin lesions, CSF studies.

PITUITARY DISORDERS

HYPOPITUITARY SYNDROMES

Panhypopituitarism (*Lancet 2016;epub*)
- Etiologies
  Primary: surgery, radiation (develops after avg 4–5 y), tumors (primary or metastatic), infection, infiltration (sarcoid, hemochromatosis), autoimmune, ischemia (including Sheehan's syndrome caused by pituitary infarction intrapartum), carotid aneurysms, cavernous sinus thrombosis, trauma, medications (eg, ipilimumab)
  Secondary (hypothalamic dysfunction or stalk interruption): tumors (including craniopharyngioma), infection, infiltration, radiation, surgery, trauma
- Clinical manifestations
  Hormonal: acute → weakness, easy fatigability, hypotension, polyuria and polydipsia; chronic → bradycardia, sexual dysfxn, loss of axillary & pubic hair, wt loss, amenorrhea
  Mass effect: headache, visual field Δs, cranial nerve palsies, galactorrhea
  Apoplexy (pituitary hemorrhage or infarction, usually w/ underlying pituitary adenoma): sudden headache, N/V, visual field Δs, cranial nerve palsies, meningismus, Δ MS, hypoglycemia, hypotension
- Diagnostic studies
  Hormonal studies
    chronic: ↓ target gland hormone + ↓ or normal trophic pituitary hormone
    acute: target gland hormonal studies may be *normal*
    partial hypopituitarism is more common than panhypopituitarism
  Pituitary MRI
- Treatment
  Replace deficient target gland hormones
  Most important deficiencies to recognize and treat in inpatients are *adrenal insufficiency* and *hypothyroidism*; if both present, treat with glucocorticoids first, then replace thyroid hormone so as not to precipitate adrenal crisis

↓ ACTH
- Sx similar to 1° adrenal insufficiency (see "Adrenal Disorders") *except:*
  no salt cravings or hypokalemia (b/c aldo preserved)
  no hyperpigmentation (b/c ACTH/MSH is not ↑)

↓ TSH
- Sx of central hypothyroidism similar to 1° (see "Thyroid Disorders") *except* absence of goiter
- Dx with free T_4 in addition to TSH, as TSH may be low or *inappropriately normal*

↓ PRL
- Inability to lactate

↓ GH
- ↑ chronic risk for osteoporosis, fatigue, weight gain
- Dx with failure to ↑ GH w/ appropriate stimulus (eg, insulin tolerance test, glucagon stimulation)
- GH replacement in adults controversial (*Annals 2003;35:419*)

↓ FSH & LH
- Clinical manifestations: ↓ libido, impotence, oligomenorrhea or amenorrhea, infertility, ↓ muscle mass, osteoporosis
- Physical exam: ↓ testicular size; loss of axillary, pubic and body hair
- Dx with: ↓ a.m. testosterone or estradiol (also assess SHBG, esp. in obese) and ↓ or normal FSH/LH (all levels ↓ in acute illness, ∴ do not measure in hospitalized Pts)
- Treatment: testosterone or estrogen replacement *vs.* correction of the underlying cause

↓ ADH (hypothalamic or stalk disease): diabetes insipidus
- Typically from mass lesion extrinsic to sella; pituitary tumor does not typically present w/ DI
- Clinical manifestations: *severe* polyuria, *mild* hypernatremia (*severe* if ↓ access to H_2O)
- Diagnostic studies: see "Sodium and Water Homeostasis"

HYPERPITUITARY SYNDROMES

Pituitary tumors
- Pathophysiology: adenoma → excess of trophic hormone (if tumor fxnal, but 30–40% not) and potentially *deficiencies* in other trophic hormones due to compression; cosecretion of PRL and growth hormone in 10% of prolactinomas
- Clinical manifestations: syndromes due to oversecretion of hormones (see below) ± mass effect: headache, visual Δs, diplopia, cranial neuropathies
- Workup: MRI, hormone levels, ± visual field testing
  if <10 mm, no mass effect, no hormonal effects, can f/up q3–6mo

Hyperprolactinemia (*NEJM* 2010;362:1219 and *JCEM* 2011;96:273)

- Etiology
  prolactinoma (50% of pituitary adenomas)
  stalk compression due to nonprolactinoma → ↓ inhibitory dopamine → ↑ PRL (mild)
- Physiology: PRL induces lactation and inhibits GnRH → ↓ FSH & LH
- Clinical manifestations: **amenorrhea, galactorrhea, infertility**, ↓ libido, impotence
- Diagnostic studies
  ↑ **PRL** (✓ *fasting* levels), but elevated in many situations, ∴ r/o pregnancy or exogenous
  estrogens, hypothyroidism, dopamine agonists (eg, psych meds, antiemetics), renal
  failure (↓ clearance), cirrhosis, stress, ↑ carb diet. Watch for *hook effect*: assay artifact
  yielding falsely low PRL if very high serum PRL levels; retest with sample dilution.
  MRI to evaluate for tumor
- Treatment
  If asx (no HA, galactorrhea, hypogonadal sx) & microadenoma (**<10 mm**), follow w/ MRI
  If sx or macroadenoma (**≥10 mm**) options include:
  medical with dopamine agonist such as cabergoline (70–100% success rate) or
  bromocriptine (not as well tol); side effects include N/V, orthostasis, nasal congestion
  surgical: transsphenoidal surgery (main indications: failed or cannot tolerate medical Rx,
  GH cosecretion or neurologic sx not improving); 10–20% recurrence rate
  radiation: if medical or surgical therapy have failed or are not tolerated

Acromegaly (↑ GH; 10% of adenomas; *NEJM* 2006;355:2558 & *JCEM* 2014;99:3933)

- Physiology: stimulates secretion of insulin-like growth factor 1 (IGF-1)
- Clinical manifestations: ↑ soft tissue, arthralgias, jaw enlargement, headache, carpal tunnel
  syndrome, macroglossia, hoarseness, sleep apnea, amenorrhea, impotence, diabetes
  mellitus, acanthosis/skin tags, ↑ sweating, HTN/CMP, colonic polyps
- Diagnostic studies: *no utility in checking random GH levels because of pulsatile secretion*
  ↑ **IGF-1** (somatomedin C); ± ↑ PRL; OGTT → GH *not* suppressed to <1 (<0.3 if
  newer assay) ng/mL; pituitary MRI to evaluate for tumor
- Treatment: **surgery**, octreotide (long- and short-acting preparations), dopamine
  agonists (if PRL co-secretion), pegvisomant (GH receptor antagonist), radiation
- Prognosis: w/o Rx 2–3× ↑ mortality, risk of pituitary insufficiency, colon cancer

Cushing's disease (↑ ACTH): 10–15% of adenomas; see "Adrenal Disorders"

Central hyperthyroidism (↑ TSH, ↑ α-subunit): extremely rare; see "Thyroid Disorders"

↑ FSH & LH: usually non-fxn, presents as *hypopituitarism* b/c of compression effects

Multiple Endocrine Neoplasia (MEN) Syndromes	
Type	**Main features**
1 (*MENIN* inactiv.)	Parathyroid hyperplasia/adenomas → hypercalcemia (~100% penetrance) Pancreatic islet cell neoplasia (gastrin, VIP, insulin, glucagon) Pituitary adenomas (fxn or non-fxn)
2A (*RET* proto-oncogene)	Medullary thyroid carcinoma (MTC) Pheochromocytoma (~50%) Parathyroid hyperplasia → hypercalcemia (15–20%)
2B (*RET* proto-oncogene)	Medullary thyroid carcinoma (MTC) Pheochromocytoma (~50%) Mucosal and gastrointestinal neuromas

Autoimmune Polyglandular Syndromes (APS)	
Type	**Features**
I (children)	Mucocutaneous candidiasis, hypoparathyroidism, adrenal insufficiency
II (adults)	Adrenal insufficiency, autoimmune thyroid disease, diabetes mellitus type 1

THYROID DISORDERS

Diagnostic Studies in Thyroid Disorders	
Test	**Comments**
Thyroid-stimulating hormone (TSH)	Most sensitive test to detect 1° hypo- and hyperthyroidism May be inappropriately normal in central etiologies ↓'d by dopamine, glucocorticoids, severe illness
Free T₄ (FT₄)	Unbound T₄, not influenced by TBG
Total T₃ and T₄	Total serum concentrations (∴ influenced by TBG)
Thyroxine-binding globulin (TBG)	↑ TBG (∴ ↑ T₄): estrogen (OCP, pregnancy), hepatitis, opioids, hereditary ↓ TBG (∴ ↓ T₄): androgens, glucocorticoids, nephritic syndrome, cirrhosis, acromegaly, antiepileptics, hereditary
Reverse T₃	Inactive, ↑'d in sick euthyroid syndrome
Thyroid antibodies	Antithyroid peroxidase (TPO) seen in Hashimoto's (high titer), painless thyroiditis and Graves' disease (low titer) Thyroid-stimulating Ig (TSI) and thyrotropin-binding inhibitory immunoglobulin (TBII) seen in Graves' disease
Thyroglobulin	↑'d in goiter, hyperthyroidism and thyroiditis ↓'d in factitious ingestion of thyroid hormone Tumor marker for thyroid cancer only after total thyroidectomy and radioiodine therapy

Radioactive iodine uptake (**RAIU**) scan	Useful to differentiate causes of hyperthyroidism
	↑ **uptake**
	  homogeneous = Graves' disease
	  heterogeneous = multinodular goiter
	  1 focus of uptake w/ suppression of rest of gland = hot nodule
	no uptake = subacute painful (de Quervain's) or silent thyroiditis, exogenous thyroid hormone, recent iodine load, struma ovarii or antithyroid drugs

(Lancet 2001;357:619 & Thyroid 2003;13:19)

Figure 7-1 Approach to thyroid disorders

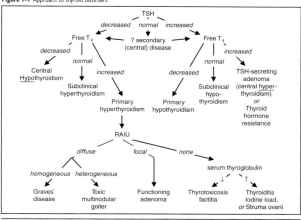

HYPOTHYROIDISM

Etiologies

- Primary (>90% of cases of hypothyroidism; ↓ free T₄, ↑ TSH)
  Goitrous: **Hashimoto's thyroiditis** (after hyperthyroid phase of thyroiditis), iodine deficiency, lithium, amiodarone

Nongoitrous: surgical destruction, s/p radioactive iodine or XRT, amiodarone
- Secondary (central): ↓ free T4; TSH low, inappropriately nl, or slightly high (although functionally inactive due to abnormal glycosylation); due to hypothalamic or pituitary failure

Hashimoto's thyroiditis
- Autoimmune destruction with patchy lymphocytic infiltration
- Associated with other autoimmune disease and may be part of APS Type II
- ⊕ antithyroid peroxidase (anti-TPO) and antithyroglobulin (anti-Tg) Abs in >90%

Clinical manifestations (Annals 2009;151:ITC61)
- **Early:** weakness, fatigue, arthralgias, myalgias, headache, depression, cold intolerance, weight gain, constipation, menorrhagia, dry skin, coarse brittle hair, brittle nails, carpal tunnel syndrome, delayed DTRs ("hung up" reflexes), diastolic HTN, hyperlipidemia
- **Late:** slow speech, hoarseness, loss of outer third of eyebrows, **myxedema** (nonpitting skin thickening due to ↓ glycosaminoglycans), periorbital puffiness, bradycardia, pleural, pericardial, & peritoneal effusions, atherosclerosis
- **Myxedema crisis:** hypothermia, hypotension, hypoventilation, Δ MS (including coma) hyponatremia, hypoglycemia; often precipitated by infection or major cardiopulmonary or neurologic illness (Med Clin North Am 2012;96:385)

Diagnostic studies
- ↓ FT4; ↑ TSH in primary hypothyroidism; ⊕ antithyroid Ab (TPO) in Hashimoto's thyroiditis
- May see hyponatremia, hypoglycemia, anemia, ↑ LDL, ↓ HDL and ↑ CK
- Screening recommended for pregnant women

Treatment of overt hypothyroidism
- Levothyroxine (1.5–1.7 μg/kg/d), re ✓ TSH q5–6wk & titrate until euthyroid (can take mos)
- *Lower starting dose* (0.3–0.5 μg/kg/d) if at risk for ischemic heart disease or elderly
- ↑ dose typically needed if:
  poor GI absorption: meds that ↓ absorption (iron, calcium, cholestyramine, sucralfate, PPI), celiac disease, IBD
  meds that accelerate T4 catabolism (eg, phenytoin, phenobarbital)
  initiation of estrogen replacement; pregnancy (~30% ↑ by wk 8): TSH goals change by trimester: 1st = 0.1–2.5 mIU/L, 2nd = 0.2–3.0 mIU/L, 3rd = 0.3–3.0 mIU/L (Thyroid 2011;21:1081)
- Myxedema coma: load 5–8 μg/kg T4 IV, then 50–100 μg IV qd; b/c peripheral conversion impaired, may also give 5–10 μg T3 IV q8h if unstable w/ bradycardia and/or hypothermia (T3 more arrhythmogenic); must give empiric *adrenal replacement therapy* first as ↓ adrenal reserves in myxedema coma

Subclinical hypothyroidism (Lancet 2012;379:1142)
- Mild ↑ TSH and **normal free T4** with only subtle or no sx
- If TSH <7 or ⊖ anti-TPO Ab, ~½ euthyroid after 2 y (JCEM 2012;97:1962)
  if ↑ titers of antithyroid Abs, progression to overt hypothyroidism is ~4%/y
- Rx controversial: follow expectantly or treat to improve mild sx or dyslipidemia
  most initiate Rx if TSH >10 mU/L, goiter, pregnancy or infertility
  if TSH 5–10 mU/L Rx if age ≤60 y (usually don't Rx if ≥60 b/c ↑ risk CV complications)

HYPERTHYROIDISM

Etiologies (Lancet 2016:epub)
- **Graves' disease** (60–80% of thyrotoxicosis)
- **Thyroiditis:** thyrotoxic phase of subacute (granulomatous) or painless (lymphocytic)
- **Toxic adenomas** (single or multinodular goiter)
- TSH-secreting pituitary tumor or pituitary resistance to thyroid hormone (↑ TSH, ↑ free T4)
- Misc: amiodarone, iodine-induced, thyrotoxicosis factitia, struma ovarii (3% of ovarian dermoid tumors and teratomas), hCG-secreting tumors (eg, choriocarcinoma), large deposits of metastatic follicular thyroid cancer

Clinical manifestations of hyperthyroidism
- Restlessness, sweating, tremor, moist warm skin, fine hair, tachycardia, AF, weight loss, ↑ frequency of stools, menstrual irregularities, hyperreflexia, osteoporosis, stare and lid lag (due to sympathetic overactivity)
- **Apathetic thyrotoxicosis:** seen in elderly who can present with lethargy as only sx
- **Thyroid storm** (extremely rare): delirium, fever, tachycardia, systolic hypertension but wide pulse pressure and ↓ MAP, GI symptoms; 20–50% mortality

Laboratory testing
- ↑ FT4 and FT3; ↓ TSH (except in TSH-secreting tumors)
- **RAIU scan** is very useful study to differentiate causes (see table on page 7-3); cannot do if recent IV contrast or amio load b/c iodine blocks uptake, so ✓ autoantibodies instead
- Rarely need to ✓ for autoantibodies except in pregnancy (to assess risk of fetal Graves')
- May see hypercalciuria ± hypercalcemia, ↑ Aφ, anemia

THYROID 7-4

Graves' disease (NEJM 2008;358:2594)

- ♀:♂ ratio is 5–10:1, most Pts between 40 and 60 y at dx
- ⊕ **thyroid antibodies:** TSI or TBII (⊕ in 80%), anti-TPO, antithyroglobulin; ANA
- Clinical manifestations in addition to those of hyperthyroidism (see above):
  goiter: diffuse, nontender, w/ thyroid bruit
  ophthalmopathy (NEJM 2010;362:726): seen in 50%; up to 90% if formally tested.
    Periorbital edema, lid retraction, proptosis, conjunctivitis, diplopia (EOM infiltration);
    associated w/ smoking. Stare and lid lag seen in any type of hyperthyroidism.
  pretibial myxedema (3%): infiltrative dermopathy

Thyroiditis (NEJM 2003;348:2646; Med Clin North Am 2012;96:223)

- **Acute:** bacterial infection (very rare in U.S. except postsurgical), typically *Staph/Strep* spp.
- **Subacute:** transient thyrotoxicosis → transient hypothyroidism → normal thyroid fxn
  painful (viral, granulomatous or de Quervain's): fever, ↑ ESR; Rx = NSAIDs, ASA, steroids
  silent (postpartum, autoimmune including Hashimoto's, or lymphocytic): painless;
    ⊕ TPO Abs; if postpartum, can recur with subsequent pregnancies
  other: meds (amiodarone, lithium, TKIs), palpation thyroiditis, post-radiation

Treatment (Thyroid 2011;21:593)

- β-blockers: control tachycardia (propranolol also ↓ T_4 → T_3 conversion)
- Graves' disease: either antithyroid drugs or radioactive iodine (JAMA 2015;314:2544)
  methimazole: 70% chance of recurrence after 1 y; side effects include pruritus,
    rash, arthralgia, fever, N/V and *agranulocytosis* in 0.5%. PTU: 2nd line (risk of
    hepatocellular necrosis; TID dosing; slower effect; JCEM 2007;92:2157).
    For both, need to ✓ LFTs, WBC, TSH at baseline and in follow-up.
  radioactive iodine (RAI) (NEJM 2011;364:542): typically done as outPt; preRx selected
    Pts w/ CV disease or elderly w/ antithyroid drugs to prevent ↑ thyrotoxicosis,
    stop 3 d before to allow RAI uptake; >75% of treated Pts become hypothyroid
  surgery: less commonly chosen for Graves', usually for Pts w/ obstructive goiter
    or ophthalmopathy
- Ophthalmopathy: can worsen after RAI; prophylax w/ prednisone in high-risk Pts;
  can be Rx'd w/ radiation and/or surgical decompression of orbits (NEJM 2009;360:994)
- Toxic adenoma or toxic multinodular goiter: RAI or surgery (methimazole preRx for surgery,
  in selected patients before RAI)
- Thyroid storm: β-blocker, PTU or methimazole, iopanoic acid or iodide (for
  Wolff-Chaikoff effect) >1 h after PTU, ± steroids (↓ T_4 → T_3)

Subclinical hyperthyroidism (Lancet 2012;379:1142)

- Mild ↓ TSH and **normal free T_4** with only subtle or no sx
- ~15% → overt hyperthyroidism in 2 y; ↑ risk of AF, CHD (Archives 2012;172:799), fracture (JAMA 2015;313:2055)
- Rx controversial: consider if TSH <0.1 mU/L and ↑ risk for CV disease or osteopenic

---

NONTHYROIDAL ILLNESS (SICK EUTHYROID SYNDROME)
(Thyroid 1997;7:125 and J Endocrinol 2010;205:1)

- TFT abnormalities in Pts w/ severe nonthyroidal illness (∴ in acute illness, ✓ TFTs only
  if ↑ concern for thyroid disease); *may* have acquired transient central hypothyroidism
- If thyroid dysfxn suspected in critically ill Pt, TSH alone not reliable; must measure total
  T_4, FT_4, & T_3
- Mild illness: ↓ T_4 → T_3 conversion, ↑ rT_3 ⇒ ↓ T_3; in severe illness: ↓ TBG & albumin, ↑↑ rT_3
  ⇒ ↓↓ **T_3**, **↓↓ T_4**, **↓ FT_4**, **↓ TSH**
- Recovery phase: ↑ TSH followed by recovery of T_4 and then T_3
- Replacement thyroxine *not* helpful or recommended for critically ill Pts w/ ↓ T_3 and T_4
  unless other s/s of hypothyroidism

AMIODARONE AND THYROID DISEASE

Overview (Annals 1997;126:63 & JCEM 2010;95:2529)

- 6 mg iodine per 200-mg tablet; risk of thyroid dysfunction lower with lower doses
- ✓ TSH prior to therapy, at 4-mo intervals on amio, and for 1 y after if amio d/c'd

Hypothyroidism (occurs in ~10%; more common in iodine-replete areas)

- Pathophysiology
  (1) Wolff-Chaikoff effect: iodine load ↓ I^- uptake, organification and release of T_4 & T_3
  (2) inhibits T_4 → T_3 conversion
  (3) ? direct/immune-mediated thyroid destruction

- Normal individuals: ↓ T_4; then escape Wolff-Chaikoff effect and have ↑ T_4, ↓ T_3, ↑ TSH; then TSH normalizes (after 1–3 mo)
- Susceptible individuals (eg, subclinical Hashimoto's, ∴ ✓ anti-TPO) do *not* escape effects
- Treatment: thyroxine to normalize TSH; may need larger than usual dose

Hyperthyroidism (3% of Pts on amio; ~10–20% of Pts *in iodine-deficient areas*)
- Type 1 = underlying multinodular goiter or autonomous thyroid tissue
  Jod-Basedow effect: iodine load → ↑ **synthesis** of T_4 and T_3 in autonomous tissue
- Type 2 = destructive thyroiditis
  ↑ **release** of preformed T_4 & T_3 → hyperthyroidism → hypothyroidism → recovery
- Doppler U/S: type 1 w/ ↑ thyroid blood flow; type 2 w/ ↓ flow
- Treatment: not absolutely necessary to d/c amio b/c amio ↓ T_4 → T_3 conversion
  methimazole for type 1; steroids (eg, 40 mg prednisone qd) for type 2
  often difficult to distinguish, so Rx for both typically initiated (*JCEM* 2001;86:3)
  consider thyroidectomy in severely ill patient

THYROID NODULES (*NEJM* 2015;373:2347 & *Thyroid* 2016;26:1)

- Prevalence 5–10% (50–60% if screen with U/S), ♀ > ♂, ~7–15% malignant
- Features associated w/ ↑ risk of malig: age <20 or >70 y, ♂, h/o neck XRT, hard & immobile mass, cervical LAN, dysphonia
- Worrisome U/S findings: hypoechoic, solid, irregular borders, microcalcifications, height > width, >20 mm (*JAMA IM* 2013;173:1788)
- Features associated w/ benign dx: cystic nodules, "spongiform" sonographic pattern
- Screening U/S recommended for those with FHx of MEN2 or medullary thyroid cancer, personal h/o neck XRT, palpable nodules or multinodular goiter
- Any evidence of tracheal deviation or compression → consider ✓ PFTs & refer to surgery
- >10-mm nodule: FNA if hypoechoic solid or solid component of cystic; ↑ suspicion of malig if irregular margins, microcalcifications, rim Ca^{2+}, height > width, or extrathyroidal extension
- >15-mm nodule: FNA if solid isoechoic, or partially cystic with mural solid component
- >20-mm nodule: FNA if spongiform/other benign solid pattern (no FNA if purely cystic)
- Molecular testing if indeterminate pattern on FNA (occurs in ~15–30%)
- Suppressive Rx w/ high-dose levothyroxine *no longer recommended* for benign nodules in iodine-sufficient regions
- Cancer very rare in asx nodules diagnosed as benign (*JCEM* 2014;99:510 & *JAMA* 2015;313:926)
- After complete surgical resection of thyroid cancer, RAI in medium- and high-risk Pts (*Lancet* 2013;381:1046 & 1058)

Figure 7-2 Approach to thyroid nodules (*NEJM* 2015;373:2347 & *Thyroid* 2016;26:1)

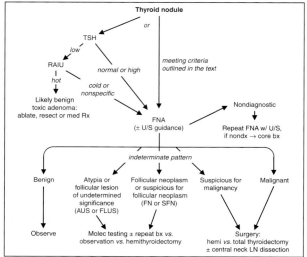

CUSHING'S SYNDROME (HYPERCORTISOLISM)

Definitions (*Lancet 2015;386:913*)
- Cushing's syndrome = cortisol excess
- Cushing's disease = Cushing's syndrome 2° to pituitary ACTH hypersecretion

Etiologies of hypercortisolism
- Most commonly iatrogenic caused by exogenous glucocorticoids (though underreported)
- **Cushing's disease** (60–70%): ACTH-secreting pituitary adenoma (usually microadenoma) or hyperplasia
- **Adrenal tumor** (15–25%): adenoma or (rarely) carcinoma
- **Ectopic ACTH** (5–10%): SCLC, carcinoid, islet cell tumors, medullary thyroid cancer, pheo

Clinical manifestations (*Lancet 2006;367:13*)
- *Nonspecific:* glucose intolerance or DM, HTN, obesity, oligo- or amenorrhea, osteoporosis
- *More specific:* central obesity w/ extremity wasting, dorsocervical fat pads, spont. bruising
- *Most specific:* proximal myopathy, rounded facies, facial plethora, wide purple striae
- Other: depression, insomnia, psychosis, impaired cognition, hypokalemia, acne, hirsutism, hyperpigmentation (if ↑ ACTH), fungal skin infxns, nephrolithiasis, polyuria

Figure 7-3 Approach to suspected Cushing's syndrome (*nb, very difficult to dx as an inPt*) (*JCEM 2008;93:1526*)

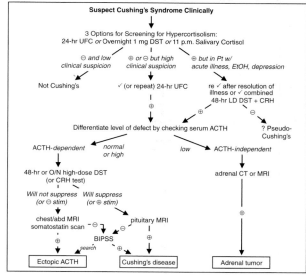

CRH, corticotropin-releasing hormone; DST, dexamethasone suppression test; UFC, urinary free cortisol

Overnight 1 mg DST = give 1 mg at 11 p.m.; ✓ 8 a.m. serum cortisol (suppression if <1.8 μg/dL); <5% false ⊕ (primarily used to evaluate subclinical Cushing's in adrenal "incidentalomas")

11 p.m. salivary cortisol = abnl if level ↑; 24-h UFC = abnl if level ↑, > 4× ULN virtually diagnostic

48-h LD DST + CRH = 0.5 mg q6h × 2 d, then IV CRH 2 h later; ✓ serum cortisol 15 min later (⊕ = >1.4 μg/dL)

48-h LD DST = 0.5 mg q6h × 2 d; ✓ 24-h UFC at base. & during last 24 h of dex (suppress if <10% of base)

48-h HD DST = 2 mg q6h × 2 d; ✓ 24-h UFC as per LD DST

O/N HD DST = 8 mg at 11 p.m.; ✓ 9 a.m. serum cortisol (suppression if <32% of baseline)

CRH test = 1 μg/kg IV; ✓ cortisol and ACTH (⊕ stim if > 35% ↑ in ACTH or >20% ↑ in cortisol above baseline)

BIPSS, bilat. inferior petrosal sinus vein sampling; ✓ petrosal:peripheral ACTH ratio (⊕ = 2 basal, >3 after CRH)

Treatment of Cushing's syndrome (*JCEM* 2015;100:2807)

- Surgical resection of pituitary adenoma, adrenal tumor or ectopic ACTH-secreting tumor
- If transsphenoidal surgery (TSS) not successful → repeat TSS. Can do pituitary XRT, but XRT not effective immediately, ∴ initiate medical Rx w/ mitotane, ketoconazole, or metyrapone to ↓ cortisol, and/or mifepristone to block cortisol action at glucocorticoid receptor, or bilat surgical adrenalectomy if med Rx fails or is contraindicated.
- Glucocorticoid replacement therapy × 6–36 mo after TSS (lifelong glucocorticoid + mineralocorticoid replacement if medical or surgical adrenalectomy)

HYPERALDOSTERONISM

Etiologies

- **Primary** (adrenal disorders, renin-independent increase in aldosterone; *JCEM* 2015;100:1) adrenal hyperplasia (60–70%), adenoma (**Conn's syndrome**, 30–40%), carcinoma glucocorticoid-remediable aldosteronism (GRA; ACTH-dep. rearranged promoter)
- **Secondary** (extra-adrenal disorders, ↑ aldosterone is renin-dependent)
  Primary reninism: renin-secreting tumor (rare)
  Secondary reninism: renovascular disease: RAS, malignant hypertension; edematous states w/ ↓ effective arterial volume: CHF, cirrhosis, nephrotic syndrome; hypovolemia, diuretics, T2D, Bartter's (defective Na/K/2Cl transporter ≈ receiving loop diuretic), Gitelman's (defective renal Na/Cl transporter ≈ receiving thiazide diuretic)
- **Nonaldosterone mineralocorticoid excess** mimics hyperaldosteronism
  11β-HSD defic. (→ lack of inactivation of cortisol, which binds to mineralocorticoid recept.)
  Black licorice (glycyrrhizinic acid inhibits 11β-HSD), extreme hypercortisolism (overwhelming 11β-HSD), exogenous mineralocorticoids
  Liddle's syndrome (constitutively activated/overexpressed distal tubular renal Na channel)

Clinical manifestations

- **Mild to moderate HTN** (11% of Pts w/ HTN refractory to 3 drugs; *Lancet* 2008;371:1921), headache, muscle weakness, polyuria, polydipsia; no peripheral edema because of "escape" from Na retention; malignant HTN is rare
- Classically **hypokalemia** (but often normal), metabolic alkalosis, mild hypernatremia

Diagnostic studies (*JCEM* 2008;93:3266)

- 5–10% of Pts w/ HTN; ∴ screen if HTN + hypoK, adrenal mass, refractory/early onset HTN
- Screening: **aldo** (>15–20 ng/dL) *and* **plasma aldo:renin ratio** (>20 if 1°) obtain 8 a.m. paired values (off spironolactone & eplerenone for 6 wk); Se & Sp >85%
- ACEI/ARB, diuretics, CCB can ↑ renin activity → ↓ PAC/PRA ratio and βBs may ↑ PAC/PRA ratio; ∴ avoid. α-blockers generally best to control HTN during dx testing.
- Confirm with **sodium suppression test** (fail to suppress aldo after sodium load)
  oral salt load (+ KCl) × 3 d, ✓ 24-h urine (⊕ if urinary aldo >12 μg/d while urinary Na >200 mEq/d) or 2L NS over 4 h, measure plasma aldo at end of infusion (⊕ if aldo >5 ng/dL)

Figure 7-4 Approach to suspected hyperaldosteronism

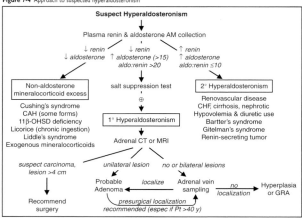

(Adapted from *JCEM* 2008;93:3266 and *Surg Clin N Am* 2014;94:643)

Treatment (Surg Clin N Am 2014;94:643)
- Adenoma → adrenalectomy vs. medical Rx w/ spironolactone or eplerenone
- Hyperplasia → spironolactone or eplerenone; GRA → glucocorticoids ± spironolactone
- Carcinoma → adrenalectomy

ADRENAL INSUFFICIENCY

Etiologies
- **Primary** = adrenocortical disease = **Addison's disease**
    autoimmune: isolated or in assoc w/ APS (see table on page 7-2)
    infection: TB, CMV, histoplasmosis, paracoccidioidomycosis
    vascular: hemorrhage (usually in setting of sepsis), adrenal vein thrombosis, HIT, trauma
    metastatic disease: (90% of adrenals must be destroyed to cause insufficiency)
    deposition diseases: hemochromatosis, amyloidosis, sarcoidosis
    drugs: azole antifungals, etomidate (even after single dose), rifampin, anticonvulsants
- **Secondary** = pituitary failure of ACTH secretion (but aldosterone **intact** b/c RAA axis)
    any cause of primary or secondary hypopituitarism (see "Pituitary Disorders")
    glucocorticoid therapy (can occur after ≤2 wk of "suppressive doses"; dose effect variable;
    even <10 mg of prednisone daily chronically can be suppressive)
    megestrol (a progestin with some glucocorticoid activity)

Clinical manifestations (Lancet 2014;383:2152)
- **Primary** or **secondary: weakness and fatigability** (99%), **anorexia** (99%),
  orthostatic hypotension (90%), nausea (86%), vomiting (75%), hyponatremia (88%)
- **Primary only** (extra s/s due to lack of aldosterone and ↑ ACTH): marked **orthostatic
  hypotension** (because volume-depleted), salt craving, **hyperpigmentation** (seen in
  creases, mucous membranes, pressure areas, nipples), **hyperkalemia**
- **Secondary only:** ± other manifestations of hypopituitarism (see "Pituitary Disorders")

Diagnostic studies (JCEM 2016;101:364)
- Early a.m. serum cortisol: <5 μg/dL virtually diagnostic; ≥18 μg/dL rules it out (except in
  severe septic shock—see below)
- Standard (250 μg) **cosyntropin stimulation test** (testing ability of ACTH → ↑ cortisol)
    normal = 60-min or (30-min) post-ACTH cortisol ≥18 μg/dL
    abnormal in *primary* b/c adrenal gland diseased and unable to give adequate output
    abnormal in *chronic secondary* b/c adrenals atrophied and unable to respond
    (very rarely, may be *normal* in *acute pituitary injury* b/c adrenals still able to respond →
    use early a.m. cortisol instead)
- Other tests (w/ guidance by endocrinologist): renin, aldosterone, insulin-induced
  hypoglycemia (measure serum cortisol response); metyrapone (blocks cortisol synthesis
  and therefore stimulates ACTH, measure plasma 11-deoxycortisol and urinary 17-
  hydroxycorticosteroid levels)
- Other lab abnormalities: hypoglycemia, eosinophilia, lymphocytosis, ± neutropenia
- ACTH: ↑ in 1°, ↓ or low-normal in 2°
- Imaging studies to consider
    pituitary MRI to detect anatomical abnormalities
    adrenal CT: small, noncalcified adrenals in autoimmune, enlarged in metastatic disease,
    hemorrhage, infection or deposition (although they may be normal-appearing)

Adrenal insufficiency & critical illness (NEJM 2003;348:727; JAMA 2009;301:2362)
- ↑ circulating cortisol despite ↓ ACTH due to ↓ clearance and possibly stimulation by
  cytokines; low cortisol binding proteins; ∴ dx of adrenal insufficiency problematic (NEJM
  2013;368:1477)
- Nonetheless, reasonable to perform ACTH stim ASAP in hypotensive Pt suspected to
  have absolute adrenal insufficiency
- Reasonable to perform 250-μg ACTH stim and initiate glucocorticoid replacement if ↑ in
  cortisol <9 μg/dL or absolute cortisol level <10 μg/dL, but decision to Rx should be based
  on clinical assessment; unlikely to require Rx if spot or post-ACTH cortisol >18 μg/dL
- Initiate corticosteroids early: use hydrocortisone 50–100 mg IV q6–8h; prior to ACTH stim
  test, use dexamethasone 2–4 mg IV q6h + fludrocortisone 50 μg daily
- Rx of *relative adrenal insufficiency* controversial (see "Sepsis")

Treatment
- *Acute* insufficiency: volume resuscitation w/ normal saline + **hydrocortisone IV** as above
- *Chronic* insufficiency
    prednisone ~5 mg PO qam, or hydrocortisone: 15–25 mg PO qd (²/₃ a.m, ¹/₃ early p.m.)
    fludrocortisone (*not* needed in 2° adrenal insufficiency): 0.05–0.1 mg PO qam
    backup dexamethasone 4-mg IM prefilled syringe given to Pt for emergency situations

Clinical manifestations (five Ps) (Lancet 2005;366:665)
- **Pressure** (hypertension, paroxysmal in 50%, severe & resistant to Rx, occ orthostatic)
- **Pain** (headache, chest pain)
- **Palpitations** (tachycardia, tremor, wt loss, fever)
- **Perspiration** (profuse)
- **Pallor** (vasoconstrictive spell)
- "Rule of 10": 10% extra-adrenal (known as paraganglioma), 10% in children,
  10% multiple or bilateral, 10% recur (↑ in paraganglioma), 10% malignant (↑ in
  paraganglioma), 10% familial, 10% incidentaloma
- Paroxysms can be triggered by meds (eg, β-blockers) abdominal manipulation
- Associated with MEN2A/2B, von Hippel Lindau, neurofibromatosis type 1, familial
  paraganglioma (mutations in succinate dehydrogenase gene B, C and D)

Diagnostic studies (JCEM 2014;99:1915)
- 24° urinary fractionated metanephrines: 85–97% Se, 69–95% Sp. Screening test of choice
  if low-risk (as false ⊕ with severe illness, renal failure, OSA, labetalol due to assay
  interference, acetaminophen, TCAs, medications containing sympathomimetics).
- Plasma-free metanephrines: 89–100% Se, 79–97% Sp (JAMA 2002;287:1427). Screening
  test of choice if high risk, but ↑ rate of false ⊕ in low-prevalence population. Draw
  blood in supine position after Pt supine for 30 min, estimated 2.8× ↑ false ⊕ if seated.
- Adrenal CT generally better than MRI; PET for known metastatic disease or to localize
  nonadrenal mass but usually easy to find; consider MIBG scintigraphy if CT/MRI ⊖
- Consider genetic testing if bilateral disease, young Pt, ⊕ FHx, extra-adrenal

Treatment
- α-blockade first (usually phenoxybenzamine) ± β-blockade (often propranolol) → surgery
- Preoperative volume expansion is critical due to possible hypotension after tumor excision

Epidemiology
- 4% of Pts undergoing abdominal CT scan have incidentally discovered adrenal mass;
  prevalence ↑ with age

Differential diagnosis
- **Nonfunctioning mass:** adenoma, cysts, abscesses, granuloma, hemorrhage, lipoma,
  myelolipoma, primary or metastatic malignancy
- **Functioning mass:** pheochromocytoma, adenoma (cortisol, aldosterone, sex hormones),
  nonclassical CAH, other endocrine tumor, carcinoma

Hormonal workup (NEJM 2007;356:601; JCEM 2010;95:4106)
- **Rule out subclinical Cushing's syndrome** in *all* Pts using 1 mg overnight DST
  (Sp 91%). Abnormal results require confirmatory testing.
- **Rule out hyperaldosteronism** *if hypertensive* w/ plasma aldo & renin (see above)
- **Rule out pheochromocytoma** in ALL Pts (b/c of morbidity unRx'd pheo) using 24-h
  urine fractionated metanephrines or plasma free metanephrines

Malignancy workup
- CT and MRI characteristics may suggest adenoma vs. carcinoma
  Benign features: size <4 cm; smooth margins, homogenous and hypodense appearance;
  unenhanced CT <10 Hounsfield units or CT contrast-medium washout >50% at
  10 min. Can follow such incidentalomas w/ periodic scans.
  Suspicious features: size >6 cm or ↑ size on repeat scan; irregular margins,
  heterogeneous, dense or vascular appearance; h/o malignancy or young age.
  Such incidentalomas warrant resection or repeat scan at short interval.
- Rule out metastatic cancer (and infection) as in Pts w/ h/o cancer, ~50% of adrenal
  incidentalomas are malignant

Follow-up
- If hormonal workup ⊖ and appearance benign, yearly fxnal testing for 4 y w/ follow-up
  imaging at 6, 12, & 24 mos reasonable approach, but controversial

Laboratory Findings in Calcium Disorders

Ca	PTH	Disease	PO4	25-(OH)D	1,25-(OH)2D
	↑↑	Hyperparathyroidism (1° and 3°)	↓	↓ to nl	↑
	↑ or nl	Familial hypocalciuric hypercalcemia	↓	nl	nl
↑	↓	Malignancy	var.	var.	var.
		Vitamin D excess	↑	↑	var.
		Milk-alkali syndrome, thiazides	↓	nl	nl
		↑ Bone turnover	↑	var.	var.
	↑↑	Pseudohypoparathyroidism	↑	nl	↓
	↑	Vitamin D deficiency	↓	↓↓	nl / ↓
↓		Chronic renal failure (2° hyperpara)	↑	var.	↓
	var.	Acute calcium sequestration	var.	var.	var.
	↓	Hypoparathyroidism	↑	nl	↓

Pitfalls in measuring calcium

- Physiologically active Ca is free or ionized (ICa). Serum Ca reflects total calcium (bound + unbound) and ∴ influenced by albumin (main Ca-binding protein).
- Corrected Ca (mg/dL) = measured Ca (mg/dL) + {0.8 × [4 − albumin (g/dL)]}
- Alkalosis will cause more Ca to be bound to albumin (∴ total Ca may be normal but ↓ ICa)
- Best to measure **ionized Ca directly** *(but accuracy is lab dependent)*

HYPERCALCEMIA

Etiologies of Hypercalcemia

Category	Etiologies
Hyperparathyroidism (HPT) *(NEJM 2011;365:2389)*	1°: adenoma (85%), hyperplasia (15–20%; spont. vs. MEN1/2A), carcinoma (<1%), meds (Lithium → ↑ PTH) 3°: after long-standing 2° hyperparathyroidism (as in renal failure) → autonomous nodule develops, requires surgery
Familial hypocalciuric hypercalcemia (FHH)	Inact. mut. in Ca-sensing receptor (FHH1), Gα11 (FHH2), AP2S1 (FHH3) → ↑ Ca set point; ± mild ↑ PTH Acquired form due to autoAb vs. Ca-sensing receptor (rare) FE$_{Ca}$ [(24-h U$_{Ca}$/serum Ca) / (24-h U$_{Cr}$/serum Cr)] <0.01
Malignancy *(JCEM 2015;100:2024)*	PTH-related peptide (PTHrP) → humoral ↑ Ca of malignancy (eg, squamous cell cancers, renal, breast, bladder) Cytokines → ↑ osteoclast activity (eg, hematologic malig) ↑ 1,25-(OH)2D (eg, rare lymphomas) Local osteolysis (eg, breast cancer, myeloma)
Vitamin D excess	Granulomas (sarcoid, TB, histo, GPA) → ↑ 1-OHase → ↑ 1,25-(OH)2D. Vitamin D intoxication.
↑ Bone turnover	Hyperthyroidism, immobilization + Paget's disease, vitamin A
Miscellaneous	Thiazides; Ca-based antacids or massive dairy consumption (milk-alkali syndrome); adrenal insufficiency
Among inPts w/ hypercalcemia: 45% have cancer, 25% 1° HPT, 10% CKD → 3° HPT	

(JCEM 2005;90:6316; NEJM 2013;368:644)

Clinical manifestations ("bones, stones, abdominal groans and psychic moans")

- **Hypercalcemic crisis** (usually when Ca >13–15): polyuria, dehydration, ∆MS
  Ca toxic to renal tubules → blocks ADH activity, causes vasoconstriction and ↓ GFR → polyuria but Ca reabsorption → ↑ serum Ca → ↑ nephrotoxicity and CNS sx
- Osteopenia, fractures and osteitis fibrosa cystica (latter seen in severe hyperpara. only → ↑ osteoclast activity → cysts, fibrous nodules, salt & pepper appearance on X-ray)
- Nephrolithiasis, nephrocalcinosis, nephrogenic DI
- Abdominal pain, anorexia, nausea, vomiting, constipation, pancreatitis, PUD
- Fatigue, weakness, depression, confusion, coma, ↓ DTRs, short QT interval
- 1° HPT: 80% asx, 20% nephrolithiasis, osteoporosis, etc.

Diagnostic studies

- Hyperparathyroidism (HPT) and malignancy account for 90% of cases of ↑ Ca; HPT more likely if asx or chronic; malignancy (usually overt) more likely if acute or sx
- Ca, alb, ICa, PTH (may be inapprop. normal in 1° HPT & FHH; JAMA 2014;312:2680), PO4; ↑ or high nl PTH: 24-h U$_{Ca}$ >200 mg → HPT; 24-h U$_{Ca}$ <100 mg & FE$_{Ca}$ <0.01 → FHH

↓ PTH: ✓ PTHrP, Aϕ, & search for malig (eg, CT, mammogram, SPEP/UPEP) and
   ✓ vit D: ↑ 25-(OH)D → meds; ↑ 1,25-(OH)$_2$D → granuloma (✓ CXR, ACE, r/o lymph)

Acute Treatment of Hypercalcemia			
Treatment	Onset	Duration	Comments
Normal saline (4–6 L/d)	h	during Rx	Natriuresis → ↑ renal Ca excretion
± Furosemide	h	during Rx	Use cautiously, only if volume overloaded
Bisphosphonates	1–2 d	var.	Inhibit osteoclasts, useful in malignancy; caution in renal failure; risk of jaw osteonecrosis
Calcitonin	h	2–3 d	Quickly develop tachyphylaxis
Glucocorticoids	days	days	? Useful in some malig, granulomatous disorders & vitamin D intox.
Denosumab (JCEM 2014;99:3144)	days	months	Monoclonal Ab against RANKL; typically used in hyperCa of malignancy; not renally cleared
Hemodialysis	min	during Rx	If other measures ineffective or contraindicated

(BMJ 2015;350:h2723)

Treatment of asymptomatic 1° HPT (JCEM 2014 99:3561)
- Surgery if: age <50 y; serum Ca >1 mg/dL >ULN; CrCl <60 mL/min, DEXA T score <−2.5
- If Rx declined/deferred, can Rx with, cinacalcet (↓ Ca & PTH but may not ↑ BMD)
- If not yet candidate for surgery: ✓ serum Ca & Cr annually and BMD q1–2y

Calciphylaxis (calcific uremic arteriopathy)
- Calcification of media of small- to med-sized blood vessels of dermis & SC fat
- Ischemia & skin necrosis. See "Chronic Kidney Disease" for further details.

HYPOCALCEMIA

Etiologies of Hypocalcemia	
Category	Etiologies
Hypoparathyroidism (NEJM 2008;359:391)	Iatrogenic (s/p thyroidectomy, rarely after parathyroidectomy); sporadic; familial (APS1, activating Ca-sensing receptor mutations; see page 7-2); Wilson's, hemochromatosis; hypoMg (↓ secretion and effect); activating Ca-sensing receptor autoAb
Pseudo-hypoparathyroidism (JCEM 2011;96:3020)	Ia and Ib: PTH end-organ resistance (∴ ↑ serum PTH) Ia: + skeletal abnormalities, short stature, & retardation Pseudopseudohypoparathyroidism = Ia syndrome but nl Ca & PTH
Vit D defic. or resist (NEJM 2011;364:248; JCEM 2012;97:1153)	Nutritional/sunlight deprivation; GI disease/fat malabs.; drugs (anticonvulsants, rifampin, ketoconazole, 5-FU/leucovorin); genetic (1α-hydroxylase, VDR mutations)
Chronic renal failure	↓ 1,25-(OH)$_2$D production, ↑ PO$_4$ from ↓ clearance
Accelerated net bone formation	Postparathyroidectomy, Rx of severe vit D deficiency or Paget's disease (NEJM 2013;368:644), osteoblastic metastases
Calcium sequestration	Pancreatitis, citrate excess (after blood transfusions), acute ↑↑ PO$_4$ (ARF, rhabdomyolysis, tumor lysis), bisphosphonates

Clinical manifestations
- **Neuromuscular irritability:** perioral paresthesias, cramps, ⊕ **Trousseau's** (inflation of BP cuff ≥3 min → carpal spasm), ⊕ **Chvostek's** (tapping facial nerve → contraction of facial muscles), laryngospasm; irritability, depression, psychosis, ↑ ICP, seizures, ↑ QT
- Rickets and/or osteomalacia: chronic ↓ vit D → ↓ Ca, ↓ PO$_4$ → ↓ bone/cartilage mineralization, growth failure, bone pain, muscle weakness
- **Renal osteodystrophy** (↓ vit D & ↑ PTH in renal failure): osteomalacia [↓ mineralization of bone due to ↓ Ca and 1,25-(OH)$_2$D] & osteitis fibrosa cystica (due to ↑ PTH)

Diagnostic studies
- Ca, alb, ICa, PTH, 25-(OH)D, 1,25-(OH)$_2$D (if renal failure or rickets), Cr, Mg, PO$_4$, Aϕ, U$_{Ca}$

Treatment (also treat concomitant vitamin D deficiency)
- Severely symptomatic: Ca gluconate (1–2 g IV over 20 min) + oral Ca + calcitriol (but takes hrs to work) ± Mg (50–100 mEq/d); 10% CaCl$_2$ in codes or via CVL
- Consider gtt or PO to follow as effect of IV bolus typically lasts only a few hours
- Chronic: oral Ca (1–3 g/d; Ca citrate better absorbed than Ca carbonate, esp. if achlorhydria or on PPI) and typically calcitriol (0.25-2 mcg/d), and replete vitamin D deficiency. Consider thiazide to ↓ urinary Ca or recombinant PTH 1-84.
- Chronic renal failure: phosphate binder(s), oral Ca, calcitriol or analogue

DIABETES MELLITUS

Definition (*Diabetes Care* 2016;39:S13)
- Either HbA_{1c} ≥6.5, fasting glc ≥126 mg/dL, or glc 2 h after OGTT ≥200 mg/dL × 2 (for any test) or single random glc ≥200 mg/dL w/ classic sx of hyperglycemia; all tests equally reasonable (n.b, may be ⊖ on one test but not another); OGTT preferred during preg
- Blood glc higher than normal, but not frank DM ("prediabetics," ~40% U.S. population) HbA_{1c} 5.7–6.4%, impaired fasting glc (IFG) 100–125 mg/dL, or 2 h prandial glc 140–199 Preventing progression to DM: diet & exercise (58% ↓), metformin (31% ↓; *NEJM* 2002;346:393), TZD (60% ↓; *Lancet* 2006;368:1096)

Categories
- **Type 1** (*Lancet* 2014;383:69): islet cell destruction; absolute insulin deficiency; ketosis in absence of insulin; prevalence 0.4%; usual onset in childhood but can occur throughout adulthood; ↑ risk if ⊕ FHx; HLA associations; anti-GAD, anti-islet cell & anti-insulin autoAb
- **Type 2** (*Annals* 2015;162:ITC1): insulin resistance + relative insulin ↓; prevalence 8%; onset generally later in life; no HLA assoc.; risk factors: age, ⊕ FHx, obesity, sedentary lifestyle
- **Type 2 DM p/w DKA** ("ketosis-prone type 2 diabetes" or "Flatbush diabetes"): most often seen in nonwhite, ± anti-GAD Ab, eventually may not require insulin (*Endo Rev* 2008;29:292)
- **Mature-Onset Diabetes of the Young (MODY)**: autosomal dom. forms of DM due to defects in insulin secretion genes; genetically and clinically heterogeneous (*NEJM* 2001;345:971)
- **Secondary causes of diabetes:** exogenous glucocorticoids, glucagonoma (3 Ds = DM, DVT, diarrhea), pancreatic (pancreatitis, hemochromatosis, CF, resection), B endocrinopathies (Cushing's disease, acromegaly), gestational, drugs (protease inhibitors, atypical antipsychotics)

Clinical manifestations
- Polyuria, polydipsia, polyphagia with unexplained weight loss; can also be asymptomatic

Diabetes Treatment Options	
Diet	Type 1: carb counting; Type 2: wt reduction diet + exercise
Metformin (biguanide) *First-line pharmacoRx for all T2D*	↓ hepatic gluconeogenesis. ↓ HbA_{1c} ~1.5%. Wt neutral, N/V & diarrhea, rare lactic acidosis Contraindic. in renal (eg, Cr >1.5) or liver failure
Sulfonylureas (SU)	↑ insulin secretion, ↓ HbA_{1c} ~1.5%. Hypoglycemia, wt gain.
Thiazolidinediones (TZD) (PPARγ agonists)	↑ insulin sens. in adipose & muscle. ↓ HbA_{1c} ~1%. Wt gain, hepatotoxicity, fluid retention & CHF, bone fractures ? ↑ MI w/ rosiglitazone; not pioglitazone (*BMJ* 2011;342:d1309) Contraindic. in liver disease and NYHA III–IV, monitor LFTs
GLP-1 agonists	↑ glc-depend insulin secretion, ↓ HbA_{1c} ~0.5%. ↓ **CV events** (*NEJM* 2016;375:311). Wt loss, N/V & diarrhea (30–45%).
DPP-4 inhibitors	Block degrad. of GLP-1 & GIP → ↑ insulin. ↓ HbA_{1c} ~0.5%. ? ↑ risk of CHF with some (*NEJM* 2013;369:1317 & 2015;373:232)
SGLT-2 inhibitors (block renal tubular glc uptake)	↓ glucosuria. ↓ HbA_{1c} ~0.6–1%. Wt loss, ↓ **CV death & HF, slows progression of kidney disease** (*NEJM* 2015;373:2117 & *NEJM* 2016;375:323). ↑ risk of normoglycemic DKA (*Diabetes Care* 2016;39:532), fungal GU infxn & UTIs, hypovolemia, ↑ LDL.
Glinides (nonsulfonylurea insulin secretagogues)	↑ insulin secretion, ↓ HbA_{1c} ~1.5% Hypoglycemia (but less than w/ SU), wt gain
α-glucosidase inhibitors	↓ intestinal CHO absorption, ↓ HbA_{1c} 0.5–0.8%. GI distress (gas).
Pramlintide	Delays gastric emptying & ↓ glucagon, ↓ HbA_{1c} 0.5%. GI sx. To be used as adjunctive Rx w/ insulin in T1D or T2D
Insulin (Additional T1D options: insulin pump, pancreatic or islet cell transplant)	Hypoglycemia, wt gain. T1D: generally combine intermed./ long-acting (NPH or glargine) & short-/rapid-acting (regular or lispro) insulin. T2D: consider if mono oral Rx not adequate (esp. if HbA_{1c} high) and start if combo oral Rx not adequate.
Gastric bypass	Can cure DM & prevent complications (*NEJM* 2014;370:2002)

(*Lancet* 2014;383:1068; *JAMA* 2015;314:1052; *Diabetes Care* 2016;39:S52; *Endocr Pract* 2016;22:84)

Insulin Preparations (*JAMA* 2014;311:2315)				
Preparation	**Onset**	**Peak**	**Duration**	**Side effects/Comments**
Lispro, aspart	5–15 min	60–90 min	2–4 h	Give immediately before meal
Regular	30–60 min	2–4 h	5–8 h	Give ~30 min before meal
NPH	1–2 h	4–8 h	12–18 h	Can cause protamine Ab prod
Glargine	2 h	No peak	20–24 h	Once daily (a.m. or p.m.)
Detemir	1–3 h	No peak	18–26 h	Once daily

Complications (NEJM 2004;351:48; 2007:356:820; 2012;366:1227)
- **Retinopathy**
  nonproliferative: "dot & blot" and retinal hemorrhages, cotton-wool/protein exudates
  proliferative: neovascularization, vitreous hemorrhage, retinal detachment, blindness
  treatment: photocoagulation, surgery, intravitreal bevacizumab injections →
- **Nephropathy:** microalbuminuria → proteinuria ± nephrotic syndrome → renal failure
  diffuse glomerular basement membrane thickening/nodular pattern (Kimmelstiel-Wilson)
  usually accompanied by retinopathy; lack of retinopathy suggests another cause
  treatment: strict BP control using ACE inhibitors or ARBs (Mayo Clin Proc 2011;86:444),
  SGLT-2 inhib (NEJM 2016;375:323), low-protein diet, dialysis or transplant
- **Neuropathy:** *peripheral:* symmetric distal sensory loss, paresthesias, ± motor loss
  autonomic: gastroparesis, constipation, neurogenic bladder, erectile dysfxn, orthostasis
  mononeuropathy: sudden-onset peripheral or CN deficit (footdrop, CN III > VI > IV)
- **Accelerated atherosclerosis:** coronary, cerebral and peripheral beds
- **Infections:** UTI, osteomyelitis of foot, candidiasis, mucormycosis, necrotizing external otitis
- **Dermatologic:** necrobiosis lipoidica diabeticorum, lipodystrophy, acanthosis nigricans

Outpatient screening and treatment goals (Diabetes Care 2015;38:S49)
- ✓ HbA1C q3–6mo, goal <7% for most Pts. Can use goal HbA1C ≤7.5–8% if h/o severe
  hypoglycemia or other comorbidities. Microvascular & macrovascular complications ↓ by
  strict glycemic control in T1D (NEJM 2005;353:2643) & T2D (NEJM 2015;372:2197).
- Microalbuminuria screening yearly with spot microalbumin/Cr ratio, goal <30 mg/g
- **BP** ≤140/90 (JAMA 2015;313:603); ≤130/80 in young or select high-risk; benefit of ACE-I
- **Lipids:** statin initiation in all diabetics age 40–75 if LDL-C >70 (see Lipids section)
- **ASA** if age >50 (♂) or 60 (♀) or other cardiac risk factors (Circ 2010;121:2694)
- Dilated retinal exam and comprehensive foot exam yearly

Management of hyperglycemia in inpatients (for ICU Pts: see "Sepsis")
- Identify reversible causes/exacerbaters (dextrose IVF, glucocorticoids, postop, ↑ carb diet)
- Dx studies: BG fingersticks (fasting, qAC, qHS; or q6h if NPO), HbA1C
- Treatment goals: avoid hypoglycemia, extreme hyperglycemia (>180 mg/dL)
- Modification of outPt treatment regimen: In T1D, do not stop basal insulin (can → DKA).
  In T2D: stopping oral DM meds generally preferred to avoid hypoglycemia or med
  interaction (except if short stay, excellent outPt cntl, no plan for IV contrast, nl diet)
- InPt insulin: can use outPt regimen as guide; if insulin naïve:
  total daily insulin = wt (kg) ÷ 2, to start; adjust as needed
  give ½ of total daily insulin as basal insulin in long-acting form to target fasting glc
  give other ½ as short-acting boluses (standing premeal & sliding scale corrective insulin)
- Discharge regimen: similar to admission regimen unless poor outPt cntl or strong
  reason for Δ. Arrange early insulin and glucometer teaching, prompt outPt follow-up.

DIABETIC KETOACIDOSIS (DKA)

Precipitants (the I's)
- **Insulin defic.** (ie, failure to take enough insulin); **Iatrogenesis** (glucocorticoids; SGLT2
  inhibitors—can be w/o marked hyperglycemia; Diabetes Care 2016;39:532)
- **Infection** (pneumonia, UTI) or **Inflammation** (pancreatitis, cholecystitis)
- **Ischemia** or **Infarction** (myocardial, cerebral, gut); **Intoxication** (alcohol, drugs)

Pathophysiology (NEJM 2015;372:546)
- Occurs in **T1D** (and in ketosis-prone T2D); ↑ glucagon and ↓ insulin
- Hyperglycemia due to: ↑ gluconeogenesis, ↑ glycogenolysis, ↓ glucose uptake in cells
- Ketosis due to: insulin deficiency → mobilization and oxidation of fatty acids,
  ↑ substrate for ketogenesis, ↑ ketogenic state of the liver, ↓ ketone clearance

Clinical manifestations (Diabetes Care 2009;32:1335 & 2016;39:S99)
- Polyuria, polydipsia, & dehydration → ↑ HR, HoTN, dry mucous membranes, ↓ skin turgor
- N/V, abdominal pain (either due to intra-abdominal process or DKA), ileus
- Kussmaul's respirations (deep) to compensate for metabolic acidosis with odor of acetone
- Δ MS → somnolence, stupor, coma; mortality ~1% even at tertiary care centers

Diagnostic studies
- ↑ **Anion gap metabolic acidosis:** can later develop nonanion gap acidosis due to
  urinary loss of ketones (HCO₃ equivalents) and fluid resuscitation with chloride
- **Ketosis:** ⊕ urine and serum ketones (predominant ketone is β-OH-butyrate, but
  acetoacetate measured by assay; urine ketones may be ⊕ in fasting normal Pts)
- ↑ Serum glc; ↑ BUN & Cr (dehydration ± artifact due to ketones interfering w/ some assays)
- Hyponatremia: corrected Na = measured Na + [2.4 × (measured glc − 100)/100]
- ↓ or ↑ K (but even if serum K is elevated, usually *total body K depleted*); ↓ total body phos
- Leukocytosis, ↑ amylase (even if no pancreatitis)

Typical DKA "Flow Sheet" Setup											
VS	**UOP**	**pH**	**HCO₃**	**AG**	**Ketones**	**Glc**	**K**	**PO₄**	**IVF**	**Insulin**

HCO_3

Note: Main ketone produced is β-OH-butyrate (βOHB), *but ketone measured by nitroprusside is acetoacetate (Ac-Ac). As DKA is treated, βOHB → Ac-Ac, ∴ AG can decrease while measured ketones can increase.*

Treatment of DKA *(Diabetes Care 2009;32:1335)*	
Rule out possible precipitants	Infection, intra-abdominal process, MI, etc. (see above)
Aggressive hydration	NS 10–14 mL/kg/h, tailor to dehydration & CV status
Insulin	10 U IV push followed by 0.1 U/kg/h Continue insulin drip until AG normal If glc <250 and AG still high → add dextrose to IVF and continue insulin to metabolize ketones AG normal → SC insulin (overlap IV & SC 2–3 h)

Electrolyte repletion	K: add 20–40 mEq/L IVF if serum K <4.5
	  insulin promotes K entry into cells → ↓ serum K
	  careful K repletion in Pts with renal failure
	HCO₃: ? replete if pH <7 or if cardiac instability
	PO₄: replete if <1

HYPEROSMOLAR HYPERGLYCEMIC STATE

Definition, precipitants, pathophysiology *(Diabetes Care 2003;26:S33)*
• Extreme hyperglycemia (w/o ketoacidosis) + hyperosm. + Δ MS in T2D (typically elderly)
• Precip same as for DKA, but also include dehydration and renal damage
• Hyperglycemia → osmotic diuresis → vol depletion → prerenal azotemia → ↑ glc, etc.

Clinical manifestations & dx studies *(Diabetes Care 2016;39:S99)*
• Volume depletion and Δ MS
• ↑ **serum glc** (usually >600 mg/dL) & ↑ **meas. serum osmolality** (>320 mOsm/L)
  effective Osm = 2 × Na (mEq/L) + glc (mg/dL)/18
• No ketoacidosis; usually ↑ BUN & Cr; [Na] depends on hyperglycemia & dehydration

Treatment (r/o possible precipitants; ~15% mortality due to precipitating factors)
• **Aggressive hydration:** initially NS, then ½ NS, average fluid loss up to 8–10 L
• **Insulin** (eg, 10 U IV followed by 0.05–0.1 U/kg/h)

HYPOGLYCEMIA

Clinical manifestations (glucose <~55 mg/dL)
• **CNS:** headache, visual Δs, Δ MS, weakness, seizure, LOC (neuroglycopenic sx)
• **Autonomic:** diaphoresis, palpitations, tremor (adrenergic sx)

Etiologies in diabetics
• Excess insulin, oral hypoglycemics, missed meals, renal failure (↓ insulin & SU clearance)
• β-blockers can mask adrenergic symptoms of hypoglycemia

Etiologies in nondiabetics
• ↑ **insulin:** exogenous insulin, sulfonylureas, insulinoma, anti-insulin antibodies
• ↓ **glucose production:** hypopituitarism, adrenal insufficiency, glucagon deficiency, hepatic failure, renal failure, CHF, alcoholism, sepsis, severe malnutrition
• ↑ **IGF-II:** non-islet tumor
• Postprandial, esp. postgastrectomy or gastric bypass: excessive response to glc load
• Low glc w/o sx can be normal

Evaluation in nondiabetics *(JCEM 2009;94:709)*
• If clinically ill: take measures to avoid recurrent hypoglycemia; ✓ BUN, Cr, LFTs, TFTs, prealbumin; IGF-I/IGF-II ratio when appropriate
• If otherwise healthy: 72-h fast w/ monitored blood glc; stop for neuroglycopenic sx
• *At time of hypoglycemia:* insulin, C peptide (↑ w/ insulinoma and sulfonylureas, ↓ w/ exogenous insulin), β-OH-butyrate, sulfonylurea levels
• At end of fast, give 1 mg glucagon IV and measure response of plasma glc before feeding

Treatment
• Glucose tablets, paste, fruit juice are first-line Rx for Pts who can take POs
• If IV access available, give 25–50 g of D₅₀ (50% dextrose)
• If no IV, can give glucagon 0.5–1 mg IM or SC (side effect: N/V)

LIPID DISORDERS

Measurements
- Lipoproteins = lipids (cholesteryl esters & triglycerides) + phospholipids + proteins include: chylomicrons, VLDL, IDL, LDL, HDL, Lp(a)
- Measure after 12-h fast; LDL typically calculated: LDL-C = TC − HDL-C − (TG/5) underestim. if TG >400 or LDL-C <70 mg/dL; ∴ directly measure LDL-C levels stable up to 24 h after ACS, then ↓ and may take 6 wk to return to nl
- PEx clues: tendon xanthomas (eg, Achilles), imply LDL >300 mg/dL; eruptive xanthomas on extensor surfaces imply TG >1000 mg/dL; xanthelasma (yellowish streaks on eyelids)
- Metabolic syndrome (≥3 of following): waist ≥40" (♂) or ≥35" (♀); TG ≥150; HDL <40 mg/dL (♂) or <50 mg/dL (♀); BP ≥130/85 mmHg; fasting glc ≥100 mg/dL (Circ 2009;120:1640)
- Lp(a) = LDL particle bound to apo(a) via apoB; genetic variants a/w MI (NEJM 2009;361:2518)

Dyslipidemias
- 1°: familial hyperchol. (FH, 1:500): defective LDL receptor; ↑↑ chol, nl TG; ↑ CAD; familial hypertrig. (FHTG, 1:500): ↑ TG, ± ↑ chol, ↓ HDL, pancreatitis; and many others
- 2°: DM (↑ TG, ↓ HDL), hypothyroidism (↑ LDL, ↑ TG), nephrotic syndrome (↑ LDL, ↑ TG), liver failure (↓ LDL), alcohol (↑ TG, ↑ HDL), thiazides (↑ LDL, ↑ TG), protease inhib (↑ TG)

Drug Treatment

Drug	↓ LDL	↑ HDL	↓ TG	Side effects/comments
Statins	20–60%	5–10%	10–25%	↑ ALT in 0.5–3%; ✓ before starting and then prn Myalgias <10%, rhabdo <0.1%, dose-dependent ↑ risk of DM; screen if risk factors
Ezetimibe	15–20%	—	—	Well tolerated
Fibrates	5–15%	5–15%	35–50%	Myopathy risk ↑ w/ statin. ↑ Cr; ✓ renal fxn q6mo.
Niacin	10–25%	~30%	40%	Flushing (ASA preRx may ↓), ↑ glc & UA. No benefit if on statin w/ low LDL-C (NEJM 2014;371:203).
Resins	20%	3–5%	↑	Bloating, binds other meds
Ω-3 FA	5% ↑	3%	25–50%	Dyspepsia, diarrhea, skin Δs, bleeding; ? effective (JAMA 2012;308:1024), definitive trials underway
PCSK9i	40–65%	5–10%	15–25%	mAb inj SC q2w or q4w (JACC 2015;65:2638)

Treatment of LDL-C (Lancet 2014;384:607)
- **Statins**: every 1 mmol (39 mg/dL) ↓ LDL-C → 22% ↓ major vascular events (CV death, MI, stroke, revasc) in individuals w/ & w/o CAD (Lancet 2010;376:1670)
- **Ezetimibe**: ↓ major vascular events incl MI & stroke when added to statin post-ACS, w/ magnitude of benefit consistent w/ LDL-statin relationship (IMPROVE-IT, NEJM 2015;372:2387)
- **PCSK9 inhibitors**: −60% ↓ LDL on top of statin, as monoRx, and in FH (EHJ 2014;35:2249); prelim data w/ encouraging ↓ CV outcomes (NEJM 2015;372:1500), definitive trials ongoing

Treatment of other lipid fractions (Lancet 2014;384:618 & 626)
- **HDL-C**: low levels a/w ↑ risk of MI, but no clinical yet benefit by raising
- **Triglycerides**: reasonable to treat levels >500–1000 mg/dL w/ fibrates or Ω-3 FA to ↓ risk of pancreatitis; genetically mediated lower levels a/w ↓ risk of CAD (NEJM 2014;371:22); modest benefit of fibrates on CV outcomes (NEJM 2010;362:1563 & 2013;368:1800)
- **Lp(a)**: consider ↓ to <50 mg/dL w/ niacin in intermed- to high-risk Pts (EHJ 2010;31:2844)

2013 ACC/AHA Guideline & 2016 Expert Consensus Decision Pathway

Population	10-y CV risk	Statin Recommendation
Clinical ASCVD	n/a	High intensity (? moderate if age >75 y)
LDL-C ≥190 mg/dL	n/a	High intensity
DM, age 40–75 y	n/a	High intensity (? moderate if risk <7.5%)
Age 40–75 y (and none of the above)	≥7.5%	High or moderate intensity
	5–<7.5%	Reasonable to offer moderate intensity
	<5%	Consider statin if additional risk factor

Consider EZE or PCKS9i if LDL-C ≥70 & h/o ACS, athero event while on statin, DM, or FH

Circ 2014;130(Suppl 2):S1 & JACC 2016;68:92. ASCVD incl h/o ACS, stable angina, art. revasc, stroke, TIA, PAD.
10-y CV Risk Score: http://my.americanheart.org/cvriskcalculator. Additional risk factors to consider: LDL-C ≥160 mg/dL, genetic hyperlipid., FHx premature ASCVD, hsCRP >2 mg/L, CAC score ≥300 or 275th %ile, ABI <0.9

Statin Doses & LDL-C Reduction (doubling of dose → 6% further ↓ LDL-C)

Intensity	↓ LDL-C	Rosuva	Atorva	Simva	Prava	Lova	Fluva	Pitava
High	≥50%	20–40	40–80	(80)				
Mod	30–50%	5–10	10–20	20–40	40–80	40	80	2–4
Low	<30%			10	10–20	20	20–40	1

Doses are in mg. Simva 80 mg has ↑ myopathy risk and should not be used unless dose already tolerated >12 mo.

Approach to patient with joint pain

- **Articular** vs. **periarticular** (bursitis, tendinitis) source of pain: typically active ROM more painful than passive ROM in periarticular process
- **Inflammatory** vs. **noninflammatory** pain: *features of inflammatory pain include swelling, warmth or redness in specific joint, prolonged morning stiffness (>30 min), improvement of pain/stiffness w/ motion/exercise*
- Physical exam (see table): localize complaint and identify objective signs of inflammation
- The physical exam is only 50–70% sensitive for detecting inflammatory arthritis

Key Physical Exam Findings in Joint Pain					
	Articular (joint) disease			*Periarticular/soft tissue*	
Physical exam	**OA**	**Inflammatory arthritis**[a]	**Arthralgia**	**Bursitis or tendinitis**	**Myofascial**
Swelling	varies	yes	no	yes	no
Erythema	no	varies	no	yes	no
Warmth	no	yes	no	yes	no
Tenderness	joint line	yes	varies	periarticular	yes
ROM[b]	limited	limited	full or limited	full, often limited by pain	full
Pain w/ active or passive	both	both	usually both	active > passive	usually both

[a]May initially present as arthralgia w/o overt arthritis. [b]Range of motion of joint or joint a/w bursa or tendon.

Figure 8-1 Approach to arthritis

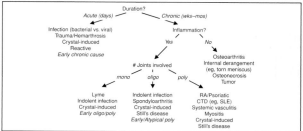

Analysis of Joint Fluid				
Test	**Normal**	**Noninflamm**	**Inflammatory**	**Septic**
Appearance	clear	clear, yellow	clear to opaque yellow-white	opaque
WBC/mm³	<200	<2000	>2000	>2000 (usually >50k*)
Polys	<25%	<25%	≥50%	≥75%
Culture	⊖	⊖	⊖	⊕
Intracellular Crystals	⊖	⊖	⊕ in some (eg, gout)	⊖

*WBC count of aspirated fluid in septic bursitis often < WBC count in septic arthritis.

Radiologic features of major arthritides

- **OA:** plain films: **osteophytes**, asym joint space narrowing (JSN), subchondral sclerosis & cysts. MRI may show early disease not seen on plain films; U/S ≈ MRI for structural damage.
- **RA:** plain films: early = periarticular **osteopenia**; late = **erosions**, symmetric JSN MRI & U/S able to detect early and subclinical disease; MRI ≈ U/S for erosions.
- **Gout:** plain films: early = nonspec swelling; late = **tophus**, joint erosions w/ overhanging edges. U/S used for detection of microtophi (double contour sign); MRI ≈ U/S for erosions.
- **Spondyloarthritis** (sacroiliac joint): plain films: pseudo-widening of joint space (early), sclerosis, erosions, **ankylosis.** MRI most Se for early Δ; U/S ≈ MRI to detect enthesitis.

Comparison of Major Arthritides

Feature	OA	RA	Gout/CPPD	Spondyloarthritis
Onset	gradual	gradual	acute	variable
Inflammation	⊖	⊕	⊕	⊕
Pathology	degeneration	pannus	microtophi	enthesitis
# of joints	poly	poly	mono to poly	oligo or poly
Typical joint involvement	hips, knees, spine, 1st CMC DIP, PIP	MCP, PIP wrists, feet, ankles, knees	MTP feet, ankles, knees	sacroiliac spine large periph
Joints often *spared*	MCP, shoulder, elbow, wrist	L & T spine, DIPs	spine	*any joint can be involved*
Special articular findings	Bouchard's & Heberden's nodes	ulnar dev. swan neck boutonnière deformities	urate/CPPD crystals tophi	dactylitis enthesitis (eg, Achilles) bamboo spine syndesmophytes
Extra-articular features		SC nodules pulmonary sicca	olec. bursitis renal stones	psoriasis IBD uveitis
Lab data	normal	often ⊕ RF & anti-CCP	↑ UA (may be nl during flare)	± HLA-B27

INFLAMMATORY MARKER & AUTOANTIBODY TESTING

Inflammatory markers (Mod Rheumatol 2009;19:469)
- **ESR:** *indirect* measure of inflammation (↑ RBC aggregation due to acute-phase proteins); slow to rise; ↑ w/ age, pregnancy, anemia, obesity
- **CRP:** *direct* measure of inflammation (protein produced by liver, part of innate immune system); *typically rises and falls before the ESR* w/ treatment/resolution of process

Autoantibody testing (Best Pract Res Clin Rheumatol 2014;28:907)
- ANA: *screening test* for Ab directed against nuclear proteins and found in autoimmune conditions, most useful in testing for suspected connective tissue diseases
- Ab against dsDNA & Ro/La/Smith/RNP are *highly specific* for various CTD and can be used to w/u ⊕ ANA further in setting of clinical suspicion
- Order ANA only when *clinical suspicion for disease* b/c nonspecific: 1:40 (low ⊕, 25–30% of healthy people); 1:80 (low ⊕, 10–15% of healthy people); ≥1:160 (⊕, 5% of healthy). May be ⊕ in Pts prior to clin manifest (NEJM 2003;349:1526; Arthritis Res Ther 2011;13:1).
- ANA does *not* correlate well w/ disease activity, ∴ no clinical value in serial testing
- RF and anti-CCP can be seen in CTD but are not specific in this clinical setting

DDx & APPROACH TO COMMON INPATIENT RHEUM PRESENTATIONS

Presentation	Rheum Ddx	Rheum Lab Workup
Fever of unknown origin	GCA/PMR, adult-onset Still's, SLE, inflammatory arthritis, Takayasu's, PAN, ANCA ⊕ vasc, cryo, HSP	ESR, CRP, ANA, RF, ANCA, ± cryo
Pulmonary hypertension	Scleroderma (limited > diffuse), MCTD, SLE, PM/DM (less common)	ANA, Scl-70, centromere, RNA Pol III, RNP
Diff alveolar hemorrhage	ANCA ⊕ vasc, Goodpasture's, SLE, APS	ANCA, GBM, ANA, C3/C4
Interstitial lung disease	Scleroderma (diffuse > limited), sarcoid, RA, DM/PM, antisynthetase syndrome, Sjögren's, MCTD, SLE (esp. pleura), ANCA ⊕ vasc (esp. MPA)	ANA, Ro/La, RF/anti-CCP, ANCA, ± myositis panel
Pleuro-pericarditis	SLE, RA, MCTD, DM/PM, ANCA ⊕ vasc, Sjögren's, PAN	ANA, dsDNA, Sm, RNP, Ro/La, RF, anti-CCP, ANCA
Acute kidney injury	SLE (GN or nephrotic), ANCA ⊕ vasc (GN), scleroderma renal crisis (diffuse), Sjögren's (RTA/TIN), PAN (infarct), HSP, Goodpasture's (GN), cryo	ANA, Ro/La (RTA/TIN) dsDNA, C3/C4, RNA Pol III (SRC), Scl-70 (SRC), ANCA, GBM, cryos
Neuropathy	ANCA ⊕ vasc, SLE, RA, PAN, Sjögren's, cryo, sarcoid	ANA, Ro/La, ANCA, cryo RF/anti-CCP, HCV, HBV

RHEUMATOID ARTHRITIS (RA)

Definition & epidemiology (Lancet 2010;376:1094; NEJM 2011;365:2205; Ann Rheum Dis 2010;69:70)
- Chronic, symmetric, debilitating and destructive inflammatory polyarthritis characterized by proliferative synovial tissue (pannus) formation in affected joints
- Pathogenesis involves over-production of TNF, IL-1, and IL-6 (∴ used as drug targets)
- Risk stems from combination of genetic (~50% of risk), environmental influences (eg, smoking, silica dust), Pt factors (periodontal disease, Δs in gut microbiome)
- HLA-DRB1 haplotype a/w disease suscept., severity & response to Rx (JAMA 2015;313:1645)
- Prevalence = 1% adults; 5% of ♀ >70 y; ♀ to ♂ ratio = 3:1; peak incidence 50–75 y

Clinical manifestations (Medicine 2010;38:167)
- Usually insidious onset **pain, swelling** and impaired function of joints (typically PIPs, MCPs, wrists, knees, ankles, MTPs and cervical spine) with **morning stiffness** for ≥1 h
- Typically polyarticular (60% small joints, 30% large joints, 10% both), may be monoarticular (knee, shoulder, wrist) early in course; nb, rheumatoid joints can become *infected*
- Joint deformities: **ulnar deviation, swan neck** (MCP flexion, PIP hyperextension, DIP flexion), **boutonnière** (PIP flexion, DIP hyperextension), **cock-up deformities** (toes)
- **C1–C2 instability** → myelopathy, ∴ ✓ C-spine flex/ext films prior to elective intubation
- Constitutional symptoms: *low-grade* fever, weight loss, malaise
- **Extra-articular manifestations** (18–41% of Pts) can occur at any time; ↑ frequency in seropositive (⊕ RF or anti-CCP) and with active disease (Autoimmun Rev 2011;11:123)

Extra-Articular Manifestations (EAMs)	
Skin	**Rheumatoid nodules** (20–30%, usually sero ⊕): extensor surface, bursae; can be in lung, heart, sclera Raynaud's, pyoderma gangrenosum, cutan. vasculitis (ulcers, purpura, etc.)
Pulm	ILD, pleuritis, effusions (low glc), nodules, airway disease, PHT 20% of the time precedes joint manifestations
CV	Pericarditis (effusions in ⅓ of sero ⊕), myocarditis, accelerated athero/MI, AF, coronary/systemic vasculitis. ↑ risk CV death (Arth Rheum 2015;67:2311).
Nervous	Mono/polyneuritis multiplex, CNS vasculitis, stroke, nerve entrapment
Ocular	Scleritis, episcleritis, keratoconjunctivitis sicca (2° Sjögren's)
Heme	Anemia of chronic disease Neutropenia Felty's syndrome (1%, typically long-standing RA): splenomegaly large granular lymphocyte leukemia: bone marrow infiltrated w/ lymphocytes ± myeloid hypoplasia NHL, amyloidosis
Renal	Glomerulonephritis (usually mesangial), nephrotic synd (2° amyloidosis) NSAIDs and MTX may also cause renal damage
Vasculitis	Small & medium vessels (usually ↑ RF titer, long-standing RA); pericarditis, ulcers, scleritis, & neuropathy most common (Curr Opin Rheum 2009;21:35)

Laboratory & radiologic studies (Annals 2007;146:797)
- **RF** (IgM/IgA/IgG anti-IgGAb) in ~70% of Pts; also seen in other rheumatic diseases (SLE, Sjögren's), infection (SBE, hepatitis, TB), types II & III cryo, 5% of healthy population
- **Anti-CCP** (Ab to cyclic citrullinated peptide): in ~80% of Pts, similar Se (~70%), more Sp (>90%) than RF particularly for early RA (Arth Rheum 2009;61:1472); a/w increased joint damage and low remission rates
- ~20% are seronegative (RF and anti-CCP negative)
- ↑ ESR/CRP but nl in ~30%; ⊕ ANA in ~40%; ↑ globulin during periods of active disease
- Radiographs of hands and wrists: periarticular osteopenia, bone erosions, joint subluxation
- Increasing use of MSK U/S to diagnosis synovitis and erosive disease

ACR/EULAR classification criteria (Arth Rheum 2010;62:2569)
- Used in clinical research, but not in clinical practice
- Relevant for Pts with ≥1 joint with synovitis not better explained by another disease
- Likelihood of RA ↑ w/ higher # (espec. ≥4) of small joints involved, ⊕ (espec. high titer) RA or anti-CCP, ANA, ↑ ESR or CRP, and duration ≥6 wk

Management (Ann Rheum Dis 2014;73:516)
- Early dx and Rx (esp. DMARD) w/ *frequent* follow-up and escalation of Rx as needed to *achieve clinical remission* or low disease activity
- ↓ time to remission ≈ ↑ length of sustained remission (Arthritis Res Ther 2010;12:R97)
- Sero-⊕ (espec. RF or anti-CCP) a/w aggressive joint disease & EAM
- At dx, start *both* rapid-acting agent (to acutely ↓ inflammation) and **D**isease-**M**odifying **A**nti-**R**heumatic **D**rug (**DMARD**) (typically take 1–3 mo to have max effect)

- Rapid-acting drugs:
  - **NSAIDs** or COX-2 inhibitors (↑ CV, GI adverse events), consider starting with PPI;
  - **glucocorticoids** [low-dose (<20 mg/d oral) or joint injection]; or
  - NSAIDs + glucocorticoids: ↑ GI adverse events, minimize long-term concurrent use
- **DMARDs**
  - **MTX** (1st line unless CKD, hepatitis, EtOH or lung disease), SAS or leflunomide; consider HCQ if seronegative and mild disease;
  - If inadequate response after 3 mo (despite DMARD dose escalation):
    - **combination Rx** w/ other DMARDs (eg, "triple therapy" w/ MTX, SAS and HCQ) or **biologic** (anti-TNF typically 1st line unless contraindication)
    - MTX/SAS/HCQ non-inferior to etanercept/MTX (NEJM 2013;369:307)
    - JAK inhibitor if fail biologics, although also promising data as initial DMARD (NEJM 2014;370:2377 & 2016;374:1243)
- Given ↑ r/o early CV morbidity/mortality, try to ↓ risk w/ lifestyle mgmt, lipid & DM screening

RA Therapeutics (Arth Rheum 2016;68:1)		
Class	**Drug**	**Side effects**
Traditional DMARDs	Methotrexate (MTX) Leflunomide Sulfasalazine (SAS)	GI distress (esp. nausea), myelo-suppression, ILD, hepatotoxicity ✓ G6PD prior to SAS Supplement MTX & SAS w/ folate
Biologic DMARDs (all anti-TNF have similar efficacy)	Anti-TNF: etanercept, infliximab, adali-mumab, certolizumab, golimumab CTLA4-Ig: abatacept IL-6R Ab: tocilizumab (studied as mono-Rx w/o MTX) Anti-CD20: rituximab IL-1R Ab: anakinra	↑ risk bacterial/fungal/viral infxn (esp. TB, zoster, hepatitis, and w/ stnd or high-dose; Lancet 2015;386: 258); ∴ ✓ for TB, Hep B/C prior to starting ? CHF & demyelinating CNS disease for anti-TNF *Never use 2 biologics together*
Other	Hydroxychloroquine (HCQ) JAK inhib: tofacitinib (TF), baricitinib Rarely: cyclosporine, azathioprine, gold	HCQ: retinopathy, rash JAK inhib: infxn, ↑ Cr, ↑ LFTs, HTN CsA: nephrotox, HTN, gum hyperplasia

(Lancet 2008;371:987; 2013;381:451,918, & 1541; NEJM 2012;367:495 & 508, & 369:307)

ADULT-ONSET STILL'S DISEASE & RELAPSING POLYCHONDRITIS

Adult-onset Still's disease (J Rheumatol 1992;19:424; Autoimmun Rev 2014;13:708)
- **Rare autoinflammatory synd;** ♂ = ♀ w/ typical onset 16–35 y; sx evolve over wks to mos
- Dx if 5 criteria are present & ≥2 major; exclude infxn, malig, other rheumatic, drug rxn
  - **major:** fever ≥39°C for ≥1 wk (usually daily or twice daily high-spiking fever); arthralgias/arthritis ≥2 wk; Still's rash (qv); ↑ WBC w/ 80% PMN
  - **minor:** sore throat; LAN; HSM; ↑ AST/ALT/LDH; negative ANA & RF
- Still's rash (>85%): nonpruritic macular or maculopapular salmon-colored rash; usually trunk or extremities; may be precipitated by trauma (Koebner phenomenon), warm water
- Plain films: soft tissue swelling (early) → cartilage loss, erosions, carpal ankylosis (late)
- Treatment: NSAIDs; steroids; steroid-sparing (MTX, **anakinra**, anti-TNF, **tocilizumab**)
- Variable clinical course: 20% w/ long-term remission; 30% remit-relapse; ~50% chronic (esp. arthritis); ↑ risk of macrophage activation syndrome (life-threatening)

Relapsing polychondritis (Rheum Dis Clin NA 2013;39:263)
- Inflammatory destruction of cartilaginous structures; onset usually age 40–60 y, ♂ = ♀
- Subacute onset of **red, painful** and **swollen cartilage;** ultimately atrophic & deformed
- Common clinical features: bilateral auricular chondritis; nonerosive inflammatory arthritis; nasal chondritis; ocular inflammation; laryngeal or tracheal chondritis; cochlear and/or vestibular dysfxn
- 40% of cases a/w immunologic disorder (eg, RA, SLE, vasc., Sjögren's), cancer or MDS
- Clinical diagnosis based on exam with multiple sites of cartilaginous inflammation
- Labs: ↑ ESR & CRP, leukocytosis, eosinophilia, anemia of chronic inflammation
- Bx (not req for dx): proteoglycan depletion, perichondrial inflammation and replacement with granulation tissue and fibrosis; immunofluorescence with Ig and C3 deposits
- Screen for pulm (PFTs, CXR/CT, ± bronch) and cardiac (ECG, TTE) involvement
- Therapy guided by disease activity and severity: **steroids** 1st line; NSAIDs, dapsone for sx control of arthralgias and mild disease; MTX, AZA, or biologics for steroid-sparing; cyclophosphamide for organ-threatening disease

CRYSTAL DEPOSITION ARTHRITIDES

Comparison of Gout and Pseudogout

	Gout (NEJM 2011;364:443)	Pseudogout (Rheum 2009;48:711)
Acute clinical	Sudden onset painful *mono-articular* arthritis (classically **podagra** [MTP of great toe]) or bursitis; freq. nocturnal *Polyarticular* in subseq flares Can mimic cellulitis (esp. in foot)	Mono- or asymmetric oligoarthritis (esp. knees, wrists & MCP joints); rare axial involvement (eg, crowned dens syndrome)
Chronic clinical	Solid crystal deposition (**tophus**) in joints (esp. toes, fingers, wrists, knees) & tissue (esp. olecranon bursa, pinna, Achilles)	"Pseudo-RA" w/ polyarticular arthritis w/ morning stiffness or "Pseudo-OA"
Assoc. conditions	Metabolic syndrome; CKD; CHF	3 H's: Hyperparathyroidism; Hypo-magnesemia; Hemochromatosis
Crystal	Monosodium urate	Calcium pyrophosphate dihydrate
Polarized microscopy*	Needle-shaped, **negatively birefringent**	Rhomboid-shaped, weakly **positively birefringent** crystals
Radio-graphic findings	Erosions w/ overhanging edge (late); "double contour sign" on MSK US	**Chondrocalcinosis**: punctate, linear densities in articular cartilage, menisci, fibrocartilage of wrist, hands, symphysis pubis
Other	a/w uric acid stones; urate nephropathy	✓ Ca, Mg, Fe, ferritin, TIBC, UA, PTH in young or severe cases

*Crystals should be intracellular; Infection can coexist with acute attacks, ∴ always ✓ Gram stain & Cx

Gout

Definition & epidemiology (Lancet 2010;375:318; Nat Rev Rheumatol 2015;11:649)
- Humans lack enzyme to metabolize urate (end-product of purine metabolism)
- Monosodium urate (MSU) crystal deposition in joints promotes inflammation
- ♂ > ♀ (9:1); peak incidence 5th decade; most common cause of inflammatory arthritis in ♂ over 30 y; *rare* in premenopausal ♀ (estrogens promote renal urate excretion)

Etiologies (Ann Rheum Dis 2012;71:1448)
- **UA underexcretion (85–90%):** meds (eg, diuretics); idiopathic; ↓ renal function; obesity
- Uric acid (UA) overproduction (10–15%): ↑ meat, seafood, EtOH, psoriasis, idiopathic, myelo- and lymphoproliferative disease, chronic hemolytic anemia, cytotoxic drugs, rare inherited enzyme defic, genetic variants (Lancet 2008;372:1953)

Diagnosis
- ↑ UA is not diagnostic: 25% of measurements nl during flare; ± ↑ WBC & ESR
- Arthrocentesis is gold standard: negatively birefringent needles (see table above)
- 2015 ACR/EULAR Classification Criteria (Ann Rheum Dis 2015;74:1789) used 1° in research

Acute treatment (Arthritis Care Res 2012;64:1447; Am Fam Physician 2014;90:831)
- No superior option; start w/in 24 h of sx onset; continue until acute flare resolves; for severe cases, consider combination therapy; rest and ice; w/o treatment self-limited in 3–10 d

Acute Treatment for Gout

Drug	Initial dose	Comments
NSAIDs (nonselect or COX-2)	Full anti-inflammatory dose → tapering	Gastritis & GIB; avoid in CKD & CVD = efficacy among NSAIDs never compared with colchicine
Colchicine (PO; IV no longer available in U.S.)	1.2 mg then 0.6 mg 1 h later → 0.6 mg bid	N/V, diarrhea (↑ w/ ↑ dose); ↓ dose in renal insufficiency (however, not nephrotoxic) a/w BM supp., myopathy, neuropathy
Corticosteroids (PO, IA, IV, IM) **or Corticotropin**	eg, prednisone ~0.5 mg/kg/d × 5–10 d ± taper	Rule out joint infection 1st Comparable to NSAID as 1st-line treatment (Annals 2016;164:464)
IL-1 inhibitors (Curr Opin Rheumatol 2015;27:156)	anakinra (100 mg SC qd × 3 d) canakinumab (150 mg SC × 1)	↑↑ cost; anakinra a/w injection site pain (Arthritis Res Ther 2007;9:R28); canakinumab approved in EU (Ann Rheum Dis 2012;71:1839; Arth Rheum 2010;62:3064)

- **Approach:** if ≥2 attacks/y, ≥1 tophus, joint erosions or urolithiasis → start urate lowering Rx & pharmacologic prophylaxis to ↓ risk of acute attacks
- **Pharmacologic prophylaxis:** continue for at least 6 mos or longer if frequent attacks: low-dose **colchicine** (~50% ↓ risk of acute flare; *J Rheum* 2004;31:2429), **NSAIDs** (less evidence; *Ann Rheum Dis* 2006;65:1312), low-dose **steroids, IL-1 inhibitors** (see above)
- **Urate-lowering Rx:** goal UA <6 mg/dL; do NOT discontinue during acute attack or acute kidney injury (unless allopurinol hypersensitivity syndrome)
- **Lifestyle** Δs (*Rheum Dis Clin NA* 2014;40:581): ↓ intake of meat, EtOH & seafood, ↑ low-fat dairy products, wt loss, avoid dehydration

Urate-Lowering Therapy (Chronic Treatment for Gout)		
Drug (route)	**Mechanism**	**Comments**
Allopurinol (PO)	Xanthine oxidase inhib	1st line; adjust starting dose in CKD; titrate ↑ q2–5wk a/w rash, hypersensitivity syndrome (see below), diarrhea, dyspepsia, BM suppression, hepatitis; monitor CBC & LFTs; not nephrotoxic max dose = 800 mg/d
Febuxostat (PO)	Nonpurine xanthine oxidase inhib	2nd line; use if allopurinol intolerant a/w LFT Δ, rash, arthralgias, nausea start 40 mg, max dose = 120 mg/d
Pegloticase (IV)	Recombinant uricase	For refractory tophaceous gout; infusion reactions (including anaphylaxis); Ab formation may limit use (*JAMA* 2011;306:711)
Probenecid (PO)	Uricosuric	Rarely used; risk of urolithiasis

- **Allopurinol hypersensitivity syndrome:** 10–25% mortality; ↓ risk by starting w/ dose 100 mg/d if eGFR >40 or 50 mg/d if eGFR ≤40; titrate up by 100 mg/d (if eGFR >40) or 50 mg/d (if eGFR ≤40) q2–5wk until UA <6 mg/dL (dose can be >300 mg/d even in CKD)
- **Associated with HLA-B5801,** esp. Han Chinese, Koreans, Thai; screen in these high-risk populations prior to initiating allopurinol (*Curr Opin Rheumatol* 2014;26:16)

CALCIUM PYROPHOSPHATE DIHYDRATE (CPPD) DEPOSITION DISEASE/PSEUDOGOUT

Definition
- Deposition of CPPD crystals w/in tendons, ligaments, articular capsules, synovium, cartilage; frequently asymptomatic

Etiologies (Rheumatology 2012;51:2070)
- Most cases **idiopathic;** consider further metabolic eval in young (<50 y) and florid forms
- Metabolic (**3 H's**): hemochromatosis; hyperparathyroidism; hypomagnesemia (esp. in Gitelman's or Bartter's syndromes)
- Joint trauma (incl. previous surgery); intra-articular hyaluronate can precipitate attacks
- Familial chondrocalcinosis (autosomal dominant disorder); early-onset, polyarticular dis.

Clinical manifestations (Rheum Dis Clin NA 2014;40:207)
- **Chondrocalcinosis:** calcification of cartilage, resulting from CPPD deposition in articular cartilage, fibrocartilage or menisci
  ↑ incidence w/ age; 20% >60 y have knee chondrocalcinosis in autopsy studies
- **Pseudogout:** acute CPPD crystal-induced mono- or asymmetric oligoarticular arthritis, indistinguishable from gout except through synovial fluid exam for crystals
  location: **knees, wrists** and MCP joints
  precipitants: surgery, trauma or severe illness
- Chronic forms: "Pseudo-RA" and pyrophosphate arthropathy (may involve axial skeleton; resembles OA)

Diagnostic studies
- Arthrocentesis is gold standard: **rhomboid-shaped, weakly positively birefringent crystals** (yellow perpendicular & blue parallel to axis on polarizer; see table above)
- Radiographs: see table above

Treatment (NEJM 2016;374:2575)
- Asymptomatic chondrocalcinosis requires no treatment
- Acute therapy for pseudogout: no RCTs, extrapolated from practice in gout; ∴ same as for gout, though colchicine not as effective
- If associated metabolic disease, Rx of underlying disorder may improve arthritis sx
- Low-dose daily colchicine or NSAID may be effective for prophylaxis or chronic arthropathy

Classification system (NEJM 2016:374:2563)
- 5 subtypes: ankylosing spondylitis (most common), reactive arthritis, psoriatic arthritis, IBD-associated arthritis and undifferentiated
- Can also distinguish axial-predominant from peripheral-predominant joint involvement
- All subtypes share common clinical manifestations: inflammatory spine disease, peripheral arthritis, enthesitis and extra-articular manifestations (primarily ocular and skin disease)

Epidemiology & pathogenesis (Nat Rev Rheumatol 2015:10:110)
- ↑ prevalence of HLA-B27; HLA-B27 accounts for ~30% of attributable genetic risk
- Environmental factors likely critical for disease, esp. reactive arthritis (eg, infection)
- Prevalence of 0.5–2% of population, worldwide

Spondyloarthritis (SpA) Epidemiology and Key Presentation Features

Disease	Epidemiology	Other
Ankylosing spondylitis	♂:♀ = 3:1; onset in teens to mid-20s (rare after 40 y)	Progressive limitation of spine motion; "bamboo spine"
Psoriatic arthritis	♂ = ♀; peak incidence 45–54 y; seen in 20–30% of Pts w/ psoriasis (Ann Rheum Dis 2005:64:ii14)	In 13–17%, arthritis precedes psoriasis by yrs. Does not correlate with psoriasis activity. A/w HIV.
Reactive arthritis	♂ >> ♀; 20–40 y; 10–30 d s/p post-GI or GU infxn* in genetically susceptible host	Previously "Reiter's syndrome": arthritis, urethritis and conjunctivitis. Most resolve w/in 12 mo.
IBD-associated	♂ = ♀; seen in 20% of IBD Pts; Crohn's > UC	Type I <5 joints: correlates w/ IBD Type II >5 joints or axial disease: does not correlate w/ IBD

*GU: Chlamydia, Ureaplasma urealyticum; GI: Shigella, Salmonella, Yersinia, Campylobacter, C. diff.

Major clinical manifestations (Lancet 2011:377:2127)
- **Inflammatory back pain:** SI joints (**sacroiliitis**), apophyseal joints of spine characterized by **IPAIN** (**I**nsidious onset, **P**ain at night, **A**ge of onset <40 y, **I**mproves w/ exercise/hot water, **N**o improvement w/ rest); a.m. stiffness, *responsive to NSAIDs*
- **Peripheral arthritis:** typically asymmetric, oligoarticular, large joints, lower > upper limb; however, can be symmetric & polyarticular (thus, mimic RA), esp. in psoriatic arthritis
- **Enthesitis:** inflammation at site of tendon/ligament insertion into bone, esp. Achilles, pre-patellar, elbow epicondyles, plantar fascia
- **Rigidity of spine:** bamboo spine by X-ray, ankylosis due to progressive growth of bony spurs which bridge intervertebral disc
- **Dactylitis** ("sausage digit"): inflammation of entire digit (joint + tenosynovial inflamm)
- **Uveitis:** anterior uveitis *most common extra-articular manifestation;* p/w pain, red eye, blurry vision, photophobia, usually unilateral

Distinguishing Features

Feature	Axial-predom Ankylosing spondylitis	Peripheral-predominant Psoriatic	Peripheral-predominant Reactive	Peripheral-predominant IBD-assoc
Axial involv.	100%	20–40%	40–60%	5–20%
Sacroiliitis	Symmetric	Asymm	Asymm	Symmetric
Periph involv.	Less common (~50%)	Frequent	Frequent	Frequent
Periph distrib.	Lower > Upper	Upper > Lower (see below)	Lower > Upper	Lower > Upper
HLA-B27	80–90%	20%	50–80%	5–30%
Enthesitis	Frequent	Frequent	Frequent	Rare
Dactylitis	Uncommon	Common	Common	Uncommon
Ocular	Uveitis in 25–40%	Conjunctivitis, uveitis, episcleritis	**Conjunctivitis** (noninfectious), uveitis, keratitis	Uveitis
Skin	None	**Psoriasis;** nail pitting and onycholysis	Circinate balanitis, keratoderma blennorrhagica	E. nodosum, pyoderma-gangrenosum
Imaging	Bamboo spine (symm syndes.)	"Pencil-in-cup" DIP deformity	*Asymmetric* syndesmophytes	Periph dis. rarely erosive
Other	↑ CAD; aortitis, AI, conduction defects	↑ CAD	**Urethritis,** AI, conduction defects	

- **Psoriasis:** erythematous plaques with sharply defined margins often w/ thick silvery scale
- **Circinate balanitis:** shallow, painless ulcers of glans penis and urethral meatus
- **Keratoderma blennorrhagica:** hyperkeratotic lesions on soles of feet, scrotum, palms, trunk, scalp
- **Erythema nodosum:** red tender nodules due to panniculitis, typically on shins; Ddx incl. idiopathic, infxn, sarcoid, drugs, vasculitis, IBD, lymphoma
- **Pyoderma gangrenosum:** neutrophilic dermatosis → painful ulcers w/ violaceous border; Ddx incl. idiopathic, IBD, RA, myelogenous leukemia

Psoriatic arthritis subtypes (Lancet 2011;377:2127)
- **Monoarticular/oligoarticular** (eg, large joint, DIP joint, dactylitic digit): most common initial manifestation
- **Polyarthritis** (small joints of the hands/feet, wrists, ankles, knees, elbows): indistinguishable from RA, but often asymmetric
- **Arthritis mutilans:** severe destructive arthritis with bone resorption, esp. hands
- **Axial disease:** unilateral/asymmetric sacroiliitis
- **DIP-limited:** good correlation with nail pitting and onycholysis

Clinical assessment (Nat Rev Rheumatol 2012;8:253)
- **Axial disease assessment**
  Nb: following not specific PEx findings but useful in monitoring disease during Rx
  Lumbar flexion deformity assessed by modified Schober's test (⊕ if <5 cm ↑ in distance between a point 5 cm below the lumbosacral jxn and another point 10 cm above, when going from standing to maximum forward flexion)
  T-spine mobility (extension) and kyphosis severity measured by occiput-to-wall distance (although occiput-to-wall distance also increased in osteoporotic kyphosis)
- **Seronegative:** notable for *absence* of rheumatoid factor or autoantibodies; ± ↑ESR/CRP
- **HLA-B27:** nonspecific, as common in general population (6–8%); most useful when high clinical suspicion w/ nl imaging; ⊕ 90% of Pts w/ AS, but only 20–80% in other SpA
- **Radiology**
  MRI preferred for *early* detection of inflammation (sacroiliitis)
  Plain films detect late structural changes (SI erosions/sclerosis)
  calcification of spinal ligaments w/ bridging symm syndesmophytes ("bamboo spine") squaring and generalized demineralization of vertebral bodies ("shiny corners")
- **Infectious evaluation for reactive arthritis** (⊖ studies do not r/o)
  U/A, PCR of urine and/or genital swab for *Chlamydia*; urethritis usually due to *Chlamydia* infxn preceding arthritis, but also can see sterile urethritis post dysentery
  ✓ stool Cx, *C. diff* toxin. Consider HIV in workup of reactive or psoriatic arthritis.

Treatment approach (Ann Rheum Dis 2012;71:319; Arth Rheum 2016;68:282)
- Untreated disease may lead to irreversible structural damage and associated ↓ function
- Early physiotherapy beneficial
- Tight control of inflammation improves joint outcomes in PsA (Lancet 2015;386:2489)
- **NSAIDs:** 1st line; rapidly ↓ stiffness and pain; prolonged, continuous administration may modify disease course but associated w/ GI and CV toxicity (Cochrane Database Syst Rev 2015;17:CD010952); may exacerbate IBD
- **Intra-articular corticosteroids** in mono- or oligoarthritis; *limited role for systemic steroids, esp. for axial disease*
- **Conventional DMARDs** (eg, MTX, SAS, leflunomide): *no efficacy for axial disease or enthesitis;* may have role in *peripheral arthritis,* uveitis and extra-articular manifestations
- **Anti-TNFs:** effective for *both axial and peripheral manifestations;* improves function (Ann Rheum Dis 2006;65:423) and may slow progression of structural changes (Curr Rheumatol Rep 2012;14:422); adalimumab or infliximab preferred if inflammatory bowel disease
- **Apremilast** (PO PDE-4 inhibitor): approved for use in PsA (Ann Rheum Dis 2014;73:1020); associated with GI side effects and significant wt loss
- **Ustekinumab** (SC IL-12/23 inhibitor): approved for use in PsA (Ann Rheum Dis 2014;73:990)
- **Secukinumab** (IL-17A inhibitor): improves signs & symptoms of PsA & ankylosing spondylitis (NEJM 2015;373:1329 & 2534; Lancet 2015;386:1137)
- **Other:**
  Abx in reactive arthritis if evidence of active infxn; consider prolonged abx for refractory *Chlamydia* ReA (Arthritis Rheum 2010;62:1298)
  Involve ophthalmologist for any evidence of inflammatory eye disease (may benefit from steroid eye drops or intravitreal steroid injections).
  Treat underlying IBD when appropriate

INFECTIOUS ARTHRITIS & BURSITIS

ETIOLOGIES & DIAGNOSIS OF INFECTIOUS ARTHRITIS

Etiologies (Curr Rheumatol Rep 2013;15:332)

- **Bacterial** (nongonococcal): early diagnosis required
- **Gonococcal** (*N. gonorrhea*): consider in sexually active young adults
- Viral: parvovirus, HCV, HBV, acute HIV; typically polyarticular, may mimic RA
- Mycobacterial: monoarticular or axial (Pott's disease)
- Fungal: *Candida* (esp. prosthetic joints), coccidiomycosis (valley fever), histoplasmosis
- Other: Lyme, *Mycoplasma*, *Salmonella* (2° to anti-TNF Rx), Brucellosis (unpast. dairy)

Diagnosis (JAMA 2007;297:1478)

- H&P w/ poor sensitivity and specificity for septic arthritis; ∴ **arthrocentesis** should be performed as soon as suspected and prior to starting antibiotics if possible
- *Take care not to tap through an infected area, thus introducing infxn into joint space*
- ✓ Synovial fluid cell count w/ differential, Gram stain, bacterial culture, crystals
  WBC >50k w/ poly predom suspicious for bact. infxn; *crystals do not r/o septic arthritis!*

BACTERIAL (NONGONOCOCCAL) ARTHRITIS

Epidemiology & risk factors

- **Immunocompromised host:** DM, EtOH use, HIV, age >80, SLE, cancer, steroid use, etc.
- **Damaged joints:** RA, OA, gout, trauma, prior surgery/prosthetic, prior arthrocentesis (rare)
- **Bacterial seeding:** bacteremia secondary to IVDU, endocarditis or skin infection direct inoculation or spread from contiguous focus (eg, cellulitis, septic bursitis, osteo)

Clinical manifestations (JAMA 2007;297:1478; Lancet 2010;375:846)

- Acute onset **monoarticular arthritis** (>80%) w/ pain (Se 85%), swelling (Se 78%), warmth
- Location: **knee** (most common), hip, wrist, shoulder, ankle. In IVDU, tends to involve other areas inc. axial joints (eg, SI, symphysis pubis, sternoclavicular, manubrial joints).
- **Constit. sx:** fevers (Se 57%), rigors (Se 19%), sweats (Se 27%), malaise, myalgias, pain
- *Septic bursitis must be differentiated from septic intra-articular effusion*

Additional diagnostic studies (JAMA 2007;297:1478)

- Synovial fluid: **WBC usually >50k** (Se 62%, Sp 92%) but can be <10k, **>90% polys**; Gram stain ⊕ in ~75% of *Staph*, ~50% of GNR; Cx ⊕ in >90%. Synovial bx most sens.
- **Leukocytosis** (Se 90%, Sp 36%); **elevated ESR/CRP** (Se >90%)
- **Blood cultures** ⊕ in >50% of cases, ~80% when more than 1 joint involved
- Conventional radiographs should be obtained but usually normal until after ~2 wk of infection when bony erosions, joint space narrowing, osteomyelitis, periostitis can be seen
- **CT & MRI** useful esp. for suspected hip infection or epidural abscess

Treatment for native joints (Curr Rheumatol Rep 2013;15:332)

- Prompt empiric antibiotics guided by Gram stain after surgical drainage. If Gram stain ⊖, empiric Rx w/ vancomycin; add anti-pseudomonal agent if elderly, immunosupp.

Common microbes (by Gram stain)		Population	Initial antibiotic regimen (tailor based on Gram stain, cx, clinical course)
GPC	*S. aureus* (most common)	Normal joints Prosthetic joints Damaged joints	Vancomycin*
	S. epidermidis	Prosthetic joints Postprocedure	Vancomycin*
	Streptococci	Healthy adults Splenic dysfunction	PCN-G or ampicillin
GN	Diplococci: *N. gonorrhea*	Sexually active young adults	Ceftriaxone or cefotaxime
	Rods: *E. coli*, *Pseudomonas*, *Serratia*	IVDU, GI infection immunosupp, trauma elderly	Cefepime or piperacillin/tazobactam + antipseudomonal aminoglycoside in IVDU

*Can later Δ to antistaphylococcal penicillin based on sensitivities

- **IV antibiotics** × ≥2 wk followed by oral antibiotics; varies by clinical course & microbiology
- Joint must be **drained**, often serially; arthroscopic drainage for larger joints and as initial treatment but may also be accomplished by arthrocentesis. Serial synovial fluid analyses should demonstrate ↓ in WBC and sterility.
- Prognosis: *10–50% mortality* depending on virulence of organism, time to Rx, host

- ↑ risk in first 2 y s/p procedure; rate generally low (0.5–2.4%); risk factors include obesity, RA, immunocompromised state, steroids, & superficial surgical site infxn
- Staphylococci (coag negative & *S. aureus*) in >50%; polymicrobial in 10–20%
- Early (<3 mo s/p surgery) or delayed (3–24 mo) onset typically acquired during implantation; early w/ virulent organisms (eg, MRSA) and delayed w/ less virulent organisms (eg, *P. acnes*, coag negative *Staph*) & more indolent presentation
- Late (>24 mo) onset typically related to secondary hematogenous seeding
- Diagnosis requires arthrocentesis by orthopedics; ESR & CRP (CRP Se 73–91%, Sp 81–86%; *NEJM* 2009; 361:787) can be helpful
- Treatment typically requires prolonged abx & 2-stage joint replacement (joint retention a/w ~40% failure rate; CID 2013;56:182) or life-long suppressive abx. *ID and orthopedics consultation required.*

DISSEMINATED GONOCOCCAL INFECTION (DGI)

Epidemiology (Infect Dis Clin North Am 2005;19:853)
- *N. gonorrhea*; most frequent type of infectious arthritis in sexually active young adults
- **Normal host** as well as Pts w/ deficiencies of terminal components of complement
- ♀:♂ = 4:1; ↑ incidence during menses, pregnancy, & postpartum period, SLE; ↑ incidence in homosexual males; rare after age 40 y

Clinical manifestations
- Preceded by **mucosal infection** (eg, endocervix, urethra or pharynx) that is often asx
- Two distinct syndromes, although Pts can have both:
  Joint localized: purulent arthritis (40%), usually 1–2 joints (knees > wrists > ankles)
  DGI: triad of **polyarthralgias, tenosynovitis, skin lesions**; purulent arthritis rare
    acute onset of tenosynovitis (60%) in wrists, fingers, ankles, toes
    rash (>50%): gunmetal gray pustules with erythematous base on extremities & trunk
- Rare complications: Fitz-Hugh-Curtis syndrome (perihepatitis), pericarditis, meningitis, myocarditis, osteomyelitis from direct extension of joint-localized infection

Additional diagnostic studies
- Synovial fluid: **WBC >50k** (but can be <10k), **poly predominant**
  Gram stain ⊕ in ~25%; culture ⊕ in up to 50% if done w/ Thayer-Martin media
- Blood culture: more likely ⊕ in DGI; rarely in joint localized disease
- Gram stain and culture of skin lesions occasionally ⊕
- Cervical, urethral, pharyngeal, rectal PCR or cx on Thayer-Martin media; ✓ *Chlamydia*

Treatment
- **Ceftriaxone or cefotaxime × 7 d w/ empiric doxycycline** for *Chlamydia* (fluoroquinolones no longer recommended due to resistance)
- Joint arthroscopy/lavage may be required if purulent arthritis; rarely >1 time

OLECRANON & PREPATELLAR BURSITIS

Epidemiology & risk factors (Infect Dis Clin North Am 2005;19:991)
- >150 bursae in the body; 2 most commonly infected are **olecranon** and **prepatellar**
- Most commonly (esp. superficial bursae) due to direct trauma, percutaneous inoculation or contiguous spread from adjacent infection (eg, cellulitis)
- Other risk factors: recurrent noninfectious inflammation (eg, gout, RA, CPPD), diabetes
- *S. aureus* (80%) most common, followed by streptococci

Diagnosis
- Physical exam: discrete bursal swelling, erythema, maximal tenderness at center of bursa with preserved joint range of motion
- Aspirate bursa if concern for infxn, ✓ cell count, Gram stain, bacterial cx, crystals
  WBC >20k w/ poly predominance suspicious for bacterial infection, but lower counts common (crystals do *not* rule out septic bursitis!)
- Assess for adjacent joint effusion, which can also be septic
- *Take care not to tap through infected skin, thus introducing infxn into bursa*

Initial therapy
- Prompt empiric coverage for staphylococci and streptococci: PO abx acceptable for mild presentation; **vancomycin** if ill-appearing; broaden spectrum based on risk factors
- Modify antibiotics based on Gram stain, culture results, & clinical course. Duration of tx is 1–4 wks. Serial aspirations every 1–3 d until sterile or no reaccumulation of fluid.
- Surgery if unable to drain bursa through aspiration, evidence of foreign body or necrosis, recurrent/refractory bursitis w/ concern for infxn of adjacent structures.

Approx Prev of Autoantibodies in Rheumatic Diseases										
Disease	**ANA**	**dsDNA**	**Sm**	**Ro/La**	**Scl-70**	**RNA PIII**	**Centr**	**Jo-1**	**U1-RNP**	**RF**
SLE	≥95	75	20	25	⊖	⊖	⊖	⊖	45	35
Sjögren's	≥95	rare	⊖	45	⊖	⊖	⊖	⊖	rare	>75
Diffuse SSc	>90	⊖	⊖	rare	40	20	rare	⊖	rare	30
Limited SSc	>90	⊖	⊖	rare	10	rare	60	⊖	rare	30
IM	75–95	⊖	⊖	⊖	rare	⊖	⊖	25	⊖	15
MCTD	≥95	⊖	⊖	rare	⊖	⊖	⊖	⊖	always	50
RA	40	⊖	⊖	⊖	⊖	⊖	⊖	⊖	⊖	70

Centr, centromere; IM, inflammatory myopathies; RF, rheumatoid factor; SSc, systemic sclerosis. (*Primer on the Rheumatic Diseases*, 12th ed., 2001; *Lancet* 2013;382:797).
- Auto-Ab testing directed by clinical findings, as auto-Ab *do not define* a particular CTD
- Overlap syndromes may be reflected by multiple autoantibodies

see "Systemic Lupus Erythematosus" and "Rheumatoid Arthritis" for those diseases

SYSTEMIC SCLEROSIS AND SCLERODERMA DISORDERS

Definition & epidemiology (*Best Pract Res Clin Rheumatol* 2010;24:857)
- **Scleroderma** refers to the presence of tight, thickened skin
- Localized scleroderma: *morphea* (plaques of fibrotic skin), *linear* (fibrotic bands), *"en coup de saber"* (linear scleroderma on one side of scalp and forehead ≈ saber scar)
- **Systemic sclerosis (SSc)** = scleroderma + internal organ involvement
  SSc w/ *limited cutaneous disease:* formerly CREST syndrome (see below)
  SSc w/ *diffuse cutaneous disease:* often rapidly progressive disorder affecting skin
  SSc *sine scleroderma* (visceral disease without skin involvement, rare)
- Peak onset of SSc between **ages 30–50**; ♀ > ♂ (7:1); African American > white
- 1–2/100,000 annual incidence of systemic disease in the U.S.
- Pathogenesis: immune damage to endothelial cells and reactive O_2 species production → persistent oxidative stress → perivascular inflammation → fibroblast activation and fibrosis. Cytokines, growth factors, genetics, environmental factors and autoantibodies (against PDGF receptor, endothelial cells and fibroblasts) all contribute (*NEJM* 2009;360:1989).

ACR/EULAR SSc classification criteria (*Ann Rheum Dis* 2013;72:1747)
- Sufficient for dx: skin thickening of fingers of both hands extending proximal to MCPs
- Other items considered in criteria: Raynaud's, SSc-related auto-Ab, PAH and/or ILD, abnormal nailfold capillaries, telangiectasia, fingertip lesions (ulcers, scars), skin thickening limited to fingers (not beyond MCPs)
- **Rule out other causes** of thickened skin: diabetes (scleredema ≠ scleroderma), toxin, hypothyroidism, nephrogenic systemic fibrosis, eosinophilic fasciitis, amyloidosis, GVHD

Diagnostic studies & monitoring (*Semin Arthritis Rheum* 2005;35:35)
- Autoantibodies: >95% Pts w/ auto-Ab; generally mutually-exclusive
  ⊕ **anti-Scl-70** (antitopoisomerase 1): a/w diffuse SSc; ↑ risk pulm fibrosis
  ⊕ **anticentromere:** a/w limited SSc; ↑ risk of severe digit ischemia and PHT
  ⊕ **anti-RNA-Pol III:** a/w diffuse SSc; ↑ risk renal crisis; a/w cancer
  ⊕ ANA (>90%), ⊕ RF (30%), ⊕ anti-U1-RNP a/w overlap syndrome
  Other: anti-Th/To (a/w limited SSc), U3-RNP (a/w ILD), PmScl (polymyositis-SSc overlap)
- CXCL4 levels reported to help diagnose disease and be correlated w/ degree of lung & skin fibrosis and disease progression but awaits validation (*NEJM* 2014;370:433)
- At baseline: ✓ BUN/Cr & UA for proteinuria, PFTs (spirometry, lung volumes, D_LCO), high-res chest CT (if diffuse disease), TTE (RVSP for PHT), RHC if ↑ RVSP or suspect PHT
- Annual PFTs; TTE q1–2y
- Skin bx not routine, but helpful to assess other possible causes for skin thickening
- ↑ risk of malignancy compared to general population, therefore must be vigilant
- Frequent (eg, daily) BP ✓ to monitor for HTN suggestive of scleroderma renal crisis

Clinical Manifestations of Systemic Sclerosis

Skin	Tightening and thickening of extremities, face, trunk (bx not req for dx) "Puffy" hands, carpal tunnel syndrome, sclerodactyly Nailfold capillary dilatation & dropout Immobile, pinched, "mouse-like" facies and "purse-string" mouth Calcinosis cutis (subcutaneous calcification), telangiectasias
Arteries	Raynaud's phenomenon (80%); digital or visceral ischemia
Renal	**Scleroderma renal crisis (SRC)** = accelerated development of HTN (*relative increase in Pt BP as compared with baseline BP*), MAHA urine sediment typically bland; path w/ "onion-skin" hypertrophy of capillaries; affects 5–10% of Pts, 66% w/in 1ˢᵗ year (*Rheum 2009;48:iii32*) ↑ risk w/ >15 mg/d of prednisone (*Arthritis Rheum 1998;41:1613*) poor prognosis w/ 50% mortality
GI (>80% of Pts)	GERD and erosive esophagitis Esophageal dysmotility → dysphagia, odynophagia, aspiration Gastric dysmotility → early satiety and gastric outlet obstruction Small intestinal dysmotility → malabsorption, bact overgrowth, bloating
Musculoskel	Arthralgias/arthritis; myositis; joint contractures; tendon friction rubs
Cardiac	Myocardial fibrosis; pericardial effusion; conduction abnormalities
Pulmonary	Pulmonary fibrosis (typically develops w/in 4 y); pulmonary arterial hypertension (typically develops after many yrs). #1 cause of mortality
Endocrine	Amenorrhea and infertility common; thyroid fibrosis ± hypothyroidism

SSc Subgroup Comparison

	Limited	Diffuse
General		Fatigue, weight loss
Skin	Thickening on extremities *distal to* elbows/knees and *face* only	Thickening of distal *and proximal* ext, face *and* trunk
Pulmonary	PAH (rapidly progressive) > fibrosis	Fibrosis > PAH
GI	PBC	
Renal	SRC later in disease course	SRC earlier & more common
Cardiac		Restrictive cardiomyopathy
Other	**CREST syndrome** = **C**alcinosis, **R**aynaud's, **E**sophageal dysmotility, **S**clerodactyly, **T**elangiectasias	Raynaud's
Antibodies	Centromere (10–40%)	Scl 70, RNA-Pol III (40%)
Prognosis	Survival >70% at 10 y	Survival 40–60% at 10 y

Treatment (*Ann Rheum Dis 2009;68:620*)
- *Minimize steroid exposure to reduce risk of renal crisis*
- Pulmonary fibrosis: **cyclophosphamide** (*NEJM 2006;354:2655; Arth Rheum 2006;54:3692*), MMF
  under investigation; improvement may be minimal (*Rheum Dis Clin NA 2015;41:237*)
  PAH: pulmonary **vasodilators** (see "Pulm Hypertension"), early Rx a/w better outcomes
- Renal crisis: **ACEI** (not ARB) for Rx, not prophylaxis (*Semin Arthritis Rheum 2015;44:687*)
- GI: PPI and/or H2-blockers for GERD; antibiotics for malabsorption
  hypomotility: metoclopramide or erythromycin; nonoperative Rx of pseudo-obstruction
- Cardiac: NSAIDs or steroids for pericarditis
- Arthritis: acetaminophen, NSAIDs, hydroxychloroquine, MTX
- Myositis: MTX, AZA, steroids
- Skin: PUVA for morphea. For pruritus: emollients, topical or oral steroids (↓ dose). MTX or
  MMF effectiveness for skin fibrosis debated (*Ann Rheum Dis 2011;70:1104*).

INFLAMMATORY MYOPATHIES

Definition & epidemiology (*JAMA 2013;305:183; NEJM 2015;372:1734*)
- All lead to skeletal muscle inflammation & weakness, variable extramuscular involvement
- **Polymyositis** (PM): idiopathic diffuse polymyopathy, onset typically 40s–50s; ♀ > ♂
- **Dermatomyositis** (DM): similar to PM; also occurs in childhood, but differentiated from
  other myopathies by skin manifestations; malignancy a/w PM (10%) & DM (24%)
- **Necrotizing autoimmune myositis** (NM): usually in adults; occurs after viral infections,
  statin exposure (⊕ anti-HMGCR)
- **Inclusion body myositis** (IBM): onset after age 50; ♂ > ♀; often *misdiagnosed as PM*

Clinical manifestations (*NEJM 2015;372:1734*)
- **Muscle weakness:** gradual (wks → mos) except in NM, progressive and painless

    DM/PM/NM: *proximal and symmetric*; difficulty climbing stairs, arising from chairs, brushing hair; fine motor skills (eg, buttoning) lost late
    IBM: *may be asymmetric and distal*

- **Dermatologic:** may precede myositis by mos to yrs (uncommon for converse)
  erythematous rash on sun-exposed skin: neck & shoulders (shawl sign), face, chest
  heliotrope rash (purplish discoloration) over upper eyelids ± periorbital edema
  Gottron's papules (in >80% & *pathognomonic*): violaceous often scaly areas symmetrically over dorsum of PIP and MCP joints, elbows, patellae, medial malleoli subungual erythema, "mechanic's hands" (skin cracks on digits), pruritus
  DM sine myositis (amyopathic DM): dermatologic features w/o myositis, in 10–20%
- Polyarthralgias or polyarthritis: usually early; nonerosive; small joints > large joints
- Raynaud's (30%, DM and overlap CTD) w/ dilatation & dropout of nail bed capillaries
- **Visceral involvement** (*J Rheumatol 2009;36:2711*)
  pulmonary: acute alveolitis; ILD; respiratory muscle weakness; aspiration
  cardiac (33%): often asx; conduction abnl; myo/pericarditis; HF uncommon; ↑ CK-MB/Tn
  GI: dysphagia, aspiration
- **Antisynthetase syndrome** (PM > DM): fever, ILD, Raynaud's, mechanic's hands, arthritis
- DDx: drug-induced myopathy (statins, cocaine, steroids, colchicine); infxn (HIV, EBV, CMV); metabolic (hypothyroid, hypo-K, hypo-Ca); neuromuscular dis. (eg, myasthenia gravis); glycogen storage disease; mitochondrial cytopathy; muscular dystrophy

Diagnostic studies

- ↑ **CK** (rarely >100,000 U/L, can be ↑↑↑ in NM), aldolase, SGOT, LDH; ± ↑ ESR & CRP
- Autoantibodies: ⊕ ANA (>75%) (*Curr Rheumatol Rep 2013;15:335*)
  ⊕ **anti-Jo-1** (25%): most common specific Ab; a/w antisynthetase syndrome
  ⊕ anti-Mi-2 (DM > PM 15-20%) is a/w disease that responds well to steroids
  ⊕ anti-SRP is a/w NM, poor Rx response; ⊕ anti-HMGCR in NM a/w statin exposure
- Consider **EMG** (↑ spontaneous activity, ↓ amplitude, polyphasic potentials w/ contraction) or **MRI** (muscle edema, inflammation, atrophy) for evaluation; may guide biopsy
- **Pathology and muscle biopsy:** all with interstitial mononuclear infiltrates, muscle fiber necrosis, degeneration & regeneration (required for definitive diagnosis)
  PM: *T cell–mediated muscle injury; endomysial* inflam. surrounds non-necrotic fibers
  DM: *immune complex deposition in blood vessels with complement* activation; perimysial, perivascular inflam (B & CD4 T cells), complement in vessels.
  NM: *necrotic fibers w/ macrophages*
  IBM: *T cell–mediated muscle injury, vacuole formation;* same as PM with eosinophilic inclusions and rimmed vacuoles (EM)

Treatment (PM & DM, *no effective treatment for IBM*) (*Autoimmun Rev 2011;11:6*)

- **Steroids** (prednisone 1 mg/kg); MTX or AZA early if mod/severe or taper fails (2–3 mo)
- For resistant (30–40%) or severe disease: AZA/MTX combo, IVIg (DM ± PM), rituximab (*Arthritis Rheum 2013;65:314*), MMF, cyclophosphamide (esp. if ILD or vasculitis)
- IVIg w/ pulse steroids acutely for life-threatening esoph or resp muscle involvement
- ✓ for occult malignancy (esp. if DM); monitor respiratory muscle strength with spirometry
- NM: discontinue statin if taking; steroids + MTX or IVIG if needed (*Muscle Nerve 2010;41:185*)

Myositides, Myopathies and Myalgias					
Disease	**Weakness**	**Pain**	**↑ CK**	**↑ ESR**	**Biopsy**
DM/PM/NM	⊕	⊖	⊕	±	as above
IBM	⊕	⊖	⊕	⊖	as above
Hypothyroidism	⊕	±	⊕	⊖	mild necrosis inflam, atrophy
Steroid-induced	⊕	⊖	⊖	⊖	atrophy
PMR	⊖	⊕	⊖	⊕	normal
Fibromyalgia (*JAMA 2014;311:1547*)	⊖	⊕ (tender points)	⊖	⊖	normal

SJÖGREN'S SYNDROME

Definition & epidemiology

- Chronic dysfxn of **exocrine glands** (eg, salivary/lacrimal) due to lymphoplasmacytic infiltration. Extraglandular manifestations common in primary form.
- Can be primary or secondary (a/w RA, scleroderma, SLE, PM, hypothyroidism, HIV)
- More prevalent in ♀ than ♂; typically presents between 40 & 60 y of age

Clinical manifestations

- **Dry eyes** (keratoconjunctivitis sicca): ↓ tear production; burning, scratchy sensation
- **Dry mouth** (xerostomia): difficulty speaking/swallowing; dental caries; xerotrachea; thrush

- **Parotid gland enlargement:** intermittent, painless, typically bilateral
- **Vaginal dryness** and **dyspareunia**
- **Recurrent nonallergic rhinitis/sinusitis** due to upper airway gland involvement
- **Extraglandular manifestations:** arthritis; interstitial nephritis (40%); type I RTA (20%); cutaneous vasculitis (25%); neuropathies (10%); PNS or CNS disease; ILD; PBC
- ↑ risk of lymphoproliferative disorders (~50× ↑ risk of lymphoma and WM in 1° Sjögren's)

Diagnostic studies
- Autoantibodies: ⊕ ANA (95%), ⊕ RF (75%)
  Primary Sjögren's: ⊕ **anti-Ro** (anti-SS-A, 56%) and/or ⊕ **anti-La** (anti-SS-B, 30%)
- **Schirmer test:** filter paper in palpebral fissures to assess tear production
- **Rose-Bengal** staining: dye that reveals devitalized epithelium of cornea/conjunctiva
- **Ocular staining score:** substitute for Rose-Bengal staining to determine degree of keratoconjunctivitis sicca using fluorescein and lissamine green
- **Biopsy** (minor salivary, labial, lacrimal or parotid gland): lymphoplasmacytic infiltration

Classification criteria (2 of 3 have 93% Se & 95% Sp; *Arthritis Care Res* 2012;64:475)
1. ⊕ anti-Ro or anti-La or RF + ANA >1:320
2. Labial salivary gland bx w/ lymphocytic sialadenitis and score >1 focus/4 mm^2
3. Keratoconjunctivitis sicca w/ ocular staining score ≥3

Treatment (*Arth Rheum* 2005;52:27 & 2007;57:310; *Arth Res Ther* 2013;15:R172)
- Ocular: artificial tears, cyclosporine eyedrops, autologous tears
- Oral: sugar-free gum, lemon drops, saliva substitute, hydration, pilocarpine, cevimeline
- Systemic: NSAIDs, steroids, DMARDs, rituximab (RCTs are needed)

MIXED CONNECTIVE TISSUE DISEASE (MCTD)

Definition (*Best Pract Res Clin Rheumatol* 2012;26:61)
- Features of **SLE, systemic sclerosis,** and/or **polymyositis** that appear gradually and often evolve to a dominant phenotype of SLE or systemic sclerosis
- Different from undifferentiated CTD (UCTD): fail to meet criteria for any CTD; 30% go on to develop CTD over 3–5 y (usually SLE)

Clinical & laboratory manifestations (variable clinical course)
- **Raynaud's phenomenon** typical presenting symptom (75–90%); see below
- Hand edema ("puffy hands"), sclerodactyly, RA-like **arthritis** w/o erosions, polyarthralgias
- Pulmonary involvement (85%) with **pulmonary hypertension,** fibrosis
- Pericarditis most frequent cardiovascular manifestation; GI: dysmotility (70%)
- Membranous & mesangial GN common (25%); low risk for renal HTN crisis or severe GN
- ⊕ ANA (>95%); ⊕ RF (50%); **anti-U1-RNP** in all but *not* specific (seen in ~50% SLE)

Treatment: As per specific rheumatic diseases detailed above

RAYNAUD'S PHENOMENON

Clinical manifestations (*NEJM* 2016;375:556)
- Episodic, reversible digital ischemia, triggered by cold temp, or stress, classically: **blanching** (white, ischemia) → **cyanosis** (blue, hypoxia) → **rubor** (red, reperfusion); color Δ usually well demarcated; affects fingers, toes, ears, nose.

Primary vs. Secondary Raynaud's Phenomenon		
	Primary (80–90%)	**Secondary** (10–20%)
Vessel wall	*Functionally* abnl	*Structurally* abnl
Etiologies	Idiopathic, however can be exacerbated by comorbid conditions, including HTN, athero, CAD, DM	SSc, SLE, PM-DM, MCTD, Sjögren's, RA Arterial dis (athero, Buerger's); trauma Heme (cryo, Waldenström's, APLAS) Drugs (ergopeptides, estrogens, cocaine)
Epidem.	20–40 y; ♀ > ♂ (5:1)	>35 y
Clinical	Mild, *symm.* episodic attacks *No PVD, tissue injury,* or *systemic sx*	**Tissue ischemia & injury** (eg, digital ulcers); can be assoc w/ systemic sx
Auto Ab	⊖	Depends on above etiology, often ⊕
Nailfold	Normal	Dropout and/or enlarged or distorted loops

Treatment (*Curr Opin Rheumatol* 2011;23:555; *BMJ* 2012;344:e289)
- All: avoid cold, maintain warmth of digits & body; avoid cigarettes, drugs, caffeine & trauma
- Mild–mod: **long-acting CCB,** topical nitrates, SSRI, ARB, α-blockers, ASA/clopidogrel
- Severe: PDE inhibitors, anti-ET-1 receptor (if ulcers esp. w/ PHT), digital sympathectomy
- Digit-threatening: IV prostaglandins, digital sympathectomy, ± anticoagulation
- Others: fish oil (1° RP only; *Am J Med* 1989;86:158), abx for infected ulceration

SYSTEMIC LUPUS ERYTHEMATOSUS (SLE)

Multisystem inflammatory autoimmune disease with a broad spectrum of clinical manifestations in association with antinuclear antibody (ANA) production

Epidemiology *(Lancet 2014;384:1878)*
- Prevalence 15–50/100,000; predominantly affects women 2nd to 4th decade
- ♀:♂ ratio = 8:1; African American:Caucasian ratio = 4:1
- Complex genetics; some HLA association; rarely C1q & C2 deficiency

Systemic Lupus International Collaborating Clinics (SLICC) Classification Criteria		
Clinical Criteria	**SLICC Classification Criteria**	**Other Clinical Features**
Constit (84%)		Fever, malaise, anorexia, ↓ wt
Cutaneous/Oral/ Ophthalmologic (81%)	**1. Acute or subacute cutaneous changes** **2. Chronic cutaneous changes** **3. Oral or nasal ulcers** **4. Nonscarring alopecia**	Malar rash (spares nasolabial folds), discoid rash (papules w/ keratosis & plugging), bullous SLE, urticaria, TEN Photosens. (n/v, rash, fever) Vasculitis, panniculitis (lupus profundus) Raynaud's, nailfold cap Δs, Sicca syndrome Conjunctivitis, episcleritis
Musculoskeletal (85–95%)	**5. Joint disease:** synovitis or tenderness & morning stiffness involving ≥2 joints	Arthralgias and myalgias Avascular necrosis of bone
Cardiopulmonary (33%)	**6. Serositis:** pleuritis (37%) or pleural effusion, pericarditis (29%) or pericardial effusion	Pneumonitis, IPF, shrinking lung, PAH, DAH Myocarditis, CAD Libman-Sacks endocarditis
Renal (77%)	**7. Proteinuria** (>0.5 g/dL) or **RBC casts**	Nephrotic syndrome Lupus nephritis (qv)
Neurologic (54%)	**8. Seizures or psychosis** w/o other cause	Cognitive dysfxn, stroke, cranial or periph neuropathies, transverse myelitis, mononeuritis multiplex
GI (~30%)		Serositis (peritonitis, ascites) Vasculitis (bleeding, perf.) Hepatitis, pancreatitis
Hematologic	**9. Hemolytic anemia** **10. Leukopenia** (<4000/mm³) or **lymphopenia** (<1000/mm³) **11. Thrombocytopenia** (<100,000/mm³)	Anemia of chronic disease Antiphospholipid synd (VTE w/ ⊕ ACL Ab, lupus anticoag, and/or B2GPI Ab) Splenomegaly, LAN
Immunologic	**12. ⊕ ANA; 13. ⊕ anti-ds-DNA** **14. ⊕ anti-Sm; 15. ⊕ APLA** **16. ↓ Complement** **17. ⊕ Direct Coombs'** (w/o #9)	↑ ESR/CRP, ⊕ anti-Ro/La, ⊕ anti-RNP, ⊕ RF, ⊕ anti-CCP

Expert opinion, not dx criteria for SLE: ≥4/17 SLICC criteria, including ≥1 clinical & ≥1 immunologic, *or* bx proven SLE nephritis w/ ⊕ ANA or anti-ds-DNA *(Arth Rheum 2012;64:2677)*

Autoantibodies in SLE *(NEJM 2008;358:929)*			
Auto-Ab	**Frequency (approx)**	**Clinical associations**	**Timeline**
ANA	95–99% if active disease 90% if in remission Homogeneous or speckled	Any or all of broad spectrum of clinical manifestations Sensitive but not specific	May appear yrs before overt disease
Ro **La**	15–35% ⊕ anti-Ro may be seen w/ ⊖ or low titer ANA	Sjögren's/SLE overlap Neonatal lupus Photosens.; subacute cutan.	
ds-DNA	70%; ~95% Sp; titers may parallel dis. activity, esp. renal	Lupus nephritis Vasculitis	Appears mos before or at dx, but may become ⊕ after dx
Sm	30%; very specific for SLE	Lupus nephritis	
U1-RNP	40%	MCTD; Raynaud's Tend *not* to have nephritis	
Histone	90% in DLE; 60–80% in SLE	Mild arthritis and serositis	At diagnosis

Workup

- Autoantibodies: ANA, if ⊕ → ✓ anti-ds-DNA, anti-Sm, anti-Ro, anti-La, anti-U1-RNP
- Lytes, BUN, Cr, U/A, urine sed, spot microalb:Cr ratio or 24-h urine for CrCl and protein
- CBC, APLA (⊕ in 20–40%; ACL, B2GP1, lupus anticoagulant), total complement, C3 & C4
- If ↓ GFR, active sediment, hematuria or proteinuria (>0.5 g/dL) → renal bx to guide Rx

Treatment of SLE (Curr Rheumatol Rep 2011;13:308; Arthritis Care 2015;67:1237)		
Drug	**Indication**	**Adverse effects**
Hydroxychloroquine (HCQ)	**All Pts as ↓ flares** (NEJM 1991;324:150); monoRx for arthritis, serositis, skin disease	Retinal damage (<1%) Stevens-Johnson; myopathy Not immunosuppressive
NSAIDs	Arthritis, myalgias, serositis	Gastritis, UGIB, renal failure
Immunosuppressive agents		
Corticosteroids	Low dose (10–15 mg) for arthritis, serositis; high-dose (1 mg/kg) or pulse (1 g × 3 d) for major dis (eg, renal, CNS, heme)	Adrenal suppression, DM, cataracts, osteopenia, avascular necrosis of bone, myopathy
Mycophenolate (MMF)	**Nephritis** (induction/maint) Nonrenal refractory to HCQ	Cytopenias, ↑ LFTs, diarrhea, teratogen
Cyclophosphamide (CYC)	**Nephritis CNS disease** (induction, minimize exposure)	Cytopenias, infertility, teratogen, myeloproliferative disorders, hemorrhagic cystitis, bladder cancer
Azathioprine (AZA)	Nephritis (maintenance) Non-renal disease refractory to HCQ	Myelosuppression (✓TPMT), hepatotoxicity, teratogen lymphoproliferative disorders
Methotrexate (MTX)	Arthritis (preferred over MMF/AZA) Skin disease & serositis	Myelosuppression, hepatotoxicity, pneumonitis, alopecia, stomatitis, teratogen
Cyclosporine (CsA)	Renal disease	Hyperplastic gums, HTN hirsutism, CKD, anemia
Belimumab (NEJM 2013;368:1528)	Arthritis, serositis, skin disease (esp. if ⊕ ds-DNA or ↓ C3/C4)	B-cell depletion (< RTX, different mechanism)
Rituximab (RTX)	Refractory SLE, ITP, AIHA	Allergic rxn; serum sickness; PML

Lupus Nephritis (Arthritis Care Res 2012;64:797)		
Class	**Presentation**	**Treatment (all benefit from HCQ)**
I: Min. mesangial	Normal U/A & creatinine	No specific treatment
II: Mesangial prolif	Micro hematuria/proteinuria	No specific treatment ± ACEI
III: Focal prolif	Hematuria/proteinuria, ± HTN, ↓ GFR, ± nephrotic	Induce: MMF or CYC + steroids
IV: Diffuse prolif	Hematuria/proteinuria and HTN, ↓ GFR, ± nephrotic	Maintenance: ? MMF > AZA
V: Membranous (Can coexist with class III or IV)	Proteinuria, nephrotic	ACEI If nephrotic range proteinuria induce w/ MMF + steroids Maint.: MMF superior to AZA
VI: Adv. sclerotic	ESRD	Renal replacement therapy

(Ann Rheum Dis 2010;69:2083; NEJM 2004;350:971 & 2005;353:2219 & 2011;365:1886)

Prognosis (Arth Rheum 2006;54:2550; Rheum [Oxford] 2016;55:252)
- 5-y survival rate >90%, 10-y survival rate >80%
- Leading causes of morbidity and mortality: **infection, renal failure,** neurologic and cardiovascular events; thrombotic complications (Medicine 2003;82:299)

Drug-induced lupus (DLE) (Drug Saf 2011;34:357; Curr Opin Rheumatol 2012;24:182)
- Many drugs: **procainamide, hydralazine,** penicillamine, minocycline, INH, methyldopa, quinidine, chlorpromazine, diltiazem, **anti-TNF** (esp. infliximab), interferons
- Idiosyncratic onset; generally mild disease with arthritis, serositis, skin disease
- ⊕Anti-histone (95%) (may be ⊖ in anti-TNF); ⊖ anti-ds-DNA (often ⊕ in anti-TNF even w/o manifestations of DLE) & anti-Sm; normal complement levels
- Usually reversible w/in 4–6 wk after stopping medication

VASCULITIS

Overview

- Inflammation w/in blood vessel walls causing end-organ damage often a/w systemic sx; may be primary or secondary (eg, infection, malignancy) in etiology
- Classified by size of *predominant* vessel affected *(Arthritis Rheum 2013;65:1)*; overlap of vessel size affected is common
- Clinical manifestations based on size of vessels involved; constitutional sx (low-grade fever, fatigue, weight loss, myalgias, anorexia) common to all

	Distinguishing Characteristics of Vasculitis Subtypes				
	Large vessel		*Medium vessel*	*Small vessel*	
	TAK	**GCA**	**PAN**	**ANCA-assoc.**	**IC**
Epidem	Young, ♀ > ♂	Elderly, ♀ > ♂	Middle-aged to older	Variable	Variable
Renal	Arteries	None	Microaneurysms	GN	GN
Pulm	Rare	None	Rare	Frequent	Cryo > HSP
Periph Neurop	No		Yes	Yes	Yes
GI	Uncommon		Yes	Yes	HSP > Cryo
Skin	Rare	None	Common	Common	Common
Granul.	Yes		No	Yes, except MPA	No
Other			Mesenteric aneurysms, testicular involv.	GPA: upper airway EGPA: asthma	HSP: IgA-dep Cryo: HCV

TAK, Takayasu's arteritis; GCA, giant cell arteritis; PAN, polyarteritis nodosa; ANCA-assoc. is GPA, EGPA, & MPA; IC, immune complex small vessel vasculitis (eg, HSP, cryoglobulinemia); GN, glomerulonephritis.

Large-Vessel Vasculitis

Takayasu's arteritis ("pulseless disease")
- **Arteritis of aorta and its branches → stenosis/aneurysm** → claudication; onset <50 y
- Pattern of involvement: aorta and branches; most often **subclavian and innominate arteries** (>90%), as well as carotid, coronary, renal, pulmonary (~50%)
- Epidemiology: Most common in **Asia**; ♀:♂ ~9:1; **age <50 y**
- Clinical manifestations and physical findings *(Circ 2015;132:1701)*
  Systemic inflamm with **fever, arthralgias,** wt loss
  Vessel inflamm w/ pain & tenderness, ↓ **& unequal pulses/BPs in extremities, bruits,** limb claudication, renovascular HTN (>50%), neurogenic syncope; Ao aneurysm ± AI
  "Burnt out" or fibrotic period (eg, vascular stenosis)
- Dx studies: ↑ ESR (75%), CRP; **arteriography** → occlusion, stenosis, irregularity and aneurysms; carotid U/S Doppler studies; PET-CT; MRA; **pathology** → focal panarteritis, cellular infiltrate with *granulomas* and giant cells (bx not required for dx)
- Treatment: **steroids** ± MTX or AZA; anti-TNF (2nd line, *Autoimmun Rev 2012;11:678*), ASA, surgical/endovascular revasc *(Circ 2008;69:70)*
- Monitoring: MRA or PET-CT *(Arth Rheum 2012;64:866)*; ESR/CRP *(Ann Rheum Dis 2009;68:318)*

Giant cell arteritis (GCA) *(JAMA 2016;315:2442)*
- **Granulomatous arteritis of aorta/branches** w/ predilection for **temporal artery,**
- Pattern of involvement: **extracranial branches of carotid artery,** esp. temporal artery (thus also called **temporal arteritis**); aorta and/or its branches in 10–80%
- 90% of Pts w/ GCA are >60 y, peak incidence at 70–80 y, extremely rare <50 y; ♀:♂ = 3:1
- Clinical manifestations *(NEJM 2014;371:50)*
  constitutional sx: **fevers, fatigue,** wt loss, PMR sx (see below)
  temporal artery (TA) → **headache, tender TAs** and scalp; absent TA pulse
  ophthalmic artery (20%) → optic neuritis, diplopia, amaurosis fugax, blindness
  facial arteries → **jaw claudication**
  large vessel vasculitis → intermittent claudication of extremities; thoracic Ao aneurysm
  ~50% of Pts w/ GCA ultimately also diagnosed w/ PMR
- Dx studies: ↑ **ESR** (Se 84%, Sp 30%), ↑ CRP (Se 86%, Sp 30%), anemia
  (ESR related to fibrinogen & Ig in blood; Ddx for >100: malignancy esp. multiple myeloma, lymphoma; GCA or other vasculitis; ESRD; endocarditis, TB, osteomyelitis)
  temporal artery bx *whenever GCA suspected* (Se ≤85%); 1–2 cm ± bilat to ↑ yield (3–7% discordance) *(Ann Rheum Dis 2009;68:318)* → vasculitis & *granulomas*
  if suspect aortitis or lg vessel involvement (BP Δ or bruits) → MRI/MRA or PET-CT

000

- **Polymyalgia rheumatica** (*Lancet* 2013;381:63; *JAMA* 2016;315:2442)
  - seen in 50% of GCA Pts; 15% of Pts w/ PMR develop GCA
  - age ≥50 y; ESR >40 mm/h (and/or ↑ CRP); *bilateral pain & morning stiffness* (>30 min), involving 2 of 3 areas: neck or torso, shoulders or prox. arms, hips or prox. thighs; nighttime pain; ± subdeltoid bursitis on U/S; exclude other causes of sx (eg, RA); nl CK
- Rx: **steroids** (*do not await bx/path results to begin steroids, have at least 2 wk to bx*)
  - GCA: 40–60 mg/d w/ slow taper, ASA daily; consider IV pulse if vision threatened. Adding tocilizumab to steroid may be beneficial (*Lancet* 2016;387:1921); await phase III results.
  - PMR: 12.5–25 mg/d; if clinical improvement, initiate slow taper. If no improvement, ↑ dose. Consider MTX if at high risk for steroid side effects (*Ann Rheum Dis* 2015;74:1799).
- Follow clinical status & ESR/CRP (*Ann Rheum Dis* 2009;68:318); ~1/3 relapse over 2 y (*J Rheum* 2015;42:1213)

MEDIUM-VESSEL VASCULITIS

Polyarteritis nodosa ("classic" PAN) (*Arth Rheum* 2010;62:616)

- **Necrotizing nongranulomatous vasculitis of medium and small arteries** (w/ muscular media) w/o glomerulonephritis or capillary involvement (ie, DAH), not a/w ANCA
- Epidemiology: ♂ > ♀; average age of onset ~50 y; primary or **HBV-associated** (~10%)
- Clinical manifestations
  - constitutional sx (80%): wt loss, **fever**, fatigue
  - neuro (79%): **mononeuritis multiplex,** peripheral neuropathies, stroke
  - musculoskeletal (64%): **extremity pain,** myalgias, arthralgias, arthritis
  - renal (51%): **HTN,** hematuria, proteinuria, renal failure, *glomerulonephritis unusual*
  - GI (38%): **abd pain,** GIB/infarction, cholecystitis; GU (25%): ovarian or testicular pain
  - skin (50%): **livedo reticularis,** purpura, nodules, ulcers, Raynaud's
  - ophthalmic (9%): retinal vasculitis, retinal exudates, conjunctivitis, uveitis
  - cardiac (22%): coronary arteritis, cardiomyopathy, pericarditis
  - *if lung involvement, suspect other vasculitis*
- Dx studies: ↑ ESR/CRP, ⊖ ANCA; ✓ HBs Ag; ↓ C3/C4 if HBV-associated
  - **angiogram** (mesenteric or renal vessels) → **microaneurysms** & focal vessel narrowing
  - CTA may be adequate to make dx, but conventional angiogram is most sensitive
  - **biopsy** (sural nerve, skin or affected organ) → vasculitis of small and medium vessel arteries with fibrinoid necrosis *without granulomas*
- Treatment: **steroids** ± CYC (if severe or failure to induce remission); antivirals if a/w HBV

ANCA-ASSOCIATED SMALL-VESSEL VASCULITIS

Microvascular vasculitis (eg, capillaries, postcapillary venules, & arterioles)

Disease	Gran	Renal	Pulm	Asthma	ANCA Type[a]	ANCA ⊕
Granulomatosis with polyangiitis[b]	⊕	80%	90% (+ ENT)	—	anti-PR3 (c-ANCA)	90%
Microscopic polyangiitis	—	90%	50%	—	anti-MPO (p-ANCA)	70%
Eosinophilic granulomatosis with polyangiitis[b]	⊕	45%	70%	⊕	anti-MPO (p-ANCA)	50%

[a]Predominant ANCA type; either p- or c-ANCA can be seen in all three diseases (*NEJM* 2012;367:214).
[b]GPA is formerly Wegener's granulomatosis and EGPA is formerly Churg-Strauss.

Differential diagnosis of ANCA (*Lancet* 2006;368:404)

- **anti-PR3 (c-ANCA):** granulomatosis w/ polyangiitis, eosinophilic granulomatosis and polyangiitis, microscopic polyangiitis (rarely)
- **anti-MPO (p-ANCA):** microscopic polyangiitis, eosinophilic granulomatosis and polyangiitis, granulomatosis w/ polyangiitis, drug-induced vasculitis, nonvasculitic rheumatic diseases
- **Atypical ANCA patterns:** drug-induced vasculitis, nonvasculitic rheumatic diseases, ulcerative colitis, primary sclerosing cholangitis, endocarditis, cystic fibrosis

Granulomatosis with polyangiitis (GPA, formerly Wegener's granulomatosis)

- **Necrotizing granulomatous systemic vasculitis** frequently affecting nose, sinuses and/or upper respiratory tract in addition to kidneys, lungs, etc.
- Epidemiology: any age, but ↑ incidence in young and middle-aged adults; ♂ = ♀
- Clinical manifestations
  - **respiratory** (90%): *upper:* sinusitis, rhinitis, oral/nasal ulcers, saddle-nose deformity, otitis, hearing loss, subglottic stenosis; *lower:* pulmonary infiltrates, nodules, pulmonary hemorrhage, hemoptysis, pleurisy

renal (80%): **RPGN** (pauci-immune), RBC casts, dysmorphic RBCs, hematuria
ocular (50%): episcleritis, scleritis, uveitis, orbital granulomas → proptosis, corneal ulcer
neurologic: cranial and peripheral neuropathies, mononeuritis multiplex
skin (50%): palpable purpura, livedo reticularis
hematologic: ↑ incidence DVT/PE (20×) when disease active (Ann Intern Med 2005;142:620)
- Dx studies: **90%** ⊕ **ANCA** (80% PR3, 20% MPO), less Se in limited upper airway disease
CXR or CT → nodules, infiltrates, cavities; sinus CT → sinusitis ± bone erosions
↑ BUN & Cr, proteinuria, hematuria; sediment w/ RBC casts, dysmorphic RBCs
Biopsy → necrotizing granulomatous inflammation of arterioles, capillaries, veins
- Treatment: assess disease severity with BVAS/WG score (Arth Rheum 2001;44:912)
  Mild disease (no end-organ dysfxn; BVAS 0-3): **MTX** + **steroids** (Arth Rheum 2012;64:3472)
  Severe disease (end-organ damage incl. pulm hemorrhage, RPGN etc.; BVAS >3):
    Induction: [**RTX** 375 mg/m²/wk × 4 wk or **CYC** 2 mg/kg/d × 3–6 mo or pulse
    15 mg/kg q2–3wk] + **steroids** 1 g IV × 3 d → 1–2 mg/kg/d (NEJM 2005;352:351,
    2010;363:211, & 2013;369:417; Annals 2009;150:670; Ann Rheum Dis 2015;74:1178)
    If RPGN: ± plasma exchange to ? ↓ risk of ESRD (Am J Kidney Dis 2011;57:566)
    Maintenance: RTX q6mo superior to AZA or watchful waiting (Arth Rheum
    2012;64:3760; NEJM 2014;371:1771)
  Relapse: mild → steroids ± MTX or AZA; severe → reinduce w/ steroids + RTX or CYC
  ↑ ANCA w/o clinical evidence of flare should not prompt Δ Rx (Annals 2007;147:611)

Microscopic polyangiitis (MPA) (Rheum Dis Clin North Am 2010;36:545)
- Similar to GPA, but **w/o ENT/airway involvement & nongranulomatous**
- Epidemiology: ♂ > ♀; avg onset 50–60 y
- Clinical manifestations: similar to GPA *w/o upper respiratory involvement;*
  renal (80–100%): glomerulonephritis
  pulmonary (25–50%): pulmonary capillary alveolitis, pulmonary fibrosis
  constitutional and neuro sx similar to GPA; skin lesions (eg, palpable purpura) in 30–60%
- Dx studies: **70%** ⊕ **ANCA** (almost all anti-MPO)
  biopsy → necrotizing, **nongranulomatous** inflammation of small vessels, pauci-immune
  (minimal deposition of complement or Ig; contrast w/ HSP, cryoglobulinemia, etc.)
  urine sediment and CXR findings similar to those seen in GPA
- Treatment: as for GPA; ↓ relapse rate compared to GPA

Eosinophilic granulomatosis with polyangiitis (EGPA, formerly Churg-Strauss)
- Similar to GPA w/ more frequent **cardiac involvement, a/w asthma and eosinophilia**
- Epidemiology: rare; can present at any age (typically 30–40 y); a/w HLA-DRB4
- Clinical manifestations (Curr Rheumatol Rep 2011;13:489)
  initial sx: **asthma,** sinusitis, allergic rhinitis (new asthma in adult raises suspicion)
  eosinophilic infiltrative phase: transient **pulm infiltrates,** gastroenteritis, or esophagitis
  systemic small-vessel vasculitis: **neuropathy** (mononeuritis multiplex), renal
    (glomerulonephritis), skin (palpable purpura, petechial, nodules)
  cardiac: coronary arteritis, myocarditis, CHF, valvular insufficiency (Medicine 2009;88:236)
- Dx studies: 50% ⊕ ANCA (MPO > PR3), **eosinophilia** (5–10 k/μL, 80–100%),
  biopsy → microgranulomas, fibrinoid necrosis and thrombosis of small arteries and
  veins w/ eosinophilic infiltrates
- Treatment: high-dose **corticosteroids** + cyclophosphamide (if severe)

Renal-limited vasculitis
- Small vessel pauci-immune vasculitis causing RPGN w/o other organ involvement
- Dx studies: 80% ⊕ ANCA (MPO > PR3); biopsy w/ pauci-immune GN ± granulomas
- Treatment identical to that for GPA/MPA

IMMUNE COMPLEX (IC)–ASSOCIATED SMALL-VESSEL VASCULITIS

Henoch-Schönlein purpura (HSP)
- **IgA-mediated** vasculitis w/ predilection for **skin, GI tract** and **kidneys**
- Epidemiology: ♂ > ♀, children > adults, onset in winter > summer
- May develop after upper respiratory tract infection (esp. *Strep*) or drug exposure
- Clinical manifestations
  palpable purpura on extensor surfaces (lower extremity first) & buttocks
  polyarthralgias (nondeforming) involving hips, knees, & ankles
  colicky **abdominal pain** ± GIB or intussusception
  nephritis ranging from **microscopic hematuria** & proteinuria to ESRD
- Dx studies: **skin bx w/ immunofluorescence → leukocytoclastic vasculitis w/ IgA**
  and **C3** deposition in vessel wall; renal bx → mesangial IgA deposition
- Treatment: often self-limiting over 4 wk; steroids ± DMARDs for renal or severe disease

Connective tissue disease–associated vasculitis
- Small vessel vasculitis a/w **RA, SLE** or **Sjögren's syndrome**
- Clinical manifestations
  distal arteritis: digital ischemia, livedo reticularis, palpable purpura, cutaneous ulceration
  visceral arteritis: pericarditis and mesenteric ischemia
  peripheral neuropathy
- Dx studies: skin/sural nerve bx, angiography, EMG; ↓ C′ in SLE; ⊕ RF or anti-CCP in RA
- Treatment: steroids, cyclophosphamide, MTX (other DMARDs)

Cutaneous leukocytoclastic angiitis
- Most common type of vasculitis; heterogeneous group of clinical syndromes due to **IC deposition** in capillaries, venules and arterioles; includes **hypersensitivity vasculitis**
- Etiologies
  drugs: PCN, ASA, amphetamines, levamisole, thiazides, chemicals, immunizations
  infections: *Strep, Staph,* endocarditis, TB, hepatitis
  malignancy (paraneoplastic)
- Clinical manifestations: abrupt onset of **palpable purpura** and **transient arthralgias** after exposure to the offending agent; visceral involvement rare but can be severe
- Dx studies: ↑ ESR, ↓ complement levels, eosinophilia; ✓ U/A; **skin biopsy** → leukocytoclastic vasculitis *w/o IgA deposition* in skin (to distinguish from HSP); if etiology not clear, consider ANCA, cryoglobulins, hepatitis serologies, ANA, RF
- Treatment: withdrawal of offending agent ± rapid prednisone taper

Behçet's syndrome (Curr Rheum Opin 2010;12:429)
- **Systemic vasculitis** affecting all vessel sizes, a/w **oral and/or genital ulcers**
- Epidemiology: usually young adults (25–35 y); a/w HLA-B51 in areas of highest prevalence on the old Silk Road (Turkey, Middle East, and other Asian countries)
- Classification criteria (#1 + ≥2 others is 91% Se & 96% Sp; Lancet 1990;335:1078)
  1. recurrent **oral aphthous ulceration** (≥3× in 1 y, usually 1st manifestation)
  2. recurrent **genital ulceration** (labia in females, scrotum in males)
  3. **eye** lesions: uveitis, scleritis, retinal vasculitis, optic neuritis (may threaten vision)
  4. **skin** lesions: pustules, papules, folliculitis, erythema nodosum (scarring)
  5. ⊕ pathergy test (prick forearm w/ sterile needle → pustule) (not sensitive in Caucasians)
- Other clinical manifestations: most recur but are not chronic
  arthritis: mild, ± symmetric, nondestructive, involving knees and ankles
  neurologic: usually involvement of midbrain parenchyma; peripheral neuropathy rare
  vascular: superficial or deep vein thrombosis (25%); arterial stenosis, occlusion and aneurysm can also occur; low incidence of thromboembolism
- Dx studies: ↑ ESR/CRP; ulcer swab to r/o HSV; ulcer bx nonspecific; ophtho eval if sx
- Treatment (Rheumatology 2007;46:736; Ann Rheum Dis 2008;67:1656 & 2009;68:1528)
  mucocutaneous
    mild: **topical steroids, colchicine** (esp. for erythema nodosum), dapsone, apremilast (PDE-4 inhib) for oral ulcers and ? genital ulcers (NEJM 2015;372:1510),
    severe: oral steroids, steroid-sparing agents
  arthritis: NSAIDs, colchicine, steroids, steroid-sparing agents
  ocular: **topical and/or systemic steroids** ± steroid-sparing agents
  steroid-sparing: AZA, anti-TNF, CYC (large vessel and CNS ds), CsA, MTX, IFNα-2A,
  venous thrombosis: steroids and anticoagulation (careful if aneurysm present)

IgG4-RELATED DISEASE

Definition & etiology (NEJM 2012:366:539; Ann Rev Pathol 2014;9:315)
- Characterized by tumor-like inflammatory lesions that can affect nearly any organ
- Etiology unclear: ? autoimmune; unclear role of IgG4 Ab; Pt may have h/o atopy

Clinical manifestations (Lancet 2015;385:1460; Arth Rheum 2015;67:2466)
- Commonly pancreatitis, aortitis, cholangitis, sialadenitis, thyroiditis, orbital myositis ± pseudotumor, retroperitoneal fibrosis
- Multiple lesions may be present synchronously or metachronously

Diagnosis (Ann Rheum Dis 2015;74:1 & 14)
- **Biopsy** w/ specific histopathology & immunohistochemistry findings: lymphoplasmacytic infiltrate w/ significant IgG4+ plasma cell infiltrate, fibrosis, obliterative phlebitis
- ↑ serum IgG4 (Se 90%, Sp 60%); *not specific* seen in GPA, bronchiectasis (Ann Rheum Dis 2014;74:14)

Treatment (Arth Rheum 2015;67:1688)
- **Prednisone** vs. rituximab (Ann Rheum Dis 2015;74:1171)

CRYOGLOBULINEMIA

Definition & types (Lancet 2012;379:348; Oncology 2013;37:1098)
- **Proteins** due to chronic immune stimulation and/or lymphoproliferation that **precipitate on exposure to cold and redissolve on rewarming,** characterized by their composition
- **Cryoglobulins** = proteins that precipitate from *serum and plasma* when cooled
- Distinguish from *cryofibrinogenemia* = proteins (eg, fibrin, fibrinogen) that precipitate only from *plasma;* found in autoimmune dis, malignancies, infxns; unclear clinical significance

Types of Cryoglobulinemia			
Feature	**Type I (monoclonal)**	**Type II (mixed)**	**Type III (mixed)**
Frequency	10–15%	50–60%	25–30%
Cryoglobulin composition	*monoclonal* Ig (usually IgM or IgG)	*monoclonal* IgM w/ RF activity + *polyclonal* IgG	*polyclonal* IgG and IgM
Common etiologies	Plasma cell dyscrasias	Infection, malignancy, autoimmune syndromes	Autoimmune synd., infxn
Primary manifestations	**Hyperviscosity** ± thrombosis → ischemia	IC-mediated vasculitis, w/ multiorgan involvement. Can be asx.	

Etiologies
- Hematologic diseases
  - type I: multiple myeloma, MGUS, Waldenström's, chronic lymphocytic leukemia
  - type II: B-cell lymphomas, solid organ malignancies
- Infections (types II & III): viral (**HCV** [>80% RNA ⊕], HBV, HIV, HAV, EBV, CMV), bacterial (endocarditis, strep, etc.), fungal (coccidiomycosis, etc.), parasitic (malaria, amoebiasis)
- Autoimmune syndromes (type III > II): **Sjögren's syndrome,** SLE, RA, PAN
- Renal transplant recipients (Clin Nephrol 2008;69:239)
- Essential (idiopathic) in 10% of cases

Pathophysiology
- Type I: cryo precipitation in microcirculation → **hyperviscosity & vascular occlusion**
- Types II/III: defective/insufficient immune complex (IC) clearance → IC-mediated inflammation of blood vessels w/ complement activation → **vasculitis**

Clinical manifestations
- Most patients with circulating cryoglobulins are asx
- Type I: hyperviscosity (cold worsens sx) → H/A, visual disturbance, livedo, digital ischemia
- Type II/III: vasculitis (sx not affected by cold exposure)
  - "Meltzer's triad" (purpura, arthralgias, weakness) seen in 25–30% of Pts
  - General: **weakness,** low-grade fever
  - Dermatologic (54–80%): lower extremity **purpura,** livedo reticularis, leg ulcers
  - Joint (44–70%): symmetric, migratory **arthralgias** of small or medium joints
  - Renal (50%): **glomerulonephritis** (proteinuria, hematuria, ARF, HTN, edema)
  - Neurologic (17–60%): **peripheral neuropathy** (polyneuropathy > mononeuritis multiplex)
  - Hematologic: anemia, thrombocytopenia, ↑ risk of B-cell lymphoma
  - GI (5%): abdominal pain, hepatosplenomegaly, abnormal LFTs

Diagnostic studies
- ✓ Cryoglobulins; must keep blood *warmed to 37°C at all times* en route to lab; early cooling causes false ⊖ cryoglobulin, loss of RF and ↓↓ complement
- *Cryocrit* is quantification of cryoprotein, does not always correlate w/ disease activity
- False ↑ in WBC or plt on automated CBC, due to cryoprecipitation
- Type I: ✓ serum viscosity, symptomatic if ≥4.0 centipoise; complement levels normal
- Type II: ↓ **C4 levels,** variable C3 levels, ↑ ESR, ⊕ rheumatoid factor (RF)
  - ✓ **HCV, HBV, & HIV serologies** in all Pts w/ mixed cryoglobulinemia
  - Bx of affected tissue: hyaline thrombi; vasculitis w/ mixed inflammatory infiltrates of small vessels; leukocytoclastic vasculitis in purpuric lesions

Treatment (Blood 2012;119:5996; Medicine 2013;92:61)
- **Treat underlying disorder:**
  - Lymphoproliferative disease: chemotherapy and/or radiation
  - HCV: antivirals ± immunosuppression for severe disease (NEJM 2013;369:1035)
  - Connective tissue-related disease: DMARD/steroids ± rituximab
- Type I: Plasma exchange if hyperviscosity; steroids, alkylating agents, rituximab, chemo
- Type II: NSAIDs for control of mild symptoms for Pts w/ normal renal function.
  - Rituximab or cyclophosphamide for major organ involvement. For mixed cryo, plasmapheresis or plasma exchange only in severe, life-threatening disease.

AMYLOIDOSIS

Deposition of misfolded and insoluble fibrous proteins in normal organs and tissues

Classification of Amyloidosis			
Type	**Precursor**	**Causative diseases**	**Main organs affected**
AL (Primary) Most common ~2000 cases/y	Monoclonal Ig light chain	MM Light chain disease ($\lambda > \kappa$) MGUS, WM	**Renal, cardiac, GI, neuro,** cutaneous, hepatic, pulmonary
AA (Secondary)	Serum amyloid A (SAA)	Inflam: RA, IBD, FMF Chronic infxns: osteo, TB	**Renal, GI, hepatic,** neuro, cutaneous
Hereditary ↑ incid Afr Am	Mutant TTR, etc.	*Mutant proteins*	**Neurologic, cardiac**
Senile	Normal TTR	*Normal proteins;* 2° aging	**Cardiac,** aorta, GI
Aβ_2M	β_2-microglobulin	Dialysis-associated β_2m (normally renally excreted)	Musculoskeletal
Localized	β-amyloid protein Peptide hormones	Localized production and processing	Neurologic Endocrine

TTR, transthyretin (prealbumin). Adapted from *NEJM* 1997;337:898; 2003;349:583; 2007;356:2361.

Clinical Manifestations of Amyloidosis *(Lancet 2016;387:2641)*		
System	**Manifestations**	**Amyloid**
Renal	Proteinuria or nephrotic syndrome	AL, AA
Cardiac	CMP (either restrictive or dilated); orthostatic hypoTN ↓ QRS amplitude, conduction abnormalities, AF	AL, hereditary, senile
GI	Diarrhea, malabsorption, protein loss Ulceration, hemorrhage, obstruction Macroglossia → dysphonia and dysphagia	all systemic
Neurologic	Peripheral neuropathy with painful paresthesias Autonomic neuro → impotence, dysmotility, ↓ BP Carpal tunnel syndrome	hereditary, AL, organ-specific, Aβ_2M
Cutaneous	Waxy, nonpruritic papules; periorbital ecchymoses "Pinch purpura" = skin bleeds with minimal trauma	AL
Hepatic & splenic	Hepatomegaly, usually *without* dysfunction Splenomegaly, usually *without* leukopenia or anemia	all systemic
Endocrine	Deposition with rare hormonal insufficiency	organ-specific
Musculoskel	Arthralgias and arthritis (especially shoulder)	AL, Aβ_2M
Pulmonary	Airway obstruction; pleural effusions	AL, AA
Hematologic	Factor X deficiency	AL

Diagnostic studies
- Biopsy (abdominal SC fat pad, rectal or affected tissue) → apple-green birefringence on **Congo red stain;** fat pad bx Se 60–85%, Sp 90–100%
- If suspect AL → ✓ SIEP & UIEP (↑ Se vs. SPEP & UPEP) & free light chains, ± BM bx
- If suspect renal involvement ✓ U/A for proteinuria
- If suspect cardiac involvement ✓ ECG (↓ voltage, conduction abnl), TTE (biventricular thickening w/ *granular sparkling* appearance; ↑ wall w/o ↑ volt 75% Se, 95% Sp), MRI
- Genetic testing for hereditary forms

Treatment of Amyloidosis	
AL	Limited involvement: high-dose **melphalan** → auto **HSCT** *(NEJM 2007;357:1083)* Not HSCT candidate: [low-dose melphalan + dexamethasone] or [cyclophosphamide + bortezomib + dexamethasone] *(Blood 2015;126:612)* Relapsed: lenalidomide, thalidomide, or bortezomib *(Blood 2010;116:1990 & 2014;124:2498)*
AA	**Rx underlying disease.** Colchicine for FMF, esp. to prevent renal disease. Eprodisate promising for renal disease *(NEJM 2007;356:2349)* ? Biologics (anakinra, tocilizumab) for rheum associated disease *(Arth Rheum 2003;48:2019; Clin Exp Rheumatol 2015;33:46)*
ATTR	Liver Tx prevents further protein deposition *(Muscle Nerve 2013;47:157)* Small interfering RNA under study *(NEJM 2013;369:819; JACC 2015;66:2451)*

- Clearance of amyloid by Ab against serum amyloid P under study *(NEJM 2015;373:1106)*
- Cardiac involvement: diuretics; avoid dig, CCB, and vasodilators; ? ICD for 1° prevention
- Heart, kidney and liver Tx may be considered in those w/ advanced disease
- Median survival: 12–18 mos for AL (~6 if cardiac); 11 y for AA; variable for others

CHANGE IN MENTAL STATUS

Consciousness/Arousal (description of patient & timing is most helpful)
- Spectrum from awake/alert → drowsy → stupor → coma. Vague terms, thus most useful to simply describe response to increasing stimulation (eg, voice → noxious stimuli).
- **Coma:** lack of response to external stimuli. Degree formalized in Glasgow Coma Scale. Caused by focal lesions in upper brainstem (eg, reticular activating system, thalami) or diffuse dysfxn of cerebral hemispheres bilaterally. Mimics: locked-in synd., catatonia.
- Nb, quality of thought can be disturbed w/o affecting level of consciousness (eg, disorient.)
- **Delirium/acute confusional state:** altered attention & awareness, develops over hrs to days, often fluctuating, accompanied by cognitive Δs (eg, disorientation, memory loss, perceptual Δs); sometimes w/ sleep–wake dysregulation, autonomic Δs, emotionality
- **Dementia:** progressive cognitive impairment beyond baseline, develops over mos to yrs, often affecting memory, language, and executive function

Etiologies of Decreased Responsiveness

1° neurologic (usually with focal signs)	Systemic (esp. in elderly or prior CNS injury)
Vasc: ischemic stroke, ICH, ven. thromb	Cardiac: global ischemia, CHF, HTN enceph
Seizure: postictal, status, nonconvulsive	Pulmonary: ↓ P$_a$O$_2$, ↑ P$_a$CO$_2$
Infxn: meningitis, encephalitis, abscess	GI: liver failure, ↑ NH$_3$
Traumatic brain injury/concussion	Renal: uremia, dialysis, ↓ or ↑ Na
↑ intracranial pressure: mass, hydrocephalus, herniation	Endo: ↓ glc, DKA/HHNS, hypothyr., Addisonian
Transient global amnesia	ID: pneumonia, UTI, sepsis
Autoimmune/paraneoplastic encephalitis	Hypothermia & hyperthermia
Neurodeg: late-stage (eg, Alzheimer's); or rapidly progressive (eg, CJD) dementia	Intoxication or withdrawal: EtOH, sedatives, opiates, carbon monoxide, anticholinergic
	Psychiatric: catatonia

Initial evaluation
- **History** (witness & background *crucial*): tempo, premorbid sx (eg, focal neuro deficits, HA, infxn, pain, falls), medical conditions (eg, dementia, epilepsy, onc, cardiac, psych, infection/immune status), accompanied by head trauma, current meds (eg, sedatives, opioids, anticoag, anticonvulsants, immunosuppressants), drug/alcohol use
- **General exam:** VS, nuchal rigidity (may be present in meningitis or SAH, *do not test if possible trauma/cervical spine fx*), breathing pattern (eg, Cheyne-Stokes), ecchymoses, rash, signs of head trauma (eg, Battle's, raccoon eyes, hemotympanum, CSF rhinorrhea), asterixis, liver disease stigmata, embolic phenomena/endocarditis, signs of drug use
- **Neuro exam** (see below): perform off sedatives/paralytics if possible, look for deficits that suggest structural cause (eg, stroke, herniation syndrome), s/s of ↑ ICP (eg, HA, vomiting, papilledema, abducens nerve palsy, unilateral dilated pupil, ↑ BP/↓HR, fixed downgaze)

Neuro Exam in Patients with Decreased Responsiveness

Mental status	Arousal (behavioral response to ↑ intensity of stimulation, GCS)
Cranial nerves	Pupils: *pinpoint* → opiates, pontine lesion; *midposition & fixed* → midbrain lesion; *fixed & dilated* → severe anoxic enceph, hern., anti-cholin. Extraocular movements / vestibulo-ocular reflex tests: oculocephalic maneuver ("doll's eyes"): nl = eyes move opposite head movement (*do not test if possible cervical spine trauma*) vestibular (cold) caloric stimulation: in coma, nl = eyes move slowly to lavaged ear, then quickly away Corneal reflex, facial grimace to nasal tickle Gag & cough reflexes (with ET tube manipulation if necessary)
Motor	Tone, spont movements, flexor/extensor posturing of arms/legs, strength
Sensory	Response to painful stimuli: purposeful vs. reflexive/posturing
Reflexes	Deep tendon reflexes, Babinski, "triple" flexion (ankle, knee, & hip flexion to noxious stimulation → not suggestive of intact cortical function)

Glasgow Coma Scale (sum points from each of 3 categories to calculate score)

Eye opening	Best verbal response	Best motor response	Points
		Follows commands	6
	Oriented	Localizes pain	5
Spontaneous	Confused	Withdraws from pain	4
To voice	Inappropriate words	Flexor posturing	3
To painful stimuli	Unintelligible sounds	Extensor posturing	2
None	None (intubated = 1T)	None	1

Initial treatment

- Immobilization of C-spine if concern for cervical trauma
- Thiamine 100 mg IV → dextrose 50 g IVP (order to prevent exacerbation of Wernicke's)
- If opiates suspected: naloxone 0.01 mg/kg; supportive care important in nearly all tox cases
- If concern for ↑ ICP ± herniation: ↑ head of bed; osmotherapy w/ mannitol or hypertonic saline; ↑ ventilation; dexamethasone for tumor edema; c/s neurosurgery (? decompress)

Diagnostic studies (Continuum 2011;17:967)

- All patients: check CBC, electrolytes, BUN/Cr, tox screen, tox screen, U/A
- *Based on clinical suspicion:*
  labs: NH_3, TSH, am cortisol, B_{12}, ABG, ESR, ANA, TPO, thyroglobulin, BCx
  imaging: head CT, then MRI; radiographs to r/o C-spine fracture
  lumbar puncture to r/o meningitis, SAH, or noninfectious inflammation (eg, autoimmune)
  EEG to evaluate for nonconvulsive seizures, toxic/metabolic encephalopathy

Further treatment of delirium (Annals 2011;154:746)

- Treat underlying acute illness, eliminate precipitating factors, & provide supportive care
- Address sensory & cognitive impairments (frequent reorientation, etc.)
- Decrease/prevent infection/restraints if possible, remove lines/catheters if unnecessary
- Promote good sleep: reduce noise & nighttime interventions; sedative med if necessary
- Meds: consider antipsychotics; avoid benzos except for alcohol withdrawal or seizures

---

ANOXIC BRAIN INJURY (at risk if ≥5 min cerebral hypoxia)

Initial evaluation (Circulation 2010:S768)

- Neuro exam: arousal/verbal, eyes & other cranial nerves, motor response to pain
- Imaging: CT usually not informative w/in first day after arrest, but should be done prior to initiating hypothermia if patient found down or has had head trauma

Temperature management (Circulation 2015;132:2448)

- Indications: comatose (eg, no meaningful response to verbal stimuli) <6 h following cardiac arrest (not isolated resp. arrest). Fully studied only in VT/VF, but consider after asystole or PEA arrest or 6–12 h after cardiac arrest.
- Exclusion: preg, CV instability despite pressors/assist devices, other cause of coma, persistent ↓ O_2
- Relative contraindications: major head trauma, coagulopathy/bleeding, major surgery <14 d, systemic infection/sepsis
- Target temp: 32–36°C × ≥24 h. Initial studies showing benefit targeted 32–34°C, but subsequent study showed ≈ outcomes for 36°C vs. 33°C (NEJM 2013;369:2197). Some still target 32–34°C and reserve 36°C for Pts w/ contraindic to more aggressive cooling.
- Method: can use cold saline infusions; ice packs to head, neck & torso; cooling blankets; cooling vest or endovascular catheter if available. Goal to achieve target temp <6 h (but no benefit to prehosp cooling; JAMA 2014;311:45). Start rewarming 24 h after cooling is initiated (rewarm ≤0.5°C per h).
- Complications
  dysrhythmias (brady most common): if signif or hemodynamic instability, rewarm
  coagulopathy (can receive lytics, GP IIb/IIIa inhibitors, etc.); ✓ PT and PTT.
  infection: ✓ surveillance blood cultures during cooling
  hyperglycemia during cooling, hypoglycemia w/ rewarming; stop insulin if glc <200 mg/dL
  hypokalemia during cooling, hyperkalemia w/ rewarming; keep K 4–5 mEq/L

Ongoing evaluation

- Neuro exam: daily focus on coma exam. No exam finding is reliable <24 h or on sedation. Pt needs to be off sedation for an adequate time to evaluate (depends on doses used, duration of Rx, metabolic processes in the individual Pt).
- Labs: daily CBC, PT/PTT, electrolytes. Serum neuron-specific enolase (NSE) on days 1–3
- Imaging: noncontrast CT 24 h after arrest; if unrevealing, consider MRI around days 3–5
- EEG: consider in all to exclude seizures; greatest risk during rewarming
- Somatosensory evoked potentials (SSEP): helpful for prediction of poor outcome if cortical responses are absent bilaterally; perform 48 h after arrest (72 h if cooled)

Prognosis (Nat Rev Neuro 2014;10:190)

- For inPt arrest, ~20% survive, ~70% of Pts who survive have good long-term prognosis
- Prior to cooling era, uniformly poor prognosis could be predicted at 72 h only in Pts who have absent pupillary and corneal reflexes, and no motor response to pain; or with absent SSEPs at 48 h. With cooling, it is less clear if the prior measures are as reliable.
- Otherwise, prognosis requires multifactorial approach considering exam, age, comorbid diseases, ancillary data (NSE, EEG, SSEP; imaging is less reliable for poor outcome)
- When in doubt, err on giving more time (esp. if younger or induced hypothermia)

SEIZURES

Definitions (*Epilepsia* 2014;55:475)
- **Seizure:** transient neurologic symptoms due to excessive synchronous neuronal activity; may be *provoked* by a reversible factor lowering the seizure threshold, or *unprovoked*
- **Epilepsy:** ≥2 unprovoked seizures occurring >24 h apart *or* 1 unprovoked seizure w/ ≥60% probability of further seizures over the next 10 yr (see below for prognostication)
- **Generalized seizures** (involves brain diffusely)
    Tonic-clonic (grand mal): tonic phase (10–20 sec) with contraction of muscles (causing expiratory moan, cyanosis, pooling of secretions, tongue biting) → clonic phase (~30 sec) with intermittent relaxing and tensing of muscles
    Absence (petit mal): transient lapse of consciousness w/o loss of postural tone, usu pedi
    Myoclonic (infantile spasms & juvenile myoclonic epilepsy): sudden, brief contraction
- **Focal seizures** (involves discrete brain area, implies a structural lesion)
    w/o impaired consciousness: focal motor/sensory sx (formerly "simple partial seizure") or focal sensory/psychic symptoms (eg, aura)
    w/ impaired consciousness: dyscognitive features (formerly "complex partial seizure") evolving to bilateral, convulsive seizure (formerly "secondarily generalized seizure")
- **Status epilepticus:** continuous convulsive seizure ≥5 min or >2 seizures w/o resolution of postictal encephalopathy; *life-threatening*
- **Nonconvulsive status epilepticus:** alteration of awareness (ranging from confusion to coma) w/o motor manifestations of seizure; dx with EEG.

Differential diagnosis
- **Syncope** (*Lancet Neurol* 2006;5:171)

Feature	Seizure	Syncope
Aura	Unusual behavior/automatisms	Diaphoresis, nausea, tunnel vision
Convulsions	Variable duration	Usually <10 sec
Postictal state	Yes; can be ≥30 min	None or short
Other clues	Tongue biting, incontinence	Skin pallor, clamminess

- **Nonepileptic seizure** (aka "psychogenic"): may see side-to-side head turning, asymmetric large-amplitude limb movements, diffuse shaking w/o LOC, crying/talking during event
- **Other:** metabolic disorders (eg, alcoholic blackouts, hypoglycemia), migraine, TIA, transient global amnesia, narcolepsy (cataplexy), nonepileptic myoclonus, tics, asterixis

Etiologies of seizures (vary strongly by age)
- **Without focal lesion:** genetic predisposition to seizures or epilepsy syndrome; alcohol withdrawal, illicit drugs;
    meds (eg, β-lactams, bupropion, tramadol, MNZ, meperidine, CsA, antidepressants); electrolyte (hyponatremia) & other metabolic (eg, uremia, liver failure, hypoglycemia); autoimmune encephalitis, idiopathic (~60%)
- **With focal lesion:** tumor, trauma, stroke, subdural hematomas, posterior reversible encephalopathy syndrome, mesial temporal sclerosis, focal cortical dysplasia

Clinical manifestations
- **Aura** (sec to mins): premonition with paresthesias, focal motor contractions, abnormal smells/tastes, fear, depersonalization, déjà vu, autonomic changes, automatisms
- **Ictal period** (sec to mins): tonic and/or clonic movements of head, eyes, trunk or extrem.
- **Postictal period** (mins to h): slowly resolving period of confusion, disorientation, and lethargy. May be accompanied by focal neurologic deficits (Todd's paralysis).

Clinical evaluation
- *History key in differentiating seizure from other causes of transient loss of consciousness.* Must talk to witnesses. Ask about prodrome, unusual behavior before spell, type & pattern of abnl movements incl. head turning & eye deviation (gaze preference usually *away* from seizure focus), loss of responsiveness
- Recent events: illnesses/fevers, head trauma, sleep deprivation
- PMH: prior seizures or ⊕ FHx, prior meningitis/encephalitis, prior stroke or head trauma
- Medications (new or noncompliance), alcohol and illicit drug use
- General physical exam should include the skin, looking for neuroectodermal disorders (eg, neurofibromatosis, tuberous sclerosis) that are a/w seizures
- Neurologic exam should look for focal abnormalities → underlying structural abnormality

Diagnostic studies (*Neurology* 2007;69:1996)
- Lab: full lytes, BUN, Cr, glc, LFTs, tox screen, med levels (if on valproic acid, phenytoin; consider for other AEDs but may take days; levetiracetam level rarely useful unless? noncompliance)

- Routine EEG (~30 min): useful in workup of 1st-time unprovoked seizure, as may determine risk of seizure recurrence. Caveat: interictal EEG nl in 50% of Pts w/ epilepsy, and interictal epileptiform activity (spikes or sharp waves) may be seen in up to 2% of nl population; sleep deprivation and repeated studies ↑ dx yield of EEG.
- Long-term EEG monitoring (hrs to days): useful for differentiating epileptic from non-epileptic spells; video monitoring may help w/ nonepileptic seizures
- MRI to r/o structural abnormalities; ↑ Se w/ fine coronal imaging of frontal & temporal lobes
- LP (if no space-occupying lesion on imaging): if suspect meningitis (eg, fever, ↑ WBC, nuchal rigidity) or encephalitis and in all HIV ⊕ Pts

Treatment (Neurology 2015;84:1705; Lancet 2015;385:884)
- Treat any underlying precipitants, including CNS infections, intoxication, withdrawal, etc.
- Antiepileptic drug (AED) Rx usually reserved for Pts w/ ≥2 unprovoked seizures, single seizure w/ high risk of recurrence (see below), or underlying structural abnormality. Provoked seizures generally treated by addressing underlying cause; consider AED if status epilepticus on presentation, focal neuro exam, postictal Todd's paralysis.
- After 1st unprovoked sz, weigh risks of recurrence vs AED. ↑ risk of recurrence if abnl EEG, MRI, or nocturnal sz. If EEG & MRI nl → 65% sz-free at 5 y (Lancet Neurol 2006;5:317)
- Immediate treatment w/ AED after 1st unprovoked seizure ↓ risk of recurrence over 2 y, but does not Δ long-term prognosis
- If AED Rx indicated, choice dependent on type of seizure, side effects, cost, mechanism of elimination (if hepatic or renal insufficiency), teratogenesis and drug interactions
- Introduce gradually, monitor carefully
- May consider withdrawal if seizure-free (typically for at least 1 y) and normal EEG
- Individual state laws mandate seizure-free duration before being allowed to drive

Antiepileptic Drugs and Side Effects			
Medication	**Avg daily dose**	**Common side effects**	
		Systemic	*Neurologic (all: sedation)*
Carbamazepine	400–1600 mg	Aplastic anemia, ↓ WBC, rash, hepatotoxicity, ↓ Na	Diplopia, confusion, ataxia
Ethosuximide	500–1500 mg	Rash, BM suppression	Behavioral Δs
Gabapentin	900–3600 mg	GI upset, wt gain	Nystagmus, ataxia
Lacosamide	200–400 mg	Prolonged PR interval	Dizziness, diplopia
Lamotrigine	100–300 mg	Rash (Stevens-Johnson)	Tremor, HA, blurred vision, insomnia
Levetiracetam	1000–3000 mg	GI upset (rare)	Emotional lability
Oxcarbazepine	600–2400 mg	Hyponatremia, rash	Diplopia, dizziness
Phenobarbital	50–200 mg	Rash	Cognitive slowing
Phenytoin	200–400 mg	Gum hyperplasia	Dizziness, ataxia
Topiramate	100–400 mg	↓ wt, hypohidrosis, kidney stones, glaucoma, met acid	Cognitive slowing
Valproic acid	500–2500 mg	Hepatotox, ↑ NH₃, ↑ wt, ↓ hair	Tremor
Zonisamide	200–600 mg	↓ wt, hypohidrosis, nephrolith	Cog slowing, fatigue

(NEJM 2008;359:166; Lancet Neurol 2011;10:446)

Status epilepticus (Neurocrit Care 2012;17:3)
- ABCs: vital signs, oral airway or endotracheal intubation. Place Pt in semiprone position to ↓ risk of aspiration. Obtain IV access. Give thiamine, dextrose, IV normal saline.
- STAT glc, metabolic panel, CBC, tox screen, lactate, AED levels, consider head CT, LP
- Start standing AED after loading dose

Treatment of Status Epilepticus			
Time (min)	**Antiepileptic**	**Dosing regimen**	**Typical adult dose**
<5	**Lorazepam** or **Midazolam** or **Diazepam***	0.1 mg/kg IV 0.2 mg/kg IM 0.2 mg/kg PR	Successive 2–4 mg IV pushes Up to 10 mg IM
<10	**Phenytoin** or **Fosphenytoin** or **Valproate** or **Levetiracetam**	20 mg/kg 20 mg PE/kg 20–30 mg/kg 1000 mg	1.0–1.5 g IV over 20 min 1.0–1.5 g PE IV over 5–10 min 1.0–1.5 g IV over 5–10 min IV over 10–15 min
	Subsequent steps mandate intubation, EEG monitoring and ICU admission		
<30–60	General anesthesia with continuous midazolam, pentobarbital, or propofol		

PE, phenytoin equivalents. *Consider PR diazepam if no IV access and IM midazolam is contraindicated.

ALCOHOL WITHDRAWAL

Pathophysiology
- Alcohol is a CNS depressant
- Chronic use → insensitivity to inhibitory neurotransmitter γ-aminobutyric acid (GABA)
- Abrupt alcohol cessation → CNS overactivity

Clinical manifestations
- Minor withdrawal sx (6–48 h after last drink): mild anxiety, tremulousness, HA
- **Withdrawal seizures:** typically w/in 48 h after last drink; if unRx'd, 1/3 → delirium tremens
- **Alcoholic hallucinosis:** isolated hallucinations (typically visual) 12–48 h after last drink
- **Delirium tremens (DT):** disorientation, agitation, hallucinations, ↑ HR & BP, fever, diaphoresis; begins 48–96 h after last drink, lasts 5–7 d
- Consider other dx: CNS infxn or bleed, sz, drug O/D, coingestions, acute liver failure, GIB

Clinical Institute Withdrawal Assessment scale for alcohol (CIWA-Ar)
- Assign points for each of the 10 criteria; each criteria is scored 0–7, except orientation, which is scored 0–4; add points to calculate score

CIWA-Ar Scale					
Points	**Anxiety**	**Agitation**	**Tremor**	**HA**	**Orientation**
0	None	None	None	None	Oriented
1	Somewhat		Not visible, but felt at fingertips	Very mild	Cannot do serial additions
2				Mild	Disorient. by ≤2 d
3				Moderate	Disorient. by >2 d
4	Guarded	Restless	Moderate w/ hands extended	Mod severe	Disoriented to person or place
5				Severe	n/a
6				Very severe	n/a
7	Panic	Pacing or thrashing	Severe	Extremely severe	n/a
Points	**N/V**	**Sweats**	**Auditory halluc.**	**Visual halluc.**	**Tactile disturb**
0	None	None	None	None	None
1		Moist palms	Very mild	Very mild photosens.	Very mild paresthesias
2			Mild	Mild photosens.	Mild paresth.
3			Moderate	Mod photosens.	Mod paresth.
4	Intermit. w/ dry heaves	Beads	Mod severe	Mod severe visual halluc.	Mod severe hallucinations
5			Severe	Severe	Severe
6			Very severe	Very severe	Very severe
7	Constant	Drenching	Cont.	Continuous	Continuous
SCORE: <8 none to minimal withdrawal; 8–15 mild; 16–20 moderate; >20 severe					

Treatment (NEJM 2003;348:1786)
- **Benzodiazepines (BDZ)**
  Drug: diazepam (long-acting w/ active metab; ↓ risk of recurrent withdrawal), lorazepam (short half-life), chlordiazepoxide, oxazepam (no active metab; good if cirrhosis)
  Route: start IV, transition to PO
  Dosing: typically start w/ diazepam 10–15 mg IV q10–15min (or lorazepam 2–4 mg IV q15–20min) until appropriate sedation achieved, then titrate to CIWA-Ar scale, evaluating q1h until score <8 × 8 h, then q4h × 72 h, then q4h (if stable, then q4h) (JAMA 1994;272:519)
- If refractory to BDZ prn → BDZ gtt, phenobarb, dexmedetomidine, or propofol (& intubation)
- *Avoid* βB (mask sx)
- Mechanical restraints as needed until chemical sedation achieved
- Volume resuscitation as needed; thiamine *then* glc to prevent *Wernicke's* encephalopathy (ataxia, ophthalmoplegia, short-term memory loss); replete K, Mg, PO_4
- Prophylaxis: if min sx or asx (ie, CIWA score <8) but prolonged heavy EtOH consumption or h/o withdrawal seizures or DTs → chlordiazepoxide 25–100 mg (based on severity of EtOH use) q6h × 24 h, then 25–50 mg q6h × 2 d

STROKE

ISCHEMIC STROKE

Etiologies
- Embolic (~75%): artery → artery, cardioembolic, paradoxical, cryptogenic (AF found in ~12%)
- Thrombotic (~25%): large vessel (atherosclerosis) vs. small vessel ("lacunar," lipohyalinosis of small arteries, often related to HTN, hyperlipidemia, & DM)
- Other: dissection, vasculitis, vasospasm, prothrombotic states, hypoperfusion, genetic

Clinical Manifestations
- Timing: embolic → sudden onset; thrombotic → stuttering course

Stroke syndromes by vascular territory	
Artery	**Deficits**
ICA → Ophth	Amaurosis fugax (transient monocular blindness)
ACA	Hemiplegia (leg > arm), abulia, urinary incontinence, primitive reflexes
MCA	Hemiplegia (face & arm > leg); hemianesthesia; homonymous hemianopia Aphasia if dom. hemisphere: sup. div. → expressive; inf. div → receptive Apraxia & neglect if nondom. hemisphere
PCA	Macular-sparing homonymous hemianopia; alexia w/o agraphia Thalamic syndromes with contralateral hemisensory disturbance
Vertebral, PICA	Wallenberg syndrome = numbness of ipsilateral face and contralateral limbs, diplopia, dysarthria, ipsilateral Horner's, hiccups
Basilar	Pupillary Δs (midbrain=dilated, pons=pinpoint), long tract signs (quadriplegia, sensory loss), CN abnl, cerebellar dysfxn. Top of basilar → "locked in" synd.
Cerebellar	Vertigo, N/V, diplopia, dysarthria, nystagmus, ipsilateral limb ataxia
Lacunar (arterioles)	5 major syndromes: pure hemiplegia, pure hemianesthesia, ataxic hemiparesis, dysarthria + clumsy hand, mixed sensorimotor

Transient ischemic attack (TIA)
- Sudden deficit due to cerebral ischemia; **no stroke on imaging**; sx resolve <24 h (most <1 h)
- Ddx: seizure, migraine, hypoglycemia, amyloid spells, TGA, anxiety
- Risk of subsequent stroke ~2% by 1 wk (NEJM 2016;374;1533). Can stratify based on **ABCD²**: **A**ge ≥60 y (+1); **B**P ≥140/90 (+1); **C**lin features: unilat. weak. (+2), speech impair. w/o weakness (+1); **D**uration ≥60 (+2) or 10–59 min (+1); **D**M (+1)

Physical exam
- General: murmurs, carotid & subclavian bruits, peripheral emboli, endocarditis sequelae
- Neurologic exam, NIH stroke scale (http://www.ninds.nih.gov/doctors/NIH_Stroke_Scale.pdf)

Acute workup
- Electrolytes, Cr (relevant for contrast); glc, CBC, coags (see exclusion criteria for lysis)
- Cardiac biomarkers, 12-lead ECG, tox screen
- **STAT CT** to r/o ICH prior to lysis (Se ≈ MRI, faster, more widely available)
  early signs: hyperdense artery, loss of gray-white differentiation, edema, insular ribbon
  CT can be nl in 1st hrs after sx onset, not Se for small strokes & brainstem strokes
  obtain CT-angio head & neck if endovascular intervention indicated

Acute treatment of ischemic stroke (JAMA 2015;313:1451 & 314:1832)
- **Thrombolysis (IV):** tPA 0.9 mg/kg (max 90 mg), w/ 10% as bolus over 1 min, rest over 1 h consider if onset w/in 4.5 h, ∅ Ⓧ contraindic. (incl. current/prior ICH; head trauma or stroke w/in 3 mo; intracranial neoplasm, AVM or aneurysm; recent intracranial/intraspinal surgery; active internal bleeding; noncompressible arterial puncture; ↑ BP; multilobar infarct; plt <100k, INR >1.7, on Xa inhib, PTT >40, glc <50)
  - 0–3 h: 12% absolute ↑ in good neuro outcome (min/no disability), 5.8% absolute ↑ in ICH, trend toward 4% absolute ↓ mortality
  - 3–4.5 h: 7.4% absolute ↑ in good neuro outcome, 1.8% absolute ↑ in ICH, ∅ mortality benefit (nb, trial excluded patients with previous strokes + DM)
  - 0.6 mg/kg (tested 1° in Asians): ? slightly ↓ efficacy but ½ ICH rate (NEJM 2016;374:2313)
- BP: lower to <185/110 to consider lysis; if lyse keep <180/105 × 24 h (consider labetalol or nicardipine), o/w permissive HTN unless >220/120 or sx; if sx HoTN consider vasopressors
- Initiate ASA w/in 24–48 h; avoid anticoagulation w/in 24 h of lysis; see below for long-term Rx
- Cerebral edema → herniation: often occurs 1–5 d post large MCA or cerebellar strokes, ↑ risk in young. Temporize: elevate HOB >30°; mannitol ± 23% NaCl. Hemicraniectomy ↓ mortality (Lancet Neurol 2007;6:215). Neurosurgery consult in select MCA and all large cerebellar strokes.
- **Endovascular thrombectomy** (JACC Intv 2016;9:307): if anterior circulation prox cutoff (mostly MCA) and w/in ~6 h of sx onset, addition of thrombectomy to IV tPA ↑ odds of fxnal independence by 71%, w/ no Δ in ICH or mortality (NEJM 2015;372:11, 1009, 1019, 2285 & 2296; Lancet 2016;387:1723)

Workup to assess for etiology/modifiable risk factors

- Cardiac: Holter to assess for AF (found in ~12%; NEJM 2014;370:2467 & 2478;374:2065); echo to r/o thrombus/vegetation, w/ bubble study to r/o PFO/atrial septal aneurysm if suspect embolic
- Vessel imaging: carotid U/S and Doppler (if no vessel imaging obtained in acute eval)
- Labs: lipids, HbA1c, TSH, homocysteine, Lp(a), hypercoag w/u (if <65 y or cryptogenic stroke; ideally drawn before starting anticoag); ESR/CRP; blood cx if s/s systemic infection
- **MRI** helpful if dx of stroke unclear (esp. post circ) or to define stroke subtype, age, exact size
  DWI bright/ADC dark = earliest finding in acute ischemia (~w/in mins, up to days)
  T2-FLAIR: hyperintense w/in hrs, persists for wks; PWI differentiates irreversibly infarcted core vs. viable penumbra; T1 fat-sat (neck vessels) if suspicious for dissection

Secondary stroke prevention (NEJM 2012;366:1914)

- Antiplatelet therapy: different agents likely have similar efficacy
  ASA ↓ death & repeat stroke; equal to warfarin in nonembolic stroke (NEJM 2001;345:1444)
  clopidogrel: marginally superior to ASA, slightly ↑ ICH (Lancet 1996;348:1329)
  ticagrelor: trend toward 13% ↓ ischemic stroke vs. ASA (NEJM 2016;375:35)
  clopidogrel + ASA (vs.ASA alone): × 90 d in minor strokes/TIA → 32% ↓ risk of stroke, no Δ ICH (NEJM 2013;369:11); extended Rx not more effective & ↑ ICH (Lancet 2004;364:331)
- **Anticoagulation (AC):** consider only if: AF (qv; cardiac/paradoxical emboli (except bacterial endocarditis); long segment extra-dural dissections; hypercoag state; bridge to CEA in sx carotid stenosis w/ongoing TIAs.
  Hold off on AC in large strokes for ~2–4 wk given risk of hemorrhagic conversion.
- Long-term SBP target 120–139 mmHg (JAMA 2011;306:2137)
- Statin: ↓ recurrent stroke w/ atorvastatin 80 mg, LDL goal <70 (NEJM 2006;355:549)
- Fluoxetine: ? improved motor recovery after 3 mo (Lancet Neurol 2011;10:123)
- Pioglitazone: 24% ↓ risk of stroke in Pts w/ stroke/TIA + insulin resist. (NEJM 2016;374:1321)
- **Carotid revascularization** (NEJM 2013;369:1143)
  CEA (if surgical morbidity & mortality ≤6%) indicated for:
    sx stenosis 70–99% (benefit ↑ for males, >75 y, ≤2 wk from stroke) → 65% ↓ RR of repeat stroke, slight benefit for 50–69% stenosis (NEJM 1991;325:445; Lancet 2004;363:915)
    asx stenosis 70–90%, <79 y: 50% ↓ RR of repeat stroke (Lancet 2004;363:1491 & 2010;376:1074)
  stenting: c/w CEA, periprocedural risk of stroke ↑ (esp. in elderly) & MI ↓ (but many asx), subsequent rates of stroke similar (NEJM 2016;374:1011 & 1021; Lancet 2016;387:1305)

Patent foramen ovale (PFO; in ~27% of population) (NEJM 2005;353:2361)

- ↑ stroke risk: ≥4 mm separation, R→L shunting at rest, ↑ septal mobility, atrial septal aneurysm
- If PFO & stroke/TIA: no benefit of warfarin over ASA (Circ 2002;105:2625), but consider if at high risk for or has DVT/PE. No sig benefit shown for PFO closure so far, albeit studies small & w/ favorable trends (NEJM 2012;366:991; 2013:1083 & 1092).

INTRACRANIAL HEMORRHAGE (ICH)

Classification by location

- Hemorrhagic strokes: intraparenchymal hemorrhage (IPH) & subarachnoid hemorrhage (SAH)
- Other ICH: epidural hematoma (EDH) & subdural hematoma (SDH)

Etiologies

- AVM, aneurysm, cerebral venous sinus thrombosis → IPH or SAH
- HTN (basal ganglia, cerebellum, brainstem), cerebral amyloid (lobar), tumor (esp. w/ melanoma, renal cell CA, chorio-CA, thyroid CA) → IPH
- Trauma → all locations (nb, IPH or SAH caused by trauma technically not a stroke)

Clinical manifestations (Lancet Neurol 2005;4:662; BMJ 2010;341:c5204)

- ↓ consciousness, N/V, HA, progressive focal neurologic deficits
- SAH: thunderclap HA, onset w/ exertion; nuchal pain/rigidity; LOC. EDH: initial lucid interval.

Workup (Acad Emerg Med 2016:doi: 10.1111/acem.12984)

- STAT CT brain, angio (CT-A or conventional) if suspicious for vascular source
- ? LP for xanthochromia if no evid of ICH on CT (although ⊖ LR 0.01) & suspicious for SAH
- Coags (PT, PTT, INR)

Management

- Reverse coagulopathies (qv), goal INR <1.4. Plt goal >100k. No benefit to plt transfusion if on antiplt Rx (Lancet 2016;387:2605), but ? consider if expanding ICH; DDAVP if uremic.
- Strict BP control w/ art line, use nicardipine or labetalol gtt. SBP goal ~160 (NEJM 2013;368:2355 & ATACH-2, NEJM 2016:doi: 10.1056/NEJMoa1603460).
- SAH: endovasc coiling vs. surg clipping (depends on location, comorbid.; Lancet 2015;385:691) of aneurysm/AVM; nimodipine to ↓ risk of vasospasm (monitor w/ TCDs), seizure Ppx
- Surg evac: EDH; SDH if >1 cm or rapid ↑; IPH: no obvious benefit (Lancet 2013;382:397)
- Venous sinus thrombosis: start anticoagulation, manage ↑ ICP and seizures as needed

Feature	Upper motor neuron	Lower motor neuron	Neuromuscular junction	Myopathy
Distribution of weakness	UE Ext, LE Flex, hip abductors	Distal, segmental	Ocular, bulbar, proximal limb	Proximal, symmetric
Atrophy	None	Severe	None	Mild
Fasciculations	None	Common	None	None
Tone	↑	↓	Normal	Normal or ↓
Reflexes (DTRs)	↑	↓	Normal	Normal or ↓
Babinski	Present	Absent	Absent	Absent

PERIPHERAL NEUROPATHIES

Etiologies based on presentation
- **Mononeuropathy** (1 nerve): if acute → trauma; if chronic → entrapment, compression, DM, Lyme. Commonly seen: median n. (carpal tunnel synd.); ulnar n. (at elbow or wrist); common peroneal n. (at knee w/ habitual leg crossing); lat femoral cutan. n. (at inguinal lig).
- **Mononeuropathy multiplex** (axonal loss of multiple, separate, noncontig. nerves): vasculitic synd. (eg, PAN, Churg–Strauss, Wegener's, cryo, SLE, RA, Sjögren's), DM, Lyme, leprosy, HIV, hereditary neuropathy w/ pressure palsies; sarcoid, lymphoma, leukemia
- **Polyneuropathy** (multiple symmetric nerves, generally length dependent). 50% idiopathic.
  W/ autonomic features: DM, EtOH, paraneoplastic, B₁₂ def, amyloid, chemo, 1° dysauto.
  Painful (small fiber neuropathies): DM, EtOH, amyloid, chemo, heavy metals, porphyria
  Demyelinating. Acute inflam demyelinating polyneuropathy (AIDP) = Guillain-Barré
    Subacute: meds (taxanes), paraneoplastic
    Chronic: idiopathic, DM, CIDP, hypothyroidism, toxins, paraproteinemia, hereditary
  Axonal. Acute: acute motor axonal neuropathy (AMAN), porphyria, vasculitis, uremia
    Subacute: DM, meds (cisplatin, paclitaxel, vincristine, INH, ddI), EtOH, sepsis, paraneo.
    Chronic: DM, uremia, lead, arsenic, HIV, paraproteinemia, B₁₂ defic

Clinical manifestations
- Weakness, fasciculations, numbness, dysesthesias (burning/tingling), allodynia
- ± Autonomic dysfxn (orthostasis, bowel/bladder retention/incontinence, impotence)
- Depressed or absent DTRs (may be normal in small fiber neuropathy)

Diagnostic studies
- Distal symmetric polyneuropathy: CBC, lytes, BUN/Cr, HbA₁C, B₁₂, TSH, ESR, SPEP + IF
- EMG & NCS (often no change in 1ˢᵗ 10–14 d or in small fiber neuropathy)
- Based on H&P: LFTs, ANA, anti-Ro/La, HIV, Cu, Lyme titers, RPR, UA, UPEP+IF, ACE, ANCA, genetic testing, heavy metal screen, LP (AIDP, CIDP), cryo, paraneoplastic panel
- Autonomic testing/skin bx (small fiber), nerve bx (mononeuropathy multiplex)
- MRI if possible radiculopathy or plexopathy (after EMG)

Pharmacologic treatment of neuropathic pain (Lancet Neurol 2015;14:162)
- Pregabalin, gabapentin, TCAs (nortriptyline, amitriptyline), SNRIs (duloxetine, venlafaxine)
- 2ⁿᵈ line: tramadol, topicals (lidocaine, capsaicin); 3ʳᵈ line: opiates, botulinum toxin A

GUILLAIN-BARRÉ SYNDROME (GBS)

Definition & epidemiology (Nat Rev Neurol 2014;10:469)
- AIDP (60–80%); acute motor axonal neuropathy (AMAN; 7–30%; w/o sensory loss; a/w anti-GM1, GD1a Ab); Miller Fisher synd. (ophthalmoplegia & ataxia; a/w anti-GQ1b Ab).
- Incidence 1–2 per 100,000; most common acute/subacute paralysis
- Precipitants in 60%: viral illness (CMV, EBV, HIV), URI (Mycoplasma), gastroenteritis (Campylobacter), Lyme, immunizations (no proven risk w/ current), surgery

Clinical manifestations (Lancet 2016;388:717)
- Pain (55–90%), distal sensory dysesthesias & numbness often 1ˢᵗ sx, back pain common
- Progressive sym paralysis in legs and arms over hrs to days; plateau in 1–4 wk
- Hypoactive then absent reflexes. <10% w/ reflexes on presentation, but all develop hypo/areflexia during course. Minority of AMAN w/ preserved reflexes throughout.
- Resp failure requiring mech vent occurs in 25%; autonomic instability & arrhythmias in 60%

Diagnostic studies (results may be normal in first several days)
- LP: albuminocytologic dissociation = ↑ protein w/o pleocytosis (<10 WBCs) seen in up to 64% of Pts. ↑ protein in ½ in 1ˢᵗ wk, ¾ by 3ʳᵈ wk of sx. Unlikely to be GBS if WBC >50.
- EMG & NCS: ↓ nerve conduction velocity, conduction block; can be nl in 1ˢᵗ 2 wks
- FVC & NIF: to assess for risk of resp. failure (cannot rely on P₄O₂ or S₄O₂).

Treatment

- Plasma exchange or IVIg of equal efficacy *(Neuro 2012;78:1009)*; steroids not beneficial
- Supportive care with monitoring in ICU setting if rapid progression or resp. failure
- Watch for autonomic dysfunction: labile BP, dysrhythmias (telemetry)
- Most recover near baseline in 1 y; 3–5% mortality. Residual deficits: pain, fatigue.

MYASTHENIA GRAVIS

Definition & epidemiology *(Lancet Neurol 2015;14:1023)*

- Autoimmune disorder with Ab against acetylcholine receptor (AChR, 80%), muscle specific kinase (MusK, 4%), lipoprotein-related protein 4 (LRP4, 2%), or other NMJ proteins
- Prevalence: 1 in 7500; affects all ages, peak incidence 20s–30s (women), 60s–70s (men)
- 15% of AChR MG a/w thymoma; 30% of Pts w/ thymoma develop AchR MG

Clinical manifestations

- Fluctuating weakness w/ *fatigability* (worse w/ repetitive use, relieved by rest)
- Cranial muscles involved early → 60% present initially w/ ocular sx (ptosis, diplopia); 20% will only have ocular sx; 15% w/ bulbar (difficulty chewing, dysarthria, dysphagia). Often later progresses to generalized weakness.
- Limb weakness proximal > distal; DTRs preserved; minimal/no atrophy
- MusK MG (F >> M): mostly cranial/bulbar, neck, and resp weakness.
- LRP4 MG: mostly ocular and limb weakness. Resp failure rare.
- Exacerbations triggered by stressors such as URI, surgery, pregnancy or postpartum, meds (eg, aminoglycosides, macrolides, fluoroquinolones, procainamide, phenytoin, D-penicillamine). Prednisone can *worsen* sx acutely.
- Myasthenic crisis = exacerbation → need for respiratory assistance
- Cholinergic crisis = weakness due to *overtreatment* with anticholinesterase meds; may have excessive salivation, abdominal cramping and diarrhea; rare at normal doses

Diagnostic studies

- Bedside: ptosis at baseline or after >45 sec of sustained upgaze; improved ptosis with ice pack over eyes for 2–5 min, Se 77%, Sp 98%
- Neostigmine test: temporary ↑ strength; false ⊕ & ⊖ occur; premedicate w/ atropine
- EMG: ↓ response with repetitive nerve stimulation (vs. ↑ response in Lambert-Eaton)
- Anti-AChR Ab: Se 80%, 50% if ocular disease only; Sp >90%; muscle specific receptor tyrosine kinase (MuSK) Ab, AchR modulating Ab.
- CT or MRI of thorax to evaluate thymus (65% hyperplasia, 10% thymoma)

Treatment

- Thymectomy if thymoma; may lead to improvement in up to 85% Pts w/o thymoma
- Cholinesterase inhib (eg, pyridostigmine) most rapid acting (benefit in 30–60 min). Less effective for MusK MG. Side effects: cholinergic stim (brady, diarrhea, drooling).
- Immunosuppression: prednisone (benefit in wks) + AZA (benefit in 6–15 mo). If no response: mycophenolate, rituximab, MTZ, CsA.
- Myasthenic crisis: treat precipitant; consider d/c cholinesterase inhib. if suspect cholinergic crisis. IVIg or plasmapheresis; if no response, high-dose glucocorticoids (in monitored setting as risk for initial worsening). ICU if rapid or severe (follow FVC, NIF).

NEUROMUSC 9-9

MYOPATHIES

Etiologies

- Hereditary: Duchenne, Becker, limb-girdle, myotonic, metabolic, mitochondrial
- Endocrine: hypothyroidism, hyperparathyroidism, Cushing syndrome
- Toxic: statins, fibrates, glucocorticoids (incl. critical illness myopathy), zidovudine, alcohol, cocaine, antimalarials, colchicine, penicillamine
- Infectious: HIV, HTLV-1, trichinosis, toxoplasmosis
- Inflammatory (see "Rheumatology"): polymyositis, dermatomyositis, inclusion body myositis

Clinical manifestations

- Progressive or episodic weakness (not fatigue)
- Weakness most often symmetric, proximal > distal (stairs, rising from sitting, etc.)
- ± Myalgias (though not prominent or frequent), cramps, myotonia (impaired relaxation)
- May develop either pseudohypertrophy (dystrophies) or mild muscle atrophy
- Assoc. organ dysfxn: cardiac (arrhythmia, CHF), pulmonary (ILD), dysmorphic features

Diagnostic studies

- CK, aldolase, LDH, electrolytes, ALT/AST, PTH, TSH, ESR, HIV
- Autoantibodies (anti-Jo1, antisynthetase, anti-Mi-2, anti-SRP, ANA, RF)
- EMG/NCS: low-amp, polyphasic units w/ early recruitment, ± fibrillation potentials
- Muscle biopsy, molecular genetic testing (where indicated)

HEADACHE

Primary headache syndromes (International Headache Society Classification)
- **Tension-type:** bilateral, pressure-like pain of mild–mod intensity, not throbbing or aggravated by physical activity. A/w photophobia or phonophobia, not N/V. Freq a/w myofascial sensitivity in neck/head. Triggers: stress, sleep deprivation, dehydration, hunger. Rx: NSAIDs, acetaminophen (risk of med overuse HA) if episodic; TCAs if chronic.
- **Cluster HA** and other trigeminal autonomic cephalalgias (TACs) (Continuum 2015;21:1041)
  Characterized by unilateral rhinorrhea, red/tearing eye, miosis/ptosis, lid edema, sweating, pain is orbital or temporal, differentiated by timing
  Cluster: ♂ > ♀, unilateral eye pain, restlessness, attacks 15 min–3 h, worsened by EtOH.
  Ppx: CCB (verapamil). Rx: high-flow O_2 via non-rebreather, sumatriptan IN/SC.
  Paroxysmal hemicrania: similar to cluster, but ♀ > ♂, attacks 2–30 min. Rx: indomethacin.
  Hemicrania continua: ♀ > ♂, ice pick–like pain lasting >3 mo. Rx: indomethacin.
  Short-lasting unilateral neuralgiform HA (SUNA/SUNCT): ♂ > ♀, excruciating, stabbing, electrical pain, 5 sec–4 min, up to 200×/d. Rx: lamotrigine, gabapentin, topiramate.
- **Migraine:** see below

Secondary causes of headaches
- Traumatic: postconcussion, SAH, SDH, postcraniotomy
- ↑ ICP: mass (tumor, abscess, vascular malformations, ICH), hydrocephalus, idiopathic intracranial hypertension (pseudotumor cerebri), altitude associated cerebral edema
- ↓ ICP: post-LP headache, CSF leak/dural tear, overshunting
- Vascular causes: stroke (esp. posterior circ), dissection, vasculitis (incl. temporal arteritis), reversible cerebral vasoconstriction syndrome (RCVS), ICH, venous sinus thrombosis
- Meningeal irritation: meningitis, SAH
- Extracranial: sinusitis, TMJ syndrome, glaucoma
- Systemic causes: hypoxia, hypercapnia, dialysis HA, HTN, hypoglycemia, ↓TSH
- Medication overuse (analgesics), withdrawal (caffeine, opioids, estrogen)

Clinical evaluation (JAMA 2006;296:1274 & 2013;310:1248)
- History: onset (sudden vs. gradual), quality, severity, location, duration, triggers, alleviating factors, positional component, hormonal triggers (menstruation), preceding trauma, associated sx (visual Δs, "floaters," N/V, photophobia, focal neurologic sx)
- Medications (analgesics), substance abuse (opioids, caffeine)
- General and neurologic exam (funduscopic exam, visual fields)
- **Warning signs (should prompt neuroimaging)**
  explosive onset (vasc); "worst HA of my life" (SAH, RCVS); *meningismus* (SAH, infxn)
  positional: lying > standing (↑ ICP); *N/V* (↑ ICP; migraines)
  visual sx: diplopia, blurring, ↓ acuity (GCA, glaucoma, ↑ ICP); *eye pain* (glaucoma, trigeminal autonomic cephalalgia)
  abnl neuro exam (struct. lesion, poss. in migraine); ↓ *consciousness* (± fever): infxn, ICH
  age >50 y; immunosuppression (CNS infections, PRES)
- LP if ? SAH (✓ for xanthochromia), idiopathic intracranial HTN (✓opening press); image first!

MIGRAINE

Epidemiology: affects 15% of women and 6% of men; onset usually by 30 y

Definition & clinical manifestations
- **Migraine w/o aura** (most common): ≥5 attacks lasting 4–72 h and with both (a) N/V or photophobia & phonophobia, and (b) ≥2 of following: unilat., pulsating, mod–severe intensity, aggravated by routine activity
- **Migraine w/ aura:** ≥2 attacks w/: (a) aura defined as ≥1 fully reversible sx: visual Δs (flickering spots, visual loss), sensory sx (paresthesias, numbness), speech disturbance; *and* (b) unilateral progression of sx(s) over ≥5 but ≤60 min; *and* (c) HA w/in 60 min of aura
- Aura may occur w/o HA ("acephalgic migraine"), must r/o TIA/stroke (typically rapid onset)
- If motor weakness, consider **sporadic hemiplegic migraine:** aura of fully reversible motor weakness lasting up to 24 hr, also w/visual and sensory aura + typical migraine HA
- Precipitants: stress, hunger, foods (cheese, chocolate) and food additives (MSG), fatigue, alcohol, menstruation, exercise

Treatment (Cephalalgia 2015;35:271)
- Abortive Rx: 5-HT$_1$ agonists ("triptans") effective if given early in migraine attack, contraindic if motor aura, CAD, prior stroke. Also consider acetaminophen, caffeine, NSAIDs, steroids; IV options include Mg, metoclopramide, prochlorperazine, valproate, dihydroergotamine (caution if CAD, recent triptan use). Avoid butalbital, opioids
- Prophylaxis: valproic acid, topiramate, βB, TCAs, butterbur, NSAIDs, magnesium, riboflavin
  (Neurology 2012;78:1337 & 1346)

BACK AND SPINAL CORD DISEASE

Differential diagnosis of back pain

- **Musculoskeletal:** involving spine (vertebra, facet joints), paraspinal muscles and ligaments, sacroiliac joint, or hip joint. Spondylolisthesis, vertebral fx, OA, inflam. spondyloarthritis (RA, ankylosing spondylitis, reactive, psoriatic), musculoligamentous "strain," myofascial pain syndrome, trochanteric bursitis.
- **Spinal cord** (myelopathy)/**nerve root** (radiculopathy):
  Degenerative/traumatic: disc herniation, foraminal or lumbar stenosis, spondylolisthesis
  Neoplastic: lung, breast, prostate, RCC, thyroid, colon, multiple myeloma, lymphoma
  Infectious (also see ID section): osteomyelitis, epidural abscess, zoster, Lyme, CMV, HIV
- **Referred pain from visceral disease:**
  GI: PUD, cholelithiasis, pancreatitis, pancreatic cancer
  GU: pyelonephritis, nephrolithiasis, uterine or ovarian cancer, salpingitis
  Vascular: aortic dissection, leaking aortic aneurysm

Initial evaluation

- **History:** location, radiation, trauma, wt loss, cancer hx, fever, immunocompromised, neurologic symptoms, saddle anesthesia, incontinence, urinary retention, IV drug use
- **General physical exam:** local tenderness, ROM, signs of infection or malignancy; paraspinal tenderness or spasm in musculoskeletal strain
- **Signs of radiculopathy** (sharp/lancinating pain radiating to limb):
  Spurling sign (cervical radiculopathy): radicular pain w/ downward force to extended & ipsilaterally rotated head; 30% Se, 93% Sp
  Straight leg raise (sciatica or lumbosacral radiculopathy): radicular pain at 30–70°; ipsilateral: 92% Se, 28% Sp; crossed (contralateral leg raised): 28% Se, 90% Sp
  Patrick/FABER test (sacroiliac joint syndrome): severe pain on hip external rotation; 70% Se, 100% Sp
  Neurogenic claudication in lumbar stenosis (see table on next page)
- **Neurologic exam:** full motor (including sphincter tone), sensory (including perineal region) and reflexes including bulbocavernous, anal wink (S4), and cremasteric (L2)
- **Red flags:** upper motor neuron signs (hyperreflexia, upgoing toes), cauda equina or conus medullaris syndromes (saddle anesthesia, bowel or bladder dysfunction, reduced rectal tone, loss of sacral reflexes)
- **Laboratory** (depending on suspicion): CBC, ESR, Ca, PO_4, CSF
- **Neuroimaging:** low yield if nonradiating pain, high false ⊕ rate (incidental spondylosis) depending on suspicion: X-rays, CT or CT myelography, MRI, bone scan
- **EMG/NCS:** may be useful to distinguish root/plexopathies from peripheral neuropathies

SPINAL CORD COMPRESSION

Clinical manifestations

- Acute: flaccid paraparesis and absent reflexes ("spinal shock")
- Subacute–chronic: spastic paraparesis and hyperactive reflexes
- Posterior column dysfunction in legs (loss of vibratory sense or proprioception)
- Sensory loss below level of lesion
- ⊕ Babinski responses ± ankle clonus

Evaluation & treatment

- Empiric spine immobilization (collar, board) for all trauma patients
- STAT MRI (at and above clinical spinal level, with gadolinium) or CT myelogram
- Emergent neurosurgical and/or neurology consultation
- Urgent radiation therapy ± surgery for compression if due to metastatic disease
- High-dose steroids depending on cause:
  Tumor: dexamethasone 16 mg/d IV (usually 4 mg q6h) with slow taper over wks
  Trauma: methylprednisolone 30 mg/kg IV over 15 min then 5.4 mg/kg/h × 24 h (if started w/in 3 h of injury) or × 48 h (if started 3–8 h after injury) *(Cochrane 2012:CD001046)*

NERVE ROOT COMPRESSION

Clinical manifestations

- Radicular pain aggravated by activity (esp. bending, straining, coughing), relieved by lying
- Sciatica = radicular pain radiating from buttocks down lateral aspect of leg, often to knee or lateral calf ± numbness and paresthesias radiating to lateral foot. Caused by compression of nerve roots, plexus, or sciatic nerve.

Disc Herniation: Cervical and Lumbar Radiculopathy

Disc	Root	Pain/paresthesias	Sensory loss	Motor loss	Reflex loss
C4–C5	C5	Neck, shoulder, upper arm	Shoulder, lateral arm	Deltoid, biceps, infraspinatus	Biceps
C5–C6	C6	Neck, shoulder, lat. arm, radial forearm, thumb & index finger	Radial forearm, thumb & index finger	Biceps brachioradialis	Biceps, brachio-radialis, supinator
C6–C7	C7	Neck, lat. arm, ring & index fingers	Index & middle fingers	Triceps, extensor carpi ulnaris	Triceps, supinator
C7–T1	C8	Ulnar forearm and hand	Ulnar half of ring finger, little finger	Intrinsic hand muscles, flexor dig profundus	Finger flexion
L3–L4	L4	Anterior thigh, inner shin	Anteromedial lower leg, inner foot	Quadriceps	Patella
L4–L5	L5	Lat. thigh & calf, dorsum of foot, great toe	Lat. calf & great toe	Foot dorsiflexion, invers. & evers., toe extension	Medial hamstring
L5–S1	S1	Back of thigh, lateral posterior calf, lat. foot	Lateral foot & toes, sole of foot	Gastrocnemius	Achilles

Nb, lumbar disc protrusion tends to compress the nerve root that exits 1 vertebral level below the protrusion.

Neurogenic vs. Vascular Claudication

Features	Neurogenic claudication	Vascular claudication
Cause	Lumbar spinal stenosis (with nerve root compression)	Peripheral artery disease (with limb ischemia)
Pain	Radicular back/buttock pain Radiating down legs	Cramping leg pain Mostly in calves; radiating up legs
Worse with	Walking & standing Hyperextension/lying prone	Walking Biking
Better with	Bending forward, sitting	Rest (standing or sitting)
Other sx	Numbness/paresthesias	Pale, cool extremity
Exam	± Focal weakness, ↓ reflexes ↓ Lumbar extension Preserved pulses	Diminished/absent pulses (dorsalis pedis/posterior tibialis) Pallor
Diagnostic studies	MRI lumbar spine CT myelogram (if no MRI) EMG/NCS	Arterial Doppler studies Ankle-brachial index (ABI) Arteriography
Treatment	PT (flexion exercise), NSAIDs, steroid injections (ESI) Surgery (if other Rx fails)	Modify vascular risk factors, exercise rehab, antiplatelet Rx, revascularization

Nb, diagnosis complicated by overlap between presentations & possibility of both diagnoses in the same patient. (NEJM 2007;356:1241 & 2008;358:818)

Treatment of nerve root compression (NEJM 2016;374:1763)

- Conservative: avoid bending/lifting; soft cervical collar (cervical radiculopathy); NSAIDs; muscle relaxants; Rx neuropathic pain (see "Peripheral Neuropathies"); physical therapy.
- Spinal epidural steroid injections (ESI): limited short-term relief of refractory radicular pain (Pain 2013;154:2249)
- Surgery: cord compression or cauda equina syndrome; progressive motor dysfunction; bowel/bladder dysfunction; failure to respond to conservative Rx after 3 mo (NEJM 2007;356:2245)

Visceral Pain		
Anatomic division	**Viscera**	**Area to which pain referred**
Foregut	Esophagus & duodenum	Epigastrium
Midgut	Jejunum to mid-transverse colon	Umbilicus
Hindgut	Mid-transverse colon to rectum	Hypogastrium

Pain due to pancreatitis and nephrolithiasis commonly radiates to the back

Figure 10-1 Etiologies of abdominal pain based on location

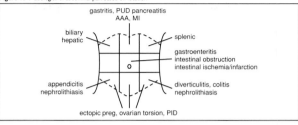

gastritis, PUD pancreatitis
AAA, MI

biliary
hepatic

splenic

gastroenteritis
intestinal obstruction
intestinal ischemia/infarction

appendicitis
nephrolithiasis

diverticulitis, colitis
nephrolithiasis

ectopic preg, ovarian torsion, PID

Initial evaluation
- History: onset of pain, location, exacerbating/relieving factors
- Assoc. sx: fevers/chills, N/V, Δ in bowel habits (diarrhea/constipation, stool diam. or color, hematochezia, melena), jaundice, Δ in urine color, Δ in wt, menstrual hx in women
- PMHx: previous incisions or abdominal surgeries; Ob/Gyn hx
- Exam: VS; general posture of Pt; comprehensive abdominal exam looking for signs of peritonitis, which include rebound tenderness and involuntary guarding, abdominal wall rigidity, pain w/ percussion/minimal palpation; presence of hernias; rectal/pelvic
- Labs: CBC, electrolytes, LFTs, amylase/lipase, pregnancy test
- Imaging: depends on suspected etiology, may include RUQ U/S for biliary/hepatic disease, KUB for intestinal obstruction, CT for pancreatitis or intestinal disease. Do not delay resuscitation or surgical consultation for ill Pt while waiting for imaging.

ACUTE ABDOMEN

Definition
- Acute onset abdominal pain that portends need for urgent surgery

Etiologies
- Perforated viscous → peritonitis (perforated ulcer, complicated diverticulitis, trauma)
- Intraperitoneal bleed
- Bowel obstruction (adhesions from previous surgeries, malignancies, hernias)
- Mimics: severe pancreatitis can resemble peritonitis; renal colic causes severe abdominal pain but not abdominal rigidity

Initial evaluation
- H&P as above
- Labs as above plus: PT/INR, PTT, type, & screen
- Imaging: KUB (upright) or if stable, CT abomen/pelvis w/ IV contrast (IV/PO if suspect obstruction)

Initial management
- Immediate surgical consultation for suspected acute abdomen
- NPO, start IV fluids (NS or LR)
- Broad spectrum abx if perforation suspected

EXTREMITY EMERGENCIES

Acute limb ischemia (see "Peripheral Artery Disease" for details)
- Definition: sudden ↓ in perfusion causing threat to limb viability

- Evaluation: detailed vascular exam; CT angiography or arteriography
- Initial management: anticoag for embolism/thrombosis; immediate surgical consultation

Compartment syndrome (Clin Orthop Relat Res 2010;468:940)
- Definition: ↑ intracompartmental pressure w/ compressive closure of venules → ↑ hydrostatic force resulting in further increases in compartment pressure
- Etiologies: orthopedic (fracture), vascular (ischemia-reperfusion), iatrogenic (eg, vascular injury in anticoagulated Pt), soft tissue injury (eg, prolonged limb compression)
- Clinical manifestations: pain esp. on passive movement, swollen/tense compartment, paraesthesia, pallor, pulselessness, paralysis (late)
- Evaluation: surgical evaluation of compartment pressures; intracompartment pressure >30 or difference between diastolic & intracompartment pressure of >10–30 is diagnostic
- Treatment: fasciotomy

SURGICAL TUBES, DRAINS, WOUNDS

Tracheostomy (Otolaryngol Head Neck Surg 2013;148:6)
- Typically a cuffed tube, which creates a tight seal to facilitate ventilation throughout tube
- Speaking valve (eg, Passy-Muir): 1-way valve that allows inhalation through tube, but exhalation around tube through vocal cords (nb, cuff should not be inflated)
- 1st routine tube Δ for *percutaneously* placed tubes should be ~10 d postop; *surgically* placed tubes can be Δ'd >5 d postop; first Δ should be overseen by experienced person
- Accidental dislodgement: intubate from above (if airway/vent nec & anatomically possible) w/in 7 d of placement: emergent surgical consultation
  >7 d after placement: replace with a similar size tube or smaller

Chest tubes (Eur J Cardiothorac Surg 2011;40:291)
- Inserted for PTX, chest trauma or after thoracic surg for drainage of air/ fluid from thoracic cavity. Range from small (8-10 Fr for spont PTX) to large (28-32 Fr after pulm resections)
- Connected to 3-chamber chest drainage system:
  1st: collection chamber for pleural fluid
  2nd: water seal chamber used to allow air to exit pleural space on exhalation and prevent air from entering on inhalation
  3rd: suction control chamber which regulates suction transmitted to pleural space
- Monitor for output and presence of air leak (indicated by bubbling in *water seal chamber*)
- Removal determined by overall daily outputs and presence of air leak
- If accidentally removed or dislodged, tube should be completely removed and an occlusive dressing (eg, 4 × 4 covered w/ Tegaderm or silk tape) should be placed *rapidly* over site. CXR STAT; new tube should be placed if persistent PTX.

Gastrostomy/jejunostomy tubes (Paediatr Child Health 2011;16:281)
- Placed for tube feedings, hydration and delivery of medications
- Securely anchor to skin to prevent inadvertent removal
- Should not be removed for ≥6–8 wk to allow establishment of mature gastrocutaneous tract
- Obstructed tubes can be cleared by flushing with agents such as carbonated water, meat tenderizer, & pancreatic enzymes. ↓ obstruction by flushing before & after meds and flushing q4–6h when receiving continuous feeds.
- Inadvertent removal: place Foley catheter of similar size or smaller into tract *immediately* to prevent stoma from closing. Tube then replaced and confirmed via fluoro study.

Suture/staple removal
- Should be done in consultation w/ surgical team; timing depends on location of wound
- *Should not be removed if there is evidence of wound separation during removal!*
- After removal, wound should be reapproximated w/ Steri-Strips

Decubitus ulcers (J Wound Ostomy Continence Nurs 2012;39:3)
- Sores in dependent areas exposed to repeated pressure (commonly sacrum, heels)
- Risk factors: immobility, poor nutritional status
- Stage I (non-blanchable erythema); Stage II (partial thickness); Stage III (full thickness skin loss); Stage IV (full thickness tissue loss)
- Treatment: offload area, air mattress, pillows and/or support boots
- Surgical consultation for debridement of ulcers with necrotic or infected tissue, may require plastic surgical reconstruction for advanced ulcers once clean
- Wound vac (negative pressure vacuum dressing) therapy may accelerate healing

MAXIMIZING A SURGICAL CONSULT

- For ill Pt, call surgical consult early, do not wait for labs & imaging results
- If potential surgical emergency, make Pt NPO, start IVF, ✓ coags, type, & screen
- Have appropriate-level MD who knows & has examined Pt call consult

VAGINAL BLEEDING

Abnormal bleeding from lower (vulva, vagina, cervix) or upper genital tract (uterus)

Etiologies
- Premenopausal
  <u>Not pregnant</u>: menses, dysfunctional uterine bleeding (menorrhagia), leiomyoma, polyp, trauma, cervical dysplasia/cancer (rare), endometrial hyperplasia/cancer (rare)
  <u>Pregnant</u>
    <u>1st trimester</u>: threatened abortion, spont. abortion (missed, incomplete or complete), ectopic pregnancy, molar pregnancy (partial or complete hydatidiform mole)
    <u>2nd or 3rd trimester</u>: preterm labor, placenta previa, placental abruption
- Postmenopausal: atrophy, polyp, leiomyoma, endometrial hyperplasia/cancer, cervical dysplasia/cancer

History & exam
- Age, menopausal status, gestational age if preg; volume & duration of current bleeding
- If premenopausal: menstrual hx including age of onset, interval between & duration of menses, any assoc. sx and LMP to assess timing of menstrual cycle
- Past Ob/Gyn hx (any structural abnl, STD, and contraception)
- Health maint. (Pap smear, HPV screening); domestic violence; anticoag or antiplt meds
- General physical & abdominal exam (incl. tenderness, masses)
- Pelvic exam: external (bleeding seen on vulva, any lesions, any trauma); also, w/ assistance from Ob/Gyn, speculum exam (quantity of bleeding; cervical os open or close and if open, dilation; any polyps), & bimanual exam (uterine size and tenderness, adnexal mass and tenderness)

Laboratory evaluation & imaging
- Urine (rapid test) & serum pregnancy test (beta-hCG); Hct/hemoglobin
- Pelvic U/S: visualize intrauterine preg to r/o ectopic; if preg, intrauterine not seen, & βHCG > discrim. zone → ? ectopic; if βHCG < discrim. zone → follow βHCG; nl placental position to r/o placenta previa and likely severe abruption
- *Ectopic pregnancy is life-threatening dx, ∴ must rule out if Pt pregnant (JAMA 2013;309:1722)*

VAGINAL DISCHARGE

Fluid or mucus from vagina, cervix, or uterus

Etiologies
- Infectious: bacterial vaginosis, candida vulvovaginitis, trichomoniasis
- Noninfectious: physiologic (in preg or non-preg), rupture of membranes, foreign-body rxn

Initial evaluation
- Age, LMP, gestational age if preg. or menopausal status
- Discharge quantity, color, consistency, odor, assoc. sx (itchiness, redness, abd/pelvic pain)
- Past gyn hx incl STD and contraception usage (condoms ↓ STD risk)
- Tampon or condom use as risk factors for retained foreign body
- Pelvic exam: external (quantity & quality of discharge on vulva, any lesions); speculum (discharge, appearance of cervix), bimanual (cervical motion tenderness)
- Laboratory: pH of discharge; microscopy (saline & KOH wet mounts); urine pregnancy test

Treatment
- Bacterial vaginosis: oral or vaginal metronidazole or clindamycin
- Candida vulvovaginitis: oral or topical antimycotic medications
- Trichomoniasis: oral metronidazole

ADNEXAL MASS IN NON-PREGNANT WOMAN

Mass arising from ovary, fallopian tube, or surrounding connective tissue

Etiologies
- Ovarian: functional (follicular and corpus luteum) or hemorrhagic cyst, endometriomas, ovarian torsion, tubo-ovarian abscess, benign & malignant ovarian tumors
- Fallopian tube: paratubal cyst, hydrosalpinx, ovarian torsion, tubo-ovarian abscess

Initial evaluation
- LMP/menopausal status; associated sx of abd/pelvic pain, FHx of gyn cancers
- Abd exam (distension, tenderness, masses); bimanual (uterine or adnexal masses)
- Preg test if premenopausal (if ⊕, then mass likely pregnancy); CA-125 if postmenopausal
- Pelvic U/S (even if mass 1st identified on CT, as U/S is best modality); U/S appearance of mass most important factor used to determine risk of malignancy

OPHTHALMIC ISSUES

INITIAL EVALUATION

- Ocular symptom: onset (sudden or progressive) & duration of sx; unilateral vs. bilateral; pain; photophobia; discharge; Δ in near (eg, book) or far (eg, TV across room) vision
- Pre-existing ocular conditions, eye meds (incl any Δs), recent h/o ocular surgery, trauma
- Ocular exam: vision (✓ with Pt's correction [glasses/contacts]) w/ each eye; pupillary exam; EOM; confrontation visual fields (important if suspect CNS problem)
- Overall: VS, immunocomp., s/s of infxn, h/o malig, CNS issues, Δ in meds, CBC, coags

COMMON VISUAL SYMPTOMS

- **Fluctuation in vision (ie, blurry):** med-induced refractive error (eg, systemic steroids, chemoRx), hyperglycemia, dry eye (common). **Visual defect** may p/w "blurred vision." Bilateral: glaucoma (common), homonymous contral. CNS lesion: bitemporal: pituitary; toxic/nutritional. Unilateral: ipsilateral orbital, retinal, or optic nerve lesion.
- **Red eye:**
  Bilateral: viral conjunct., (starts in 1 eye; also w/ lid swelling, discharge); chronic inflammation (dry eyes, rosacea, autoimmune disease)
  Unilateral: subconj. hemorrhage, iritis, or inflam (eg, episcleritis, iritis, uveitis, scleritis); acute angle closure (qv). Scleritis & acute angle closure p/w severe pain, H/A, nausea.
- **Double vision (diplopia):** fixed double vision w/ ophthalmoplegia from orbital process or cranial nerve palsy (III, IV, VI). Transient "diplopia" due to fatigue or sedation.
- **Flashing lights/floaters:** vitreous detach. (common, benign); retinal detach. (unilateral visual field defect; urgent ophthalmology consult); hemorrhage; intraocular lymphoma

ACUTE VISUAL CHANGES

	Etiologies of Acute Vision Loss *(italics indicates a/w pain)*	
	Unilateral	**Bilateral**
Transient (<24 h, often <1 h)	Ret. art. embolism, impending retinal artery or vein occlusion (amaurosis fugax), vasospasm, carotid disease	Ocular surface dis. (dry eye), bilat. carotid dis., TIA, migraine, high ICP (papilledema)
Prolonged (>24 h)	Retinal art/vein occl, retinal detach., retina/vitreous heme, retinitis, ant. optic neurop./*corneal ulcer, GCA, acute angle closure glaucoma*	Visual cortex stroke, post. ischemic neuropathy (profound hypotension during surgery), post. reversible enceph. synd., *GCA*

COMMON OCULAR CONDITIONS (FRONT TO BACK)

Orbit: **orbital cellulitis** (fever, proptosis, ↓ EOM; *emergent abx & referral*)

Lids: hordeolum or chalazion (stye); preseptal cellulitis; **ptosis** (age; Horner's; **CN III palsy:** EOM restricted in all directions except laterally [eye is "down & out"], a/w ptosis & mydriasis, seen w/ uncal herniation, aneurysm of post com art., GCA, HTN, DM); incomplete lid closure (**CN 7th palsy**)

Conjunctiva: conjunctivitis (**red eye**); subconj. hemorrhage (HTN, blood thinner); ocular surface disease (dry eyes); episcleritis/scleritis (deep vessels of sclera)

Cornea: **contact lens related ulcer;** herpetic keratitis/scarring/neurotropic ulcers (**CN V paresis**); pterygium; keratoconus; corneal dystrophy

Ant. chamber: iritis (inflam. cells); hyphema (blood, post trauma); hypopyon (inflam./infxn)

Pupil: Anisocoria (physiologic); Horner's; CN III

Lens: cataract (age, trauma, medication, radiation, congenital); post cataract surgery infxn

Vitreous/Retina/Macula: diabetic retinopathy; macular degen.; retinal detachment; retinal ± vitreous hemorrhage; retinitis (infectious)

Optic nerve (CN II): ischemic neuropathy p/w acute unilat. visual loss, altitudinal field defect; a/w GCA; nonarteritic a/w HTN, hyperchol., DM, thrombophilia. Optic neuritis: often p/w unilat. central scotoma, pain w/ EOM, ↑ visual loss over days; a/w demyelinating disease (eg, MS), also seen w/ sarcoidosis & CTD. Optic neuropathy (glaucoma common).

OCULAR EMERGENCIES

- **Chemical splash:** alkali worse than acid; immediate eye flush; pH 7.3–7.4 normal
- **Acute angle closure glaucoma:** fixed mid-dilated pupil, corneal edema, high intraocular pressure (typically >50; normal 8–21). Rx w/ topical drops; may require AC tap/laser.
- **Penetrating eye injury:** protect eye (no patching), IV antibiotics, NPO, surgical prep

Drug	Class	Dose	
		per kg	**average**
Pressors, Inotropes and Chronotropes			
Phenylephrine	α_1	10–300 µg/min	
Norepinephrine	$\alpha_1 > \beta_1$	1–40 µg/min	
Vasopressin	V_1	0.01–0.1 U/min (usually <0.04)	
Epinephrine	$\alpha_1, \alpha_2, \beta_1, \beta_2$	2–20 µg/min	
Isoproterenol	β_1, β_2	0.1–10 µg/min	
Dopamine	D	0.5–2 µg/kg/min	50–200 µg/min
	β, D	2–10 µg/kg/min	200–500 µg/min
	α, β, D	>10 µg/kg/min	500–1000 µg/min
Dobutamine	$\beta_1 > \beta_2$	2–20 µg/kg/min	50–1000 µg/min
Milrinone	PDE	± 50 µg/kg over 10 min then 0.25–0.75 µg/kg/min	3–4 mg over 10 min then 20–50 µg/min
Vasodilators			
Nitroglycerin	NO	10–1000 µg/min	
Nitroprusside	NO	0.25–10 µg/kg/min	10–800 µg/min
Labetalol	α_1, β_1 and β_2 blocker	20–80 mg q10min or 10–120 mg/h	
Fenoldopam	D	0.1–1.6 µg/kg/min	10–120 µg/min
Clevidipine	CCB	1–16 mg/h	
Epoprostenol	vasodilator	2–20 ng/kg/min	
Antiarrhythmics			
Amiodarone	K et al. (Class III)	150 mg over 10 min, then 1 mg/min × 6 h, then 0.5 mg/min × 18 h	
Lidocaine	Na channel (Class IB)	1–1.5 mg/kg then 1–4 mg/min	100 mg then 1–4 mg/min
Procainamide	Na channel (Class IA)	17 mg/kg over 60 min then 1–4 mg/min	1 g over 60 min then 1–4 mg/min
Ibutilide	K channel (Class III)	1 mg over 10 min, may repeat × 1	
Propranolol	β blocker	0.5–1 mg q5min then 1–10 mg/h	
Esmolol	$\beta_1 > \beta_2$ blocker	500 µg/kg then 50–200 µg/kg/min	20–40 mg over 1 min then 2–20 mg/min
Verapamil	CCB	2.5–5 mg over 1–2′, repeat 5–10 mg in 15–30′ prn 5–20 mg/h	
Diltiazem	CCB	0.25 mg/kg over 2 min reload 0.35 mg/kg × 1 prn then 5–15 mg/h	20 mg over 2 min reload 25 mg × 1 prn then 5–15 mg/h
Adenosine	purinergic	6 mg rapid push; if no response: 12 mg → 12–18 mg	
Sedation			
Morphine	opioid	1–30 (in theory, unlimited) mg/h	
Fentanyl	opioid	50–100 µg then 50–800 (? unlimited) µg/h	
Propofol	anesthetic	1–3 mg/kg then 0.3–5 mg/kg/h	50–200 mg then 20–400 mg/h
Dexmedetomidine	α_2 agonist	1 µg/kg over 10 min → 0.2–0.7 µg/kg/h	
Diazepam	BDZ	1–5 mg q1–2h then q6h	
Midazolam	BDZ	0.5–2 mg q5min prn; 0.02–0.1 mg/kg/h or 1–10 mg/h	
Lorazepam	BDZ	0.01–0.1 mg/kg/h	
Naloxone	opioid antag.	0.4–2 mg q2–3min to total of 10 mg	
Flumazenil	BDZ antag.	0.2 mg over 30 sec then 0.3 mg over 30 sec prn may repeat 0.5 mg over 30 sec to total of 3 mg	

Drug	Class	Dose per kg	Dose average
Miscellaneous			
Aminophylline	PDE	5.5 mg/kg over 20 min then 0.5–1 mg/kg/h	250–500 mg then 10–80 mg/h
Octreotide	somatostatin analog	50 µg then 50 µg/h	
Glucagon	hormone	3–10 mg IV slowly over 3–5 min then 3–5 mg/h	
Mannitol	osmole	1.5–2 g/kg over 30–60 min repeat q6–12h to keep osm 310–320	

Figure 11-1 ACLS pulmonary edema, hypotension or shock algorithm

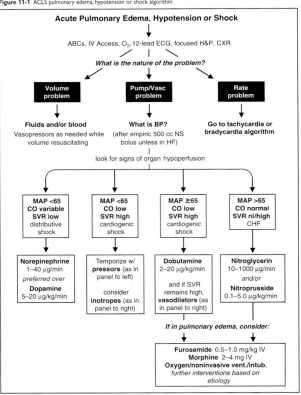

(Adapted from ACLS 2005 Guidelines)

ANTIBIOTICS

The following tables of spectra of activity for different antibiotics are generalizations.
Sensitivity data at your own institution should be used to guide therapy.

Penicillins

Generation	Properties	Spectrum
Natural (eg, penicillin)	Some GPC, GPR, GNC, most anaerobes (except *Bacteroides*)	Group A streptococci Enterococci, *Listeria, Pasteurella Actinomyces,* Syphilis
Anti-staph (eg, nafcillin)	Active vs. PCNase-producing Staph Little activity vs. Gram ⊖	Staphylococci (except MRSA) Streptococci
Amino (eg, ampicillin)	Penetrate porin channel of Gram ⊖ Not stable against PCNases	*E. coli, Proteus, H. influenzae Salmonella, Shigella* Enterococci, *Listeria*
Extended (eg, piperacillin)	Penetrate porin channel of Gram ⊖ More resistant to PCNases	Most GNR incl. *Enterobacter, Pseudomonas, Serratia*
Carbapenems (eg, imipenem)	Resistant to most β-lactamases	Most Gram ⊕ & ⊖, including anaerobes; *not* MRSA or VRE
Monobactams (aztreonam)	Active vs. Gram ⊖ but not Gram ⊕	Gram ⊖ bacterial infxn in Pt w/ PCN or Ceph allergy
β-lact. Inhib. (eg, sulbactam)	Inhibit plasma-mediated β-lactamases	Adds staph, *B. fragilis* & some GNR (*H. flu, M. cat,* some *Klebs*); intrinsic activity against *Acinetobacter* (sulbactam only)

Cephalosporins

Resistant to most β-lactamases. No activity vs. enterococci.

Gen.	Spectrum	Indications
1st (eg, cefazolin)	Most GPC (incl. staph & strep, not MRSA) Some GNR (incl. *E. coli, Proteus, Klebsiella*)	Used for surgical Ppx & skin infxns
2nd (eg, cefuroxime, cefotetan)	↓ activity vs. GPC, ↑ vs. GNR. 2 subgroups: Respiratory: *H. influenzae* & *M. catarrhalis* GI/GU: ↑ activity vs. *B. fragilis*	PNA/COPD flare Abdominal infxns
3rd (eg, ceftriaxone)	Broad activity vs. GNR & some anaerobes Ceftazidime active vs. *Pseudomonas*	PNA, sepsis, meningitis
4th (eg, cefepime)	↑ resistance to β-lactamases (incl. of staph and *Enterobacter*)	Similar to 3rd gen. MonoRx for nonlocalizing febrile neutropenia
5th (eg, ceftaroline)	Only class of cephalosporin with MRSA activity. NOT active vs *Pseudomonas*	MRSA. Not 1st line for MRSA bacteremia.

Other Antibiotics

Antibiotic	Spectrum
Vancomycin	Gram ⊕ bacteria incl. MRSA, PCNase-producing pneumococci and enterococci (except VRE)
Linezolid	
Daptomycin	GPC incl. MRSA & VRE (check susceptibility for VRE)
Quinupristin/ Dalfopristin	
Quinolones	Enteric GNR & atypicals. 3rd & 4th gen. ↑ activity vs. Gram ⊕.
Aminoglycosides	GNR. Synergy w/ cell-wall active abx (β-lactam, vanco) vs. GPC. ↓ activity in low pH (eg, abscess). No activity vs. anaerobes.
Macrolides	GPC, some respiratory Gram ⊖, atypicals
TMP/SMX	Some enteric GNR, PCP, *Nocardia, Toxoplasma,* most community-acquired MRSA
Clindamycin	Most Gram ⊕ (except enterococci) & anaerobes (incl. *B. fragilis*)
Metronidazole	Almost all anaerobic Gram ⊖, most anaerobic Gram ⊕
Doxycycline	*Rickettsia, Ehrlichia, Chlamydia, Mycoplasma, Nocardia,* Lyme
Tigecycline	Many GPC incl. MRSA & VRE; some GNR incl. ESBL but not *Pseudomonas* or *Proteus.* Approved for abdominal or skin/soft tissue infections. Check susceptibility if organism isolated.

CARDIOLOGY

Hemodynamic parameters	Normal value
Mean arterial pressure (MAP) $= \dfrac{SBP + (DBP \times 2)}{3}$	70–100 mmHg
Heart rate (HR)	60–100 bpm
Right atrial pressure (RA)	≤6 mmHg
Right ventricular (**RV**)	systolic 15–30 mmHg diastolic 1–8 mmHg
Pulmonary artery (PA)	systolic 15–30 mmHg mean 9–18 mmHg diastolic 6–12 mmHg
Pulmonary capillary wedge pressure (PCWP)	≤12 mmHg
Cardiac output (CO)	4–8 L/min
Cardiac index (CI) $= \dfrac{CO}{BSA}$	2.6–4.2 L/min/m^2
Stroke volume (SV) $= \dfrac{CO}{HR}$	60–120 mL/contraction
Stroke volume index (SVI) $= \dfrac{CI}{HR}$	40–50 mL/contraction/m^2
Systemic vascular resistance (SVR) $= \dfrac{MAP - mean\ RA}{CO} \times 80$	800–1200 dynes × sec/cm^5
Pulmonary vascular resistance (PVR) $= \dfrac{mean\ PA - mean\ PCWP}{CO} \times 80$	120–250 dynes × sec/cm^5

"Rule of 6s" for PAC: RA ≤6, RV ≤30/6, PA ≤30/12, WP ≤12. Nb 1 mmHg = 1.36 cm water or blood.

Fick cardiac output
Oxygen consumption (L/min) = CO (L/min) × arteriovenous (AV) oxygen difference
CO = oxygen consumption/AV oxygen difference
Oxygen consumption must be measured (can estimate w/ 125 mL/min/m^2, but inaccurate)
AV oxygen difference = Hb (g/dL) × 10 (dL/L) × 1.36 (mL O$_2$/g of Hb) × (S$_a$O$_2$–S$_{Mv}$O$_2$)
  S$_a$O$_2$ is measured in any arterial sample (usually 93–98%)
  S$_{Mv}$O$_2$ (mixed venous O$_2$) is measured in RA, RV or PA (assuming no shunt) (nl ~75%)
∴ **Cardiac output** (L/min) $\approx \dfrac{\text{Oxygen consumption}}{\text{Hb (g/dL)} \times 13.6\ (S_aO_2 - S_vO_2)}$

Shunts
$Q_p = \dfrac{\text{Oxygen consumption}}{\text{Pulm. vein O}_2\ \text{sat} - \text{Pulm. artery O}_2\ \text{sat}}$ (if no R → L shunt, PV O$_2$ sat ≈ S$_a$O$_2$)

$Q_s = \dfrac{\text{Oxygen consumption}}{S_aO_2 - \text{mixed venous O}_2\ \text{sat}}$ (MVO$_2$ drawn proximal to potential L → R shunt)

$\dfrac{Q_p}{Q_s} = \dfrac{S_aO_2 - \text{MV O}_2\ \text{sat}}{\text{PV O}_2\ \text{sat} - \text{PA O}_2\ \text{sat}} \approx \dfrac{S_aO_2 - \text{MVO}_2\ \text{sat}}{S_aO_2 - \text{PA O}_2\ \text{sat}}$ (if only L → R and no R → L shunt)

Valve equations
Simplified Bernoulli: Pressure gradient (ΔP) $= 4 \times v^2$ (where v = peak flow velocity)
Continuity (conservation of flow): Area$_1$ × Velocity$_1$ = A$_2$ × V$_2$ (where 1 & 2 different points)

or AVA (unknown) $= A_{LV\ outflow\ tract} \times \left(\dfrac{V_{LVOT}}{V_{AoV}} \right)$ (all of which can be measured on echo)

Gorlin equation: Valve area $= \dfrac{CO/(DEP\ or\ SEP) \times HR}{44.3 \times constant \times \sqrt{\Delta P}}$ (constant = 1 for AS, 0.85 for MS)

Hakki equation: Valve area $\approx \dfrac{CO}{\sqrt{\Delta P}}$

Chest Imaging (CXR & CT) Patterns

Pattern	Pathophysiology	Ddx
Consolidation	Radiopaque material in air space & interstitium patent airway → "air bronchograms"	*Acute:* water **(pulm edema)**, pus **(PNA)**, blood *Chronic:* neoplasm (BAC, lymphoma), aspiration, inflammatory (BOOP, eosinophilic PNA), PAP, granuloma (TB/fungal, alveolar sarcoid)

Ground glass (CT easier than CXR)	Interstitial thickening or partial filling of alveoli (but vessels visible)	*Acute:* pulm edema, infxn (PCP, viral, resolving bact. PNA)
		Chronic: ILD
		  w/o fibrosis: acute hypersens., DIP/RB, PAP
		  w/ fibrosis: IPF

Septal lines Kerley A & B	Radiopaque material in septae	**Cardiogenic pulm edema**, interstitial PNA viral, mycoplasma), lymphangitic tumor
Reticular	Lace-like net (ILD)	**ILD** (esp. IPF, bleomycin, asbestos)
Nodules	Tumor Granulomas Abscess	*Cavitary:* **Primary or metastatic cancer**, **TB** (react. or miliary), **fungus**, Wegener's, RA septic emboli, PNA *Noncavitary:* any of above + **sarcoid**, hypersens. pneum., HIV, Kaposi's sarcoma
Wedge opac.	Peripheral infarct	**PE**, cocaine, angioinv. aspergillus, Wegener's
Tree-in-bud (best on CT)	Inflammation of small airways	**Bronchopneumonia**, endobronchial TB/MAI, viral PNA, aspiration, ABPA, CF, asthma, BOOP
Hilar fullness	↑ LN or pulm arteries	**Neoplasm** (lung, mets, lymphoma) **Infxn** (AIDS); **Granuloma** (sarcoid/TB/fungal) Pulmonary hypertension
Upper lobe	n/a	**TB**, fungal, sarcoid, hypersens. pneum., CF, XRT
Lower lobe	n/a	**Aspiration**, bronchiect., IPF, RA, SLE, asbestos
Peripheral	n/a	BOOP, IPF & DIP, eos PNA, asbestosis

CXR in heart failure
- ↑ cardiac silhouette (in systolic dysfxn, not in diastolic)
- Pulmonary venous hypertension: cephalization of vessels (vessels size > bronchi in upper lobes), peribronchial cuffing (fluid around bronchi seen on end → small circles), Kerley B lines (horizontal 1–2-cm lines at bases), ↑ vascular pedicle width, loss of sharp vascular margins, pleural effusions (~75% bilateral)
- Pulmonary edema: ranges from ground glass to consolidation; often dependent and central, sparing outer third ("bat wing" appearance)

Dead space = lung units that are ventilated but not perfused

Intrapulmonary shunt = lung units that are perfused but not ventilated

Alveolar gas equation: $P_AO_2 = [F_IO_2 \times (760 - 47)] - \dfrac{P_aCO_2}{R}$ (where R ≈ 0.8)

$$P_AO_2 = 150 - \dfrac{P_aCO_2}{0.8} \text{ (on room air)}$$

A-a gradient = $P_AO_2 - P_aO_2$ [normal A-a gradient ≈ 4 + (age/4)]

Minute ventilation (V_E) = tidal volume (V_T) × respiratory rate (RR)(nl 4–6 L/min)

Tidal volume (V_T) = alveolar space (V_A) + dead space (V_D)

Fraction of tidal volume that is dead space $\left(\dfrac{V_D}{V_T}\right) = \dfrac{P_aCO_2 - P_{expired}CO_2}{P_aCO_2}$

$$P_aCO_2 = k = \times \dfrac{CO_2 \text{ Production}}{\text{alveolar ventilation}} = k \times \dfrac{V_{CO_2}}{RR \times V_T \times \left(1 - \dfrac{V_D}{V_T}\right)}$$

NEPHROLOGY

Anion gap (AG) = $Na - (Cl + HCO_3)$ (normal = [alb] × 2.5; typically 12 ± 2 mEq)

Delta-delta ($\Delta\Delta$) = [Δ AG (ie, calc. AG − expected) / Δ HCO₃ (ie, 24 − measured HCO₃)]

Urine anion gap (UAG) = $(U_{Na} + U_K) - U_{Cl}$

Calculated osmoles = $(2 \times Na) + \left(\dfrac{glc}{18}\right) + \left(\dfrac{BUN}{2.8}\right) + \left(\dfrac{EtOH}{4.6}\right)$

Osmolal gap (OG) = measured osmoles − calculated osmoles (normal <10)

Estimated creatinine clearance = $\dfrac{[140 - \text{age (yes)}] \times \text{wt (kg)}}{\text{serum Cr (mg/dL)} \times 72}$ (× 0.85 in women)

Fractional excretion of Na (FE$_{Na}$, %) = $\left[\dfrac{\dfrac{U_{Na}(mEq/L)}{P_{Na}(mEq/L)} \times 100\%}{\dfrac{U_{Cr}(mg/mL)}{P_{Cr}(mg/dL)} \times 100 \ (mL/dL)}\right] = \dfrac{U_{Na}/P_{Na}}{U_{Cr}/P_{Cr}}$

Corrected Na in hyperglycemia

estimate in all Pts: corrected Na = measured Na + $\left[2.4 \times \dfrac{(\text{measured glc} - 100)}{100}\right]$

however, Δ in Na depends on glc *(Am J Med 1999;106:399)*
Δ is 1.6 mEq per each 100 mg/dL ↑ in glc ranging from 100−440
Δ is 4 mEq per each 100 mg/dL ↑ in glc beyond 440

Total body water (TBW) = $0.60 \times IBW$ (× 0.85 if female and × 0.85 if elderly)

Free H$_2$O deficit = TBW $\times \left(\dfrac{[Na]_{serum} - 140}{140}\right) \approx \left(\dfrac{[Na]_{serum} - 140}{3}\right)$ (in 70-kg Pt)

Trans-tubular potassium gradient (TTKG) = $\dfrac{U_K/P_K}{U_{Osm}/P_{Osm}}$

HEMATOLOGY

Peripheral Smear Findings (also see Photo Inserts)	
Feature	**Abnormalities and diagnoses**
Size	normocytic vs. microcytic vs. macrocytic → see below

Shape	**anisocytosis** → unequal RBC size; **poikilocytosis** → irregular RBC shape
	  acanthocytes = **spur** cells (irregular sharp projections) → liver disease
	  bite cells (removal of Heinz bodies by phagocytes) → G6PD deficiency
	  echinocytes = **burr** cells (even, regular projections) → uremia, artifact
	  pencil cell → long, thin, hypochromic - very common in adv. iron deficiency
	  rouleaux → hyperglobulinemia (eg, multiple myeloma)
	  schistocytes, helmet cells → MAHA (eg, DIC, TTP/HUS), mechanical valve
	  spherocytes → HS, AIHA; **sickle** cells → sickle cell anemia
	  stomatocyte → central pallor appears as curved slit → liver disease, EtOH
	  target cells → liver disease, hemoglobinopathies, splenectomy
	  tear drop cells = dacryocytes → myelofibrosis, myelophthisic anemia,
	   megaloblastic anemia, thalassemia

Intra-RBC findings	**basophilic stippling** (ribosomes) → abnl Hb, sideroblastic, megaloblastic **Heinz bodies** (denatured Hb) → G6PD deficiency, thalassemia **Howell-Jolly bodies** (nuclear fragments) → splenectomy or functional asplenia (eg advanced sickle cell) **nucleated** RBCs → hemolysis, extramedullary hematopoiesis
WBC findings	**blasts** → leukemia, lymphoma; **Auer rods** → acute myelogenous leukemia **hypersegmented** (>5 lobes) PMNs: megaloblastic anemia (B₁₂/folate def.) **pseudo-Pelger-Huët anomaly** (bilobed nucleus, "pince-nez") → MDS **toxic granules** (coarse, dark blue) and **Döhle bodies** (blue patches of dilated endoplasmic reticulum) → (sepsis, severe inflammation)
Platelet	**clumping** → artifact, repeat plt count **#** → periph blood plt count ~10,000 plt for every 1 plt seen at hpf (100×) **size** → MPV (mean platelet volume) enlarged in ITP

(NEJM 2005;353:498)

Heparin for Thromboembolism	
80 U/kg bolus	
18 U/kg/h	
PTT	Adjustment
<40	bolus 5000 U, ↑ rate 300 U/h
40–49	bolus 3000 U, ↑ rate 200 U/h
50–59	↑ rate 150 U/h
60–85	no Δ
86–95	↓ rate 100 U/h
96–120	hold 30 min, ↓ rate 100 U/h
>120	hold 60 min, ↓ rate 150 U/h

(Modified from *Chest* 2008;133:141S)

Heparin for ACS	
60 U/kg bolus (max 4000 U)	
12 U/kg/h (max 1000 U/h)	
PTT	Adjustment
<40	bolus 3000 U, ↑ rate 100 U/h
40–49	↑ rate 100 U/h
50–75	no Δ
76–85	↓ rate 100 U/h
86–100	hold 30 min, ↓ rate 100 U/h
>100	hold 60 min, ↓ rate 200 U/h

(Modified from *Circ* 2007;116:e148 & *Chest* 2008;133:670)

✓ PTT q6h after every Δ (t½ of heparin ~90 min) and then qd or bid once PTT is therapeutic
✓ CBC qd (to ensure Hct and plt counts are stable)

Warfarin Loading Nomogram					
	INR				
Day	<1.5	1.5–1.9	2–2.5	2.6–3	>3
1–3	5 mg (7.5 mg if >80 kg)	2.5–5 mg	0–2.5 mg	0 mg	
4–5	10 mg	5–10 mg	0–5 mg		0–2.5 mg
6	Dose based on requirements over preceding 5 d				

(*Annals* 1997;126:133; *Archives* 1999;159:46) or, go to www.warfarindosing.org

Warfarin-heparin overlap therapy
- Indications: when failure to anticoagulate carries ↑ risk of morbidity or mortality
  (eg, DVT/PE, intracardiac thrombus)
- Rationale: (1) Half-life of factor VII (3–6 h) is shorter than half-life of factor II (60–72 h);
  ∴ warfarin can elevate PT *before achieving a true antithrombotic state*
  (2) Protein C also has half-life less than that of factor II;
  ∴ theoretical concern of *hypercoagulable state* before antithrombotic state
- Method: (1) Therapeutic PTT is achieved using heparin
  (2) Warfarin therapy is initiated
  (3) Heparin continued until INR therapeutic for ≥2 d and ≥4–5 d of warfarin
  (roughly corresponds to ~2 half-lives of factor II or a reduction to ~25%)

Common Warfarin-Drug Interactions	
Drugs that ↑ PT	**Drugs that ↓ PT**
Amiodarone	Antimicrobials: rifampin
Antimicrobials: erythromycin, ? clarithro, ciprofloxacin, MNZ, sulfonamides	CNS: barbiturates, carbamazepine, phenytoin (initial transient ↑ PT)
Antifungals: azoles	Cholestyramine
Acetaminophen, cimetidine, levothyroxine	

OTHER

Ideal body weight (IBW) = [50 kg (men) or 45.5 kg (women)] + 2.3 kg/inch over 5 feet

Body surface area (BSA, m²) = $\sqrt{\dfrac{\text{height (cm)} \times \text{weight (kg)}}{3600}}$

		Disease	
		present	absent
Test	⊕	a (true ⊕)	b (false ⊕)
	⊖	c (false ⊖)	d (true ⊖)

Sensitivity = $\dfrac{\text{true positives}}{\text{all diseased}} = \dfrac{a}{a + c}$ **Specificity** = $\dfrac{\text{true negatives}}{\text{all healthy}} = \dfrac{d}{b + d}$

⊕ **Predictive value** = $\dfrac{\text{true positives}}{\text{all positives}} = \dfrac{a}{a + b}$

⊖ **Predictive value** = $\dfrac{\text{true negatives}}{\text{all negatives}} = \dfrac{d}{c + d}$

5'-NT	5'-nucleotidase		**AVB**	atrioventricular block
6-MP	6-mercaptopurine		**AVNRT**	AV nodal reentrant tachycardia
a/w	associated with		**AVR**	aortic valve replacement
AAA	abdominal aortic aneurysm		**AVRT**	AV reciprocating tachycardia
AAD	antiarrhythmic drug		**AZA**	azathioprine
Ab	antibody		**Aφ**	alkaline phosphatase
ABE	acute bacterial endocarditis			
ABG	arterial blood gas		**βB**	beta-blocker
abnl	abnormal		**b/c**	because
ABPA	allergic bronchopulmonary		**BAL**	bronchoalveolar lavage
	aspergillosis		**BBB**	bundle branch block
abx	antibiotics		**BCx**	blood culture
AC	assist control		**BD**	bile duct
ACE	angiotensin-converting enzyme		**BDZ**	benzodiazepines
ACEI	ACE inhibitor		**bili.**	bilirubin
ACI	anemia of chronic inflammation		**BiPAP**	bilevel positive airway pressure
ACL	anticardiolipin antibody		**BiV**	biventricular
ACLS	advanced cardiac life support		**BM**	bone marrow
ACS	acute coronary syndrome			bowel movement
ACTH	adrenocorticotrophic hormone		**BMD**	bone mineral density
ACV	acyclovir		**BMI**	body mass index
ADA	adenosine deaminase		**BMS**	bare metal stent
ADH	antidiuretic hormone		**BNP**	B-type natriuretic peptide
ADL	activities of daily living		**BOOP**	bronchiolitis obliterans with
AF	atrial fibrillation			organizing pneumonia
AFB	acid-fast bacilli		**BP**	blood pressure
AFL	atrial flutter		**BPH**	benign prostatic hypertrophy
AFP	α-fetoprotein		**BRBPR**	bright red blood per rectum
AFTP	ascites fluid total protein		**BS**	breath sounds
AG	aminoglycoside anion gap		**BT**	bleeding time
Ag	antigen		**BUN**	blood urea nitrogen
AGN	acute glomerulonephritis		**bx**	biopsy
AI	aortic insufficiency		**BYCE**	buffered charcoal yeast extract
	aromatase inhibitor			
AIDS	acquired immunodefic. synd.		**C'**	complement
AIH	autoimmune hepatitis		**c/s**	consult
AIHA	autoimmune hemolytic anemia		**c/w**	compared with
AIN	acute interstitial nephritis			consistent with
AIP	acute interstitial pneumonia		**CABG**	coronary artery bypass grafting
AKI	acute kidney injury		**CAD**	coronary artery disease
ALF	acute liver failure		**CAH**	congenital adrenal hyperplasia
ALL	acute lymphoblastic leukemia		**CALLA**	common ALL antigen
ALS	amyotrophic lateral sclerosis		**CAPD**	chronic ambulatory peritoneal
ALT	alanine aminotransferase			dialysis
AMA	anti-mitochondrial antibody		**CBC**	complete blood count
AMI	anterior myocardial infarction		**CBD**	common bile duct
AML	acute myelogenous leukemia		**CCB**	calcium channel blocker
amy	amylase		**CCl₄**	carbon tetrachloride
ANA	antinuclear antibody		**CCP**	cyclic citrullinated peptide
ANCA	antineutrophilic cytoplasmic Ab		**CCS**	Canadian Cardiovascular
AoD	aortic dissection			Society
AoV	aortic valve		**CCY**	cholecystectomy
APAP	acetyl-para-aminophenol		**CD**	Crohn's disease
APC	activated protein C		**CEA**	carcinoembryonic antigen
APL	acute promyelocytic leukemia			carotid endarterectomy
APLA	antiphospholipid Ab		**ceph.**	cephalosporin
APS	antiphospholipid Ab synd.		**CF**	cystic fibrosis
ARB	angiotensin receptor blocker		**Cftx**	ceftriaxone
ARDS	acute resp distress synd.		**CFU**	colony forming units
ARV	antiretroviral		**CHB**	complete heart block
ARVC	arrhythmogenic RV CMP		**CHD**	congenital heart disease
AS	aortic stenosis		**CHF**	congestive heart failure
ASA	aspirin		**CI**	cardiac index
ASD	atrial septal defect		**CIAKI**	contrast-induced AKI
AST	aspartate aminotransferase		**CIDP**	chronic inflammatory
asx	asymptomatic			demyelinating
AT	atrial tachycardia			polyneuropathy
ATII	angiotensin II		**CJD**	Creutzfeldt-Jakob disease
ATIII	antithrombin III		**CK**	creatine kinase
ATN	acute tubular necrosis		**CKD**	chronic kidney disease
ATRA	all-*trans*-retinoic acid		**CLL**	chronic lymphocytic leukemia
AV	atrioventricular		**CMC**	carpometacarpal (joint)
AVA	aortic valve area		**CML**	chronic myelogenous leukemia

CMML	chronic myelomonocytic leukemia
CMP	cardiomyopathy
CMV	cytomegalovirus
CN	cranial nerve
CNI	calcineurin inhibitor
CO	carbon monoxide
	cardiac output
COP	cryptogenic organizing PNA
COPD	chronic obstructive pulm dis.
COX	cyclo-oxygenase
CP	chest pain
CPAP	continuous positive airway pressure
CPP	cerebral perfusion pressure
CPPD	calcium pyrophosphate dihydrate
Cr	creatinine
CrAg	cryptococcal antigen
CRC	colorectal cancer
CrCl	creatinine clearance
CRP	C-reactive protein
CRT	cardiac resynchronization therapy
CsA	cyclosporine A
CSF	cerebrospinal fluid
CSM	carotid sinus massage
CT	computed tomogram
CTA	CT angiogram
CTD	connective tissue disease
CV	cardiovascular
CVA	cerebrovascular accident
CVD	cerebrovascular disease
	collagen vascular disease
CVID	common variable immunodefic.
CVP	central venous pressure
CVVH	continuous veno-venous hemofiltration
CW	chest wall
cx	culture
CXR	chest radiograph
CYC	cyclophosphamide
d	day
D	death
ΔMS	change in mental status
DA	dopamine
DAD	diffuse alveolar damage
DAH	diffuse alveolar hemorrhage
DAT	direct antiglobulin test
DBP	diastolic blood pressure
d/c	discharge discontinue
DCCV	direct current cardioversion
DCIS	ductal carcinoma in situ
DCMP	dilated cardiomyopathy
Ddx	differential diagnosis
DES	drug-eluting stent
DFA	direct fluorescent antigen detection
DI	diabetes insipidus
DIC	disseminated intravascular coagulation
diff.	differential
DIP	desquamative interstitial pneumonitis
	distal interphalangeal (joint)
DKA	diabetic ketoacidosis
D$_L$CO	diffusion capacity of the lung
DLE	drug-induced lupus
DM	dermatomyositis
	diabetes mellitus
DMARD	disease-modifying anti-rheumatic drug
DOE	dyspnea on exertion
DRE	digital rectal exam
DRESS	drug reaction w/ eosinophilia & systemic symptoms
DSE	dobutamine stress echo
DST	dexamethasone suppression test
DTRs	deep tendon reflexes
DU	duodenal ulcer
DVT	deep vein thrombosis
dx	diagnosis
EAD	extreme axis deviation
EAV	effective arterial volume
EBV	Epstein-Barr virus
ECG	electrocardiogram
ECMO	extracorporeal membrane oxygenation
ED	emergency department
EDP	end-diastolic pressure
EDV	end-diastolic volume
EEG	electroencephalogram
EF	ejection fraction
EGD	esophagogastroduodenoscopy
EGFR	epidermal growth factor receptor
EGPA	eosinophilic granulomatosis with polyangiitis
EI	entry inhibitor
EIA	enzyme-linked immunoassay
ELISA	enzyme-linked immunosorbent assay
EM	electron microscopy
EMB	ethambutol
ENT	ears, nose, & throat
EOM	extraocular movement/muscles
EP	electrophysiology
Epo	erythropoietin
EPS	electrophysiology study
ERCP	endoscopic retrograde cholangiopancreatography
ERV	expiratory reserve volume
ESP	end-systolic pressure
ESR	erythrocyte sedimentation rate
ESRD	end-stage renal disease
ESV	end-systolic volume
ET	endotracheal tube
	essential thrombocythemia
EtOH	alcohol
ETT	endotracheal tube
	exercise tolerance test
EUS	endoscopic ultrasound
EVAR	endovascular aneurysm repair
FDP	fibrin degradation product
FEV$_1$	forced expir. vol in 1 sec
FFP	fresh frozen plasma
FHx	family history
FI	fusion inhibitor
FMD	fibromuscular dysplasia
FMF	familial Mediterranean fever
FNA	fine-needle aspiration
FOB	fecal occult blood
FOBT	fecal occult blood testing
FQ	fluoroquinolone
FRC	functional residual capacity
FSGS	focal segmental glomerulosclerosis
FSH	follicle stimulating hormone
FTI	free thyroxine index
FUO	fever of unknown origin
f/up	follow-up
FVC	forced vital capacity
G6PD	glc-6-phosphate dehydrogenase
GB	gallbladder
GBM	glomerular basement membrane

GBS	Guillain-Barré syndrome	ICa	ionized calcium
GCA	giant cell arteritis	ICD	implantable cardiac defibrillator
GCS	Glasgow coma scale	ICH	intracranial hemorrhage
G-CSF	granulocyte colony stimulating factor	ICP	intracranial pressure
		ICU	intensive care unit
GE	gastroesophageal	IE	infective endocarditis
gen.	generation	IGF	insulin-like growth factor
GERD	gastroesophageal reflux disease	IGRA	interferon-γ release assay
GFR	glomerular filtration rate	II	integrase inhibitor
GGT	γ-glutamyl transpeptidase	IIP	idiopathic interstitial PNA
GH	growth hormone	ILD	interstitial lung disease
GIB	gastrointestinal bleed	IMI	inferior myocardial infarction
GIST	gastrointestinal stromal tumor	infxn	infection
glc	glucose	inh	inhaled
GMCSF	granulocyte-macrophage colony-stimulating factor	INH	isoniazid
		INR	international normalized ratio
GN	glomerulonephritis	IPAA	ileal pouch-anal anastomosis
GNR	gram-negative rods	IPF	idiopathic pulmonary fibrosis
GnRH	gonadotropin-releasing hormone	ITP	idiopathic thrombocytopenic purpura
GPA	granulomatosis w/ polyangiitis	IVB	intravenous bolus
GPC	gram-positive cocci	IVC	inferior vena cava
GPI	glycoprotein IIb/IIIa inhibitor	IVDU	intravenous drug use(r)
GRA	glucocorticoid-remediable aldosteronism	IVF	intravenous fluids
		IVIg	intravenous immunoglobulin
GU	gastric ulcer		
GVHD	graft-versus-host disease	JVD	jugular venous distention
		JVP	jugular venous pulse
h	hour		
H2RA	H2-receptor antagonist	KS	Kaposi's sarcoma
HA	headache	KUB	kidney-ureter-bladder (radiography)
HACA	human antichimeric antibody		
HAV	hepatitis A virus	LA	left atrium long-acting lupus anticoagulant
Hb	hemoglobin		
HBIG	hepatitis B immunoglobulin	LABA	long-acting β2-agonist
HBV	hepatitis B virus	LAD	left anterior descending coronary artery
HCC	hepatocellular carcinoma		
HCMP	hypertrophic cardiomyopathy	LAE	left atrial enlargement
Hct	hematocrit	LAN	lymphadenopathy
HCV	hepatitis C virus	LAP	left atrial pressure leukocyte alkaline phosphatase
HCW	health care worker		
HD	hemodialysis	LBBB	left bundle branch block
HDL	high-density lipoprotein	LCA	left coronary artery
HDV	hepatitis D virus	LCIS	lobular carcinoma *in situ*
HELLP	hemolysis, abnl LFTs, low plts	LCx	left circumflex cor. art.
HEV	hepatitis E virus	LDH	lactate dehydrogenase
HF	heart failure	LDL	low-density lipoprotein
HGPRT	hypoxanthine-guanine phosphoribosyl transferase	LE	lower extremity
		LES	lower esophageal sphincter
HHS	hyperosmolar hyperglycemic state	LFTs	liver function tests
HIT	heparin-induced thrombocytopenia	LGIB	lower gastrointestinal bleed
		LH	luteinizing hormone
HK	hypokinesis	LLQ	left lower quadrant
HL	Hodgkin lymphoma	LM	left main coronary artery
h/o	history of	LMWH	low-molecular-weight heparin
HOB	head of bed	LN	lymph node
HoTN	hypotension	LOC	loss of consciousness
hpf	high-power field	LOS	length of stay
HPT	hyperparathyroidism	LP	lumbar puncture
HR	heart rate	lpf	low-power field
HRT	hormone replacement therapy	LQTS	long QT syndrome
HS	hereditary spherocytosis	LR	lactated Ringer's
HSCT	hematopoietic stem cell transplantation	LUSB	left upper sternal border
		LV	left ventricle
HSM	hepatosplenomegaly	LVAD	LV assist device
HSP	Henoch-Schönlein purpura	LVEDP	LV end-diastolic pressure
HSV	herpes simplex virus	LVEDV	LV end-diastolic volume
HTN	hypertension	LVH	left ventricular hypertrophy
HUS	hemolytic uremic syndrome	LVOT	left ventricular outflow tract
hx	history	LVSD	LV systolic dimension
I&D	incision & drainage	mAb	monoclonal antibody
IABP	intra-aortic balloon pump	MAC	mitral annular calcification
IBD	inflammatory bowel disease		*Mycobacterium avium* complex
IBS	irritable bowel syndrome		
IC	inspiratory capacity		

MAHA	microangiopathic hemolytic anemia
MALT	mucosa-assoc. lymphoid tissue
MAO	monoamine oxidase
MAP	mean arterial pressure
MAT	multifocal atrial tachycardia
MCD	minimal change disease
MCP	metacarpal phalangeal (joint)
MCS	mechanical circulatory support
MCTD	mixed connective tissue dis.
MCV	mean corpuscular volume
MDI	metered dose inhaler
MDMA	3,4-methylenedioxymethamphetamine (Ecstasy)
MDR	multidrug resistant
MDS	myelodysplastic syndrome
MEN	multiple endocrine neoplasia
MG	myasthenia gravis
MGUS	monoclonal gammopathy of uncertain significance
MI	myocardial infarction
min	minute
min.	minimal
MM	multiple myeloma
MMEFR	max. mid-expir. flow rate
MMF	mycophenolate mofetil
MN	membranous nephropathy
MNZ	metronidazole
mo	month
mod.	moderate
MODS	multiple organ dysfxn synd.
MPA	microscopic polyangiitis
MPGN	membranoproliferative glomerulonephritis
MPN	myeloproliferative neoplasm
MR	magnetic resonance / mitral regurgitation
MRA	magnetic resonance angiography
MRCP	MR cholangiopancreatography
MRI	magnetic resonance imaging
MRSA	methicillin-resistant S. aureus
MS	mitral stenosis
MSA	multisystem atrophy
MTb	Mycobacterium tuberculosis
mTOR	mechanistic target of rapamycin
MTP	metatarsal phalangeal (joint)
MTX	methotrexate
MV	mitral valve
MVA	mitral valve area
MVP	mitral valve prolapse
MVR	mitral valve replacement
Mϕ	macrophage
NAC	N-acetylcysteine
NAFLD	non-alcoholic fatty liver disease
NASH	non-alcoholic steatohepatitis
NG	nasogastric
NGT	nasogastric tube
NHL	non-Hodgkin lymphoma
NIDCM	non-ischemic dilated CMP
NIF	negative inspiratory force
NJ	nasojejunal
nl	normal
NM	neuromuscular
NMJ	neuromuscular junction
NNRTI	non-nucleoside reverse transcriptase inhibitor
NNT	number needed to treat
NO	nitric oxide
NPJT	nonparoxysmal junctional tachycardia
NPO	nothing by mouth
NPPV	noninvasive positive pressure ventilation
NPV	negative predictive value

NRTI	nucleoside reverse transcriptase inhibitor
NS	normal saline
NSAID	nonsteroidal anti-inflam. drug
NSCLC	non-small cell lung cancer
NSF	nephrogenic systemic fibrosis
NTG	nitroglycerin
N/V	nausea and/or vomiting
NVE	native valve endocarditis
NYHA	New York Heart Association
O/D	overdose
o/w	otherwise
O&P	ova & parasites
OA	osteoarthritis
OCP	oral contraceptive pill
OG	osmolal gap
OGT	orogastric tube
OGTT	oral glucose tolerance test
OI	opportunistic infection
OM	obtuse marginal cor. art.
OSA	obstructive sleep apnea
OTC	over-the-counter
p/w	present(s) with
PA	pulmonary artery
PAC	pulmonary artery catheter
PAD	peripheral artery disease
PAN	polyarteritis nodosa
PASP	PA systolic pressure
PAV	percutaneous aortic valvuloplasty
pb	problem
PBC	primary biliary cholangitis
PCI	percutaneous coronary intervention
PCN	penicillin
PCP	Pneumocystis jiroveci pneumonia
PCR	polymerase chain reaction
PCT	porphyria cutanea tarda
PCWP	pulmonary capillary wedge pressure
PD	Parkinson's disease peritoneal dialysis
PDA	patent ductus arteriosus posterior descending cor. art.
PE	pulmonary embolism
PEA	pulseless electrical activity
PEEP	positive end-expiratory pressure
PEF	peak expiratory flow
PET	positron emission tomography
PEx	physical examination
PFO	patent foramen ovale
PFT	pulmonary function test
PGA	polyglandular autoimmune syndrome
PHT	pulmonary hypertension
PI	protease inhibitor
PID	pelvic inflammatory disease
PIF	prolactin inhibitory factor
PIP	peak inspiratory pressure proximal interphalangeal (joint)
PKD	polycystic kidney disease
PM	polymyositis
PMF	primary myelofibrosis
PMHx	past medical history
PMI	point of maximal impulse
PML	progressive multifocal leukoencephalopathy
PMN	polymorphonuclear leukocyte
PMR	polymyalgia rheumatica
PMV	percutaneous mitral valvuloplasty

PMVT	polymorphic ventricular tachycardia	**RDW**	red cell distribution width	
PNA	pneumonia	**RE**	reticuloendothelial	
PND	paroxysmal nocturnal dyspnea	**RF**	rheumatoid factor risk factor	
PNH	paroxysmal nocturnal hemoglobinuria	**RHD**	rheumatic heart disease	
		RI	reticulocyte index	
PNS	peripheral nervous system	**RIBA**	recombinant immunoblot assay	
PO	oral intake	**RMSF**	Rocky Mountain spotted fever	
POTS	postural orthostatic tachycardia syndrome	**ROS**	review of systems	
		RPGN	rapidly progressive glomerulonephritis	
PPD	purified protein derivative	**RR**	respiratory rate	
PPH	primary pulmonary HTN	**RRT**	renal replacement therapy	
PPI	proton pump inhibitors	**RT**	radiation therapy	
Pplat	plateau pressure	**RTA**	renal tubular acidosis	
PPM	permanent pacemaker	**RTX**	rituximab	
PPV	positive predictive value	**RUQ**	right upper quadrant	
Ppx	prophylaxis	**RUSB**	right upper sternal border	
PR	PR segment on ECG	**RV**	residual volume	
	pulmonary regurgitation		right ventricle	
PRBCs	packed red blood cells	**RVAD**	RV assist device	
PRL	prolactin	**RVH**	right ventricular hypertrophy	
PRPP	phosphoribosyl-I-pyrophosphate	**RVOT**	RV outflow tract	
		RVSP	RV systolic pressure	
PRWP	poor R wave progression	**Rx**	therapy	
PS	pressure support	**RYGB**	roux-en-Y gastric bypass	
	pulmonic stenosis			
PSA	prostate specific antigen	**SA**	sinoatrial	
PsA	Pseudomonas aeruginosa	**SAAG**	serum-ascites albumin gradient	
PSC	primary sclerosing cholangitis	**SAH**	subarachnoid hemorrhage	
PSGN	post streptococcal glomerulonephritis	**SAS**	sulfasalazine	
		SBE	subacute bacterial endocarditis	
PSHx	past surgical history	**SBO**	small bowel obstruction	
PSV	pressure support ventilation	**SBP**	spontaneous bacterial peritonitis	
Pt	patient			
PT	prothrombin time		systolic blood pressure	
PTA	percutaneous transluminal angioplasty	**SBT**	spontaneous breathing trial	
		SC	subcutaneous	
PTH	parathyroid hormone	**SCD**	sudden cardiac death	
PTH-rP	PTH-related peptide	**SCID**	severe combined immunodefic.	
PTT	partial thromboplastin time	**SCLC**	small-cell lung cancer	
PTU	propylthiouracil	**s/e**	side effect	
PTX	pneumothorax	**Se**	sensitivity	
PUD	peptic ulcer disease	**sec**	second	
PUVA	psoralen + ultraviolet A	**SERM**	selective estrogen receptor modulator	
PV	polycythemia vera			
	portal vein	**sev.**	severe	
PVD	peripheral vascular disease	**SHBG**	steroid hormone binding globulin	
PVE	prosthetic valve endocarditis			
PVR	pulmonary vascular resistance	**SIADH**	synd. of inappropriate ADH	
PZA	pyrazinamide	**SIBO**	small intestine bacterial overgrowth	
		SIEP	serum immunoelectrophoresis	
qac	before every meal	**SIMV**	synchronized intermittent mandatory ventilation	
qhs	every bedtime			
QoL	quality of life	**SIRS**	systemic inflammatory response syndrome	
Qw	Q wave			
		SJS	Stevens-Johnson syndrome	
r/i	rule in	**SLE**	systemic lupus erythematosus	
r/o	rule out	**SMA**	superior mesenteric artery	
RA	refractory anemia	**SMV**	superior mesenteric vein	
	rheumatoid arthritis	**SMX**	sulfamethoxazole	
	right atrium	**SOS**	sinusoidal obstructive synd.	
RAA	renin-angiotensin-aldosterone	**s/p**	status post	
RAD	right axis deviation	**Sp**	specificity	
RAE	right atrial enlargement	**SPEP**	serum protein electrophoresis	
RAI	radioactive iodine	**SR**	sinus rhythm	
RAIU	radioactive iodine uptake	**s/s**	signs and symptoms	
RAS	renal artery stenosis	**SSCY**	Salmonella, Shigella, Campylobacter, Yersinia	
RAST	radioallergosorbent test			
RBBB	right bundle branch block	**SSRI**	selective serotonin reuptake inhibitor	
RBC	red blood cell			
RBF	renal blood flow	**SSS**	sick sinus syndrome	
RBV	ribavirin	**ST**	sinus tachycardia	
RCA	right coronary artery	**STD**	sexually transmitted disease	
RCMP	restrictive cardiomyopathy		ST-segment depression	
RCT	randomized controlled trial			

STE	ST-segment elevation	
SV	stroke volume	
SVC	superior vena cava	
SVR	systemic vascular resistance	
SVT	supraventricular tachycardia	
sx	symptom(s) or symptomatic	

T1D	type 1 diabetes mellitus
T2D	type 2 diabetes mellitus
T₃RU	T_3 resin uptake
TAA	thoracic aortic aneurysm
TB	tuberculosis
TBG	thyroid binding globulin
TCA	tricyclic antidepressant
TCD	transcranial Doppler
TCN	tetracycline
Tdap	tetanus, diphtheria, pertussis
TdP	torsades de pointes
TdT	terminal deoxynucleotidyl transferase
TEE	transesophageal echo
tfn	transfusion
TFTs	thyroid function tests
TG	triglycerides
TGA	transposition of the great arteries
TIA	transient ischemic attack
TIBC	total iron binding capacity
TINU	tubulointerstitial nephritis and uveitis
TIPS	transjugular intrahepatic portosystemic shunt
TKI	tyrosine kinase inhibitor
TLC	total lung capacity
TMP	trimethoprim
Tn	troponin
TP	total protein
TPMT	thiopurine methyltransferase
TPN	total parenteral nutrition
Tpo	thrombopoietin
TPO	thyroid peroxidase
TR	tricuspid regurgitation
TRALI	transfusion-related acute lung injury
TRH	thyrotropin-releasing hormone
TRS	TIMI risk score
TRUS	transrectal ultrasound
TS	tricuspid stenosis
TSH	thyroid-stimulating hormone
TSI	thyroid-stimulating immunoglobulin
TSS	toxic shock syndrome
TTE	transsphenoidal surgery
TTE	transthoracic echo
TTKG	transtubular potassium gradient
TTP	thrombotic thrombocytopenic purpura
TV	tricuspid valve
Tw	T wave
TWF	T-wave flattening

TWI	T-wave inversion
Tx	transplant
TZD	thiazolidinediones

U/A	urinalysis
UA	unstable angina uric acid
UAG	urine anion gap
UC	ulcerative colitis
UCx	urine culture
UES	upper esophageal sphincter
UFH	unfractionated heparin
UGIB	upper gastrointestinal bleed
UIP	usual interstitial pneumonitis
ULN	upper limit of normal
UOP	urine output
UPEP	urine protein electrophoresis
UR	urgent revascularization
URI	upper resp. tract infxn
U/S	ultrasound
UTI	urinary tract infection

V/Q	ventilation-perfusion
VAD	ventricular assist device
VAP	ventilator-associated PNA
VATS	video-assisted thoracoscopic surgery
VBI	vertebrobasilar insufficiency
VC	vital capacity
VD	vessel disease
VDRL	venereal disease research laboratory (test for syphilis)
VEGF	vascular endothelial growth factor
VF	ventricular fibrillation
VLDL	very-low-density lipoproteins
VOD	veno-occlusive disease
VS	vital signs
VSD	ventricular septal defect
V$_T$	tidal volume
VT	ventricular tachycardia
VTE	venous thromboembolus
vWD	von Willebrand's disease
vWF	von Willebrand's factor
VZV	varicella zoster virus

w/	with
WBC	white blood cell (count)
WCT	wide-complex tachycardia
WHO	World Health Organization
wk	week
WM	Waldenström's macroglobulinemia
WMA	wall motion abnormality
w/o	without
WPW	Wolff-Parkinson-White syndrome
w/u	workup

XRT	radiation therapy

INDEX

Figure ACLS-1 ACLS Tachycardia Algorithm

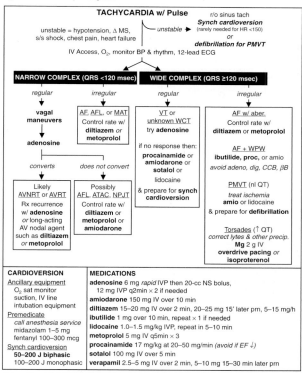

TACHYCARDIA w/ Pulse

r/o sinus tach

unstable = hypotension, Δ MS, s/s shock, chest pain, heart failure ─── **unstable** ▶ *Synch cardioversion* (rarely needed for HR <150)
or
defibrillation for PMVT

IV Access, O₂, monitor BP & rhythm, 12-lead ECG

NARROW COMPLEX (QRS <120 msec) | **WIDE COMPLEX (QRS ≥120 msec)**

regular

vagal maneuvers

↓

adenosine

converts / *does not convert*

Likely <u>AVNRT</u> or <u>AVRT</u>	Possibly <u>AFL</u>, <u>ATAC</u>, <u>NPJT</u>
Rx recurrence w/ **adenosine** *or* long-acting AV nodal agent such as **diltiazem** *or* **metoprolol**	Control rate w/ **diltiazem** *or* **metoprolol** *or* **amiodarone**

irregular

<u>AF, AFL,</u> or <u>MAT</u>
Control rate w/ **diltiazem** *or* **metoprolol**

regular

<u>VT</u> or unknown WCT
try **adenosine**

if no response then:
procainamide *or* **amiodarone** *or* **sotalol** *or* **lidocaine**
& prepare for **synch cardioversion**

irregular

<u>AF w/ aber.</u>
Control rate w/ **diltiazem** *or* **metoprolol**

<u>AF + WPW</u>
ibutilide, proc, or **amio**
avoid adeno, dig, CCB, βB

<u>PMVT</u> (nl QT)
treat ischemia
amio *or* **lidocaine**
& prepare for **defibrillation**

<u>Torsades</u> (↑ QT)
correct lytes & other precip.
Mg 2 g IV
overdrive pacing *or* **isoproterenol**

CARDIOVERSION

<u>Ancillary equipment</u>
O₂ sat monitor
suction, IV line
intubation equipment

<u>Premedicate</u>
call anesthesia service
midazolam 1–5 mg
fentanyl 100–300 mcg

<u>Synch cardioversion</u>
50–200 J biphasic
100–200 J monophasic

MEDICATIONS

adenosine 6 mg *rapid* IVP then 20-cc NS bolus, 12 mg IVP q2min × 2 if needed
amiodarone 150 mg IV over 10 min
diltiazem 15–20 mg IV over 2 min, 20–25 mg 15′ later prn, 5–15 mg/h
ibutilide 1 mg over 10 min, repeat × 1 if needed
lidocaine 1.0–1.5 mg/kg IVP, repeat in 5–10 min
metoprolol 5 mg IV q5min × 3
procainamide 17 mg/kg at 20–50 mg/min *(avoid if EF ↓)*
sotalol 100 mg IV over 5 min
verapamil 2.5–5 mg IV over 2 min, 5–10 mg 15–30 min later prn

(Adapted from ACLS 2015 *Guidelines* & *Circ* 2016;133:e506)

Figure ACLS-2 ACLS Bradycardia Algorithm

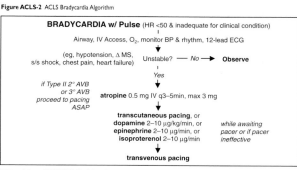

BRADYCARDIA w/ Pulse (HR <50 & inadequate for clinical condition)

Airway, IV Access, O₂, monitor BP & rhythm, 12-lead ECG

(eg, hypotension, Δ MS, s/s shock, chest pain, heart failure) **Unstable?** ── No ▶ **Observe**

↓ *Yes*

if Type II 2° AVB or 3° AVB *proceed to pacing ASAP*

atropine 0.5 mg IV q3–5min, max 3 mg

transcutaneous pacing, or
dopamine 2–10 μg/kg/min, or
epinephrine 2–10 μg/min, or
isoproterenol 2–10 μg/min

while awaiting pacer or if pacer ineffective

transvenous pacing

(Adapted from ACLS 2015 Guidelines)

PULSELESS ARREST

1. CPR
- **C**ompressions
  - **Push hard (2–2.4 inches) & fast (100–120/min)**
  - Minimize interruptions; rotate compressor q2min
- **A**irway: open airway (eg, head tilt-chin lift)
- **B**reathing: 10–12 breaths/min; 2 breaths q 30 compressions
  - Bag-mask acceptable; supplemental O_2

Attach monitor/defibrillator ASAP

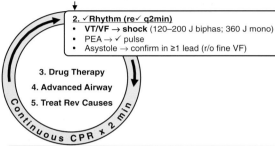

2. ✓Rhythm (re✓ q2min)
- **VT/VF → shock** (120–200 J biphas; 360 J mono)
- PEA → ✓ pulse
- Asystole → confirm in ≥1 lead (r/o fine VF)

3. Drug Therapy

4. Advanced Airway

5. Treat Rev Causes

Continuous CPR x 2 min

3. Drug Therapy
- Establish IV/IO access *(do not interrupt CPR)*
- **Epinephrine 1 mg IV q3–5min** (or 2 mg via ETT)
- **Amiodarone 300 mg IVB** ± 150 mg IVB 3–5 min later
  - ? lidocaine 1–1.5 mg/kg IVB (~100 mg) then
    0.5–0.75 mg/kg (~50 mg) q5–10min, max 3 mg/kg
  - magnesium 1–2 g IV for TdP

4. Consider Advanced Airway
- Endotracheal intubation or supraglottic advanced airway
- Clinical assessment: bilat. chest expansion & breath sounds
- Device to ✓ tube placement
  - Continuous waveform capnography (~100% Se & Sp)
  - Colorimetric exhaled CO_2 detection (≈ clinical assess.); false
    neg w/ ineffective CPR, PE, pulm edema, etc.
- 10 breaths/min w/ continuous compressions

5. Treat Reversible Causes
- Hypovolemia: volume
- Hypoxia: oxygenate
- H+ ions (acidosis): $NaHCO_3$
- Hypo/hyper K: KCl/Ca et al.
- Hypothermia: warm
- Tension PTX: needle decomp.
- Tamponade: pericardiocent.
- Toxins: med-specific
- Thromb. (PE): lysis, thrombect.
- Thromb. (ACS): PCI or lysis

(Adapted from ACLS 2015 *Guidelines* & *Circ* 2015;132(Suppl 2):S444)

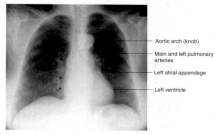

— Aortic arch (knob)

— Main and left pulmonary arteries

— Left atrial appendage

— Left ventricle

1 Normal PA CXR. The convex right cardiac border is formed by the right atrium (straight arrows), and the curved arrows indicate the location of the superior vena cava. The left cardiac and great vessels border what might be considered as 4 skiing moguls. From cephalad to caudad, the moguls are the aortic arch, the main and left pulmonary arteries, the left atrial appendage, and the left ventricle. (*Radiology 101*, 3rd ed, 2009.)

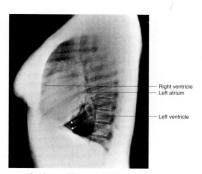

— Right ventricle
— Left atrium

— Left ventricle

2 Normal lateral CXR. (*Radiology 101*, 3rd ed, 2009.)

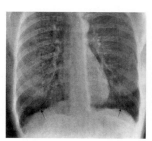

3 COPD: with hyperlucent, overinflated lungs and flat diaphragms. (*Radiology 101*, 3rd ed, 2009.)

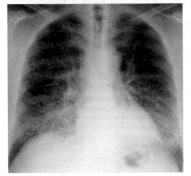

4 Interstitial pulmonary edema: with Kerley A, B, and C lines and cephalization of the vascular markings. (*Fund. Diag. Radiology* 3rd ed, 2006.)

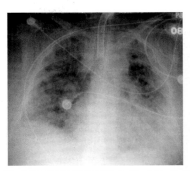

5 Alveolar pulmonary edema. (*Fund. Diag. Radiology* 3rd ed, 2006.)

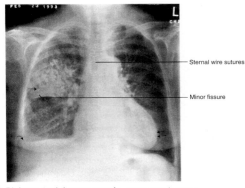

6 Right upper lobe pneumonia. (*Radiology 101,* 3rd ed, 2009.)

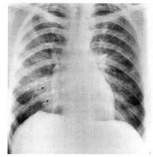

7 Right middle lobe pneumonia. *(Radiology 101, 3rd ed, 2009.)*

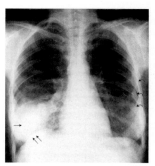

8 Right lower lobe pneumonia (PA). *(Radiology 101, 3rd ed, 2009.)*

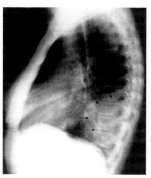

9 Right lower lobe pneumonia (lateral). *(Radiology 101, 3rd ed, 2009.)*

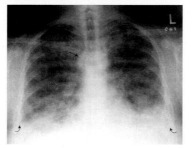

10 Bilateral pleural effusions (curved arrows) and enlarged azygous vein (straight arrow) (PA). (*Radiology 101*, 3rd ed, 2009.)

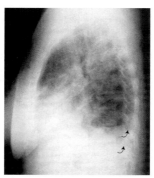

11 Bilateral pleural effusions (curved arrows) (lateral). (*Radiology 101*, 3rd ed, 2009.)

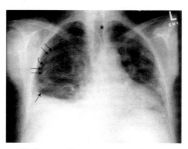

12 Pneumothorax. (*Radiology 101*, 3rd ed, 2009.)

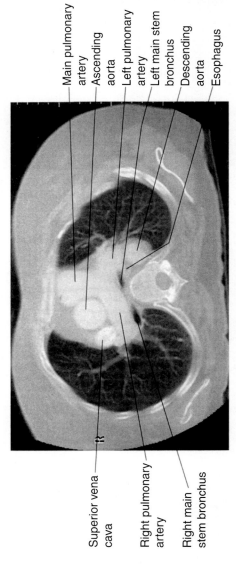

Main pulmonary artery

Ascending aorta

Left pulmonary artery

Left main stem bronchus

Descending aorta

Esophagus

Superior vena cava

Right pulmonary artery

Right main stem bronchus

13 Normal chest CT at level of pulmonary arteries (parenchymal windows).
(*Radiology 101*, 3rd ed, 2009.)

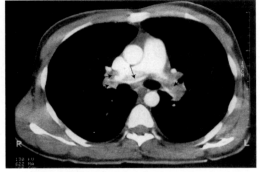

14 Bilateral PE (mediastinal windows). *(Radiology 101, 3rd ed, 2009.)*

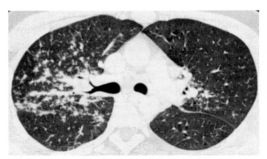

15 Sarcoidosis with perilymphatic nodules. *(Fund. Diag. Radiology 3rd ed, 2006.)*

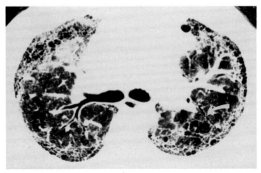

16 Idiopathic pulmonary fibrosis. *(Fund. Diag. Radiology 3rd ed, 2006.)*

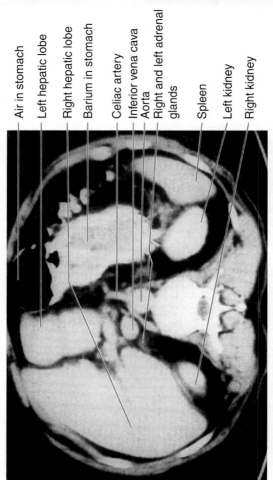

Air in stomach

Left hepatic lobe

Right hepatic lobe

Barium in stomach

Celiac artery

Inferior vena cava

Aorta

Right and left adrenal glands

Spleen

Left kidney

Right kidney

17 Normal abdomen CT at level of liver & spleen. (*Radiology 101*, 3rd ed, 2009.)

Stomach air
Right hepatic lobe
Duodenum second portion
Pancreas head and body
Superior mesenteric artery
Aorta
Pancreas tail
Diaphragm crura
Inferior vena cava
Psoas muscle
Right and left kidneys

Superior mesenteric vein-portal vein confluence

18 Normal abdomen CT at level of pancreas. (*Radiology 101*, 3rd ed, 2009)

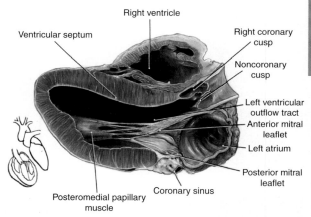

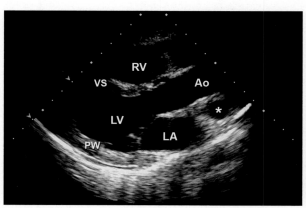

1 Parasternal long-axis view allows visualization of the right ventricle (RV), ventricular septum (VS), posterior wall (PW) aortic valve cusps, left ventricle (LV), mitral valve, left atrium (LA), and ascending thoracic aorta (Ao). *Pulmonary artery. (Top: From *Mayo Clinic Proceedings.* [Tajik AJ, Seward JB, Hagler DJ, et al. Two-dimensional real-time ultrasonic imaging of the heart and great vessels: Technique, image orientation, structure identification, and validation. *Mayo Clinic Proceedings,* 1978;53:271–303], with permission. Bottom: From Oh JK, Seward JB, Tajik AJ. *The Echo Manual, 3rd ed.* Philadelphia: Lippincott Williams & Wilkins, 2006. By permission of Mayo Foundation for Medical Education and Research. All rights reserved.)

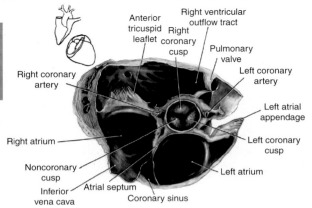

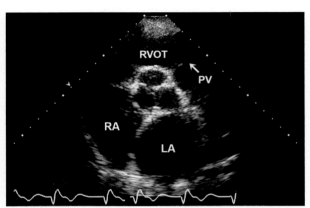

2 Parasternal short-axis view at the level of the aorta: LA, left atrium; PV, pulmonary valve; RA, right atrium; RVOT, right ventricular outflow tract. (Top: From *Mayo Clinic Proceedings.* [Tajik AJ, Seward JB, Hagler DJ, et al. Two-dimensional real-time ultrasonic imaging of the heart and great vessels: Technique, image orientation, structure identification, and validation. *Mayo Clinic Proceedings,* 1978;53:271–303], with permission. Bottom: From Oh JK, Seward JB, Tajik AJ. *The Echo Manual, 3ʳᵈ ed.* Philadelphia: Lippincott Williams & Wilkins, 2006. By permission of Mayo Foundation for Medical Education and Research. All rights reserved.)

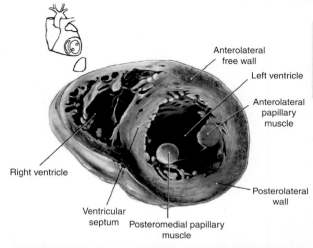

Anterolateral
free wall

Left ventricle

Anterolateral
papillary
muscle

Right ventricle

Posterolateral
wall

Ventricular
septum

Posteromedial papillary
muscle

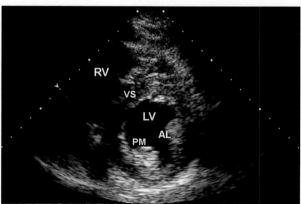

3 Parasternal short-axis view at the level of the papillary muscles: AL, anterolateral papillary muscle; PM, posteromedial papillary muscle; RV, right ventricle; VS, ventricular septum; LV, left ventricle. (Top: From *Mayo Clinic Proceedings*. [Tajik AJ, Seward JB, Hagler DJ, et al. Two-dimensional real-time ultrasonic imaging of the heart and great vessels: Technique, image orientation, structure identification, and validation. *Mayo Clinic Proceedings*, 1978;53:271–303], with permission. Bottom: From Oh JK, Seward JB, Tajik AJ. *The Echo Manual*, 3rd ed. Philadelphia: Lippincott Williams & Wilkins, 2006. By permission of Mayo Foundation for Medical Education and Research. All rights reserved.)

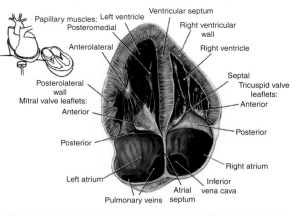

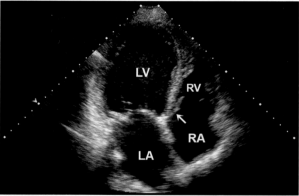

4 Apical four-chamber view: Note that at some institutions the image is reversed so that the left side of the heart appears on the right side of the screen. LA, left atrium; LV, left ventricle; RA, right atrium; RV, right ventricle. (Top: From *Mayo Clinic Proceedings.* [Tajik AJ, Seward JB, Hagler DJ, et al. Two-dimensional real-time ultrasonic imaging of the heart and great vessels: Technique, image orientation, structure identification, and validation. *Mayo Clinic Proceedings*, 1978;53:271–303], with permission. Bottom: From Oh JK, Seward JB, Tajik AJ. *The Echo Manual, 3rd ed.* Philadelphia: Lippincott Williams & Wilkins, 2006. By permission of Mayo Foundation for Medical Education and Research. All rights reserved.)

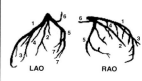
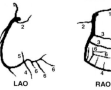

LEFT CORONARY ARTERY

1. **Left anterior descending artery (LAD)**
2. Ramus medianus artery
3. Diagonal branches
4. Septal branches
5. **Left circumflex artery (LCx)**
6. Left atrial circumflex artery
7. Obtuse marginal branches

RIGHT CORONARY ARTERY

1. Conus artery
2. SA node artery
3. Acute marginal branches
4. Posterior descending artery (PDA)
5. AV node artery
6. Posterior left ventricular artery (PLV)

Coronary arteries. (From Grossman WG. *Cardiac Catheterization and Angiography*, 4th ed. Philadelphia: Lea & Febiger, 1991, with permission.)

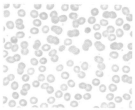

1 Normal smear.

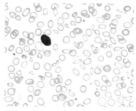

2 Hypochromic, microcytic anemia due to iron-deficiency.

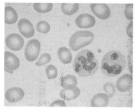

3 Macrocytic anemia due to pernicious anemia; note macro-ovalocytes and hypersegmented neutrophils.

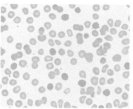

4 Spherocytes due to autoimmune hemolytic anemia.

Peripheral Blood Smears

PHOTO INSERT · P-13

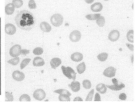

5 Sickle cell anemia.

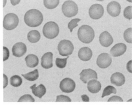

6 Schistocytes.

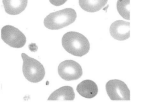

7 Teardrop shaped RBC (dacrocyte).

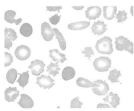

8 Acanthocytes.

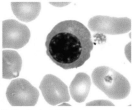

9 Nucleated RBC.

10 Rouleaux.

Leukemias

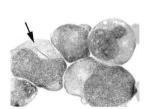

1 AML with Auer rod.

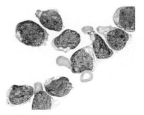

2 ALL.

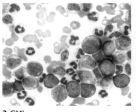

3 CML.

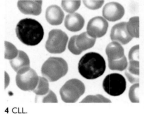

4 CLL.

All photos excluding Leukemias Fig. 4: From Wintrobe's *Clin. Hematol.* 12th ed, 2009; Leukemias Fig. 4 From Devita, Hellman, and Rosenberg's *Cancer: Princip. & Prac. of Oncol.* 8th ed, 2008.

Urinalysis

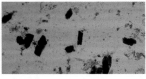

1 "Muddy brown" or granular cast (courtesy Nicholas Zwang, MD)

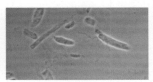

2 Hyaline cast (courtesy Nicholas Zwang, MD)

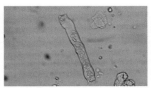

3 "Waxy broad" cast (courtesy Nicholas Zwang, MD)

4 Renal tubular epithelial cell (courtesy Nicholas Zwang, MD)

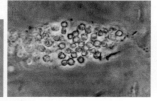

5 RBC cast. (*Dis. of Kidney & Urinary Tract*, 8th ed, 2006.)

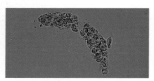

6 WBC cast. (*Clin. Lab. Medicine*, 2nd ed, 2002.)

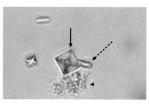

7 Calcium oxalate crystals (courtesy Mallika Mendu, MD). Calcium monohydrate (arrow), calcium dihydrate (dashed arrow), and amorphous calcium crystals (arrowhead)

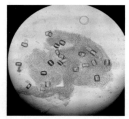

8 "Struvite" magnesium ammonia phosphate crystals (courtesy Brett Carroll, MD)

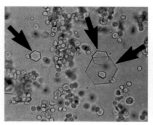

9 Cystine crystals (*Clin. Lab. Medicine*, 1994.)

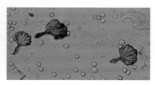

10 Sulfadiazine "shock of wheat" crystals (courtesy Nicholas Zwang, MD)